T0383541

Diagnostic and Behavioral Assessment in Children and Adolescents

A CLINICAL GUIDE

EDITED BY

BRYCE D. MCLEOD

AMANDA JENSEN-DOSS

THOMAS H. OLLENDICK

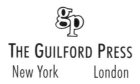

THE GUILFORD PRESS

New York   London

© 2013 The Guilford Press
A Division of Guilford Publications, Inc.
72 Spring Street, New York, NY 10012
www.guilford.com

Printed in the United States of America

This book is printed on acid-free paper.

Last digit is print number: 9 8 7 6 5 4 3 2 1

The authors have checked with sources believed to be reliable in their efforts to provide information that is complete and generally in accord with the standards of practice that are accepted at the time of publication. However, in view of the possibility of
human error or changes in behavioral, mental health, or medical sciences, neither the
authors, nor the editors and publisher, nor any other party who has been involved in
the preparation or publication of this work warrants that the information contained
herein is in every respect accurate or complete, and they are not responsible for any
errors or omissions or the results obtained from the use of such information. Readers
are encouraged to confirm the information contained in this book with other sources.

Library of Congress Cataloging-in-Publication Data

Diagnostic and behavioral assessment in children and adolescents: a clinical guide / edited
by Bryce D. McLeod, Amanda Jensen Doss, Thomas H. Ollendick.
    pages cm
Includes bibliographical references and index.
ISBN 978-1-4625-0861-7 (hardback)
1. Child psychopathology—Diagnosis. 2. Adolescent psychopathology—Diagnosis.
3. Behavioral assessment of children. 4. Diagnostic and statistical manual of mental
disorders. I. McLeod, Bryce D., editor of compilation. II. Doss, Amanda Jensen,
1976–editor of compilation. III. Ollendick, Thomas H., editor of compilation.
RJ503.5.D47 2013
618.92′89075—dc23

                                                         2012051198

To our families, with love

To Rose, Isabela, and Gabriela
—B. D. M.

To Brian, Abby, and Matthew
—A. J.-D.

To Mary, daughters Laurie and Kathleen, sons-in-law David and Billy, and grandchildren Braden, Ethan, Calvin, Addison, and Victoria
—T. H. O.

About the Editors

Bryce D. McLeod, PhD, is Associate Professor of Psychology at Virginia Commonwealth University, where he is Director of the child/adolescent track in the Clinical Psychology Program. He is the author or coauthor of numerous scientific articles and book chapters. Dr. McLeod has served on a number of committees of the Association for Behavioral and Cognitive Therapies. His clinical and research interests include youth diagnostic and behavioral assessment, child anxiety disorders, therapy process and treatment integrity research, and the implementation of evidence-based practices in community mental health settings.

Amanda Jensen-Doss, PhD, is Assistant Professor of Psychology at the University of Miami. She is the author or coauthor of numerous research publications and book chapters on youth diagnostic assessment and the implementation of evidence-based practices in community mental health settings. Dr. Jensen-Doss has served on the board of the Society of Clinical Child and Adolescent Psychology and on other committees of the American Psychological Association and the Association for Behavioral and Cognitive Therapies.

Thomas H. Ollendick, PhD, is University Distinguished Professor in Clinical Psychology and Director of the Child Study Center at Virginia Polytechnic Institute and State University. He is the editor of *Behavior Therapy* and founding coeditor of *Clinical Child and Family Psychology Review.* Dr. Ollendick has authored or coauthored numerous books and research publications. His clinical and research interests include diverse forms of child psychopathology and their assessment, treatment, and prevention from the perspective of social learning/social cognitive theory.

Contributors

Thomas M. Achenbach, PhD, Department of Psychiatry, University of Vermont, Burlington, Vermont

Sherilynn Chan, BA, Department of Psychology, University of Miami, Coral Gables, Florida

Christine L. Cole, PhD, Department of Education and Human Services, Lehigh University, Bethlehem, Pennsylvania

Patrice S. Crisostomo, MA, Department of Psychology, University of Denver, Denver, Colorado

Mark R. Dadds, PhD, School of Psychology, University of New South Wales, Sydney, New South Wales, Australia

Andy P. Field, PhD, School of Psychology, University of Sussex, Falmer, East Sussex, United Kingdom

Bruce H. Friedman, PhD, Department of Psychology, Virginia Polytechnic Institute and State University, Blacksburg, Virginia

Nancy A. Gonzales, PhD, Department of Psychology, Arizona State University, Tempe, Arizona

David J. Hawes, PhD, School of Psychology, University of Sydney, Sydney, New South Wales, Australia

Whitney Herge, MA, Department of Psychology, University of Miami, Coral Gables, Florida

Lindsay E. Holly, MS, Department of Psychology, Arizona State University, Tempe, Arizona

Amanda Jensen-Doss, PhD, Department of Psychology, University of Miami, Coral Gables, Florida

Catherine A. Kunsch, PhD, Department of Education and Human Services, Lehigh University, Bethlehem, Pennsylvania

Annette M. La Greca, PhD, Department of Psychology, University of Miami, Coral Gables, Florida

Betty Lai, PhD, Department of Psychology, University of Miami, Coral Gables, Florida

Kathryn J. Lester, PhD, MRC Social, Genetic and Developmental Psychiatry Centre, Institute of Psychiatry, King's College London, London, United Kingdom

Carla E. Marin, PhD, Department of Psychology, Florida International University, Miami, Florida

Stacey McGregor, MS, Center for Psychological Studies, Nova Southeastern University, Fort Lauderdale, Florida

Bryce D. McLeod, PhD, Department of Psychology, Virginia Commonwealth University, Virginia

Thomas H. Ollendick, PhD, Department of Psychology, Virginia Polytechnic Institute and State University, Blacksburg, Virginia

Michelle A. Patriquin, MS, Department of Psychology, Virginia Polytechnic Institute and State University, Blacksburg, Virginia

Armando A. Pina, PhD, Department of Psychology, Arizona State University, Tempe, Arizona

David Reitman, PhD, Center for Psychological Studies, Nova Southeastern University, Fort Lauderdale, Florida

Alexis Resnick, MS, Center for Psychological Studies, Nova Southeastern University, Fort Lauderdale, Florida

Yasmin Rey, PhD, Department of Psychology, Florida International University, Miami, Florida

John Paul M. Reyes, MA, Department of Psychology, University of Denver, Denver, Colorado

Angela Scarpa, PhD, Department of Psychology, Virginia Polytechnic Institute and State University, Blacksburg, Virginia

Stephen R. Shirk, PhD, Department of Psychology, University of Denver, Denver, Colorado

Wendy K. Silverman, PhD, Department of Psychology, Florida International University, Miami, Florida

Henry Wynne, MA, Department of Psychology, Arizona State University, Tempe, Arizona

Argero A. Zerr, PhD, Department of Psychology, Arizona State University, Tempe, Arizona

Preface

The evidence-based practice movement has had an enormous impact on the field of clinical child and adolescent psychology over the past two decades. This movement has primarily focused on promoting evidence-based treatments. However, more attention has recently been paid to the importance of evidence-based assessment—defined as an approach to clinical evaluation that utilizes science and theory to guide the assessment process (Hunsley & Mash, 2007)—and to the central role assessment plays in informing the treatment process.

A goal of the evidence-based assessment movement is to develop and promote a set of guidelines to steer assessment research, practice, and training. Recent publications have sought to delineate guidelines for assessment practices (e.g., Hunsley & Mash, 2008); however, until now few resources have been available for training the next generation of clinicians in the application of these new guidelines. The purpose of this book is to fill this gap. Specifically, the main goal of this book is to illustrate how and when diverse diagnostic and behavioral assessment tools can be used to inform each step of treatment, from intake to termination.

The development of this book began in 2007, when the first editor (Bryce D. McLeod) was asked to develop a graduate assessment course based on emerging trends in the field. The overarching goal was to introduce students to the principles, knowledge, skills, and values embodied within the evidence-based assessment movement (see Hunsley & Mash, 2008). The course was to cover the theory and practice of diagnostic and behavioral assessment, including the conceptual underpinnings and major methods associated with these assessment approaches, in order to teach students how diagnostic and behavioral assessment approaches can be used in tandem to guide diagnostic formulation, case conceptualization, treatment selection, treatment planning, and monitoring of treatment progress and outcome. Ultimately, the course was designed to help students learn how to critically apply evidence-based assessment strategies to guide clinical work from intake to termination.

The three editors corresponded about the course as it was being prepared. During this correspondence, we discovered that few courses covering these materials were being taught at other universities. Furthermore, it became evident that no textbooks then available focused on both diagnostic and behavioral assessment approaches or showed how these approaches could be used together to inform diagnostic formulation, case conceptualization, treatment selection, treatment planning, and treatment progress and outcome monitoring. Following discussions among us about the need to fill this gap, we decided to put together this volume. We hope that it will address a critical training need in the field.

ORGANIZATION OF THE VOLUME

This book is organized into two sections. In Part I, "Fundamental Issues," the historical, theoretical, and conceptual underpinnings of the diagnostic and behavioral assessment approaches are presented. Emphasis is placed on providing readers with the background they will need to know when and how to apply different diagnostic and behavioral assessment tools throughout treatment. Chapter 1, "Overview of Diagnostic and Behavioral Assessment," sets the stage for the following chapters by presenting the assessment principles that are used to guide the selection, use, and interpretation of assessment methods with children, adolescents, and their families. Chapter 2, "Diagnostic Assessment," and Chapter 3, "Behavioral Assessment," focus specifically on the theory, methods, and issues related to diagnostic and behavioral assessment tools, respectively; they also describe how these methods are typically used to inform the treatment process with children and their families. The final chapter in Part I, "Case Conceptualization, Treatment Planning, and Outcome Monitoring," provides a practical guide for readers to use when applying the principles of diagnostic and behavioral assessment to generate a case conceptualization that can guide the treatment process. In this chapter, two sample cases are presented. These sample cases are used throughout the remainder of the book to help illustrate how the different assessment concepts, strategies, and tools can be applied in clinical practice.

In Part II, "Assessment Tools," we present the key diagnostic and behavioral assessment tools typically used to inform the treatment process from intake to termination. Each chapter provides a description of its assessment method, the theory underlying the method, psychometric properties of the method, and implications for using the method in treatment planning and outcome evaluation. Each chapter also describes how its assessment method might be applied to the sample cases presented in Chapter 4 of Part I. Readers working with children and adolescents in a variety of settings will find the guidance provided in this section sufficiently detailed to cover the use of these assessment methods with a wide range of young clients. The chapters provide details on the rationale and the principles underlying each type of assessment tool, in order to help ensure that readers are well equipped to use these methods with the populations they serve.

The final chapter in the volume, "Diagnostic and Behavioral Assessment in Action," is designed to demonstrate how the themes and methods presented in Parts I and II can be utilized in clinical practice. Namely, we demonstrate in Chapter 15 how the various diagnostic and behavioral assessment methods can be used to inform the treatment process and develop a case conceptualization. We also apply the concepts presented in Chapter 4 to the two sample cases and share the case conceptualizations for both. Overall, we think we have produced a volume that will be highly informative and clinically useful.

REFERENCES

Hunsley, J., & Mash, E. J. (2007). Evidence-based assessment. *Annual Review of Clinical Psychology, 3*, 29–51.

Hunsley, J., & Mash, E. J. (Eds.). (2008). *A guide to assessments that work*. New York: Oxford University Press.

Contents

I. FUNDAMENTAL ISSUES

1. Overview of Diagnostic and Behavioral Assessment   3
   Bryce D. McLeod, Amanda Jensen-Doss,
   and Thomas H. Ollendick

2. Diagnostic Assessment   34
   Amanda Jensen-Doss, Bryce D. McLeod,
   and Thomas H. Ollendick

3. Behavioral Assessment   56
   Thomas H. Ollendick, Bryce D. McLeod,
   and Amanda Jensen-Doss

4. Case Conceptualization, Treatment Planning,   77
   and Outcome Monitoring
   Bryce D. McLeod, Amanda Jensen-Doss,
   and Thomas H. Ollendick

II. ASSESSMENT TOOLS

5. Interviews   103
   Carla E. Marin, Yasmin Rey, and Wendy K. Silverman

6. Checklists and Rating Scales   133
   Thomas M. Achenbach

7. Direct Observation   164

   David Reitman, Stacey McGregor, and Alexis Resnick

8. Self-Monitoring   196

   Christine L. Cole and Catherine A. Kunsch

9. Physiological Assessment   219

   Michelle A. Patriquin, Angela Scarpa,
   and Bruce H. Friedman

10. Laboratory-Based Cognitive Methodologies   240

   Kathryn J. Lester and Andy P. Field

11. Peer Assessment Strategies   277

   Annette M. La Greca, Betty Lai, Sherilynn Chan,
   and Whitney Herge

12. Parent and Family Assessment Strategies   316

   David J. Hawes and Mark R. Dadds

13. Toward Evidence-Based Clinical Assessment   348
    of Ethnic Minority Youth

   Armando A. Pina, Nancy A. Gonzales, Lindsay E. Holly,
   Argero A. Zerr, and Henry Wynne

14. Assessment of Therapy Processes   377

   Stephen R. Shirk, John Paul M. Reyes,
   and Patrice S. Crisostomo

15. Diagnostic and Behavioral Assessment in Action   417

   Amanda Jensen-Doss, Thomas H. Ollendick,
   and Bryce D. McLeod

   Author Index   449

   Subject Index   465

Part I

FUNDAMENTAL ISSUES

1

Overview of Diagnostic and Behavioral Assessment

Bryce D. McLeod, Amanda Jensen-Doss, and Thomas H. Ollendick

"Assessment" is the process by which information is gathered, interpreted, and used to produce a clinical description of an individual (Hunsley, 2002). In clinical practice, assessment of the individual can help inform the treatment process from initial intake to progress during treatment until termination. Indeed, assessment techniques can be used for a variety of purposes in psychotherapy, which include (but are not limited to) diagnosing disorders, informing treatment planning, building a case conceptualization, and monitoring and evaluating treatment outcomes. When assessment is used to arrive at an accurate description of the individual, then the treatment itself is presumably made more efficient and effective. However, a clinician needs to use the "right" assessment tools during the different phases of treatment to produce an accurate description of the individual. No single assessment technique can be used to guide every phase of treatment. Instead, a clinician must rely upon a number of tools pulled from both the diagnostic and behavioral assessment traditions.

The time is ripe for a book focused on using assessment to inform treatment. The past two decades have witnessed the rise of the evidence-based assessment movement, which has focused attention upon assessment training and practice (Ollendick, 1999). "Evidence-based assessment" is defined as an approach to clinical evaluation that utilizes science and theory to guide the assessment process (Hunsley & Mash, 2007). A goal of this movement is to develop and promote a set of assessment guidelines to direct research, structure training, and inform clinical practice.

Assessment is a complex process, and the assessment literature is voluminous. In the past, the large number of instruments and practices has made it difficult to compare instruments and to select psychometrically sound assessment tools. To address this problem, Hunsley and Mash (2008) outlined psychometric criteria for judging assessment tools and organized the assessment literature around particular disorders. These efforts represent important advances for the field, as it is now easier for clinicians to identify psychometrically strong assessment tools for routine clinical use.

Despite these recent advances, research on how best to employ and interpret assessment tools to improve treatment is lacking. Very few studies have examined the validity of assessment tools across different populations, or have considered whether incorporating assessment into treatment can improve treatment outcomes (Hunsley & Mash, 2007; Youngstrom, 2008). This means that there is little empirical evidence to guide the assessment process during treatment.

The goal of this book is to provide readers with the knowledge and skills needed to guide the assessment process from intake to termination. Other resources are available to help readers identify particular assessment tools for specific disorders (see Hunsley & Mash, 2008). Our purpose here is to cover areas of knowledge—such as the basics of psychometric theory; the connection between assessment and treatment; and the assessment of target behaviors and other key factors (cognitive, affective, behavioral, contextual)—that are needed to use assessment tools effectively over the course of treatment (Krishnamurthy et al., 2004). We also cover key skill areas, such as target behavior identification, case conceptualization, and tool selection and interpretation, which are relevant to using assessment tools to inform treatment. To gain the right combination of knowledge and skills, clinicians are advised to take graduate-level courses in developmental psychopathology, developmental psychology, psychometric theory, child and family intervention, and culture and diversity, as well as in evidence-based assessment.

TRENDS IN ASSESSMENT TRAINING AND PRACTICE

Assessment in clinical practice falls clearly under the domain of psychology. However, assessment does not presently represent a central focus of the field (Youngstrom, 2008). The past two decades have witnessed an explosion of treatment research resulting from the evidence-based practice movement. These efforts have generated a number of treatments for a wide range of youth emotional and behavioral problems (Barrett & Ollendick, 2004; McLeod & Weisz, 2004; Weisz, Jensen-Doss, & Hawley, 2005). However, research on assessment has not kept pace. As a result, assessment and treatment have become disconnected processes (Youngstrom, 2008).

Unfortunately, in our opinion, this disconnection has adversely affected graduate training in clinical psychology. At present, few graduate programs provide courses on the interrelationship between assessment and treatment (Childs & Eyde, 2002). Most assessment training required by graduate programs focuses on intellectual and personality testing, and sometimes behavioral assessment; relatively few programs require courses on clinical assessment (Childs & Eyde, 2002). Assessment training has been criticized for not adjusting to the new assessment trends. Graduate programs differ in their coverage of the knowledge and skills related to using assessment to inform treatment (Carama, Nathan, & Puente, 2000; Krishnamurthy et al., 2004). As a result, not all graduate students learn how assessment can be used to tailor evidence-based treatments to meet the unique needs of a particular child and her or his family.

This volume is intended to illustrate how assessment can be used to inform treatment for children and adolescents. Our basic premise is that effective treatment depends upon accurate assessment rather than solely subjective decision making. To do this, clinicians must know *when* to utilize various diagnostic and behavioral assessment tools at the various phases of treatment, and *why* these assessment tools are helpful for treatment selection and delivery. Next, we turn to the role assessment plays in the different phases of treatment.

WHAT ROLE DOES ASSESSMENT PLAY IN TREATMENT?

Assessment should directly inform choices about treatment, and different assessment tools are more or less relevant at various treatment stages (see Table 1.1). At each stage, clinicians must select the appropriate "nomothetic" and "idiographic" assessment tools available to them. Nomothetic tools (e.g., diagnostic interviewing and parent rating scales) provide data about where an individual child falls relative to the larger population on a domain of interest. For example, a clinician trying to determine whether a child needs services might use an anxiety rating scale to establish whether that child falls above a clinical cutoff. If the child's score is above this cutoff, this would indicate that the child's level of anxiety exceeds what is considered typical for children of similar age and gender, and treatment may be warranted. On the other hand, idiographic tools (e.g., direct observation and self-monitoring) provide individualized information that is more useful for case conceptualization, treatment planning, and outcome monitoring. For example, a clinician seeking to design an exposure hierarchy for a given child might design a behavioral avoidance activity tailored to the child's specific fears, to determine the exact type of situations most likely to elicit anxiety in that child. As we note below in more detail, nomothetic and idiographic tools play important, and complementary, roles in the different phases of treatment.

TABLE 1.1. The Role Assessment Plays in Different Phases of Treatment

Treatment phase	Definition and purpose
Screening	Brief assessment designed to identify children who have a problem or are at risk for developing a problem without intervention. Screening is used to determine the need for treatment, generate a prognosis, and gather baseline data on symptom severity and potential causal factors.
Diagnosis	Determining whether a child meets formal criteria for a psychiatric disorder. Diagnosis is used to establish treatment need and facilitates case conceptualization, treatment planning, and treatment selection.
Prognosis	A prediction regarding the course of an illness or the likelihood of developing of a problem given the presence of specific risk factors. A prognosis helps determine the need for treatment and informs treatment planning.
Case conceptualization	A set of hypotheses about the causes, antecedents, and maintaining factors of a client's target behaviors. Case conceptualization is a critical component of treatment that informs treatment planning, treatment selection, outcome monitoring, and treatment evaluation.
Treatment planning and selection	Using the case conceptualization to identify therapeutic interventions designed to address produce change in the target behaviors.
Treatment monitoring	Ongoing assessment of core symptoms, causal factors, and maintaining processes, in order to monitor treatment response and to identify changes needed to the treatment plan.
Treatment evaluation	Assessment conducted at the end of treatment, in order to evaluate the impact of treatment.

Screening

Screening is primarily used to identify areas in need of more detailed assessment. It can also be used to determine the need for treatment, generate a prognosis, and gather baseline data on symptom severity and potential causal factors. Brief nomothetic measures can be used to screen for possible diagnoses. Such measures can be used to generate an estimate about the likelihood a child meets diagnostic criteria for one or more diagnoses, and/or to ascertain whether symptoms are above a clinical cutoff. Screening can also be used to gather data to formulate a prognosis. Noting the presence of certain risk factors (e.g., trauma, child abuse, poverty) can help a clinician determine whether a child is likely to develop future problems. Sometimes screening may indicate that treatment is not needed (e.g., the child's score is below a clinical cutoff); however, when screening indicates the need for treatment, then the assessment data can serve as baseline data as well as help identify targets for in-depth assessment.

Diagnosis

Generating an accurate diagnosis is a critical step in treatment. Meeting criteria for a disorder indicates a need for treatment and provides a starting point for identifying target behaviors. In many instances, the actual symptoms of disorders can be operationalized and selected for change. In addition, the developmental psychopathology, treatment, and assessment literatures are all organized around diagnoses, so an accurate diagnosis is frequently fundamental to case conceptualization and treatment planning.

Prognosis

Youngstrom (2008) defines "prognosis" as "the course of illness or the longitudinal outcomes that are likely for individuals affected by a particular condition or showing a particular marker or trait" (p. 46). To formulate a prognosis, a clinician must assess for the presence of risk factors that are associated with particular outcomes and use knowledge from the developmental psychopathology literature to determine the likely outcome for a child. A prognosis may indicate a need for treatment if it is determined that a child will probably develop a disorder without intervention. For example, a young child with an inhibited temperament may not meet diagnostic criteria for a disorder, but may be at increased risk for developing an anxiety disorder. Or a prognosis may guide treatment planning by helping to identify the most important treatment targets for a child experiencing multiple problems. For example, when a child presents with multiple problems, it is often important to give problems that have the greatest potential for adverse long-term outcomes (e.g., symptomatology related to a trauma) the highest priority in the treatment plan.

Case Conceptualization

"Case conceptualization" is defined as a set of hypotheses about the causes, antecedents, and maintaining factors of a client's emotional, interpersonal, and behavior problems (Eells, 2007; McLeod, Jensen-Doss, Wheat, & Becker, in press; Nezu, Nezu, Peacock, & Girdwood, 2004). Case conceptualization is a critical component of treatment, as its hypotheses guide assessment and treatment. Assessment related to case conceptualization includes a focus upon "mediators," "moderators," and "therapy processes." Mediators are factors (e.g., cognitions or physiological processes) that account for change in the target behavior. Moderators are factors (e.g., developmental level, gender, ethnicity, or socioeconomic status) that might influence the course of treatment and/or a target behavior. Therapy processes include client (motivation, involvement) and therapist (treatment integrity, competence) factors that influence the effectiveness of psychotherapy (see Shirk, Reyes, & Crisostomo, Chapter 14, this volume). All assessment should inform case conceptualization and feed directly into treatment design/planning, outcome monitoring, and treatment evaluation.

Treatment Planning and Selection

Treatment planning and selection are important, and challenging, components of treatment. Children often present for treatment with multiple problems, and clinicians must determine which problems warrant treatment. Numerous evidence-based treatments designed to treat a variety of specific diagnoses (e.g., anxiety disorders, depression, conduct disorder, eating disorders) exist. Treatment planning starts with generating a diagnosis and identifying the treatments designed to treat that disorder. A clinician must then use the case conceptualization to select the "right" evidence-based treatment and then tailor the intervention to meet the needs of the individual and his or her family.

Treatment Monitoring

Once treatment begins, ongoing assessment of core symptoms, causal factors, and therapy processes can be used to monitor treatment response and to identify any changes that may be needed in the treatment plan. In adult psychotherapy, evidence indicates that continual assessment and feedback to the client can improve therapy outcomes (Lambert et al., 2003), and studies are beginning to support this benefit in child psychotherapy as well (Stein, Kogan, Hutchison, Magee, & Sorbero, 2010). Because assessment during treatment can become time-consuming, selective targeting of variables for treatment monitoring that will directly inform treatment planning is important. In some cases, this will require assessment to be focused upon the specific symptoms being treated (e.g., panic attacks), causal variables (e.g., anxiety sensitivity), or therapy processes (e.g., exposures to feared stimuli).

Treatment Evaluation

At the end of treatment, a thorough assessment is warranted. To evaluate the impact of treatment, it is important to determine whether the child still meets diagnostic criteria for the disorder that was the focus of treatment, as this represents an important indicator of clinically significant change. This assessment can also determine level of functioning, which represents another clinically meaningful category. The end-of-treatment evaluation should assess the need for further referrals or interventions as well. Clearly, it is important to select outcome assessment measures that have been demonstrated to be sensitive to change.

WHY FOCUS ON DIAGNOSTIC AND BEHAVIORAL ASSESSMENT?

We focus on both diagnostic and behavioral assessment in this volume, because the theory and tools that are part of each tradition inform different facets of treatment (see Table 1.2). These assessment traditions developed along separate paths. Each approach has different conceptual underpinnings and psychometric strengths. It is important to understand how tools from both approaches can be used to produce a complete picture of a child across treatment.

Diagnostic Assessment

For the purposes of this volume, diagnostic assessment is considered to include tools and techniques designed to generate diagnoses and classify behavior. Diagnostic assessment stems from the medical model of psychopathology, which posits that symptoms (and, by extension, diagnoses) fall into classifiable disorders that express themselves in somewhat uniform

TABLE 1.2. Diagnostic and Behavioral Assessment

	Diagnostic	Behavioral
Goals	Based upon nomothetic principles, which are concerned with the discovery of general laws as applied to a large number of individuals	Based upon idiographic principles, which are focused on mapping out the interactions among variables distinctively patterned in each individual
Uses	Classification and prediction	Monitoring target behaviors and/or antecedent, causal, and maintaining variables
Common methods	Interviews Rating scales	Functional interviews Rating scales Direct observation Self-monitoring
Treatment phases	Screening Prognosis Diagnosis Case conceptualization Treatment monitoring Treatment evaluation	Case conceptualization Treatment monitoring
Psychometric principles	Classical test theory Internal reliability Test–retest reliability Interrater reliability Construct validity Criterion validity	Generalizability theory Interrater reliability Accuracy Construct validity Criterion validity

fashion and are caused by identifiable factors that are internal to the child (e.g., genetics, biology) and external/contextual to the child (e.g., family factors, socioeconomic status, traumatic events). Consistent with this model, most diagnostic tools are based upon nomothetic principles, which are concerned with the discovery of general laws as they are applied to large numbers of individuals (Cone, 1986). The nomothetic approach is said to be variable-centered (i.e., deals with how particular characteristics or traits are distributed in the population). Measures and tools designed according to this tradition also include rating scales and interviews that provide global statements about how the behavior of a particular child compares to that of the larger population.

Nomothetic measures are used primarily for classification and prediction (Barrios & Hartmann, 1986) and are typically designed according to the tenets of classical test theory. This approach views scores on a measure as representative of an underlying construct that cannot be directly assessed. Because nomothetic measures are designed to assess individual differences, the meaning of a score produced by such a measure is derived by comparing it to norms from the general population. Indeed, diagnostic tools classify individuals along categories (diagnoses) that are posited to be consistent across time and situations (Bem & Allen, 1974). Variation in scores across situations, time, or items is considered error. Thus the development of nomothetic measures emphasizes stability, and the measures may not be most appropriate for repeated administration (e.g., weekly outcome monitoring; Foster & Cone, 1995).

Early in treatment, diagnostic tools are appropriate for screening, determining whether a child's behavior is normative, and formulating a prognosis. Once treatment begins, diagnostic tools can be used for treatment evaluation. Using diagnostic tools at the end of treatment allows a clinician to determine whether a child has experienced clinically significant change or returned to a normative developmental trajectory. Diagnostic tools therefore play a number of important roles in treatment.

Behavioral Assessment

The behavioral assessment approach is based upon idiographic principles. This person-centered approach focuses upon the uniqueness of a given individual (Cone, 1986; Ollendick & Hersen, 1984); unlike the nomothetic approach, it focuses upon mapping out the interactions among variables distinctively patterned in each individual. The point of comparison for idiographic measures is the child's own behavior across situations and/or time. As Mischel (1968, p. 190) observed over 40 years ago, "Behavioral assessment involves an exploration of the unique or idiosyncratic aspects of the single case, perhaps to a greater extent than any other approach."

Idiographic assessment focuses upon a target behavior or response class. A "response class" is defined as a group of behaviors that serve the same function within a specific context (Jackson, 1999; Johnston & Pennybacker, 1993). "Experiential avoidance," defined as the avoidance of situations and conditions eliciting certain internal experiences (emotions, cognitions) that an individual finds intolerable, is an example of a response class (see Hayes, Wilson, Gifford, Follette, & Strosahl, 1996). The assessment of behavior is guided by two key concepts. The first of these is "situational specificity," or variance in a child's behavior as situational factors surrounding the child change. This means that assessment focuses upon those variables that elicit (antecedents) and maintain (consequences) a target behavior in a particular situation (Olweus, 1979). Situational specificity necessitates that assessment samples behavior across diverse settings and time points. Hence assessment of the child's behavior at home, in school, and on the playground is important, in addition to information obtained in the clinic setting. Furthermore, the information obtained from these various settings probably will not be, and in fact should not be, expected to be the same. For instance, the child may behave aggressively in school and on the playground, but not at home or in the clinic. The second concept is "temporal instability," or variance in a child's behavior over time. Such instability in behavior dictates that a child's behavior needs to be assessed at several points in time.

Measures designed according to idiographic principles generally adhere to "generalizability theory" (Cronbach, Gleser, Nanda, & Rajaratnam, 1972). Generalizability theory is a statistical framework for investigating and designing idiographic tools that evaluates the performance of a measure across facets (i.e., sources of variation) relevant to different applications of the measure. Five facets—forms, items, observers, time, and situation—are typically considered (Barrios & Hartmann, 1986; Cronbach et al., 1972). In contrast to classical test theory, which views variability across these facets as error, generalizability theory views this variability as something to understand and something central to change. Variability in scores across the different facets is examined. If a facet is associated with significant variability, then this suggests that scores would not generalize from one condition of the facet to another. For example, if observer bias accounts for a significant proportion of the variance in direct observations of aggressive behavior, then the scores would not be considered reliable across these different observers. Generalizability theory is therefore consistent with the tenets of behavioral theory.

The underlying assumptions and psychometric strengths of idiographic tools make them uniquely suited for specific aspects of treatment. In essence, these assessment tools pick up where nomothetic tools leave off. After a diagnosis is assigned, idiographic tools are uniquely suited to assessing behavioral, cognitive, affective, and contextual variables that may serve to maintain the target behavior. These tools therefore play a critical role in generating the case conceptualization and determining the impact of treatment.

Combining Diagnostic and Behavioral Assessment

The importance of using both diagnostic and behavioral assessment tools is increasingly being recognized (Mash & Barkley, 2007). However, it is important that clinicians understand when to use diagnostic and behavioral tools during treatment. At one time, it was relatively easy to differentiate behavioral from diagnostic assessment on the basis of the methods employed. Direct observation was originally the sole assessment technique of behavioral assessment, whereas interviewing characterized diagnostic assessment. However, as both assessment traditions evolved to include a wider repertoire of methods, differentiating behavioral and diagnostic approaches simply on the use of specific methods became more difficult. Indeed, there is now considerable overlap in ongoing assessment practices between the two approaches.

Presently, the difference between the two approaches lies less in the methods employed than in the manner in which findings generated with these assessment tools can (and should) be interpreted and used. Measures designed according to nomothetic principles are designed to compare an individual child to the larger population on a domain of interest. Measures designed according to idiographic principles are designed to identify target behaviors (overt or covert), their controlling conditions, and the functions they serve for a particular individual. Because the line between diagnostic and behavioral assessment techniques has become blurred, clinicians must understand how to critically evaluate assessment tools to determine their most appropriate application. This means that they need to understand how to determine whether a measure was developed according to nomothetic or idiographic principles, and to know when assessment tools from each tradition should be used at different stages in treatment.

ASSESSMENT PRINCIPLES

As noted at the beginning of this chapter, child assessment requires knowledge and skills from several domains: developmental principles, child psychopathology, psychometric theory, diversity/cultural issues, and therapy process and outcome research. The knowledge and skills gained from these different areas are required to guide the selection and interpretation of assessment data throughout treatment. Though the field has accumulated data on a wide variety of measures, we currently lack research on how to combine and interpret findings from these various measures. In the absence of empirical findings to direct the assessment process, we recommend that clinicians adhere to a set of principles to guide this process. The following overarching principles that guide our approach to child and adolescent assessment are summarized in Table 1.3. We now turn to a more detailed description of each principle and how each applies to assessment.

TABLE 1.3. Six Assessment Principles

Number	Principle
Principle 1	Empirical evidence and developmental psychopathology theory are used in selecting the constructs to target in assessment, as well as the best methods and tools to use.
Principle 2	Assessment is an ongoing process that uses a hypothesis-testing approach to inform decision making. As such, emphasis is placed on assessment tools that inform screening, diagnosis, case conceptualization, treatment selection/planning, and evaluation of treatment progress and outcome.
Principle 3	Thorough child assessment requires a multimethod, multi-informant approach that utilizes both nomothetic and idiographic assessment tools, and that focuses on a child's behavior, cognitions, affect, and social context.
Principle 4	Selecting constructs for assessment, determining a method for gathering assessment data, and interpreting findings should be informed by knowledge of developmental norms associated with specific child and adolescent emotional and behavioral problems.
Principle 5	Selecting constructs for assessment, determining a method for gathering assessment data, and interpreting findings should be informed by knowledge of ways in which culture and diversity can influence the experience and expression of child and adolescent emotional and behavioral problems.
Principle 6	The choice of assessment tools should be based on the strength of the tools' psychometric support for the type of client being assessed and the goals of the assessment. Careful attention should also be given to the judgmental heuristics that guide the interpretation of findings.

Principle 1. Empirical evidence and developmental psychopathology theory are used in selecting the constructs to target in assessment, as well as the best methods and tools to use.

Child assessment is complex. It is challenging to choose the right methods and informants for the wide range of possible targets. To reduce the potential for bias, the selection of methods and informants needs to be guided by the most recent empirical evidence and theory. The developmental psychopathology perspective (e.g., Cicchetti & Cohen, 1995; Masten & Braswell, 1991) provides an organizational framework for understanding childhood psychopathology and identifying the mechanisms and processes implicated in the development, maintenance, and alleviation of these problems (McLeod et al., in press; Youngstrom, 2008). As the mechanisms and processes represent potential treatment targets, this literature is ideal for identifying constructs to target in assessment and treatment.

To appreciate how this research can inform child assessment, it is important to understand the foundational principles of developmental psychopathology. According to this perspective, children grow and change within the context of larger systems that can exert an influence upon child development and the expression of psychopathology. Risk and protective factors that are external (e.g., familial, social/environmental) and internal (e.g., biological, cognitive) interact to determine whether a child successfully masters each developmental stage. Mastery of the skills associated with each stage tends to leave a child better equipped to handle subsequent challenges. Failure to master the skills associated with a developmental stage leaves a child unprepared to deal with the demands of successive stages. Protective factors promote adaptation and help a child successfully negotiate a particular developmental stage. Risk factors, in contrast, decrease the likelihood that a child will achieve developmental milestones (Cicchetti & Cohen, 1995). The longer a child goes without mastering the skills of a developmental stage, the harder it is for her or him to return to normality. Ultimately, the interplay of risk and protective factors determines child outcomes; the development of a problem is more likely when the number of risk factors outweigh the protective factors.

Though certain risk factors are implicated in the development of specific disorders, developmental psychopathology considers each child unique. Two concepts explain this perspective. The first is the concept of "multifinality," or the idea that a single risk factor may lead to a variety of outcomes, depending upon the context in which it occurs. Basically, this principle suggests that a process (i.e., impact upon the individual) of any one factor (e.g., genetics, environment) varies, depending upon the context (e.g., family system) in which the factor operates (Cicchetti & Cohen, 1995). For example, some research suggests that parenting style can buffer children with behaviorally inhibited temperaments against the development of anxiety (Fox, Henderson, Marshall, Nichols, & Ghera, 2005). The second concept is "equifinality," or the idea that any given outcome (e.g., an anxiety disorder, conduct disorder) can have multiple causes. This means that a single causal pathway does not universally account for the development of specific emotional or behavioral problems. For example, an inhibited temperament (i.e., genetic pathway) and traumatic events (i.e., classical conditioning) have both been linked to social phobia (Stemberger, Turner, Beidel, & Calhoun, 1995). Together, these concepts have important implications for child assessment. Specifically, it is important to assume that although research can tell us about general risk factors for specific disorders, each child will have a unique combination of risk factors implicated in the development and maintenance of a disorder; assessment therefore needs to be highly individualized and tailored to each child.

Principle 2. Assessment is an ongoing process that uses a hypothesis-testing approach to inform decision making. As such, emphasis is placed on assessment tools that inform screening, diagnosis, case conceptualization, treatment selection/planning, and evaluation of treatment progress and outcome.

Using the developmental psychopathology literature to guide the assessment process necessitates adopting a hypothesis-testing approach to assessment. Research has identified specific risk factors that are associated with the development and maintenance of each disorder. However, each child will have a unique combination of factors implicated in the development and maintenance of a disorder. Thus the literature can be used to generate hypotheses about the mechanisms and processes at play for a particular child, which then are tested through both assessment and treatment. In other words, assessment and treatment should focus on the research-supported risk factors associated with a particular disorder and should systematically work toward identifying the specific factor(s) that play a role for a particular child. By doing so, the clinician will be able to develop and test hypotheses about which factors need to be targeted as part of treatment.

Assessment designed to inform treatment is an ongoing process that constantly evolves over the course of treatment. To guide the clinical decision-making process, and to ensure that this entire process is objective and grounded in the research literature, we advocate that the clinician's hypothesis-testing approach be rooted in the empirical principles of the behavioral assessment tradition (Ollendick & Hersen, 1984). Again, using the research literature to select targets for assessment, the clinician can generate hypotheses about the functional relation among causal, maintaining, and target behaviors. These hypotheses form the foundation of the case conceptualization, which is designed to guide treatment selection and planning as well as evaluation of treatment progress and outcome. Specific behavioral assessment tools and strategies, such as functional analysis and single-case series design, can be used to test the hypotheses during treatment. Assessment during treatment is then used to test the hypotheses, and the resulting data are used to make adjustments to the case conceptualization and treatment plan.

Principle 3. Thorough child assessment requires a multimethod, multi-informant approach that utilizes both nomothetic assessment tools, and that focuses on a child's behavior, cognitions, affect, and social context.

A multimethod, multi-informant approach is an important part of child assessment. Child assessment aims to describe multiple target behaviors accurately, including overt behavior, affective states, cognitive processes, and information about the child's context (Barry, Frick, & Kamphaus, 2013). Multiple tools are needed to assess these different facets of child behavior, because most assessment tools are designed to characterize only one aspect of child behavior. For example, some measures catalog child symptoms (e.g., parent rating scales), but do not provide information about how contextual factors may influence the symptoms. Part of a multimethod approach is blending diagnostic (nomothetic) and behavioral (idiographic) methods, as these approaches play important, complementary roles in child assessment. Psychometric issues also necessitate the use of multiple assessment tools. Every assessment tool has psychometric strengths and weaknesses. Clinicians must therefore pick measures with complementary areas of strength, so that appropriate tools are used to assess each aspect of child behavior (Barry et al., 2013). For these reasons, it is important to employ a multimethod approach to child assessment.

A multi-informant approach is also an important component of child assessment. In choosing informants, clinicians must consider a number of factors. In the following paragraphs, we discuss when and why different individuals might be asked to serve as informants in child assessment.

Children

When children present for treatment, it is important to get their perspective on the target behavior. Gathering information from children provides an opportunity to build an alliance as well as to arrive at treatment goals. Several factors must, however, be considered in collecting and interpreting data from child informants. Younger children may not provide accurate information or be able to report about certain symptoms (Kamphaus & Frick, 2005; Schroeder & Gordon, 2002). As children enter adolescence, they are able to report upon their behavior and may be better informants for certain types of problems (e.g., substance abuse, anxiety) and/or for problems that adult informants do not observe (e.g., covert behaviors, such as stealing). When clinicians are considering the accuracy of child report, however, social desirability must also be considered (see De Los Reyes & Kazdin, 2005). Some children may want to please a clinician and thus provide answers they believe the clinician wants to hear. Other children may wish to conceal certain behaviors and thus may not provide accurate answers about those. The attributions children make about the causes of their problems may also influence the information they provide (De Los Reyes & Kazdin, 2005). In particular, children may be more likely to attribute the cause of their problems to environmental factors (e.g., family relations), which may make them less likely to endorse specific symptoms of certain disorders (e.g., less likely to see their own behavior as oppositional or defiant).

Parents

Typically, parents are the primary informants in child assessment (Paikoff & Brooks-Gunn, 1991), especially if a child is young. Interviewing parents provides clinicians with an important opportunity to build an alliance and engage the parents in the clinical process (see Hawes & Dadds, Chapter 12, this volume). However, a number of factors can influence the accuracy of parent report. First, parental psychopathology (e.g., depression) can negatively influence the accuracy of parent report (Chi & Hinshaw, 2002; Richters, 1992). Second, parents may not have an accurate understanding of normative child behavior, especially compared to that of other adults (e.g., teachers; Barry et al., 2013). If so, parents may see particular child behaviors as problematic when in fact the behaviors are part of a normative developmental process. Third, parents' attributions regarding child behavior must be considered (De Los Reyes & Kazdin, 2005). Finally, parents of adolescents may not have full access to all aspects of their children's lives and thus may not be accurate reporters on certain behavior (e.g., affect, stealing, drug use).

Teachers

For certain child problems, teachers can be important informants. Certain symptoms may be observed first at school or may be particularly problematic in this setting. In such cases, a teacher can offer an important viewpoint, especially if a parent does not have the same opportunity to view the behavior. Furthermore, because teachers may have more experience with children than parents have, they may have a more developmentally sensitive view of child behavior (Barry et al., 2013). This can be helpful in deciding whether a parent's report is accurate or not. As with other informants, however, several factors may influence the accuracy of teacher data. First, teachers often do not have access to all facets of child behavior, so they are generally more accurate when reporting upon behavior they have actually observed (Loeber, Green, Lahey, & Stouthamer-Loeber, 1991). Second, a clinician must consider the amount of contact a teacher has with a student when asking the teacher to provide information on a child. Teachers typically have less contact with children as they get older, so this must be considered for children of middle school age or above (Edelbrock, Costello, Dulcan, Kalas, & Conover, 1985). Third, the attributions made by a teacher about a child's behavior must be considered in interpreting teacher report data.

Peers

Social disruptions and impairment are common problems in youth. Peer report provides a unique perspective on a child and his or her social functioning/status. However, asking peers to provide ratings raises some ethical issues (e.g., asking peers to provide ratings might violate a client's confidentiality). Thus a clinician must be careful not to be too intrusive when asking peers to report data.

Principle 4. Selecting constructs for assessment, determining a method for gathering assessment data, and interpreting findings should be informed by knowledge of developmental norms associated with specific child and adolescent emotional and behavioral problems.

The choice of assessment methods and the process of interpreting the findings should be influenced by knowledge of the developmental norms associated with specific disorders and symptoms (Holmbeck et al., 2008). Age-related constraints are numerous in child assessment and should be considered in selecting specific methods of assessment. For example, interviews may be more difficult to conduct and self-report measures less reliable with younger children, whereas self-monitoring and direct observations may be more reactive at older ages (Ollendick & Hersen, 1984). The selection of assessment instruments should therefore be guided by knowledge of cognitive and socioemotional developmental processes.

The interpretation of assessment data must also be informed by normative guidelines. As part of the assessment process, clinicians must ascertain whether a child is exhibiting developmentally adaptive or maladaptive behavior. Symptoms and behaviors that are considered normative at one developmental stage may not be considered so at a later stage. For example, it is typical for fear of separation to develop in infancy, for fear to move on to social situations in childhood, and for fear to become more generalized in adolescence (Gullone, 1996). So an intense fear of separation from caregivers is not unusual in young children, but is not considered developmentally appropriate in school-age children (Gullone, 1996; Warren & Sroufe, 2004). As another example, tantrums are considered normative at a young age, but become less so for school-age children. It is therefore important to determine whether the expression of a particular symptom is congruent with a child's developmental level or likely to represent a symptom that is interfering with functioning (Silverman & Ollendick, 2005; Warren & Sroufe, 2004).

Another factor that influences the interpretation of assessment data is knowledge of how age differences can influence the expression of behaviors and syndromes. Young children cannot manifest certain symptoms, such as guilt, hopelessness, or worry, before they achieve certain developmental milestones. For example, worry requires insight, which may not fully develop until late childhood (e.g., Dadds, James, Barrett, & Verhulst, 2004). Understanding the relation between cognitive development and the experience of certain symptoms can help a clinician avoid misattributing reports of a child's behavior to symptoms that are not consistent with the child's developmental level.

In sum, it is important for clinicians to take developmental factors into consideration when using assessment data to drive the therapy process. Developmental factors determine what assessment tools (e.g., interview, questionnaire, and direct observation) will provide accurate and valid information. Clinicians must therefore select developmentally appropriate methods of assessment and interpret the resulting data from the perspective of developmental norms.

Principle 5. Selecting constructs for assessment, determining a method for gathering assessment data, and interpreting findings should be informed by knowledge of ways in which culture and diversity can influence the experience and expression of child and adolescent emotional and behavioral problems.

"Culture" is defined as "an integrated pattern of human behavior that includes thought, language, action, and artifacts and depends on man's capacity for learning and transmitting knowledge to succeeding generations" (Frisby & Reynolds, 2005, p. 5). Culture can influence the experience and expression of distress, so an individual's nationality, ethnicity, acculturation level, socioeconomic status, and gender must all be considered during assessment. The failure to take culture into consideration when conducting an assessment can lead to interpretative errors (Edwards, 1982; Ridley & Kelly, 2007). First, a behavior may be labeled as pathological when it is in fact normative within a given culture. Second, the opposite may also occur: A child's behavior may be assumed to be explained by cultural factors when the behavior is pathological. In either case, serious errors can occur.

Therefore, it is important for clinicians to consider cultural and diversity factors when selecting assessment tools and interpreting assessment data (see, e.g., Friedberg & McClure, 2002; Ridley & Kelly, 2007). First, the available evidence suggests that the expression of psychological symptoms and/or distress may vary across cultures (Weisz, Sigman, Weiss, & Mosk, 1993). This variation may be due to value systems that find different symptoms more or less acceptable. For example, cultures that place a high value on deference to authority appear to have lower rates of externalizing problems (Weisz, Suwanlert, Chaiyasit, & Walter, 1987). As another example, some have hypothesized that the acceptability of medical symptoms (as opposed to psychological symptoms) in the Hispanic/Latino cultures explains why Hispanic/Latino children report more somatic symptoms than European American children (see, e.g., Pina & Silverman, 2004).

Second, cultural factors can influence reporting practices. Specifically, the acceptability of certain symptoms may influence what symptoms are reported as problematic. For example, families from inner-city communities may see aggressive behavior as adaptive and thus may not report aggressive behaviors to a clinician (Atkins, McKay, Talbot, & Arvanitis, 1996). This means that a clinician cannot assume that a particular symptom is present or absent just because a family does not report it as a problem. The accurate interpretation of assessment data depends, in part, upon gaining an understanding of particular families' values.

In sum, understanding how culture influences symptom expression and reporting practices is an important component of conducting a culturally sensitive assessment. In selecting assessment tools, it is important to determine whether the tools have demonstrated validity across different cultural groups (see Pina, Gonzales, Holly, Zerr, & Wynne, Chapter 13, this volume). It is also important to work with the child and family to understand whether cultural factors influence the interpretation of assessment data (e.g., by using cultural mapping techniques; Pina, Villalta, & Zerr, 2009). It is vital for clinicians to be able to distinguish between normal variations associated with culture and abnormal variations characteristic of psychopathology.

Principle 6. The choice of assessment tools should be based on the strength of the tools' psychometric support for the type of client being assessed and the goals of the assessment. Careful attention should also be given to the judgmental heuristics that guide the interpretation of findings.

Assessment procedures should not only be culturally sensitive and developmentally appropriate, but also psychometrically validated (Ollendick & Hersen, 1984). To date, the practice of child assessment has been marked by the use of assessment tools that are convenient, with far too little attention paid to the measures' psychometric properties (Hunsley & Mash, 2008; Youngstrom, 2008). However, recent commentators on assessment have argued for a technology of evidence-based assessment that includes efforts to identify important psychometric dimensions and a system for rating the quality of each metric (Hunsley & Mash, 2008). It is imperative that the selection of assessment instruments be informed by the psychometric properties of specific tools, the evidence supporting how best to interpret particular tools, and the methods used to integrate multiple sources of data. When a clinician is reviewing the data in support of a particular instrument, it is important to note that a given tool is only supported for particular types of clients and probably only for certain purposes (Hunsley & Mash, 2008). For example, a scale may be very reliable when completed by an adolescent, but much less so when completed by a younger child. Similarly, a scale may be very useful for screening, but may not be sensitive to change and therefore not useful for outcome monitoring. In other words, the selection of an assessment tool needs to be influenced by whether the psychometric properties of the tool are supported for the type of client being assessed and the goals of the assessment.

It is important to note that the psychometric concepts relevant to nomothetic tools do not directly apply to idiographic instruments (Foster & Cone, 1995). In fact, there have been debates about what psychometric categories are relevant to idiographic tools (Foster & Cone, 1995; Jackson, 1999). Perhaps for this reason, recent efforts to identify important psychometric dimensions have focused upon nomothetic tools. Hunsley and Mash (2008) recently introduced a framework for considering the psychometric properties of nomothetic tools. This framework focuses upon the following categories: standardization, norms, reliability, validity, and clinical utility. Below, we cover these domains; however, we also review domains relevant to idiographic instruments.

Standardization

"Standardization" refers to the extent to which an assessment technique is delivered in a consistent manner across various conditions of administration (Barrios & Hartmann, 1986). The goal of standardization is to improve reliability by minimizing the influence of potential sources of error—child, clinician, context—on the scores produced by a particular instrument. When clinicians do not follow a predetermined set of questions or procedures, assessment techniques are susceptible to bias. The administration of diagnostic (e.g., diagnostic interviews) and behavioral (e.g., self-monitoring activities) tools can be standardized. Unstructured clinical interviews have been criticized for producing variable results (Angold & Fisher, 1999; Garb, 1998, 2005). Similarly, idiographic tools have been criticized because they lack standardized administration (Jackson, 1999). For this reason, it is important to ensure that when idiographic instruments are used, the instructions and items used with children and their families are held constant, so that changes in scores can be clearly interpreted.

Norms

For nomothetic tools, the availability of norms provides a concrete assessment of a child's behavior relative to other children. However, the quality of a measure's norms is important to consider. Ideally, a normative sample (1) should be representative of the population under study, (2) should be large enough to provide stable estimates of the population mean and standard deviation, and (3) should include clinical and nonclinical samples (Anastasi, 1988; Hunsley & Mash, 2008). To evaluate whether the norms for a measure fit a specific client, it is necessary to compare the composition of the normative sample to specific client characteristics. If a client is very different from a measure's normative sample on characteristics that might affect the meaning of the client's scale score, it is better to find a measure with more representative norms. Idiographic tools do not typically rely upon population norms, so this psychometric dimension is not relevant when the psychometric strength of idiographic tools is being considered.

Reliability

For nomothetic instruments, "reliability" refers to the consistency and dependability of a person's score on a measure. For example, a self-report measure is considered reliable if it provides the same score across repeated assessments. When clinicians are evaluating the quality of a nomothetic tool, it is important to consider internal consistency and test–retest reliability. "Internal consistency" assesses whether all questions in a measure contribute consistently to the overall measure score. Low internal consistency indicates that the questions may not all assess the same construct (e.g., depression). According to Hunsley and Mash (2008), the accumulated evidence for a measure should suggest that the internal validity for a measure is at least .70. "Test–retest" reliability assesses the stability of scores over multiple time points. This form of reliability is used when an instrument is designed to assess a construct that is purported to be stable over time (e.g., temperament). According to Hunsley and Mash (2008), test–retest coefficients are considered acceptable if equal to or greater than .70 over a short period of time (days or weeks) and excellent if over .70 for a long period of time (1 year or longer).

The concepts of reliability and accuracy also overlap with idiographic instruments (Cone, 1998; Jackson, 1999). "Accuracy" refers to the extent to which recorded data (self-report, self-monitoring, observational) provide a good representation of a target behavior (Cone, 1998; Jackson, 1999). To determine accuracy, an incontrovertible index is required that represents a "gold-standard" measure of the target behavior. As an incontrovertible index rarely exists for most behaviors, it is difficult to determine the true accuracy of specific observations. Reliability can also be assessed within the framework of generalizability theory. Facets that result in significant variability indicate that scores on a measure are not reliable for those facets. Decision studies can be used to determine how many observations are needed from a particular facet in order to produce a reliable estimate (Brennan, 2001).

The concept of "interrater reliability" applies to both idiographic and nomothetic tools; it refers to the differences in obtained results among raters who are using the same instrument. This type of reliability estimate is useful when clinicians are using interviews (e.g., standardized interviews such as the Anxiety Disorders Interview Schedule for DSM-IV: Child and Parent Versions; Silverman & Albano, 1996) or direct observation (e.g., the Autism Diagnostic Observation Schedule; Lord et al., 2000). According to Hunsley and Mash (2008), for categorical data, acceptable interrater reliability (kappa) falls between .70 and .79 and is preferred to be above .85; an acceptable Pearson/intraclass correlation ranges from .70 to .79 and is preferred to be above .90.

Validity

"Validity" refers to whether or not an instrument assesses what it purports to measure. Foster and Cone (1995) draw a distinction between *representative* and *elaborative* validity. "Representative validity" focuses upon establishing whether a tool assesses the theoretical domain or response class it is designed to assess (e.g., depression, experiential avoidance). "Elaborative validity" refers to whether a tool has utility for measuring a construct or response class. Several different validity dimensions exist. Whether a validity dimension is relevant to a particular nomothetic or idiographic tool depends in part upon what the instrument is designed to do.

"Content validity" is an important component of representative validity for nomothetic and idiographic instruments; it means that items capture all aspects of a given domain (e.g., depression). To establish content validity, researchers must clearly define the target domain and then demonstrate that the items represent all facets of that domain. For nomothetic tools, content validity is established by demonstrating that the items on an instrument tap into all aspects of the purported construct. Ideally, test developers of nomothetic instruments should clearly define the domain of interest and have expert judges rate the fit of each item on a quantitative scale (McLeod et al., in press). For idiographic tools that focus on a response class, content validity involves ensuring that all facets of the response class are defined. Content validity for idiographic tools also includes the sampling plan. To ensure content validity, a behavior must be sampled enough times to ensure the data will generalize across time and situations (Jackson, 1999).

Accuracy is a key validity dimension for idiographic instruments. As noted above, "accuracy" is defined as the extent to which scores represent the cognitive, affective, and behavioral components of the behavior (Foster & Cone, 1995). Establishing accuracy requires the existence of an independent, incontrovertible index of the target behavior. Three different ways of assessing accuracy have been proposed. First, scores produced by an idiographic instrument can be compared to physical evidence of a target behavior, such as mechanical recordings (Foster & Cone, 1995; Johnston & Pennypacker, 1993). Second, scores produced by an idiographic instrument can be compared to direct observation of a target behavior within the natural environment (Foster & Cone, 1995; Suen & Ary, 1989). And finally, controlled stimuli to which an idiographic instrument should be sensitive can be introduced to determine whether the tool captures the manipulation (Foster & Cone, 1999). For idiographic instruments that assess covert events and/or rely upon indirect methods (self-report), it is challenging to demonstrate accuracy. For this reason, these instruments are often evaluated in terms of convergent and discriminant validity (Jackson, 1999).

"Construct validity" provides evidence that an instrument taps into the theoretical concept that it was designed to assess (Foster & Cone, 1995; Hill & Lambert, 2004). There are multiple forms of construct validity (i.e., "convergent," "discriminant," "predictive," and "concurrent"). Two important categories of construct validity are convergent and discriminant evidence, which help to establish the representative validity of an instrument. This evidence is concerned with whether an instrument converges with measures of similar constructs and diverges from measures of different constructs. Traditionally, these categories were used for nomothetic instruments. However, as idiographic tools began to assess covert behaviors and employ indirect methods, these validity dimensions were applied to idiographic instruments.

Another important category of construct validity is "test–criterion relationships" (related to the traditional concepts of "concurrent" and "predictive" validities), which helps evaluate the elaborative validity of an instrument. This evidence applies to both nomothetic and idiographic tools, and indicates whether a measure is related to some present or future outcome that is thought to be meaningfully related to the construct the measure is supposed to be assessing. In the case of tools used to inform treatment, an important test–criterion relationship might be whether people who are assigned diagnoses by the instrument also show high levels of functional impairment that would be anticipated to result from the disorder. For an instrument to demonstrate construct validity, the majority of the data collected on the measure should support the different facets of construct validity. A dimension related to test–criterion relationships is "validity generalization." This dimension relates to elaborative validity and assesses the extent to which a measure's test–criterion relationships generalize across settings and populations different from the ones in which the instrument was originally validated. Validity generalization addresses the important question of whether the tool can be used across multiple contexts (home, school, clinic) and/or populations (age, gender, ethnicity).

The final validity dimension is "treatment sensitivity," which is also related to elaborative validity. This dimension is only relevant to instruments used for treatment monitoring and evaluation. Evidence for treatment sensitivity is demonstrated when a measure evidences some sensitivity to change over the course of treatment. This is a relatively new validity dimension, so clear guidelines for assessing the strength of evidence do not exist. Important issues to consider in evaluating evidence for treatment sensitivity include whether a measure is responsive to change across different types of treatment and how often the measure can be administered (whether the measure can be administered weekly, monthly, or at longer intervals).

In sum, validity is extremely important, because it indicates whether a measure is assessing the construct or behavior of interest. Multiple studies are needed to demonstrate the different forms of validity evidence, so it can sometimes be challenging to review validity evidence for particular measures.

Clinical Utility

In order to meet evidence-based standards for assessments, measures should also provide some indicator of "clinical utility" (Hunsley & Mash, 2007; Nelson-Gray, 2003; Vasey & Lonigan, 2000). Clinical utility is a relatively new validity dimension and has not received much empirical attention. At present, it can include "diagnostic utility" (a measure's ability to lead to a correct diagnostic conclusion), "incremental utility" (what information a particular measure can provide that cannot be provided by other instruments), "treatment utility" (a measure's beneficial contribution to treatment outcome), and "feasibility" (the ease with which the measure can be integrated into clinical practice). Essentially, for an instrument to have clinical utility, empirical studies must demonstrate that the use of the tool improves the accuracy, outcome, and/or efficiency of clinical activities (Hunsley & Mash, 2007).

The practicality and cost of an instrument should also be considered in the choice of an assessment tool. A number of factors can influence cost, including the amount of time required to administer the measure, the financial cost of administering and scoring it, the amount of time spent scoring and interpreting it, and required equipment (e.g., computers to score the measure; Jensen-Doss, 2005; Yates & Taub, 2003). Cost can also include training costs and/or the level of training required to administer and score the instrument (i.e., whether a trained clinician must administer the measure). In sum, balancing practical considerations with psychometric quality can be challenging, but it is an important aspect of deciding what measures to use to inform treatment.

COMBINING DATA ACROSS INFORMANTS

As noted earlier, a multimethod, multi-informant approach is recommended in child assessment. However, very few empirical data exist about how best to combine findings across measures and informants to produce a picture of an individual child. Questions persist about when and how certain measures should be used, whether tools need to be differentially weighted in the clinical decision-making process, and how to resolve discrepant reports. Obviously, it is important to use psychometrically strong instruments; however, combining the data also represents a critical step. Unfortunately, no research exists to guide this process. In this section, we provide some general issues to consider in combining findings across informants.

Once assessment data are collected, the clinician must integrate the data and produce a treatment plan. The low rates of agreement across informants commonly seen in child assessment can make this a challenging endeavor (De Los Reyes & Kazdin, 2005). Until recently, the field offered very little guidance on how to conceptualize or address such discrepancies. Fortunately, a new model has emerged that provides a framework for understanding this important aspect of assessment with children.

De Los Reyes and Kazdin (2005) have proposed the "attributions bias context" (ABC) model. The ABC model posits three factors that may influence informant discrepancies in child assessment. First, *informant's attributions* about the causes of problems may influence their reports. Children may be more likely to view their problems as contextual (e.g., "I am being bullied"), whereas others may view them as dispositional (e.g., "He is aggressive"). These differences in attributions are then related to differences in *informant's perspectives* regarding the nature of the problem and the need for treatment. For example, children may view their problems as lying within a specific situational context (e.g., "I get into fights because I am being bullied at school") and therefore not needing treatment, whereas others may perceive a need for treatment and may be more likely to report problems to support this view (e.g., "He is aggressive"). Finally, the *goal of the clinical process*—which is often perceived as collecting negative information about the child—probably contributes to discrepancies, as children are less likely to want to provide this type of information than other informants. In addition to these perceptual differences, the model also posits that differences between informants arise from the circumstances under which they observe a child's behavior. A recent study supported this last point by demonstrating that children behaved differently in lab-based interactions with examiners than they did in interactions with their parents; their behavior with the examiners was strongly correlated with their teachers' reports of their behavior, whereas their behavior with their parents was correlated with the parents' reports (De Los Reyes, Henry, Tolan, & Wakschlag, 2009).

The ABC model provides a new lens through which to consider data gathered from multiple informants. Despite these recent advances, however, there is precious little empirical evidence to guide the combination of data across informants. As a result, it is possible for biased clinical judgment to have a negative influence on this process. This is another reason why clinicians need to take an empirical, hypothesis-testing approach: to minimize the impact of clinician bias on the assessment process. Building upon the recommendations of De Los Reyes and Kazdin (2005), along with others (Barry et al., 2013), we offer the following two recommendations for dealing with multiple informants.

First, while clinicians are gathering assessment data, it may be helpful to gather information related to the ABC model that might help explain informant discrepancies (De Los Reyes & Kazdin, 2005). For example, it is helpful to ask informants what their attributions for the causes of a child's behavior are, and whether they think the child's behavior warrants treatment. In addition, given that informants are likely to vary in their views about whether the child's behavior is contextual or dispositional, it is important to strike a balance between general questions about a child's behavior (e.g., "Is your child anxious about talking to people she does not know?") and context-specific questions (e.g., "Does your child experience anxiety about talking to people she does not know when she is at parties with other children?"; example from De Los Reyes & Kazdin, 2005). Finally, gathering data that might help clarify contextual influences on informant behaviors can help interviewers interpret assessment data. Behavioral assessment methods can be very useful in this regard; indeed, they are based upon the idea that behavior is context-specific. For example, direct observation of a child's behavior in the school and in the home can help a clinician understand whether teachers and parents are observing and reporting on the same types of behaviors.

Second, once the assessment data have been gathered, a clinician should determine which informants have reported clinically significant behaviors and whether there is convergence across informants. The clinician may have more confidence in reports that converge across informants, but variation does not mean that any of the reports are incorrect. The clinician must therefore generate theory-driven hypotheses about what factors, such as context, culture, perceptual differences, or development, might account for differences across informants. For example, a given child may exhibit behavioral problems at home because those problems are reinforced by the parents, but does not exhibit those problems at school because the consequences for doing so are consistently negative. In this case, discrepancies between parent and teacher reports of behavior problems are not only to be expected, but are helpful for treatment planning, as they suggest that interventions targeting the home environment might be more useful than interventions targeting the school. Viewed through the lens of a theoretical model like the ABC model, informant discrepancies can be considered important sources of clinical data, rather than "noise" to be removed from the clinical picture. Multiple informants can therefore help in problem identification, case conceptualization, and treatment planning.

ETHICS AND STANDARDS OF CHILD DIAGNOSTIC AND BEHAVIORAL ASSESSMENT

A number of ethical issues arise in diagnostic and behavioral assessment with children and adolescents. Many of these issues cut across areas of practice and are not unique to assessment. For example, the American Psychological Association's (2002) "Ethical Principles of Psychologists and Code of Conduct" outlines guidelines for protecting client confidentiality, setting appropriate professional boundaries, maintaining records and billing, and other general areas of professional behavior. Standard 2 of this code of conduct also discusses at length issues related to competence. When applied to assessment, Standard 2 specifies that someone who conducts assessment should stay within the boundaries of his or her education, training, and experience. For example, it would not be considered ethical for a psychologist who has never been trained in the assessment of autism spectrum disorders to conduct an assessment to determine whether a child meets criteria for one of those disorders. As such, it is important to obtain training in the assessment strategies relevant to one's clinical practice, and to refer cases with assessment questions falling outside of one's training and expertise to other clinicians.

   In addition to these general ethical principles, Standard 9 of the code details ethical issues specific to assessment. Here we highlight those most relevant to the assessment of youth psychopathology. First, the recommendations stemming from an assessment should be based on sufficient data to support those recommendations. The assessment principles described in this chapter, including the use of multimethod, multi-informant assessment, can help ensure that this is the case. Second, these data must be interpreted in a way that takes into account the test-taking and personal characteristics of the client that might influence the interpretation. Grounding an assessment in the developmental psychopathology literature and being sensitive to multicultural issues can help ensure that assessment data are interpreted in an appropriate manner.

The code also specifies that the tools used in an assessment should be used in a manner supported by research and should have established reliability and validity for the members of the population tested. As discussed by Pina et al. in Chapter 13, this often presents a challenge for clinicians working with ethnic minority youth, because few instruments have been well tested with these populations. In those cases, the ethical code indicates that clinicians must be clear about the strengths and limitations of their testing approach.

Standard 9 also details principles to guide the process of informed consent for assessment, indicating that before clients consent to an assessment, they must receive information about the nature and purpose of the assessment, the cost of the assessment, and limits to confidentiality. For child assessments, unique issues arise in relation to informed consent. Legally, only parental consent is often required for child services, including assessment. However, often it is ethical to obtain assent from child clients as well. The type of information that is developmentally appropriate to provide to children, and the correct timing of informed consent (e.g., is it ethical to conduct a behavioral observation before obtaining assent?), are among issues that are not clearly addressed in the ethical code.

Finally, Standard 9 states that the results of an assessment must be clearly explained to the individual or a "delegated representative." In the case of child assessment, this means that the results must be clearly explained to parents. Together with the parents, the clinician should also decide how much information is appropriate to provide to the child, taking into account the nature of the assessment feedback and the child's developmental level. A thorough discussion of all ethical issues related to assessment is beyond the scope of this volume. However, a detailed understanding of the entire ethical code is essential for both psychology trainees and licensed psychologists.

SUMMARY

The past two decades have witnessed exciting advances in assessment. The rise of the evidence-based assessment movement has focused attention on assessment training and practice. At the heart of the evidence-based assessment movement is the principle that science and theory should guide and inform the assessment process. Increasingly, the field is moving toward establishing a set of guidelines for assessment practice. Despite these advances, critical gaps still exist. Most notably, very little research is available to guide assessment practices during treatment. It is our hope that the evidence-based assessment movement will inspire more research that will help fill these knowledge gaps in the coming years.

Our approach to assessment is informed by this movement. The principles presented in this chapter are consistent with evidence-based assessment and are designed to help guide the assessment process from intake to termination. Both diagnostic and behavioral assessment tools are needed to inform the treatment process, and we have covered areas of knowledge (such as psychometric theory) that are needed to apply assessment tools over the course of treatment. With an overview of our assessment approach thus presented, we now turn to more detailed coverage of the knowledge and skills needed for diagnostic and behavioral assessment.

REFERENCES

American Psychological Association. (2002). Ethical principles of psychologists and code of conduct. *American Psychologist, 57,* 1060–1073.

Anastasi, A. (1988). *Psychological testing* (6th ed.). New York: Macmillan.

Angold, A., & Fisher, P. W. (1999). Interviewer-based interviews. In D. Shaffer, C. P. Lucas, & J. E. Richters (Eds.), *Diagnostic assessment in child and adolescent psychopathology* (pp. 34–64). New York: Guilford Press.

Atkins, M. S., McKay, M. M., Talbot, E., & Arvanitis, P. (1996). DSM-IV diagnosis of conduct disorder and oppositional defiant disorder: Implications and guidelines for school mental health teams. *School Psychology Review, 25,* 274–283.

Barrett, P. M., & Ollendick, T. H. (Eds.). (2004). *Handbook of interventions that work with children and adolescents.* Chichester, UK: Wiley.

Barrios, B., & Hartmann, D. P. (1986). The contributions of traditional assessment: Concepts, issues, and methodologies. In R. O. Nelson & S. C. Hayes (Eds.), *Conceptual foundations of behavioral assessment* (pp. 81–110). New York: Guilford Press.

Barry, C. T., Frick, P. J., & Kamphaus, R. W. (2013). Psychological assessment in child mental health settings. In B. Bracken, J. Carlson, J. Hansen, N. Kucel, S. Reise, & M. Rodrequez (Eds.), *APA handbook of testing and assessment in psychology.* Washington, DC: American Psychological Association.

Bem, D. I., & Allen, A. (1974). On predicting some of the people some of the time: The search for cross-situational consistencies in behavior. *Psychological Review, 81,* 506–520.

Brennan, R. L. (2001). *Generalizability theory.* New York: Springer-Verlag.

Camara, W. J., Nathan, J. S., & Puente, A. E. (2000). Psychological test usage: Implications in professional psychology. *Evaluation, 31,* 141–154.

Chi, T. C., & Hinshaw, S. P. (2002). Mother–child relationships of children with ADHD: The role of maternal depressive symptoms and depression-related distortions. *Journal of Abnormal Child Psychology, 30,* 387–400.

Childs, R. A., & Eyde, L. D. (2002). Assessment training in clinical psychology doctoral programs: What should we teach? What do we teach? *Journal of Personality Assessment, 78,* 130–144.

Cicchetti, D., & Cohen, D. J. (1995). *Developmental psychopathology: Vol. 1. Theory and methods.* New York: Wiley.

Cone, J. D. (1986). Idiographic, nomothetic, and related perspectives in behavioral assessment. In R. O. Nelson & S. C. Hayes (Eds.), *Conceptual foundations of behavioral assessment* (pp. 111–128). New York: Guilford Press.

Cone, J. D. (1998). Psychometric considerations: Concepts, contents, and methods. In M. Hersen & A. S. Bellack (Eds.), *Behavioral assessment: A practical handbook* (4th ed., pp. 22–46). Boston: Allyn & Bacon.

Cronbach, L. J., Gleser, G. C., Nanda, H., & Rajaratnam, N. (1972). *The dependability of behavioral measurements: Theory of generalizability of scores and profiles.* New York: Wiley.

Dadds, M. R., James, R. C., Barrett, P. M., & Verhulst, F. C. (2004). Diagnostic issues. In T. H. Ollendick & J. S. March (Eds.), *Phobic and anxiety disorders in children and adolescents: A clinician's guide to effective psychosocial and pharmacological interventions* (pp. 3–33). New York: Oxford University Press.

De Los Reyes, A., Henry, D. B., Tolan, P. H., & Wakschlag, L. S. (2009). Linking informant discrepancies to observed variations in young children's disruptive behavior. *Journal of Abnormal Child Psychology, 37,* 637–652.

De Los Reyes, A., & Kazdin, A. E. (2005). Informant discrepancies in the assessment of childhood psychopathology: A critical review, theoretical framework, and recommendations for further study. *Psychological Bulletin, 131,* 483–509.

Edelbrock, C., Costello, A. J., Dulcan, M. K., Kalas, R., & Conover, N. C. (1985). Age differences in the reliability of the psychiatric interview of the child. *Child Development, 56,* 265–275.

Edwards, A. W. (1982). The consequences of error in selecting treatment for blacks. *Social Casework, 63,* 429–433.

Eells, T. D. (2007). *Handbook of psychotherapy case formulation* (2nd ed.). New York: Guilford Press.

Foster, S. L., & Cone, J. D. (1995). Validity issues in clinical assessment. *Psychological Assessment, 7,* 248–260.

Fox, N. A., Henderson, H. A., Marshall, P. J., Nichols, K. E., & Ghera, M. M. (2005). Behavioral inhibition: Linking biology and behavior within a developmental framework. *Annual Review of Psychology, 56,* 235–262.

Friedberg, R., & McClure, J. (2002). Review of clinical practice of cognitive therapy with children and adolescents. *Journal of Developmental and Behavioral Pediatrics, 23,* 457–458.

Frisby, C. L., & Reynolds, C. R. (2005). *Comprehensive handbook of multicultural school psychology.* Hoboken, NJ: Wiley.

Garb, H. N. (1998). *Studying the clinician: Judgment research and psychological assessment.* Washington, DC: American Psychological Association.

Garb, H. N. (2005). Clinical judgment and decision making. *Annual Review of Clinical Psychology, 1,* 67–89.

Gullone, E. (1996). Normal fear in people with a physical or intellectual disability. *Clinical Psychology Review, 16,* 689–706.

Hayes, S. C., Wilson, K. G., Gifford, E. V., Follette, V. M., & Strosahl, K. (1996). Experiential avoidance and behavioral disorders: A functional dimensional approach to diagnosis and treatment. *Journal of Consulting and Clinical Psychology, 64,* 1152–1168.

Hill, C. E., & Lambert, M. (2004). Methodological issues in studying psychotherapy processes and outcomes. In M. J. Lambert (Ed.), *Bergin and Garfield's handbook of psychotherapy and behavior change* (5th ed., pp. 84–136). New York: Wiley.

Holmbeck, G. N., Thill, A. W., Bachanas, P., Garber, J., Miller, K. B., Abad, M., Zuckerman, J. (2008). Evidence-based assessment in pediatric psychology: Measures of psychosocial adjustment and psychopathology. *Journal of Pediatric Psychology, 33,* 958–980.

Hunsley, J. (2002). Psychological testing and psychological assessment: A closer examination. *American Psychologist, 57,* 139–140.

Hunsley, J., & Mash, E. J. (2007). Evidence-based assessment. *Annual Review of Clinical Psychology, 3,* 29–51.

Hunsley, J., & Mash, E. J. (Eds.). (2008). *A guide to assessments that work.* New York: Oxford University Press.

Jackson, J. L. (1999). Psychometric considerations in self-monitoring assessment. *Psychological Assessment, 11,* 439–447.

Jensen-Doss, A. (2005). Evidence-based diagnosis: Incorporating diagnostic instruments into clinical practice. *Journal of the American Academy of Child and Adolescent Psychiatry, 44,* 947–952.

Johnston, J. M., & Pennypacker, H. S. (1993). *Strategies and tactics of behavioral research* (2nd ed.). Hillsdale, NJ: Erlbaum.

Kamphaus, R. W., & Frick, P. J. (2005). *Clinical assessment of child and adolescent personality and behavior.* New York: Springer.

Krishnamurthy, R., VandeCreek, L., Kaslow, N. J., Tazeau, Y. N., Miville, M. L., Kerns, R., & Benton, S. A. (2004). Achieving competency in psychological assessment: Directions for education and training. *Journal of Clinical Psychology, 60,* 725–739.

Lambert, M. J., Whipple, J. L., Hawkins, E. J., Vermeersch, D. A., Nielsen, S. L., & Smart, D. W. (2003). Is it time for clinicians to routinely track patient outcome?: A meta-analysis. *Clinical Psychology: Science and Practice, 10,* 288–301.

Loeber, R., Green, S. M., Lahey, B. B., & Stouthamer-Loeber, M. (1991). Differences and similarities between children, mothers, and teachers as informants on childhood psychopathology. *Journal of Abnormal Child Psychology, 19,* 75–95.

Lord, C., Risi, S., Lambrecht, L., Cook, E. H., Jr., Leventhal, B. L., DiLavore, P. C., & Rutter, M. (2000). The Autism Diagnostic Observation Schedule—Generic: A standard measure of social and communication deficits associated with the spectrum of autism. *Journal of Autism and Developmental Disorders, 30,* 205–223.

Mash, E. J., & Barkley, R. A. (2007). *Assessment of childhood disorders* (4th ed.). New York: Guilford Press.

Masten, A. S., & Braswell, L. (1991). Developmental psychopathology: An integrative framework. In P. R. Martin (Ed.), *Pergamon general psychology series: Vol. 164. Handbook of behavior therapy and psychological science: An integrative approach* (pp. 35–56). New York: Pergamon Press.

McLeod, B. D., Jensen-Doss, A., Wheat, E., & Becker, E. M. (in press). Evidence-based assessment and case formulation for child anxiety. In C. Essau & T. H. Ollendick (Eds.), *Treatment of childhood and adolescent anxiety.*

McLeod, B. D., & Weisz, J. R. (2004). Using dissertations to examine potential bias and child and adolescent clinical trials. *Journal of Consulting and Clinical Psychology, 72,* 235–251.

Mischel, W. (1968). *Personality and assessment.* New York: Wiley.

Nelson-Gray, R. O. (2003). Treatment utility of psychological assessment. *Psychological Assessment, 15,* 521–531.

Nezu, A. M., Nezu, C. M., Peacock, M. A., & Girdwood, C. P. (2004). Case formulation in cognitive-behavior therapy. In M. Hersen (Series Ed.) & S. N. Haynes & E. M. Heiby (Vol. Eds.), *Comprehensive handbook of psychological assessment: Vol. 3. Behavioral assessment* (pp. 402–426). Hoboken, NJ: Wiley.

Ollendick, T. H. (1999). Empirically supported assessment for clinical practice: Is it possible? Is it desirable? *The Clinical Psychologist, 52,* 1–2.

Ollendick, T. H., & Hersen, M. (Eds.). (1984). *Child behavioral assessment: Principles and procedures.* New York: Pergamon Press.

Olweus, D. (1979). Stability of aggressive reaction patterns in males: A review. *Psychological Bulletin, 86,* 852–875.

Paikoff, R. L., & Brooks-Gunn, J. (1991). Do parent–child relationships change during puberty? *Psychological Bulletin, 110,* 47–66.

Pina, A. A., & Silverman, W. K. (2004). Clinical phenomenology, somatic symptoms, and distress in Hispanic/Latino and European American youths with anxiety disorders. *Journal of Clinical Child and Adolescent Psychology, 33,* 227–236.

Pina, A. A., Villalta, I. K., & Zerr, A. A. (2009). Exposure-based cognitive behavioral treatment of anxiety in youth: A culturally-prescriptive framework. *Behavioral Psychology, 17,* 111–135.

Richters, J. E. (1992). Depressed mothers as informants about their children: A critical review of the evidence for distortion. *Psychological Bulletin, 112,* 485–499.

Ridley, C. R., & Kelly, S. M. (2007). Multicultural considerations in case formulation. In T. D. Eells (Ed.), *Handbook of psychotherapy case formulation* (2nd ed., pp. 33–64). New York: Guilford Press.

Schroeder, C. S., & Gordon, B. N. (2002). *Assessment and treatment of childhood problems* (2nd ed.). New York: Guilford Press.

Silverman, W. K., & Albano, A. M. (1996). *Anxiety Disorders Interview Schedule for DSM-IV: Child and Parent Versions.* San Antonio, TX: Psychological Corporation.

Silverman, W. K., & Ollendick, T. H. (2005). Evidence-based assessment of anxiety and its disorders in children and adolescents. *Journal of Clinical Child and Adolescent Psychology, 34,* 380–411.

Stein, B. D., Kogan, J. N., Hutchison, S. L., Magee, E. A., & Sorbero, M. J. (2010). Use of outcomes information in child mental health treatment: Results from a pilot study. *Psychiatric Services, 61,* 1211–1216.

Stemberger, R. T., Turner, S. M., Beidel, D. C., & Calhoun, K. S. (1995). Social phobia: An analysis of possible developmental factors. *Journal of Abnormal Psychology, 104,* 526–531.

Suen, H. K., & Ary, D. (1989). *Analyzing quantitative behavioral observation data.* Hillsdale, NJ: Erlbaum.

Vasey, M. W., & Lonigan, C. J. (2000). Considering the clinical utility of performance-based measures of childhood anxiety. *Journal of Clinical Child Psychology, 29,* 493–508.

Warren, S. L., & Sroufe, L. A. (2004). Developmental issues. In T. H. Ollendick & J. S. March (Eds.), *Phobic and anxiety disorders in children and adolescents:*

A clinician's guide to effective psychosocial and pharmacological interventions (pp. 92–115). New York: Oxford University Press.

Weisz, J. R., Jensen-Doss, A., & Hawley, K. M. (2005). Youth psychotherapy outcome research: A review and critique of the literature. *Annual Review of Psychology, 56,* 337–363.

Weisz, J. R., Sigman, M., Weiss, B., & Mosk, J. (1993). Behavioral and emotional problems among Embu children in Kenya: Comparisons with African-American, Caucasian, and Thai children. *Child Development, 64,* 98–109.

Weisz, J. R., Suwanlert, S., Chaiyasit, W., & Walter, B. R. (1987). Over- and undercontrolled referral problems among children and adolescents from Thailand and the United States: The *wat* and *wai* of cultural differences. *Journal of Clinical and Consulting Psychology, 55,* 719–726.

Yates, B. T., & Taub, J. (2003). Assessing the costs, benefits, cost-effectiveness, and cost-benefit of psychological assessment: We should, we can, and here's how. *Psychological Assessment, 15,* 478–495.

Youngstrom, E. (2008). Evidence-based strategies for the assessment of developmental psychopathology: Measuring prediction, prescription, and process. In W. E. Craighead, D. J. Miklowitz, & L. W. Craighead (Eds.), *Psychopathology: History, diagnosis, and empirical foundations* (pp. 34–77). Hoboken, NJ: Wiley.

2

Diagnostic Assessment

Amanda Jensen-Doss, Bryce D. McLeod,
and Thomas H. Ollendick

The *Oxford English Dictionary* defines "diagnosis" as "identification of a disease by careful investigation of its symptoms and history; also, the opinion (formally stated) resulting from such investigation" ("Diagnosis," 1989). This term originated with the diagnosis of medical conditions, which often are clearly defined and measurable disease processes that differ from typical healthy functioning. The use of the term "diagnosis" in child and adolescent psychopathology therefore reflects a medical model orientation toward viewing such psychopathology as consisting of identifiable clusters of symptoms that are measurably different from typical emotional and behavioral development. Thus the purpose of diagnostic assessment of child psychopathology is to identify whether a child is experiencing a syndrome or disorder that is different from the behavior that would be expected in a typically developing child and that is interfering with the child's day-to-day functioning. Given its focus on classifying behavior relative to developmental norms, diagnostic assessment is nomothetic in nature, and must be complemented with idiographic assessment methods to formulate a full clinical picture that can inform treatment planning.

As noted in Chapter 1, diagnostic assessment serves several important purposes. Perhaps most importantly, diagnoses facilitate communication among professionals about clinical clients and research samples. The two currently prevailing diagnostic systems—those of the American Psychiatric Association (2013) and the World Health Organization (1993)—detail specific, standard symptoms that characterize mental health diagnoses. As such, diagnostic labels are designed to convey information about a specific clinical picture. Diagnoses can therefore be used by clinicians to summarize their clients' problems easily, and thus to simplify communicating with other professionals. Researchers also use them to specify the presenting problems of their research samples, facilitating integration of research findings across studies and allowing clinicians to access the research findings most relevant to their clients.

A second important purpose is to inform treatment planning and selection. The role of diagnosis in treatment planning has become more salient as the field has increasingly focused on providers' use of "evidence-based practice," defined as "the integration of the best available research with clinical expertise in the context of patient characteristics, culture, and preferences" (American Psychological Association Presidential Task Force on Evidence-Based Practice, 2006, p. 273). Diagnoses play a central role in evidence-based practice, as most guidelines for such practice are organized by diagnosis—including lists of evidence-based treatments (e.g., Silverman & Hinshaw, 2008), evidence-based assessment reviews (Hunsley & Mash, 2007), and practice parameters (Birmaher et al., 2007; Cohen et al., 2010; Connolly & Bernstein, 2007; McClellan, Kowatch, & Findling, 2007). Underlying all these guidelines is the notion that treatments should be matched to diagnosis, an assumption that is largely untested (Nelson-Gray, 2003). Research is needed to establish the treatment utility of using diagnoses to determine treatment choice (Nelson-Gray, 2003). Nevertheless, diagnoses currently serve as the main avenue for clinicians to identify researcher-developed therapies to use with their clients.

A third purpose is for service authorization. Many clinics and insurance providers require clients to meet criteria for a diagnosis, or even one of a specific set of diagnoses, to qualify for services. Diagnosis also plays a role in qualifying children for some types of special education services under the Individuals with Disabilities Education Improvement Act of 2004 (Public Law No. 108-446) or under Section 504 of the Rehabilitation Act.

Finally, diagnoses can be used to monitor treatment outcomes. Optimally, children who meet criteria for a disorder at the beginning of treatment will no longer meet those criteria when treatment is over. Traditionally, psychotherapy research has focused on determining whether symptom differences between treated and untreated children are statistically different, rather than on how meaningful treatment gains are in terms of returning clients to healthy levels of functioning. Increasingly, the field is emphasizing whether treatments produce "clinically significant" change, representing a return to, or significant progress toward, "normal" functioning (Jacobson & Truax, 1991). Determining whether someone continues to meet criteria for a diagnosis at the end of treatment is one important indicator of clinically significant change.

HISTORICAL ROOTS OF DIAGNOSTIC ASSESSMENT

The first documentation of a mental disorder was recorded in Egypt in 3000 B.C.E. and the first system for identifying psychiatric diagnoses was developed in India in 1400 B.C.E. (Mack, Forman, Brown, & Frances, 1994). Childhood psychopathology was largely neglected as an area of study prior to the 20th century (Rubinstein, 1948), and the first version of the prevailing diagnostic system in the United States, the *Diagnostic and Statistical Manual of Mental Disorders* (DSM; American Psychiatric Association, 1952), contained only two categories of childhood disorders. However, the study of childhood psychopathology has surged during the past several decades, and the current version of DSM (DSM-5; American Psychiatric Association, 2013) is organized around developmental and lifespan considerations, progressing from diagnoses that begin early in life (e.g., autism spectrum disorder), to those common in adolescence and young adulthood (e.g., depressive disorders), and ending with diagnoses that emerge later in life. Over time, the field has struggled with several issues related to the definition and measurement of child psychopathology. Here we review several key issues that continue to be sources of discussion among researchers and clinicians alike.

Categorical versus Dimensional Classification

Since Hippocrates developed his dimensional model of psychopathology based on the balance of "humors" (i.e., fluids) within the body, and Plato countered it with a categorical model of "divine madness," one of the fundamental debates about diagnosis has been the issue of dimensional versus categorical classification (Mack et al., 1994). Although the pendulum of prevailing opinion has swung back and forth between the two sides of the issue, today the prevailing model is the categorical approach. The categorical model of classification is based on the theory that mental health difficulties can be classified into distinct disorders. Categorical approaches assume that individuals either do or do not have a particular diagnosis. To determine whether someone meets criteria for a diagnosis, clinicians assess the presence or absence of the specific symptoms constituting the diagnosis, including their duration and associated impairment. The categorical approaches are at the core of the DSM-5 (American Psychiatric Association, 2013) and *International Statistical Classification of Diseases and Related Health Problems, 10th revision* (ICD-10; World Health Organization, 1993) systems of diagnosis. A description of the DSM system can serve as an illustration of how categorical systems work.

Originally developed in 1952 by the American Psychiatric Association to facilitate communication among professionals, DSM has undergone six revisions, most recently resulting in the DSM-5 (American Psychiatric Association, 2013). In DSM-I and DSM-II, diagnoses were defined according to specific theories of psychopathology, primarily psychoanalytic theory. This reliance on defining diagnoses in terms of specific theories limited the acceptance of the system (Follette & Houts, 1996). To gain a wider appeal, diagnoses in DSM-III (American Psychiatric Association, 1980) were not tied to a specific theory of psychopathology, and an emphasis was placed on creating definitions with empirical support. Subsequent versions have employed work groups of researchers and clinicians to generate diagnostic categories based on research.

Although the previous version of the DSM (DSM-IV-TR; American Psychiatric Association, 2000) included a multiaxial system to separately classify an individual's problems falling into different domains (e.g., clinical disorders, general medical conditions, etc.), DSM-5 uses a single axis system in which clinicians document any mental health and medical diagnoses. Clinicians are also instructed to use V-codes to separately document any psychosocial (e.g., relational problems, child maltreatment) or environmental (e.g., problems related to access to mental health care, housing problems) problems that might contribute to an individual's psychopathology or influence the diagnosis, course, prognosis or treatment of a disorder. For each disorder in DSM-5, the manual provides explanations of associated features; information about the prevalence, development and course of the disorder; risk and prognostic factors; culture- and gender-related diagnostic issues; information about suicide risk associated with the disorder; a description of the functional consequences of the disorder; and strategies for differential diagnosis (i.e., how to tell the difference between that disorder and other similar conditions). Diagnoses are assigned according to a "polythetic" format, in which only a subset of a larger set of symptoms is required to meet criteria for a given disorder. For example, a diagnosis of oppositional defiant disorder requires a child to have at least four of eight symptoms lasting at least 6 months (American Psychiatric Association, 2013). Importantly, this structure allows for variation in symptom presentation across individuals; however, some researchers have pointed out that this within-diagnosis heterogeneity adds confusion to the diagnostic process, and probably decreases its reliability and validity (Clark, Watson, & Reynolds, 1995).

The primary advantage of categorical models of psychopathology is that they lend themselves well to the purposes of diagnosis. Nearly all of the purposes of diagnosis discussed above relate to making categorical decisions about "clients" (whether to admit them for treatment, whether to apply a particular evidence-based treatment to a client, etc.); categorical diagnosis therefore facilitate these types of decisions. However, data increasingly suggest that categorical models may not accurately capture the structure of psychopathology. Studies in both the youth and adult literature have found that many forms of psychopathology are dimensional in nature, rather than being distinct categories that differ from "normal" functioning (e.g., Broman-Fulks et al., 2009; Hankin, Fraley, Lahey, & Waldman, 2005; Haslam et al., 2006; Kendler et al., 1996). In addition, evidence suggests that clients who are symptomatic, but fall below diagnostic cutoffs, experience functional impairment (e.g., Angold, Costello, Farmer, Burns, & Erkanli, 1999), and that the presence of subsyndromal symptoms is a risk factor for developing more severe psychopathology (Costello, Angold,

& Keeler, 1999). These findings suggest that dimensional models may be more appropriate ways of conceptualizing and measuring psychopathology.

Dimensional systems conceptualize psychopathology as existing along a continuum. Rather than considering individuals with a diagnosis to be qualitatively different from those without it, the dimensional model posits that symptoms vary naturally across the population, with low levels of symptoms being associated with lower impairment and higher levels of symptoms warranting clinical attention. Given the above-described research supporting these models, many researchers advocated for the inclusion of more dimensional models in DSM-5 (Helzer, Kraemer, & Krueger, 2006; Widiger & Samuel, 2005); some dimensional approaches were described in a section of DSM-5 on "Emerging Measures and Models," with recommendations that they be studied further (American Psychiatric Association, 2013). The National Institute of Mental Health (NIMH) is also working on developing a dimensional approach that conceptualizes psychopathology in terms of core domains (e.g., approach motivation, attention) that cut across traditional categorical disorders (Insel et al., 2010). Achenbach and his colleagues have been at the forefront of the movement to promote dimensional models of childhood psychopathology. This work has resulted in the Achenbach System of Empirically Based Assessment (ASEBA; Achenbach & Rescorla, 2001), a set of youth, parent, and teacher report measures of childhood emotional and behavioral symptoms. Though other dimensional systems have been developed, we briefly use the ASEBA to illustrate a typical dimensional approach to classification. This system is discussed in more detail by Achenbach himself in Chapter 6 of this volume.

Although some dimensional measures are based on "top-down" approaches similar to those used to develop DSM (i.e., theory or expert consensus is used to develop measures), others, including the ASEBA, are based on "bottom-up" approaches (Helzer et al., 2006). In bottom-up or "empirical" approaches, scales are statistically developed by creating items representing common symptoms, administering those items to large groups of children or the parents or teachers of those children, and then applying factor analysis or other statistical models to detect common factors of psychopathology.

Because dimensional measures such as the ASEBA are based on the notion that symptoms are distributed continuously across the population, normative samples are often used to determine what level of symptoms is considered typical within a population and what level is considered non-normative. For example, the current version of the ASEBA was administered to approximately 2,300 children from the 48 contiguous states (Achenbach & Rescorla, 2001). The means and standard deviations of scale scores obtained within normative samples can be used to create norms, which can then be utilized to compare a given child's score to scores of other children. Norms can be created either by using the entire normative sample, or by using subgroups of the sample (e.g., the ASEBA has norms based on age and gender). To compare a given client's score to a measure's norms, the client's score is converted to a standard score indicating where that score lies relative to the normative group's mean in terms of the normative group's standard deviation. Most often the T score is used in psychopathology rating scales, which has a mean of 50 and a standard deviation of 10; on most such scales, a T score of 70 (i.e., two standard deviations above the mean) is considered to be in the "clinical range."

The main disadvantage of dimensional approaches is that, used in a purely dimensional fashion, they do not lend themselves well to many of the clinical decisions that clinicians and researchers need to make. To address this limitation, the authors of dimensional measures of psychopathology typically include "clinical cutoff" scores, which essentially allow clinicians to generate categorical information from dimensional measures. Importantly, when applied in this way, dimensional measures have the added advantage of enabling clinicians to apply different cutoffs for different purposes (e.g., one cutoff to qualify for outpatient treatment and another for hospitalization)—a flexibility not found in categorical diagnoses (Widiger & Samuel, 2005).

Another advantage of dimensional measures is that they capture variability in symptom expression within the population, something that is disregarded in categorical definitions. Dimensional measures therefore have more statistical power when used in research (Helzer et al., 2006). They are also more sensitive to symptom changes occurring in treatment, making them more useful than categorical approaches for treatment outcome monitoring.

Because both categorical and dimensional approaches to classifying psychopathology seem to have their benefits, some are calling for the field to find ways to combine the two approaches (e.g., Helzer et al., 2006). As DSM-5 was being developed, some efforts were made to answer this call. For example, the Autism Spectrum Disorder definition includes both a categorical definition of the disorder and a dimensional severity rating scale (American Psychiatric Association, 2013). However, many other proposed dimensional approaches were not formally included in the diagnostic system. For example, the personality disorders work group created a model for evaluating personality pathology in terms of domains of personality functioning and pathological personality traits, with specific diagnoses defined in terms of the areas of functioning impacted and the types of traits manifested (American Psychiatric Association, 2013); however, this model was not adopted for DSM-5, but recommended for further study. Also included in the DSM-5 section of approaches in need of additional study were dimensional cross-cutting symptom measures, a clinician-rated severity measure to be used in combination with the categorical psychotic disorder diagnoses, and the World Health Organization Disability Assessment Schedule (World Health Organization, 2012), a measure that captures level of functional impairment associated with categorical diagnoses.

The Role of Clinical Judgment in Diagnosis

Another controversy linked to diagnosis relates to the role that clinical judgment must necessarily play in the diagnostic process. Traditionally, clinicians primarily used their clinical judgment to assign diagnoses: They would gather information from young clients and/or their parents about the client's symptoms and then use their clinical expertise to determine what diagnosis best described the client's behavior.

Unfortunately, research has shown that clinicians engage in several information-gathering biases that could influence the diagnostic process (Angold & Fisher, 1999; Garb, 1998, 2005). Although such biases have not been as widely examined in mental health clinicians as in medical professionals, many models of diagnostic errors among medical practitioners (e.g., Croskerry, 2009; Norman, 2009) are based on the dual-processing theory of decision making (Evans, 2008; Sloman, 1996). Developed in cognitive psychology, this theory proposes that human decision-making strategies fall into two primary categories. The first, "heuristic" or "System 1" decision making, is intuitive and based on pattern recognition. System 1 decision making allows humans to make efficient decisions without lengthy deliberative processes. The second, "analytic" or "System 2" decision making, is based on systematic data collection and deliberation. System 2 strategies allow humans to make more complex and reflective decisions.

In his "Universal Model of Diagnostic Reasoning," Croskerry (2009) proposes that both types of decision making play important roles in the diagnostic process and have relative advantages and disadvantages. He proposes that System 1 processes are engaged when an illness is easily recognized, either because it is a typical presentation or because the clinician is experienced. This is supported by data suggesting that experts in a variety of fields often use System 1 decision-making strategies with accuracy (Evans, 2008). However, System 1 strategies have several disadvantages, primarily that they are prone to a number of decision-making biases. Several of the biases observed in clinicians' diagnostic behavior suggest that the clinicians may be relying on System 1 decision making. For example, clinicians often decide on a diagnosis before collecting all relevant data, and then seek information to confirm that diagnosis while ignoring information inconsistent with the diagnosis, engaging in what has been called a "confirmation bias" (Croskerry, 2002). Research also suggests that clinicians combine information in ways that do not conform to DSM criteria, perhaps because they base decisions on whether their clients conform to a predetermined cognitive schema regarding a prototypical client with the diagnosis (Garb, 2005). Basic research on decision making also suggests that clinicians may base diagnostic judgments on the most readily available cognitive pattern (Angold & Fisher, 1999; Garb, 1998); for example, a clinician may be more likely to assign a diagnosis that is often seen than a diagnosis rarely encountered. Additional biases thought to influence clinicians' data gathering and decision making include a bias toward perceiving psychopathology over normative behavior, as well as biases based on stereotypes about gender, ethnicity, and/or age (Garb, 1998).

To date, most efforts to improve mental health diagnosis have focused on getting clinicians to gather and interpret data in ways consistent with System 2 decision making. The seminal work in this area was Meehl's (1954/1996) book *Clinical versus Statistical Prediction: A Theoretical Analysis and a Review of the Evidence*, which suggested that statistically based algorithmic models for making decisions are at least as accurate as clinicians, if not more so. Research has largely supported this proposition, with a recent meta-analysis finding a small but significant advantage of algorithmic techniques over clinical predictions (Grove, Zald, Lebow, Snitz, & Nelson, 2000).

In research on mental health diagnosis, many researchers have compared diagnoses assigned by clinicians to those generated through use of algorithmic standardized diagnostic interviews (SDIs) consisting of standard rules for information gathering (see "Standardized Interviews," below). These studies were combined in a meta-analysis that found the average agreement for youth diagnoses with these two approaches to be kappa = .39 (Rettew, Lynch, Achenbach, Dumenci, & Ivanova, 2009), which is considered "poor" agreement (Landis & Koch, 1977). Although this low agreement does not necessarily mean that algorithmic diagnostic methods are more accurate, studies examining the relative validity of the two diagnostic approaches have found stronger support for structured diagnostic interviews. Basco et al. (2000) found that such interviews had higher concordance than clinician diagnoses with diagnoses generated by experts who reviewed all available information. Other studies comparing both types of diagnoses to external validity indicators, such as daily behavior reports (Jewell, Handwerk, Almquist, & Lucas, 2004) and impaired functioning (Tenney, Schotte, Denys, van Megen, & Westenberg, 2003), have also found higher validity for the interviewers. Finally, youth whose clinician-generated diagnoses match structured diagnostic interviews have been found to have better therapy engagement and outcomes (Jensen-Doss & Weisz, 2008; Kramer, Robbins, Phillips, Miller, & Burns, 2003; Pogge et al., 2001). Taken together, these data suggest that efforts to help clinicians generate diagnoses more in line with structured diagnostic interviews might increase the validity of those diagnoses and thus have a positive impact on youth outcomes.

The Call for Evidence-Based Diagnosis

Although evidence-based assessment has not received as much attention as evidence-based treatment, researchers are increasingly focusing on studying ways to define and disseminate information about such assessment (Hunsley & Mash, 2005, 2007; Jenkins, Youngstrom, Washburn, & Youngstrom, 2011; Mash & Hunsley, 2005), in part to improve the accuracy of clinicians' diagnoses. As discussed above, these efforts might improve youth mental health care directly by improving treatment engagement and outcomes. Improving diagnostic accuracy might also improve youth mental health care indirectly by facilitating use of research findings in practice.

In response to data suggesting that the quality of "usual clinical care" might be less than optimal (e.g., Weisz & Jensen, 2001), professional organizations (e.g., American Psychological Association Presidential Task Force on Evidence-Based Practice, 2006), state mental health agencies (Chorpita & Donkervoet, 2005; Jensen-Doss, Hawley, Lopez, & Osterberg, 2009), and federal funders of mental health research (e.g., National Institute of Mental Health, 2010) have called for increased use of evidence-based practices in clinical settings.

Although the application of research in practice is urgently needed, it is extremely complex. Glasziou and Haynes (2005) have described the pipeline from research to practice as "leaky." They suggest that research can be diluted or misused at several points in the pipeline, including clinicians' *awareness* of the literature, their *acceptance* of findings as "true," their *application* of evidence to the correct patients, their *ability* to apply that evidence, their choice to *act on* it, and the degree to which patients *agree* and *adhere to* treatment. These authors recommend that efforts to improve the use of research findings in practice settings be tailored to address specific "leaks" in the pipeline.

As discussed above, diagnoses are often used to communicate about research findings and clinical clients, making them central to the *application* stage of the research–practice pipeline. This stage occurs early in the pipeline and can have cascading consequences. To the extent that clinicians are not engaged in accurate diagnosis, it is difficult to apply research findings to individual clients. Because evidence-based treatments are often designed for specific disorders, encouraging therapists to use evidence-based treatments without an associated emphasis on evidence-based diagnosis may result in their *application* to inappropriate clients, potentially leading families to be less *adherent* to treatment and reducing its efficacy. In turn, clinicians may perceive evidence-based treatments as not useful, which may make them less *accepting* of research. Improving clinicians' diagnoses could plug a major hole in the research–practice pipeline, improving overall use of research evidence in clinical practice.

THE DIAGNOSTIC PROCESS

In Chapter 1 of this book, we have laid out the overarching principles that guide our approach to assessment. Here we focus on the tools available to assist a clinician in conducting a multimethod, multi-informant diagnostic assessment grounded in empirical evidence and theory. Because later chapters in this book describe these methods in some detail, we provide only a brief overview of each type of tool and the role it plays in a comprehensive diagnostic assessment. Then we describe some of the available models for combining these data to arrive at a final diagnosis.

Diagnostic Tools

Unstructured Interviews

The unstructured interview is a foundational diagnostic tool, although one with serious limitations. In an unstructured interview, a clinician interviews a child and/or parent, guided by his or her clinical expertise, to gather information. Surveys indicate that the unstructured clinical interview is the assessment tool used most often by clinicians (e.g., Cashel, 2002), and many clinicians use this as their sole method of gathering the information needed to assign a diagnosis (Anderson & Paulosky, 2004). Given that an unstructured interview may be used as just one tool within a broader diagnostic assessment battery, or as a stand-alone diagnostic method, it is difficult to define exactly what it looks like. When such an interview is used as a stand-alone diagnostic tool, it typically takes 1–2 hours, during which the clinician asks about the presence, frequency, intensity, and duration of symptoms and about factors that might be contributing to the symptoms (the child's home situation, developmental history, academic performance, family history of psychopathology, etc).

Unstructured interviews have many advantages that make them useful in diagnosis. Unlike the standardized interviews and rating scales described below, an unstructured interview allows a clinician to tailor questioning to the individual client and apply his or her clinical expertise to probe for additional information. In addition, few standardized instruments include thorough assessment of contextual factors that may be contributing to a child's symptoms, such as individual and family history, so the unstructured interview is often useful for gathering this information.

Unstructured interviews also have several disadvantages. As described above, the clinical judgment used to guide these interviews is prone to a number of information-gathering and interpretation biases, which can limit their validity as stand-alone instruments. In terms of practical considerations, an unstructured interview also can be costly as a stand-alone diagnostic method, because it requires a considerable investment of time by a highly trained clinician.

Unstructured interviews are likely best used to complement standardized diagnostic tools. They can be a good means of gathering information not covered by standardized interviews; however, given the biases noted above, clinicians may want to consider generating a list of questions they want to cover in these areas to guide an interview. They can also be used to clarify information received through standardized tools.

Standardized Interviews

Because of the risk of bias, researchers no longer use unstructured interviews as stand-alone methods of diagnosis. The gold-standard research diagnostic tool is the standardized diagnostic interview (SDI). SDIs use standardized sets of questions and standard scoring algorithms to assess the criteria for DSM diagnoses. SDIs are discussed at length by Marin, Rey, and Silverman in Chapter 5 of this book, so we describe them here only briefly.

SDIs have traditionally been placed in two categories: "structured" and "semistructured." In a structured interview, the interviewer administers a standard set of questions guided by a strict set of rules for administration and scoring. In contrast, a semistructured interview allows interviewers to use clinical judgment to influence the interview by adding questions or clarifying the wording of the standardized questions. Semistructured interviews also often allow some level of clinical judgment in both administration and scoring. Angold and Fisher (1999) objected to the structured–semistructured terminology, arguing that the essential difference between these two classes of interviews is the role of clinical judgment, not the level of structure. They proposed the term "respondent-based interview" (RBI) for an interview that follows a set script and is scored based solely on the respondent's answers, and the term "interviewer-based interview" (IBI) for one with a standard set of questions, but in which the interviewer makes the final interpretation as to whether a symptom or diagnosis is present.

Both RBIs and IBIs typically consist of questions organized into diagnostic "modules" that cover the DSM criteria for specific diagnoses. Within each module, SDIs typically have contingency rules to guide the questioning. For example, if a parent answers "yes" to the question "Has your child felt depressed in the past year?", the interviewer then asks about the frequency, duration, and impairment associated with the symptom of depression. If the parent answers "no" to this question, then the interviewer moves on and asks about a different symptom. Because of these contingency rules, both RBIs and IBIs require a trained interviewer or, in the case of RBIs, a computer to guide the interview.

Numerous RBIs and IBIs have been developed for use with children and their parents and are reviewed by Marin et al. in Chapter 5. Many of these interviews have strong psychometric support and are included in evidence-based assessment recommendations for many childhood disorders. SDIs are considered useful for assigning a diagnosis at the beginning of treatment (Dougherty, Klein, Olino, & Laptook, 2008; Frick & McMahon, 2008; Johnston & Mah, 2008; Silverman & Ollendick, 2008), although reviews have concluded that currently available SDIs may not be as useful for diagnosing disorders such as attention-deficit/hyperactivity disorder (Pelham, Fabiano, & Massetti, 2005) or pediatric bipolar disorder (Youngstrom, Duax, & Hamilton, 2005). In addition, evidence-based assessment guidelines for some disorders suggest that SDIs can be useful for treatment planning and case conceptualization (Frick & McMahon, 2008; Silverman & Ollendick, 2008) and for treatment outcome monitoring (Dougherty et al., 2008; Silverman & Ollendick, 2008).

These interviews have some practical disadvantages, however. They can be costly to administer. They often require considerable time to administer, usually up to 2 hours per informant (although some exceptions do exist, such as the Mini International Neuropsychiatric Interview for Children and Adolescents [Sheehan et al., 2010] and the Children's Interview for Psychiatric Syndromes [Weller, Well, Fristad, Rooney, & Schecter, 2000]). Conducting a multi-informant diagnostic assessment with these instruments can therefore take an even longer time (e.g., if such interviews are administered to a child as well as her or his parents). Training to conduct these interviews reliably, particularly IBIs, can also be time-consuming.

Perhaps in part because of these practical concerns, SDIs are rarely used by practicing clinicians, although they have become nearly ubiquitous in research studies (Bruchmüller, Margraf, Suppiger, & Schneider, 2011; Jensen-Doss & Hawley, 2011). In addition to these practical concerns, many clinicians believe that SDIs are unacceptable to clients (Bruchmüller et al., 2011), although data gathered from clients do not support this concern (Suppiger et al., 2009).

Rating Scales

Rating scales figure prominently in guidelines for evidence-based assessment for youth psychopathology and are recommended for use in diagnosis, case conceptualization, treatment planning, and outcome monitoring (Dougherty et al., 2008; Frick & McMahon, 2008; Johnston & Mah, 2008; Silverman & Ollendick, 2008). A rating scale is a "measure that provides relatively rapid assessment of a specific construct with an easily derived numerical score, which is readily interpreted, whether completed by the youth or someone else, regardless of the response format and irrespective of application" (Myers & Winters, 2002, p. 115). Numerous rating scales exist—measures designed to assess one specific problem area, as well as multidimensional scales that cover a wide range of problem behaviors. Problem-specific rating scales are most useful for confirming or ruling out a diagnosis. In contrast, multidimensional scales are most useful for assessing a broad range of psychopathology. Achenbach provides an in-depth discussion of rating scales in Chapter 6.

Compared to other methods of assessment, rating scales have several advantages. First, like SDIs, rating scales provide a consistent and systematic method of assessment relative to unstructured interviews (Hart & Lahey, 1999). Second, many rating scales have normative data that allow clinicians to compare a given child's level of symptoms to other similar children, facilitating nomothetic assessment. Third, rating scales are more time-efficient than interviews; these measures can often be completed in 5–20 minutes. Finally, these measures do not require extensive training, although training is needed to interpret them.

However, rating scales also have disadvantages. Unlike IBIs, rating scales do not have procedures in place to probe for additional information about a symptom (Hart & Lahey, 1999). In addition, in settings requiring the assignment of a DSM diagnosis, most rating scales have to be augmented with further assessment to determine whether a client actually meets DSM criteria (Jensen-Doss, 2005).

Observational Methods

Although direct observational methods figure more predominantly in behavioral assessment approaches (see Ollendick, McLeod, & Jensen-Doss, Chapter 3), some standardized observational methods have good support for diagnostic assessment as well. Standardized observational measures are included in some evidence-based assessment guidelines for diagnosis (Frick & McMahon, 2008; Ozonoff, Goodlin-Jones, & Solomon, 2005), as well as for treatment planning, case conceptualization, and outcome monitoring (Frick & McMahon, 2008; Silverman & Ollendick, 2008). Observational methods are covered in depth by Reitman, McGregor, and Resnick in Chapter 7.

Standardized observational methods typically involve placing a child, and sometimes his or her parent, into standard situations and coding behavior during that situation. The types of behaviors demonstrated by the child and/or family can then be compared to normative data regarding typical behavior elicited by that situation. For example, the Autism Diagnostic Observational Schedule (ADOS; Lord et al., 2000) is a semistructured assessment tool for the diagnosis of autism spectrum disorders. During the ADOS, a child engages in a series of standardized social, communication, and play activities designed to elicit behaviors such as eye contact or a question from the child. The child's behavior is then coded by trained observers to determine whether it is developmentally typical. The ADOS has empirically defined scoring algorithms with cutoff scores for autistic disorder and for broader autism spectrum disorders (e.g., pervasive developmental disorder not otherwise specified).

Observational methods have the advantage of assessing the child's behavior within a naturalistic or analogue setting, without being filtered through the perceptions of any particular reporter. However, it can also be difficult to find standardized observational methods with good psychometric support, and they can be taxing in terms of training and administration time. In addition, in situations where the assignment of a DSM diagnosis is required, they often must be supplemented with other assessment methods.

Methods for Combining Diagnostic Assessment Data

As McLeod, Jensen-Doss, and Ollendick discussed in detail in Chapter 1, several assessment tools exist with good psychometric support for their use, but the field currently lacks good data regarding how the information generated from these tools should be combined to make clinical decisions. In Chapter 1, we have provided a list of recommendations for conducting an evidence-based assessment of youth psychopathology, according to a hypothesis-testing approach grounded in the developmental psychopathology literature. In this chapter, we briefly discuss some approaches that have been proposed to support clinical decision making when it comes specifically to assigning clinical diagnoses. The first of these, the so-called "LEAD standard" (Spitzer, 1983) is applied widely in psychopathology research; the second, rooted in the evidence-based medicine tradition, is only recently being applied to the diagnosis of youth psychopathology. The third is an approach to differential diagnosis advocated by the authors of DSM.

The LEAD Standard

As SDIs were developed to support clinical diagnosis, it became clear that they were still not sufficient to be treated as a "gold-standard" method of diagnosis (Spitzer, 1983). This becomes immediately apparent when SDIs are applied to a young client, because youth and parent report interviews often generate different sets of diagnoses for the same client. Spitzer (1983) proposed the LEAD standard for incorporating diagnostic data, and it now often serves as the gold-standard diagnostic method in research studies. LEAD stands for "longitudinal, expert, and all data."

Consistent with the iterative, hypothesis-driven approach described in Chapter 1, the first principle of the LEAD standard is that a diagnostic evaluation should not be limited to a single evaluation point; rather, it should be conducted *longitudinally*, and diagnoses should be revised as new information becomes available through further assessment or during treatment (Spitzer, 1983). Second, diagnoses should be generated by a team of *expert* clinicians who have demonstrated that they can generate reliable diagnoses. Based on information gathered via thorough interviews, these experts should make independent diagnoses, discuss any diagnostic disagreements, and then come to a consensus regarding the final diagnosis. Finally, a LEAD-standard diagnosis will be generated on *all data* available to a clinical team, including clinical records and reports from multiple informants, rather than on a single instrument like an SDI.

The LEAD standard is frequently used to generate the gold-standard diagnosis by which other diagnostic methods are evaluated in research studies. Because it involves a team of experts who discuss the diagnosis and come to consensus, it may not be feasible to utilize this method in many clinical practice settings. Nonetheless, the "longitudinal" and "all data" aspects of this approach generalize to other settings and are good principles to follow for assigning diagnoses in clinical settings.

The Evidence-Based Medicine Approach

In the evidence-based medicine tradition, diagnosis is conceptualized as gathering information to estimate the likelihood of various diagnostic possibilities (Straus, Glasziou, Richardson, & Haynes, 2011). Within this framework, diagnosis is a process of moving from a pretest probability (i.e., the initial impression of the likelihood of different diagnostic possibilities) to a posttest probability (i.e., the likelihood of a given diagnosis after appropriate tests have been conducted). In this approach, the clinician starts with a sense of the probability that a given individual has a particular diagnosis. This initial probability can be drawn from the research literature (e.g., the prevalence of major depression) and should be based on the most specific and recent data relevant to the client population within which a given client falls (e.g., the prevalence of major depression among children seeking outpatient mental health services). Then, as the clinician gathers additional data throughout the assessment process, this probability is adjusted until the clinician decides that it is unlikely that the client meets criteria for a given diagnosis (resulting in the diagnosis being "ruled out") or determines that it is very likely (resulting in probable treatment). This additional data can take the form of information about risk factors (e.g., a family history of major depression) or scores on diverse assessment measures (e.g., the client's score on a depression rating scale).

This "Bayesian" (i.e., a method of statistical inference and probability) approach to diagnosis has not received widespread attention in the child psychopathology literature, but has recently been applied to the problem of diagnosing pediatric bipolar disorder. Youngstrom and colleagues have utilized the developmental psychopathology literature to develop a Bayesian decision-making process for the assessment of pediatric bipolar disorder (Youngstrom et al., 2005; Youngstrom & Youngstrom, 2005). This work has demonstrated that clinicians can use information like family history and scores on standardized symptom checklists to estimate the probability that clients have pediatric bipolar disorder. These methods can make the diagnostic process more efficient, as clinicians can reserve lengthy SDI methods for clients who do not clearly meet criteria for a disorder, rather than using them for all clients. This research group has also demonstrated that training in Bayesian approaches can increase clinician diagnostic accuracy in diagnosing pediatric bipolar disorder (Jenkins et al., 2011). Although these methods can be statistically complex to develop, and are currently only available for pediatric bipolar disorder, technological advances should make these methods more accessible to clinicians in the future.

The DSM Approach to Differential Diagnosis

Assigning a diagnosis can often be complicated, because similar symptoms can appear across different diagnoses or may be caused by factors other than a psychological condition (e.g., substance-induced symptoms). To help clinicians work through the process of differentiating among different diagnoses, the American Psychiatric Association has published a guide to assist clinicians in differential diagnosis (First, Frances, & Pincus, 2002; First, in press). This book outlines a six-step approach for differential diagnosis and provides decision trees to assist in the diagnostic process.

First, the authors recommend determining whether a reported symptom is actually real (rather than a factitious disorder or malingering), as there may be situations in which a child or parent may be motivated to report symptoms that do not actually exist (e.g., to qualify for Social Security Disability Insurance, to gain child custody). In the second step, the clinician should rule out a substance-related cause for the symptoms (e.g., exposure to a toxin, use of psychotropic drugs, use of illicit drugs). First et al. (2002) provide a decision tree for determining the relationship between the use of any substances and the presentation of psychiatric symptoms, after which the clinician can either assign a DSM diagnosis of a substance-induced disorder, or determine that the psychiatric symptoms exist independently of any substance use. In the latter case, the clinician should move on to Step 3, which involves following a decision tree to rule out any medical cause for the symptoms. Once the clinician has ruled out substance-related and medical causes for the symptoms, Step 4 is to identify the client's primary diagnosis or diagnoses. First et al. (2002) provide a series of decision trees organized by presenting symptom (e.g., aggression, anxiety) to assist with this process.

At this point, the clinician may have arrived at a diagnostic decision. However, in cases in which a client is experiencing significant, impairing symptoms that do not conform to a clearly defined diagnosis, Step 5 involves determining whether the symptoms might best be captured by assigning an adjustment disorder diagnosis, indicating that the symptoms reflect difficulties adjusting to some identifiable event in the client's life, or whether it would be more appropriate to assign a "not otherwise specified" label. This label applies to symptoms that do not stem from a specific stressor, but rather appear to be an atypical presentation of a category of disorder (e.g., depressive disorder not otherwise specified). Finally, in Step 6, the clinician must determine whether the symptoms are "clinically significant" and warrant the assignment of a diagnosis. As First et al. (2002) point out, many of the symptoms detailed in DSM are fairly common, and do not necessarily mean that an individual experiencing them has a psychological disorder. The assignment of a DSM diagnosis requires that the symptoms be impairing. DSM does not provide a concrete definition of such impairment, so the clinician must work with the client, his or her parents, and other reporters to determine whether and how the client's specific symptoms might be impairing.

CONCLUDING THOUGHTS AND FUTURE DIRECTIONS

In sum, the classification of psychopathology in youth is an important and complex process. Diagnostic assessment methods can be extremely useful for determining whether a child is in need of treatment, selecting a treatment approach, and determining whether that treatment approach was effective. However, diagnostic methods also have limitations. For example, through diagnostic methods can point to a general treatment approach that might be effective for a given child, they often lack utility in helping clinicians tailor treatment to that child. Also, through diagnostic methods can identify the types of symptoms a youth is experiencing, a comprehensive assessment and outcome-monitoring approach must include a broader range of variables, such as academic and family functioning, many of which may be more concerning to many of the stakeholders in the treatment process (Hoagwood, Jensen, Petti, & Burns, 1996). These limitations can be addressed by using diagnostic assessment tools in combination with idiographic, behavioral assessment methods.

When diagnostic assessment tools are used to assign diagnoses, additional issues arise. As described above, categorical diagnoses can be helpful in many ways, but also may not accurately represent the dimensional nature of psychopathology. In addition, although DSM purports to be atheoretical (American Psychiatric Association, 2013), it does endorse a medical model of psychopathology that may imply to children and families that child emotional and behavioral conditions are biologically based, although many of them may not be. Many families may also be concerned about the potential negative impact of their children's being "labeled" with a disorder. It is important that clinicians providing assessment feedback provide clear explanations for any diagnoses being assigned and be prepared to support family members who may find such feedback upsetting.

Despite these limitations, diagnostic assessment methods are extremely useful in understanding and treating youth psychopathology, particularly when used in the multi-informant, multimethod approach described in this volume. Many different diagnostic assessment measures have been developed to assist clinicians, although future research is clearly needed on the best ways to combine these measures to make accurate diagnostic decisions. As described by Pina, Gonzales, Holly, Zerr, and Wynne in Chapter 13, few nomothetic measures have good norms and other psychometric support for use with ethnic minority clients; future research should test existing measures with these populations or, if necessary, develop new measures.

As the debate between dimensional and categorical models of psychopathology continues, it is likely that our systems for classifying psychopathology will change significantly in the future. As such, being an effective diagnostician requires remaining up to date on the child psychopathology and assessment literatures. By doing so, we clinicians have the best chance of meeting our primary obligation in the diagnostic assessment process, generating accurate assessment data that will contribute to clients' positive outcomes.

REFERENCES

Achenbach, T. M., & Rescorla, L. A. (2001). *Manual for the ASEBA School-Age Forms & Profiles*. Burlington: University of Vermont, Research Center for Children, Youth, & Families.

American Psychiatric Association. (1952). *Diagnostic and statistical manual of mental disorders*. Washington, DC: Author.

American Psychiatric Association. (1980). *Diagnostic and statistical manual of mental disorders* (3rd ed.). Washington, DC: Author.

American Psychiatric Association. (2000). *Diagnostic and statistical manual of mental disorders* (4th ed., text rev.). Washington, DC: Author.

American Psychiatric Association. (2013). *Diagnostic and statistical manual of mental disorders* (5th ed.). Arlington, VA: Author.

American Psychological Association Presidential Task Force on Evidence-Based Practice. (2006). Evidence-based practice in psychology. *American Psychologist, 61*, 271–285.

Anderson, D. A., & Paulosky, C. A. (2004). A survey of the use of assessment instruments by eating disorder professionals in clinical practice. *Eating and Weight Disorders, 9*, 238–241.

Angold, A., Costello, E. J., Farmer, E. M. Z., Burns, B. J., & Erkanli, A. (1999). Impaired but undiagnosed. *Journal of the American Academy of Child and Adolescent Psychiatry, 38*, 129–137.

Angold, A., & Fisher, P. W. (1999). Interviewer-based interviews. In D. Shaffer, C. P. Lucas, & J. E. Richters (Eds.), *Diagnostic assessment in child and adolescent psychopathology* (pp. 34–64). New York: Guilford Press.

Basco, M. R., Bostic, J. Q., Davies, D., Rush, A. J., Witte, B., Hendrickse, W., & Barnett, V. (2000). Methods to improve diagnostic accuracy in a community mental health setting. *American Journal of Psychiatry, 157*, 1599–1605.

Birmaher, B., Brent, D., Bernet, W., Bukstein, O., Walter, H., Benson, R. S., & Medicus, J. (2007). Practice parameter for the assessment and treatment of children and adolescents with depressive disorders. *Journal of the American Academy of Child and Adolescent Psychiatry, 46*, 1503–1526.

Broman-Fulks, J. J., Ruggiero, K. J., Green, B. A., Smith, D. W., Hanson, R. F., Kilpatrick, D. G., & Saunders, B. E. (2009). The latent structure of posttraumatic stress disorder among adolescents. *Journal of Traumatic Stress, 22*, 146–152.

Bruchmüller, K., Margraf, J., Suppiger, A., & Schneider, S. (2011). Popular or unpopular?: Therapists' use of structured interviews and their estimation of patient acceptance. *Behavior Therapy*. Retrieved from *www.sciencedirect.com/science/article/pii/S0005789411000554*

Cashel, M. L. (2002). Child and adolescent psychological assessment: Current clinical practices and the impact of managed care. *Professional Psychology: Research and Practice, 33*, 446–453.

Chorpita, B. F., & Donkervoet, C. (2005). Implementation of the Felix Consent Decree in Hawaii: The impact of policy and practice development efforts on service delivery. In R. G. Steele & M. C. Roberts (Eds.), *Handbook of mental health services for children, adolescents, and families* (pp. 317–332). New York: Kluwer Academic/Plenum.

Clark, L. A., Watson, D., & Reynolds, S. (1995). Diagnosis and classification of psychopathology: Challenges to the current system and future directions. *Annual Review of Psychology, 46,* 121–153.

Cohen, J. A., Bukstein, O., Walter, H., Benson, R. S., Chrisman, A., Farchione, T. R., & Medicus, J. (2010). Practice parameter for the assessment and treatment of children and adolescents with posttraumatic stress disorder. *Journal of the American Academy of Child and Adolescent Psychiatry, 49,* 414–430.

Connolly, S. D., & Bernstein, G. A. (2007). Practice parameter for the assessment and treatment of children and adolescents with anxiety disorders. *Journal of the American Academy of Child and Adolescent Psychiatry, 46*(2), 267–283.

Costello, E. J., Angold, A., & Keeler, G. P. (1999). Adolescent outcomes of childhood disorders: The consequences of severity and impairment. *Journal of the American Academy of Child and Adolescent Psychiatry, 38,* 121–128.

Croskerry, P. (2002). Achieving quality in clinical decision making: Cognitive strategies and detection of bias. *Academic Emergency Medicine, 9,* 1184–1204.

Croskerry, P. (2009). A universal model of diagnostic reasoning. *Academic Medicine, 84,* 1022–1028.

Diagnosis. (1989). *The Oxford English Dictionary* (2nd ed.). OED Online. Retrieved October 25, 2011, from *www.oed.com/view/Entry/51836.*

Dougherty, L. R., Klein, D. N., Olino, T. M., & Laptook, R. S. (2008). Depression in children and adolescents. In J. Hunsley & E. J. Mash (Eds.), *A guide to assessments that work* (pp. 69–95). New York: Oxford University Press.

Evans, J. S. B. T. (2008). Dual-processing accounts of reasoning, judgment, and social cognition. *Annual Review of Psychology, 59,* 255–278.

First, M. B. (in press). *DSM-5 handbook of differential diagnosis.* Arlington, VA: American Psychiatric Association.

First, M. B., Frances, A. F., & Pincus, H. A. (2002). *DSM-IV-TR handbook of differential diagnosis.* Arlington, VA: American Psychiatric Publishing.

Follette, W. C., & Houts, A. C. (1996). Models of scientific progress and the role of theory in taxonomy development: A case study of the DSM. *Journal of Consulting and Clinical Psychology, 64,* 1120–1132.

Frick, P. J., & McMahon, R. J. (2008). Child and adolescent conduct problems. In J. Hunsley & E. J. Mash (Eds.), *A guide to assessments that work* (pp. 41–66). New York: Oxford University Press.

Garb, H. N. (1998). *Studying the clinician: Judgment research and psychological assessment.* Washington, DC: American Psychological Association.

Garb, H. N. (2005). Clinical judgment and decision making. *Annual Review of Clinical Psychology, 1,* 67–89.

Glasziou, P., & Haynes, B. (2005). The paths from research to improved health outcomes. *Evidence-Based Medicine, 10,* 4–7.

Grove, W. M., Zald, D. H., Lebow, B. S., Snitz, B. E., & Nelson, C. (2000). Clinical versus mechanical prediction: A meta-analysis. *Psychological Assessment, 12*(1), 19–30.

Hankin, B. L., Fraley, R. C., Lahey, B. B., & Waldman, I. D. (2005). Is depression best viewed as a continuum or discrete category?: A taxometric analysis of childhood and adolescent depression in a population-based sample. *Journal of Abnormal Psychology, 114,* 96–110.

Hart, E. L., & Lahey, B. B. (1999). General child behavior rating scales. In D. Shaffer (Ed.), *Diagnostic assessment in child and adolescent psychopathology* (pp. 65–87). New York: Guilford Press.

Haslam, N., Williams, B., Prior, M., Haslam, R., Graetz, B., & Sawyer, M. (2006). The latent structure of attention-deficit/hyperactivity disorder: A taxometric analysis. *Australian and New Zealand Journal of Psychiatry, 40,* 639–647.

Helzer, J. E., Kraemer, H. C., & Krueger, R. F. (2006). The feasibility and need for dimensional psychiatric diagnoses. *Psychological Medicine, 36,* 1671–1680.

Hoagwood, K., Jensen, P. S., Petti, T., & Burns, B. J. (1996). Outcomes of mental health care for children and adolescents: I. A comprehensive conceptual model. *Journal of the American Academy of Child and Adolescent Psychiatry, 35,* 1055–1063.

Hunsley, J., & Mash, E. J. (2005). Introduction to the special section on developing guidelines for the evidence-based assessment (EBA) of adult disorders. *Psychological Assessment, 17,* 251–255.

Hunsley, J., & Mash, E. J. (2007). Evidence-based assessment. *Annual Review of Clinical Psychology, 3,* 29–51.

Insel, T., Cuthbert, B., Garvey, M., Heinssen, R., Pine, D. S., Quinn, K., et al. (2010). Research domain criteria (RDoC): Toward a new classification framework for research on mental disorders. *American Journal of Psychiatry, 167,* 748–751.

Jacobson, N. S., & Truax, P. (1991). Clinical significance: A statistical approach to defining meaningful change in psychotherapy research. *Journal of Consulting and Clinical Psychology, 59,* 12–19.

Jenkins, M. M., Youngstrom, E. A., Washburn, J. J., & Youngstrom, J. K. (2011). Evidence-based strategies improve assessment of pediatric bipolar disorder by community practitioners. *Professional Psychology: Research and Practice, 42,* 121–129.

Jensen-Doss, A. (2005). Evidence-based diagnosis: Incorporating diagnostic instruments into clinical practice. *Journal of the American Academy of Child and Adolescent Psychiatry, 44,* 947–952.

Jensen-Doss, A., & Hawley, K. M. (2011). Understanding clinicians' diagnostic practices: Attitudes toward the utility of diagnosis and standardized diagnostic tools. *Administration and Policy in Mental Health and Mental Health Services Research, 38,* 476–485.

Jensen-Doss, A., Hawley, K. M., Lopez, M., & Osterberg, L. D. (2009). Using evidence-based treatments: The experiences of youth providers working under a mandate. *Professional Psychology: Research and Practice, 40,* 417–424.

Jensen-Doss, A., & Weisz, J. R. (2008). Diagnostic agreement predicts treatment process and outcomes in youth mental health clinics. *Journal of Consulting and Clinical Psychology, 76,* 711–722.

Jewell, J., Handwerk, M., Almquist, J., & Lucas, C. (2004). Comparing the validity of clinician-generated diagnosis of conduct disorder to the Diagnostic Interview Schedule for Children. *Journal of Clinical Child and Adolescent Psychology, 33,* 536–546.

Johnston, C., & Mah, J. W. T. (2008). Child attention-deficit hyperactivity disorder. In J. Hunsley & E. J. Mash (Eds.), *A guide to assessments that work* (pp. 17–40). New York: Oxford University Press.

Kendler, K. S., Eaves, L. J., Walters, E. E., Neale, M. C., Heath, A. C., & Kessler, R. C. (1996). The identification and validation of distinct depressive syndromes in a population-based sample of female twins. *Archives of General Psychiatry, 53,* 391–399.

Kramer, T. L., Robbins, J. M., Phillips, S. D., Miller, T. L., & Burns, B. J. (2003). Detection and outcomes of substance use disorders in adolescents seeking mental health treatment. *Journal of the American Academy of Child and Adolescent Psychiatry, 42*, 1318–1326.

Landis, J. R., & Koch, G. G. (1977). The measurement of observer agreement for categorical data. *Biometrics, 33*, 159–174.

Lord, C., Risi, S., Lambrecht, L., Cook, E. H., Jr., Leventhal, B. L., DiLavore, P. C., & Rutter, M. (2000). The Autism Diagnostic Observation Schedule—Generic: A standard measure of social and communication deficits associated with the spectrum of autism. *Journal of Autism and Developmental Disorders, 30*, 205–223.

Mack, A. H., Forman, L., Brown, R., & Frances, A. (1994). A brief history of psychiatric classification: From the ancients to DSM-IV. *Psychiatric Clinics of North America, 17*, 515–523.

Mash, E. J., & Hunsley, J. (2005). Evidence-based assessment of child and adolescent disorders: Issues and challenges. *Journal of Clinical Child and Adolescent Psychology, 34*, 362–379.

McClellan, J., Kowatch, R., & Findling, R. L. (2007). Practice parameter for the assessment and treatment of children and adolescents with bipolar disorder. *Journal of the American Academy of Child and Adolescent Psychiatry, 46*, 107–125.

Meehl, P. E. (1996). *Clinical versus statistical prediction: A theoretical analysis and a review of the evidence.* Northvale, NJ: Aronson. (Original work published 1954)

Myers, K., & Winters, N. C. (2002). Ten-year review of rating scales: I. Overview of scale functioning, psychometric properties and selection. *Journal of the American Academy of Child and Adolescent Psychiatry, 41*, 114–122.

National Institute of Mental Health. (2010). The National Institute of Mental Health strategic plan. Retrieved February 17, 2010, from *www.nimh.nih.gov/about/strategic-planning-reports/index.shtml.*

Nelson-Gray, R. O. (2003). Treatment utility of psychological assessment. *Psychological Assessment, 15*, 521–531.

Norman, G. (2009). Dual processing and diagnostic errors. *Advances in Health Sciences Education, 14*, 37–49.

Ozonoff, S., Goodlin-Jones, B. L., & Solomon, M. (2005). Evidence-based assessment of autism spectrum disorders in children and adolescents. *Journal of Clinical Child and Adolescent Psychology, 34*, 523–540.

Pelham, W. R., Fabiano, G. A., & Massetti, G. M. (2005). Evidence-based assessment of attention deficit hyperactivity disorder in children and adolescents. *Journal of Clinical Child and Adolescent Psychology, 34*(3), 449–476.

Pogge, D. L., Wayland-Smith, D., Zaccario, M., Borgaro, S., Stokes, J., & Harvey, P. D. (2001). Diagnosis of manic episodes in adolescent inpatients: Structured diagnostic procedures compared to clinical chart diagnoses. *Psychiatry Research, 101*, 47–54.

Rettew, D. C., Lynch, A. D., Achenbach, T. M., Dumenci, L., & Ivanova, M. Y. (2009). Meta-analyses of agreement between diagnoses made from clinical evaluations and standardized diagnostic interviews. *International Journal of Methods in Psychiatric Research, 18*(3), 169–184.

Rubinstein, E. A. (1948). Childhood mental disease in America: A review of the literature before 1900. *American Journal of Orthopsychiatry, 18*, 314–321.

Sheehan, D. V., Sheehan, K. H., Shytle, R. D., Janavs, J., Bannon, Y., Rogers, J. E., & Wilkinson, B. (2010). Reliability and validity of the Mini International Neuropsychiatric Interview for Children and Adolescents (MINI-KID). *Journal of Clinical Psychiatry, 71*, 313–326.

Silverman, W. K., & Hinshaw, S. P. (Eds.). (2008). The second special issue on evidence-based psychosocial treatments for children and adolescents: A 10-year update [Special issue]. *Journal of Clinical Child and Adolescent Psychology, 37*(1).

Silverman, W. K., & Ollendick, T. H. (2008). Child and adolescent anxiety disorders. In J. Hunsley & E. J. Mash (Eds.), *A guide to assessments that work* (pp. 181–206). New York: Oxford University Press.

Sloman, S. A. (1996). The empirical case for two systems of reasoning. *Psychological Bulletin, 119*, 3–22.

Spitzer, R. L. (1983). Psychiatric diagnosis: Are clinicians still necessary? *Comprehensive Psychiatry, 24*, 399–411.

Straus, S. E., Glasziou, P., Richardson, W. S., & Haynes, R. B. (2011). *Evidence-based medicine: How to practice and teach EBM* (4th ed.). New York: Churchill Livingstone.

Suppiger, A., In-Albon, T., Hendriksen, S., Hermann, E., Margraf, J., & Schneider, S. (2009). Acceptance of structured diagnostic interviews for mental disorders in clinical practice and research settings. *Behavior Therapy, 40*, 272–279.

Tenney, N. H., Schotte, C. K. W., Denys, D. A. J. P., van Megen, H. J. G. M., & Westenberg, H. G. M. (2003). Assessment of DSM-IV personality disorders in obsessive–compulsive disorder: Comparison of clinical diagnosis, self-report questionnaire, and semi-structured interview. *Journal of Personality Disorders, 17*, 550–561.

Weisz, J. R., & Jensen, A. L. (2001). Child and adolescent psychotherapy in research and practice contexts: Review of the evidence and suggestions for improving the field. *European Child and Adolescent Psychiatry, 10*, I12–I18.

Weller, E. B., Weller, R. A., Fristad, M. A., Rooney, M. T., & Schecter, J. (2000). Children's Interview for Psychiatric Syndromes (ChIPS). *Journal of the American Academy of Child and Adolescent Psychiatry, 39*, 76–84.

Widiger, T. A., & Samuel, D. B. (2005). Diagnostic categories or dimensions? A question for the *Diagnostic and Statistical Manual of Mental Disorders—Fifth Edition. Journal of Abnormal Psychology, 114*, 494–504.

World Health Organization. (1993). *The ICD-10 classification of mental and behavioural disorders: Diagnostic criteria for research.* Geneva: Author.

World Health Organization (2012). *Measuring health and disability: Manual for Who disability assessment schedule* (WHODAS 2.0). Geneva: Author.

Youngstrom, E. A., Duax, J., & Hamilton, J. (2005). Evidence-based assessment of pediatric bipolar disorder: Part I. Base rate and family history. *Journal of the American Academy of Child and Adolescent Psychiatry, 44*, 712–717.

Youngstrom, E. A., & Youngstrom, J. K. (2005). Evidence-based assessment of pediatric bipolar disorder: Part II. Incorporating information from behavior checklists. *Journal of the American Academy of Child and Adolescent Psychiatry, 44*, 823–828.

3

Behavioral Assessment

Thomas H. Ollendick, Bryce D. McLeod, and Amanda Jensen-Doss

As first described by Mash and Terdal (1981) and expanded on by Ollendick and Hersen (1984, p. 6), child behavioral assessment can best be viewed as an "exploratory, hypothesis-testing process in which a range of specific procedures is used in order to understand a given child, group, or social ecology, and to formulate and evaluate specific intervention strategies." As such, it entails more than the identification of discrete target behaviors. Although the importance of direct behavioral observation of target behaviors should not be underestimated, advances in behavioral assessment over the years have incorporated a large range of assessment procedures, including behavioral interviews, self-reports, ratings by significant others, self-monitoring, physiological measurement, *and* behavioral observations. An approach combining these procedures can best be described as a multimethod one that is informed by multiple informants, through which a composite "picture" of a child or adolescent is obtained. This snapshot is designed to be not only descriptive, but also clinically useful in the understanding, modification, and measurement of specific behavior problems (Ollendick & Cerny, 1981; Ollendick & Hersen, 1984, 1993).

Two other important features characterize child behavioral assessment procedures. First, as we have noted in Chapter 1, they should be sensitive to rapid developmental changes; second, they should be validated empirically. Probably the most distinguishing characteristic of children and adolescents is change. Whether such change is based on hypothetical stages of growth or assumed principles of learning, it has direct implications for the selection of specific assessment procedures and for their use in the understanding of behavior problems and in the evaluation of treatment outcomes.

Behavioral interviews, self-reports, other-reports, self-monitoring, physiological assessment, and behavioral observation are all affected by rapidly changing developmental processes. Further, some of these procedures may be more useful at one age than another. For example, interviews may be more difficult to conduct and self-reports less reliable with younger children, whereas self-monitoring and behavioral observations may be more reactive with older children and adolescents (Ollendick & Hersen, 1984). Age-related constraints are numerous, and clinicians should consider them when selecting specific methods of assessment.

Just as child behavioral assessment procedures should be developmentally sensitive, they should also be validated empirically (as we have emphasized in Chapter 1). All too frequently, mental health professionals working with children and adolescents have used assessment methods of convenience without sufficient regard for their psychometric properties, including their reliability, validity, and clinical utility (Cone, 1981). Although child behavior assessors have fared somewhat better in this regard, they too have tended to design and use highly idiosyncratic tools for assessment. As noted elsewhere (Ollendick & Hersen, 1984), comparison across studies is extremely difficult, if not impossible, and the advancement of an assessment technology is not realized with such an individualized approach. Recent advances in evidence-based assessment have acknowledged and addressed some of these issues and have argued for a technology of evidence-based assessment (Haynes, Smith, & Hunsley, 2011; Hunsley & Mash, 2008; Ollendick, 1999).

Although a multimethod, multi-informant approach that is based on developmentally sensitive and empirically validated procedures is recommended, it should be clear that a "test battery" approach is not being espoused here. The specific assessment tools to be used depend on a careful case conceptualization surrounding a host of factors, including the age, gender, and ethnicity of the young client; the nature of the referral question; and the personnel, time, and resources available for the assessment process. Nonetheless, given the inherent limitations of the different assessment tools, as well as the desirability of obtaining as complete a picture of the child or adolescent as possible, we recommend a multimethod, multi-informant approach whenever it is feasible. Any single procedure, including direct behavioral observation, is not sufficient to provide a composite view. The multimethod, multi-informant approach is helpful not only in assessing specific target behaviors and in determining response to behavior change, but also in understanding child behavior disorders and advancing our database in this area of study (Ollendick & Shirk, 2011).

Based on these initial considerations, we offer the following overarching principles that guide the substance of this chapter:

1. Young clients are a special population. The automatic extension of adult behavioral assessment methods to them is not warranted

and is often inappropriate. Age-related variables affect the choice of methods, the informants, as well as the procedures employed.

2. Given the rapidity of developmental change, normative comparisons are required to ensure that appropriate target behaviors are selected and that change in behavior is related to treatment, not to normal developmental change. Such comparisons require identification of suitable reference groups and information about the "natural course" of child behavior problems.

3. Thorough child behavioral assessment involves multiple targets of change, including overt behaviors, affective states, and cognitive processes. Furthermore, such assessment entails determining the context (e.g., familial, social, cultural) in which the behaviors occur, their antecedents and consequences, and the function(s) that the target behaviors serve.

4. Given the wide range of targets for change, multimethod, multiinformant assessment is desirable. This approach, however, should not be viewed as a test battery approach; rather, the choice of methods and informants should be based on their appropriateness to the referral question. As such, an idiographic approach to assessment is espoused.

5. The end product of a child behavioral assessment is a careful description of the target behaviors and the derivation of a functional analysis of those behaviors which will in turn lead to selection of specific treatment strategies and efficacious outcomes.

HISTORY OF BEHAVIORAL ASSESSMENT

As emphasized above, adequate assessment of a child's behavior problems requires a multimethod, multi-informant approach in which data are gathered from both the child and significant others. In this manner, important information from cognitive and affective modalities can be combined with behavioral observations to provide a more complete picture. In addition, a multimethod, multi-informant approach provides the clinician with necessary information regarding the perceptions and reactions of significant others in the child's environment (e.g., parents, teachers, and peers). It should be noted, however, that this comprehensive approach is of relatively recent origin in the area of child behavioral assessment.

In its earliest stages, behavioral assessment of children relied almost exclusively on the identification and specification of discrete and highly observable target behaviors (see Ullmann & Krasner, 1965). As such, assessment was limited to gathering information from the motoric response modality. This early assessment approach followed logically from the theoretical assumptions of the operant model of behavior, which was in vogue at the time. Early behaviorally oriented psychologists posited that the only appropriate behavioral domain for empirical study was that which was directly observable (Skinner, 1953). Contending that the objective demonstration of behavior change following intervention was of utmost importance, behaviorists relied upon data that could be measured objectively. Hence frequency, intensity, and duration measures of the behaviors of interest were obtained. Although the existence of cognitions and affective states was not denied, they were not deemed appropriate subject matter for experimental behavioral analysis.

As treatment approaches with children were broadened to include cognitive and self-control techniques in the 1970s (e.g., Bandura, 1971; Kanfer & Phillips, 1970; Meichenbaum, 1977), it became apparent that assessment strategies would have to be expanded into the cognitive and affective domains as well. Furthermore, even though operant techniques were shown to be highly effective in producing behavior change under controlled experimental conditions, the clinical significance and social validity of these changes were questioned (Ollendick & Cerny, 1981). This state of affairs prompted behaviorists to expand their coverage and to pursue information from a variety of sources (e.g., significant others), even though these sources provided only indirect measures of behavior (Cone, 1978). The issue of the clinical significance of behavior change is especially crucial in child behavioral assessment, because children are invariably referred for treatment by others (e.g., parents, teachers). Once treatment goals have been identified adequately, the ultimate index of treatment efficacy lies in the referral source's perceptions of change. Hence other-report measures become as important as direct observational ones. Subsequently, the scope of behavioral assessment was broadened to incorporate the impact of large-scale social systems (e.g., schools, communities) on a child's behavior (Patterson, 1976; Wahler, 1976; Wahler, House, & Stambaugh, 1976). Although inclusion of these additional factors served to complicate the assessment process, it was an indispensable aspect of the evolution of child behavioral assessment. The ideologies and expectations of these seemingly distal social systems often have immediate and profound effects on individual behavior (see Prinz, 1986, and Winett, Riley, King, & Altman, 1989, for discussions of these issues).

In sum, child behavioral assessment has progressed from sole reliance on measurement of discrete target behaviors to a broader approach that takes into account cognitive and affective processes that mediate behavior change, as well as the social contexts in which the target behaviors occur. The assessment techniques that accompany this approach include indirect behavioral measures (e.g., behavioral interviews, self- and other-report measures). These measures are utilized in addition to direct behavioral observation, which remains the hallmark of behavioral assessment (Mash & Terdal, 1981, 1987; Ollendick & Hersen, 1984).

THEORETICAL UNDERPINNINGS

Although behavioral assessment has had a historical development of its own, it is fair to state that the increased popularity of this approach was at least partially generated by dissatisfaction with the "traditional" approaches to assessment in vogue at that time (i.e., projective assessment, objective personality assessment of traits). An index of this dissatisfaction is that virtually all early discussions of adult and child behavioral assessment were carried out through comparison and contrast with the traditional assessment approaches (e.g., Bornstein, Bornstein, & Dawson, 1984; Cone & Hawkins, 1977; Evans & Nelson, 1977; Goldfried & Kent, 1972; Hayes, Nelson, & Jarrett, 1986; Mash & Terdal, 1981; Mischel, 1968; Nelson, 1977; O'Leary & Johnson, 1979; Ollendick & Hersen, 1984). Though such comparisons often resulted in an oversimplification of both approaches, they were nevertheless useful and served to elucidate the theoretical underpinnings of the behavioral approach.

The most fundamental difference between traditional and behavioral assessment approaches lies in the conceptions of personality and behavior. In the traditional assessment approach, personality was viewed as a reflection of underlying and enduring traits, and behavior was assumed to be caused by these internal personality characteristics ("personolgism"). In contrast, behavioral approaches generally avoided references to underlying personality constructs, focusing instead on what an individual does under specific conditions. From the behavioral perspective, the term "personality" refers more to patterns of behavior than to attributes of the person or causes of behavior (Staats, 1975, 1986). Furthermore, behavior is viewed as a result of current environmental factors ("situationalism") or of current environmental factors interacting with organismic or "person" variables ("interactionism"). Thus the role of the environment is stressed more in behavioral assessment than in traditional assessment. The focus of child assessment is more on what a child does in a given situation than on what the child "is" (Mischel, 1968). As a result, a lower level of inference is required in behavioral assessment than in traditional assessment.

It is important not to oversimplify the behavioral view of the causes of behavior, however. It has often been erroneously asserted that the behavioral approach focuses on external determinants of behavior, to the exclusion of organismic states or internal cognitions and affects. To be sure, as we have noted above, early behavioral views of childhood disorders emphasized the primary role of current environmental factors in the manifestation of behavior. However, intraorganismic variables that influence behavior were not ignored (Skinner, 1957). Today this is evidenced by the array of self-report instruments tapping cognitive and affective modalities that are used in behavioral assessment (see Hunsley & Mash, 2008). A thorough behavioral assessment should attempt to identify controlling variables, whether these are environmental or organismic in nature. As Mash and Terdal (1981) noted, "the relative importance of organismic and environmental variables and their interaction ... should follow from a careful analysis of the problem" (p. 23). Such an analysis also informs case formulation and treatment planning.

The traditional conception of personality as made up of stable and enduring traits implies that behavior is relatively consistent across situations and stable over time (Bem & Allen, 1974). The behavioral view, in contrast, is one of situational specificity; that is, because behavior is in large part a function of situational determinants, a child's behavior will change as situational factors change. Similarly, stability of behavior across time is not necessarily expected. Hence an aggressive act, such as a child's hitting another child, would be seen from the traditional viewpoint as a reflection of some underlying construct such as hostility, which in turn might be hypothesized to be related to early life experiences and intrapsychic conflict. In such a conception, little or no attention would be given to specific situational factors or to the environmental context in which the aggressive acts occur. In contrast, from the behavioral perspective, an attempt is made to identify those variables that elicit and maintain the aggressive act in that particular situation (Olweus, 1979). That the child may aggress in a variety of situations is explained in terms of a learning history in which reinforcing consequences have been obtained for past aggressive acts, and not in terms of an underlying personality trait of hostility. From this analysis, it is clear that actual behavior is of primary importance to behaviorists, because it represents a *sample* of the child's behavioral repertoire in a given situation. From the traditional viewpoint, the behavior assumes importance only insofar as it is a *sign* of some hypothesized underlying cause.

These differing assumptions have direct implications for the assessment process. In behavioral assessment, the emphasis on situational specificity necessitates an assessment approach that samples behavior across settings. Hence assessment of the child's behavior at home, in school, and on the playground is important, in addition to information obtained in the clinic setting. Furthermore, the information obtained from these various settings probably will not be, and in fact should not be expected to be, the same. The child may behave aggressively in school and on the playground, but not at home or in the clinic. This lack of consistent findings would be more problematic for the traditional approach, which would hypothesize consistency across situations. Similarly, the notion of temporal instability (see Chapter 1) requires that the child's behavior be assessed at several points in time, whereas this would not be required from the traditional assessment standpoint.

In brief, traditional approaches interpret assessment data as signs of underlying personality functioning. These data are then used to diagnose and classify the child and to make prognostic statements, as we have described in Chapter 2. From the behavioral perspective, assessment data are utilized to identify target behaviors (overt or covert), their controlling conditions, and the functions they serve. From this perspective, information obtained from the assessment process serves as a sample of the child's behavior under specific circumstances. This information guides the selection of appropriate treatment procedures. Because behavioral assessment is ongoing, such information serves as an index enabling the clinician to continually evaluate the effects of treatment and to make appropriate modifications in treatment. Furthermore, because assessment data are viewed as samples of behavior, the level of inference is low, whereas a high level of inference is required when one attempts to make statements about personality functioning from responses to interview questions or specific test items.

In addition to these differences, Cone (1986) has expanded on the nomothetic and idiographic distinction between traditional and behavioral assessment (see also our discussion of this distinction in Chapter 1). Stated briefly, the nomothetic approach is concerned with the discovery of general laws as they are applied to large numbers of individuals. Usually these laws provide heuristic guidelines as to how certain variables are related to one another. Such an approach can be said to be variable-centered, because it deals with particular characteristics (traits) such as intelligence, achievement, diagnoses, aggression, and so on. In contrast, the idiographic approach is concerned more with the uniqueness of a given individual and is said to be person-centered rather than variable-centered (Cone, 1986; Ollendick & Hersen, 1984). Unlike the nomothetic approach, the idiographic perspective emphasizes the discovery of relationships among variables uniquely patterned in each person. The idiographic approach is more consistent with a behavioral perspective, whereas the nomothetic approach is more closely related to the traditional approach. Cone (1986) illustrates how the idiographic–nomothetic distinction relates to the general activities of behavioral assessors by exploring five basic questions: (1) What is the purpose of assessment? (2) What is its specific subject matter? (3) What general scientific approach guides this effort? (4) How are differences accounted for? (5) To what extent are currently operative environmental variables considered? Although further discussion of these important questions is beyond the scope of this chapter, Cone's schema helps us recognize the pluralistic nature of behavioral assessment and calls our attention to meaningful differences in the diverse practices contained therein. As Cone (1986) concludes, "There is not one behavioral assessment, there are many" (p. 126). We agree.

In sum, traditional and behavioral assessment approaches operate under different assumptions regarding a child's behavior. These assumptions in turn have clear implications for the assessment process. Of paramount importance for child behavioral assessment is the need to tailor the assessment approach to the specific child, in order to identify the target problems accurately, specify treatment, and evaluate treatment outcome. Such tailoring requires ongoing assessment from a number of methods and sources under appropriately diverse stimulus situations.

Finally, although we have highlighted differences between traditional and behavioral assessment, they need not be mutually exclusive. Some behaviors are more consistent across time and situations, whereas others are not. Given this, when appropriate, the two approaches can be combined to provide a rich glimpse into the functioning of the child from different perspectives—an approach that we espouse in this volume (see also Nelson-Gray & Paulson, 2004, for a similar approach).

DESCRIPTION OF ASSESSMENT PROCEDURES

Multimethod, multi-informant behavioral assessment of children entails the use of a wide range of specific procedures. As we have noted above, in recent years the identification of discrete target behaviors has been expanded to include cognitions and affects, as well as large-scale social systems affecting a child (e.g., families, schools, communities). Information regarding these additional areas can be obtained most efficiently through behavioral interviews, self-reports, and other-reports. Cone (1978) has described these assessment methods as indirect ones; that is, though they may be used to measure behaviors of relevance, they are obtained at a time and place different from those in which the actual behaviors occur. In clinical and diagnostic interviews as well as self-report questionnaires, a verbal report of the behaviors of interest is obtained. Reports of significant others are also included in the indirect category, because they involve retrospective descriptions of behavior. Generally a significant person in a child's environment (e.g., parent, teacher) is asked to rate the child's behaviors based on previous observations (recollections).

As noted by Cone (1978), ratings such as these should not be confused with direct observation methods, which assess the behaviors of interest at the time and place of their occurrence. Of course, information regarding cognition and affects, as well as overt behaviors, can be obtained through direct behavioral observations—either by self-monitoring, physiological recordings, or coding of actual behaviors. These direct and indirect measures are presented in detail in the chapters that follow.

FUNCTIONAL ANALYSIS AND ITS ROLE IN BEHAVIORAL ASSESSMENT

Functional analysis is at the core of behavioral assessment and is the cornerstone of effective cognitive-behavioral treatment (Cone, 1997; Haynes, Leisen, & Blaine, 1997; Haynes, O'Brien, & Kaholokula, 2011; Ollendick & Cerny, 1981; Yoman, 2008). It can guide the clinician to effective interventions by informing a case conceptualization of an individual child and her or his family, based on the data obtained about the targets of change, their controlling variables, and the functions they serve. It can also be useful in the selection and use of evidence-based interventions (Haynes et al., 2011; Heyne et al., 2002; Kearney & Albano, 2007; Kearney & Silverman, 1999; King, Heyne, Tonge, Gullone, & Ollendick, 2001; King et al., 1998).

In general, a functional analysis requires the description of the target behaviors and their controlling variables in observable, measurable terms. As such, attempts are made to measure the frequency, intensity, and duration of the target behaviors (commonly referred to as the "topography" of the behaviors), as well as the contexts in which they occur and the functions they serve. Topographic features of behavior vary considerably. For some behaviors their frequency is more salient, whereas for others their intensity and duration may be more problematic. Consider a child who does not get angry often but who explodes into a tantrum that lasts hours when he or she does get angry, versus a child who gets mildly angry frequently but whose anger does not last long and does not persist over time. It is important to note that the target behaviors can include not only overt and directly measurable behaviors, but also thoughts and feelings associated with those behaviors. Thus it is possible to monitor and record thoughts of "danger" or "loss" or "anger," as well as the affect associated with those thoughts. Sometimes these thoughts and feelings are also "controlling" variables that serve as antecedents or consequences to the observed behaviors; at other times, the overt behaviors themselves may serve as controlling variables and set the stage for certain thoughts and feelings. The important points here are that thoughts, feelings, and behaviors are all measurable, are intricately related to one another, and exist in a dynamic, transactive manner.

In a functional analysis, the first order of business is to define and measure the behaviors of interest (by conducting a thorough behavioral assessment as described above). For a child who is shy and socially anxious, for example, the target behaviors might include overt behaviors such as speaking in class, eating in public, and being assertive with peers; thoughts of being rejected by peers; and feelings of loneliness. For a child who is oppositional, the targets might include overt behaviors such as argumentativeness and defiance toward authority figures; thoughts of "I am a failure"; and feelings of jealousy or anger toward siblings or peers. Importantly, it would be necessary to obtain measures of the frequency, intensity and duration of these behaviors, thoughts, and feelings. A variety of measures—including behavioral interviews, self-monitoring, parent and teacher reports, physiological indices during behavioral tests, laboratory measures of inhibition and arousal, and behavioral observation in a variety of situations—might be enlisted.

In defining target behaviors, although we are not driven or restrained by diagnostic systems (see Chapter 2), we have found these systems to be useful in making sure that relevant and frequently co-occurring behaviors are identified. For example, with a boy who is anxious about separating from his parents, the eight *Diagnostic and Statistical Manual of Mental*

Disorders, Fourth Edition (DSM-IV-TR) symptoms of separation anxiety disorder (American Psychiatric Association, 2000) can be operationalized and examined in detail.[1] Does the child express developmentally inappropriate and excessive anxiety concerning separation from home or from those to whom the child is attached, as evidenced by three (or more) of the following behaviors?

1. Recurrent excessive distress when separation from home or major attachment figures occurs or is anticipated
2. Persistent and excessive worry about losing, or about possible harm befalling, major attachment figures
3. Persistent and excessive worry that an untoward event will lead to separation from a major attachment figure (e.g., getting lost or being kidnapped)
4. Persistent reluctance or refusal to go to school or elsewhere because of fear of separation
5. Persistently and excessively fearful or reluctant to be alone or without major attachment figures at home or without significant adults in other settings
6. Persistent reluctance or refusal to go to sleep without being near a major attachment figure or to sleep away from home
7. Repeated nightmares involving the theme of separation
8. Repeated complaints of physical symptoms (such as headaches, stomachaches, nausea, or vomiting) when separation from major attachment figures occurs or is anticipated[2]

As may be evident, these behaviors may take the form of thoughts, feelings, or motor behaviors. For example, "reluctance or refusal" to go to school might take the form of outright school refusal, but might also take the form of thoughts of impending doom or catastrophe when at school and feelings of panic while away from major caregivers. As with all target behaviors, multiple informants and multiple methods of assessment are necessary to obtain a complete picture of the child's "anxiety" in separation situations. Such assessment is especially useful in operationalizing the behaviors and in determining whether they are "excessive," "persistent," or "repeated" over time. When viewed in this manner, diagnostic "symptoms"

---

[1]Reprinted with permission from *Diagnostic and Statistical Manual of Mental Disorders, Fourth Edition, Text Revision*. Copyright 2000 by the American Psychiatric Association.

[2]The symptoms of separation anxiety disorder listed in the *Diagnostic and Statistical Manual of Mental Disorders, Fifth Edition* (DSM-5; American Psychiatric Association, 2013) can also be used for this purpose. In the DSM-5, the symptoms of separation anxiety disorder remain unchanged, save for minor wording changes in the symptoms that reflect changes in the criteria (e.g., the DSM-5 does not require onset before age 18).

can be quite useful and integrated quite readily into a functional behavioral analysis system (see also Nelson-Gray & Paulson, 2004).

After identifying the behaviors of interest, a functional analysis next turns to the events that are associated with those behaviors—both "antecedent" and "consequent" events. Antecedent events precede the behaviors of interest and set the stage for those behaviors to occur. These events are also known as "discriminative stimuli," because they signal the child when to respond and inform the child that a certain consequence is likely to occur. In our school refusal example, the boy might associate facial cues (e.g., stern facial cues vs. more conciliatory ones) from his parents as signals for when his refusal behaviors (verbal complaints, headaches, statements of worry, looks of dread) are likely to result in his being able to stay home from school and when they are not. He might also learn that certain facial cues may mean different things when they are exhibited by his father versus his mother. Of course, school refusal might also be more likely on certain days of the week when the child has to make a presentation in class or to take a test—especially so if the child is socially anxious and wary of the evaluation of others. These various conditions or contexts also serve as discriminative stimuli for the child.

Consequent stimuli follow the behavior of interest. There are two main types of consequences: "reinforcers" and "punishers," which are distinguished by their effects on behavior. They either increase behavior (reinforcers) or decrease it (punishers). Consequent stimuli are defined by their effect on the target behaviors, *not* by the expectation or intention of the concerned parent, teacher, peer, or clinician. Praise, for example, is often delivered with the expectation that it will reinforce the behavior it follows, but this in fact is often not the case. Similarly, a child is often reprimanded or scolded with the intent that this will punish the behavior it follows, but it often does not. Whether praise or criticism serves as reinforcers or punishers is a function of their demonstrated effects on behaviors, not their intended consequences.

Although functional analysis emerged from the principles of operant conditioning, it is also informed by the principles of respondent conditioning. The behaviors involved in respondent or classical conditioning differ from those in operant conditioning in several important ways: They are said to occur "within the skin" of the child, and they are elicited by stimuli that occur prior to the behavior, rather than controlled by stimuli that occur after the behavior. Such learning principles are especially important in understanding emotional responses and more instinctive behaviors such as heart rate and salivation. This form of conditioning is concerned with how stimuli come to control such involuntary or instinctive behaviors through their relations with other stimuli that elicit these responses. As such, respondent conditioning can shed some light on how certain stimuli are established as reinforcers or punishers.

In regard to functional analysis, it is crucial to comment briefly on the "function" of the target behaviors as well as their form or topography (i.e., frequency, intensity, and duration, as noted above; see also King, Ollendick, & Tonge, 1995; Ollendick & Mayer, 1984). To continue with our example of school refusal, we are interested in determining not only how frequently it occurs, how intense the emotional response is, how long the behavior has been a problem, and in which contexts it occurs, but also what *functions* the school refusal behavior serves (regardless of its topography and context). The work of Kearney and Silverman illustrates this approach (Kearney, 2001; Kearney & Silverman, 1999). Basically, these authors have proposed a model of school refusal behavior that classifies youth on the basis of what reinforces school absenteeism. They suggest that children refuse school for one or more of the following primary reasons or functions: (1) to avoid school-related objects and situations (stimuli) that provoke negative emotional responses (e.g., symptoms of anxiety or depression); (2) to escape aversive social or evaluative situations in school; (3) to receive or pursue attention from significant others outside of school; and (4) to obtain or pursue tangible rewards outside of school. Examples of school-related objects and situations include having to ride on the school bus, unexpected or loud fire alarms, being in noisy or chaotic hallways, and having to dress for and participate in gymnastic or other activities. Examples of school-related social and evaluative situations include meeting new teachers or students, being ridiculed or bullied by students, taking tests, putting on recitals, and speaking or writing in front of others. In Kearney and Silverman's model, the first two functions pertain to children who refuse school for negative reinforcement reasons (i.e., to get away from something unpleasant at school). In a two-process model, they may also reflect a classical conditioning process in which school-related cues have become associated with pain or discomfort (as in classical conditioning), which is then followed by escape and negative reinforcement. The second two functions pertain to children who refuse school for positive reinforcement reasons (i.e., to pursue or obtain something attractive outside of school). Here, examples include having parents provide extra attention and be close to them, as well as tangible rewards such as watching television at home, playing computer games during the day, lazing around the home, and perhaps even socializing with others who are not in school. Of course, some children refuse school for multiple reasons.

To assess these sometimes disparate functions of the target behavior—in this case, school refusal—Kearney and colleagues recommend use of a structured diagnostic interview such as the Anxiety Disorders Interview Schedule for DSM-IV: Child and Parent Versions (ADIS-IV: C/P; Silverman & Albano, 1996), in addition to the behavioral assessment tools reviewed above. Importantly, the ADIS-IV: C/P not only assesses for most disorders present in childhood, but also contains a special section on school-refusal-related problems that can provide invaluable information on both the topography and the function of the targeted behaviors.

Illustrative questions include "Do you get nervous or scared about having to go to school?", "Has your mother, father, or someone else ever picked you up early from school because you were nervous or scared?", and "Have you ever stayed home from school because you like it better at home?" Responses to these questions can be followed up with additional questions to determine the "function" of these behaviors, as well as their antecedents and consequences. This clinical interview can then be supplemented by a questionnaire designed specifically to test further functional hypotheses about the school refusal: the School Refusal Assessment Scale—Revised (SRAS-R; Kearney, 2002, 2006). The SRAS-R is a 24-item questionnaire that measures the relative contribution of the four functional conditions for school refusal behavior. The items are scored on a 0–6 scale ranging from "never" to "always." Child and parent versions are available. Representative items for each function include "How often do you have bad feelings about going to school because you are afraid of something related to school (for example, tests, school bus, teacher, fire alarm)?", "How often do you stay away from school because you feel embarrassed in front of other people at school?", "How often do you feel you would rather be with your parents than go to school?", and "When you are not in school during the week, how often do you leave the house and do something fun?"

Importantly, information from the clinical interview and the SRAS-R can be further supplemented by behavioral observations conducted in the home and the school. These observations help define the topography of the school refusal behavior and help determine the controlling variables that maintain it. More specifically, the clinician can schedule a time to meet with the family members in their home on a school day. The clinician arranges to arrive at the home 15 minutes before the child arises and, using a stopwatch, records the amount of time the child fails to engage in behaviors that would prepare him for school attendance. The clinician also records behaviors specific to the school refusal: (1) resistance to arising from bed at the specified time; (2) resistance to dressing, washing, and eating breakfast; (3) resistance to riding in the family car or school bus to school; (4) resistance to entering the school building; and (5) resistance to entering the classroom and attending classes. Quite obviously, these behavioral observations are extensive and time-consuming; however, most importantly, they provide a rich description of the child's behavior and, along with the interview and SRAS-R, a rich description of the function of the school-refusing behavior (Kearney & Albano, 2007).

The utility of behavioral assessment in naturalistic and simulated settings is illustrated in an early case study of a girl who also refused to attend school (Ayllon, Smith, & Rogers, 1970). In this case study, observers in the child's home monitored the stream of events occurring on school days, in order to delineate better the actual school-refusing behaviors and to determine the antecedent and consequent events associated with them. In this single-parent family, it was noted that the mother routinely left for work about 1 hour after the targeted girl (Valerie) and her siblings were to leave for school. Although the siblings left for school without incident, Valerie was observed to cling to her mother and refuse to leave the house and go to school. As described by Ayllon et al. (1970), "Valerie typically followed her mother around the house, from room to room, spending approximately 80 percent of her time within 10 feet of her mother. During these times, there was little or no conversation" (p. 128). Given her refusal to go to school, the mother took Valerie to a neighbor's apartment for the day. However, when the mother attempted to leave for work, Valerie followed her at a 10-foot distance. Frequently, the mother had to return to the neighbor's apartment with Valerie in hand. This daily pattern was observed to end with the mother "literally running to get out of sight of Valerie" so that she would not follow her to work. During the remainder of the day, it was observed that Valerie could do whatever she pleased: "Her day was one which would be considered ideal by many grade-school children—she could be outdoors and play as she chose all day long. No demands of any type were placed on her" (p. 129). Based on these observations, it appeared that Valerie's refusal to attend school were related to her mother's attention and to the reinforcing environment of the neighbor's apartment where she could play all day.

However, because Valerie was also reported to be afraid of school itself, Ayllon et al. (1970) designed a simulated school setting in the home to determine the extent of anxiety or fear toward specific school-related tasks. (Obviously, observation in the school itself would have been desirable, but this was impossible because she refused to attend school.) Unexpectedly, little or no fear was evinced in the simulated setting; in fact, Valerie performed well and appeared to enjoy the school-related setting and tasks. In this case, these detailed behavioral observations were useful in ruling in or out differential hypotheses related to the "function" of her school refusal. They led directly to a specific and efficacious treatment program based on shaping and differential reinforcement principles.

A major disadvantage of behavioral assessment in the natural environment is that the target behavior may not occur during the designated observation periods. In such instances, simulated settings that occasion the target behaviors can be used (as well as the reports of caregivers and the child him- or herself). Simulated observations are especially helpful when the target behavior is of low frequency, when the target behavior is not observed in the naturalistic setting due to reactivity effects of being observed (although see Reitman, McGregor, & Resnick, Chapter 7, this volume, for a discussion about how to decrease and measure reactivity effects), or when the target behavior is difficult to observe in the natural environment due to practical constraints. Ayllon et al.'s (1970) use of a simulated school setting illustrates this approach under the latter conditions. A study by Matson and Ollendick (1976) illustrates this approach for low-frequency behaviors. In this study, parents reported that their children would often bite and hit their parents or siblings when the children "were unable to get their way or were frustrated" (p. 411). Direct behavioral observations in the home confirmed parental reports, but it was necessary to observe the children for several hours before one incident of the behavior was actually observed. Furthermore, the parents reported that their children were being "nice" while the observers were present, and that the frequency of the biting and hitting behaviors was much lower than usual. Accordingly, the parents were trained in observation procedures and instructed to engage their children in play for four structured play sessions per day. During these sessions, the parents were instructed to attempt to elicit biting and hitting behaviors by removing a preferred toy. As expected, the removal of favored toys in the structured situations resulted in increases in target behaviors, which were then possible to reduce through differential reinforcement and mild punishment procedures. The structured, simulated play settings maximized the probability that biting and hitting would occur and that it could be observed and treated under controlled conditions.

SUMMARY

Direct behavioral observation—in either the natural or controlled simulated environment—provides valuable information for child behavioral assessment. When combined with information gathered through behavioral interviews, self- and other-reports, self-monitoring, and (if appropriate) physiological and laboratory-based measurement, a comprehensive picture of the child and her or his behaviors, as well as the behaviors' controlling variables, can be obtained. Moreover, following a functional analysis, the specific function of the behavior can be hypothesized and empirically tested. Although we have illustrated the multimethod, multi-informant approach to assessment with school-refusing behavior, this approach is equally applicable to the other "symptoms" of separation anxiety disorder. One could readily develop behavioral assessment strategies for measuring "worry about losing, or about possible harm befalling, major attachment figures," "distress when separation from home or major attachment figures occurs or is anticipated," and "repeated complaints of physical symptoms (such as headaches, stomachaches, nausea, or vomiting) when separation from major attachment figures occurs or is anticipated." So, too, could one expand these strategies to the assessment of other problematic behaviors that characterize other child and adolescent disorders. In fact, several authors have shown the applicability of this approach to other anxiety and depressive disorders (Albano & Morris, 2008; Ollendick, Allen, Benoit, & Cowart, 2011), as well as to oppositional defiant disorder and conduct disorder (Rhodes & Dadds, 2010; Scotti, Mullen, & Hawkins, 1998). They have also shown its suitability for large-scale use in school settings (Umbreit, Ferro, Liaupsin, & Lane, 2007).

FUTURE DIRECTIONS

A number of directions for future research and development in child behavioral assessment may be evident. What follows is our attempt to highlight those areas that appear most promising and in need of greater attention.

First, it seems to us that greater attention must be given to developmental factors as they affect the selection and evaluation of child behavioral assessment procedures. Although we have argued that these procedures should be developmentally sensitive, child behavioral assessors have frequently not attended to this suggestion. As we have noted earlier, the most distinguishing characteristic of children is developmental change. Such change encompasses basic biological growth and maturity, as well as affective, behavioral, and cognitive fluctuations that characterize children at different age levels and in different settings. Although the importance of accounting for developmental level in assessing behavior may be obvious, ways of integrating developmental concepts and principles into child behavioral assessment are less clear. In an early publication, Edelbrock (1984) noted three areas for the synthesis of developmental and behavioral principles: (1) use of developmental fluctuations in behavior to establish normative baselines of behavior; (2) determination of age and gender differences in the expression and covariation of behavioral patterns; and (3) study of stability and change in behavior over time, as related to such variables as age of onset and situational influences. Clearly, these areas of synthesis and integration are in need of considerably greater articulation even now—almost 30 years after his recommendations.

Our second point is somewhat related to the first: Greater attention must be focused on the incremental validity of the multimethod, multi-informant approach for youth of varying ages. Throughout this chapter (and this book), we espouse an approach consisting of interviews, self- and other-reports, self-monitoring, physiological assessment, behavioral observations and other evidence-based strategies. Quite obviously, some of these procedures may be more appropriate at certain age levels than at others. Furthermore, the psychometric properties of these procedures may vary with age. If certain procedures are found to be less reliable or valid at different age levels, their indiscriminate use with children should not be endorsed. Inasmuch as these strategies are found to be inadequate, the combination of them in a multimethod approach would serve only to compound their inherent limitations (Ollendick & Hersen, 1984). The sine qua non of child behavioral assessment is that the procedures be empirically validated. Finally, the different procedures may vary in their treatment utility. As noted by Hayes, Nelson, and Jarrett (1987), "treatment utility" refers to the degree to which assessment strategies are shown to contribute to beneficial treatment outcomes. More specifically, treatment utility addresses issues related to the selection of specific target behaviors and to the choice of specific assessment strategies. For example, we might wish to examine the treatment utility of using self-report questionnaires to guide treatment planning, above and beyond that provided by direct behavioral observation of children who are wary of social encounters. All children could complete a fear schedule and be observed in a social situation, but the self-report data for only half of the children could be made available for treatment planning. If the children for whom self-reports were made available improved more than those whose treatment plans were based solely on behavioral observations, then the treatment utility of using self-report data principles would be established (for this problem with children of this age). In a similar fashion, the treatment utility of interviews, role plays, laboratory-based measures, and other devices could be evaluated (Hayes et al., 1987; Haynes et al., 2011). Although the concept of treatment utility has been with us for some time, it has not been fully investigated. We should not necessarily assume that more assessment is better assessment.

Third, more effort must be directed toward the development of developmentally sensitive and empirically validated procedures for the assessment of cognitive and affective processes in children. In recent years, child behavioral assessors have become increasingly interested in the relation of children's cognitive processes to observed behaviors and affective experiences. The need for assessment in this area is further evidenced by the increase in cognitive-behavioral treatment procedures with children (see Kendall, 2011). There is a particularly pressing need to develop procedures for examining the very cognitions and processes that are targeted for change in these intervention efforts (Prins & Ollendick, 2003). For example, the reliable and valid assessment of self-statements made by children in specific situations would facilitate the empirical evaluation of cognitive-behavioral procedures such as cognitive restructuring.

Fourth, we must concentrate additional effort on the role of the child in child behavioral assessment. All too frequently, "tests are administered *to* children, ratings are obtained *on* children, and behaviors are observed *in* children" (Ollendick & Hersen, 1984, p. 17; emphasis in original). This process views the child as a relatively passive responder—someone who is largely incapable of actively shaping and determining the behaviors of clinical relevance. Although examination of these organismic variables is evolving, systematic effort must be directed to their description and articulation. The process described above also implies that child behavior (problematic or otherwise) occurs in a vacuum, and that the perceptions and behaviors of referral sources (parents, teachers) and characteristics of the environments in which behavior occurs are somehow less critical to assess. Recent efforts to develop reliable methods for assessing parent–child interactions indicate an increased awareness of the need to broaden the scope of assessment to include the specific individuals with whom, and environments in which, child behavior problems commonly occur. However, much additional work remains to be done in this area.

Fifth, and finally, we must continue to focus our attention on ethical issues in child behavioral assessment (see also Chapter 1). Various ethical issues regarding children's rights, proper and legal consent, professional judgment, and social values are raised in the routine practice of child behavioral assessment. Are children capable of granting full and proper consent to a behavioral assessment procedure? At what age are children competent to give such consent? Is informed consent necessary? Or might not informed consent be impossible, impractical, or countertherapeutic in some situations? What ethical guidelines surround the assessment procedures to be used? Current professional guidelines suggest that our procedures should be reliable, valid, and clinically useful. Do the procedures suggested in this chapter and in this book meet these professional guidelines? What are the rights of parents? Of society? It should be evident from these questions that numerous ethical questions exist. Striking a balance among the rights of parents, society, and children is no easy matter, but is one that takes on added importance in our increasingly litigious society.

In short, the future directions of child behavioral assessment are rich and numerous. Even though a technology for child behavioral assessment has evolved, we need to begin exploring the issues raised in this chapter and throughout our book before we can conclude that the procedures are maximally productive and in the best interests of children and their families. We are at an exciting juncture in this field of inquiry.

REFERENCES

Albano, A. M., & Morris, T. M. (1998). Childhood anxiety, obsessive–compulsive disorder, and depression. In J. J. Plaud & G. H. Eifert (Eds.), *From behavior theory to behavior therapy* (pp. 203–222). Boston: Allyn & Bacon.

American Psychiatric Association (2000). *Diagnostic and statistical manual of mental disorders* (4th ed., text rev.). Washington, DC: Author.

American Psychiatric Association. (2013). *Diagnostic and statistical manual of mental disorders* (5th ed.). Arlington, VA: Author.

Ayllon, T., Smith, D., & Rogers, M. (1970). Behavioral management of school phobia. *Journal of Behavior Therapy and Experimental Psychiatry, 1,* 125–138.

Bandura, A. (1971). *Social learning theory.* Englewood Cliffs, NJ: General Learning Press.

Bem, D. I., & Allen, A. (1974). On predicting some of the people some of the time: The search for cross-situational consistencies in behavior. *Psychological Review, 81,* 506–520.

Bornstein, P. H., Bornstein, M. T., & Dawson, B. (1984). Integrated assessment and treatment. In T. H. Ollendick & M. Hersen (Eds.), *Child behavioral assessment: Principles and procedures* (pp. 223–243). New York: Pergamon Press.

Cone, J. D. (1978). The behavioral assessment grid (BAG): A conceptual framework and taxonomy. *Behavior Therapy, 9,* 882–888.

Cone, J. D. (1986). Idiographic, nomothetic, and related perspectives in behavioral assessment. In R. O. Nelson & S. C. Hayes (Eds.), *Conceptual foundations of behavioral assessment* (pp. 111–128). New York: Guilford Press.

Cone, J. D. (1997). Issues in functional analysis in behavioral assessment. *Behaviour Research and Therapy, 35*, 259–275.

Cone, J. D., & Hawkins, R. P. (Eds.). (1977). *Behavioral assessment: New directions in clinical psychology.* New York: Brunner/Mazel.

Edelbrock, C. S. (1984). Developmental considerations. In T. H. Ollendick & M. Hersen (Eds.), *Child behavioral assessment: Principles and procedures* (pp. 20–37). New York: Pergamon Press.

Evans, I. M., & Nelson, R. O. (1977). Assessment of child behavior problems. In A. R. Ciminero, K. S. Calhoun, & H. E. Adams (Eds.), *Handbook of behavioral assessment* (pp. 603–682). New York: Wiley-Interscience.

Goldfried, M. R., & Kent, R. N. (1972). Traditional versus behavioral personality assessment: A comparison of methodological and theoretical assumptions. *Psychological Bulletin, 77*, 409–420.

Hayes, S. C., Nelson, R. O., & Jarrett, R. B. (1986). Evaluating the quality of behavioral assessment. In R. O. Nelson & S. C. Hayes (Eds.), *Conceptual foundations of behavioral assessment* (pp. 463–503). New York: Guilford Press.

Hayes, S. C., Nelson, R. O., & Jarrett, R. B. (1987). The treatment utility of assessment: A functional approach to evaluating assessment quality. *American Psychologist, 42*, 963–974.

Haynes, S. N., Leisen, M. B., & Blaine, D. D. (1997). Design of individualized behavioral treatment programs using functionally analytic clinical case models. *Psychological Assessment, 9*, 334–348.

Haynes, S. N., O'Brien, W. H., & Kaholokula, J. K. (2011). *Behavioral assessment and case formulation.* Baltimore, MD: Johns Hopkins University Press.

Haynes, S. N., Smith, G., & Hunsley, J. (2011). *Scientific foundations of clinical assessment.* New York: Routledge/Taylor & Francis.

Heyne, D., King, N. J., Tonge, B., Rollings, S., Young, D., Pritchard, M., & Ollendick, T. H. (2002). Evaluation of child therapy and caregiver training in the treatment of school refusal. *Journal of the American Academy of Child and Adolescent Psychiatry, 41*, 687–695.

Hunsley, J., & Mash, E. (Eds.). (2008). *A guide to assessments that work.* New York: Oxford University Press.

Kanfer, F. H., & Phillips, J. S. (1970). *Learning foundations of behavior therapy.* New York: Wiley.

Kearney, C. A. (2001). *School refusal behavior in youth: A functional approach to assessment and treatment.* Washington, DC: American Psychological Association.

Kearney, C. A. (2002). Identifying the function of school refusal behavior: A revision of the School Refusal Assessment Scale. *Journal of Psychopathology and Behavioral Assessment, 28*, 235–245.

Kearney, C. A. (2006). Confirmatory factor analysis of the School Refusal Assessment Scale—Revised: Child and parent versions. *Journal of Psychopathology and Behavioral Assessment, 28*(3), 139–144.

Kearney, C. A., & Albano, A. M. (2007). *When children refuse school: A cognitive-behavioral therapy approach* (2nd ed.). New York: Oxford University Press.

Kearney, C. A., & Silverman, W. K. (1999). Functionally-based prescriptive and nonprescriptive treatment for children and adolescents with school refusal behavior. *Behavior Therapy, 30*, 673–695.

Kendall, P. C. (Ed.). (2011). *Child and adolescent therapy: Cognitive-behavioral procedures* (4th ed.). New York: Guilford Press.

King, N. J., Heyne, D., Tonge, B., Gullone, E., & Ollendick, T. H. (2001). School refusal: Categorical diagnoses, functional analysis and treatment planning. *Clinical Psychology and Psychotherapy, 8,* 352–360.

King, N. J., Tonge, B. J., Heyne, D., Pritchard, M., Rollings, S., Young, D., & Ollendick, T. H. (1998). Cognitive-behavioral treatment of school refusing children: A controlled evaluation. *Journal of the American Academy of Child and Adolescent Psychiatry, 37,* 395–403.

King, N. J., Ollendick, T. H., & Tonge, B. J. (1995). *School refusal: Assessment and treatment.* Boston: Allyn & Bacon.

Mash, E. J., & Terdal, L. G. (1981). Behavioral assessment of childhood disturbance. In E. J. Mash & L. G. Terdal (Eds.), *Behavioral assessment of childhood disorders* (pp. 3–76). New York: Guilford Press.

Mash, E. J., & Terdal, L. G. (Eds.). (1987). *Behavioral assessment of childhood disorders* (2nd ed.). New York: Guilford Press.

Matson, J. L., & Ollendick, T. H. (1976). Elimination of low-frequency biting. *Behavior Therapy, 7,* 410–412.

Meichenbaum, D. H. (1977). *Cognitive-behavior modification.* New York: Plenum Press.

Mischel, W. (1968). *Personality and assessment.* New York: Wiley.

Nelson, R. O. (1977). Methodological issues in assessment via self-monitoring. In J. D. Cone & R. P. Hawkins (Eds.), *Behavioral assessment: New directions in clinical psychology* (pp. 217–240). New York: Brunner/Mazel.

Nelson-Gray, R. O., & Paulson, J. F. (2004). Behavioral assessment and the DSM system. In S. N. Haynes & E. H. Heiby (Eds.), *Behavioral assessment* (pp. 470–489). Hoboken, NJ: Wiley.

O'Leary, K. D., & Johnson, S. B. (1979). Psychological assessment. In H. C. Quay & J. S. Werry (Eds.), *Psychopathological disorders of children* (pp. 210–246). New York: Wiley.

Ollendick, T. H. (1999). Empirically supported assessment for clinical practice: Is it possible? Is it desirable? *The Clinical Psychologist, 52,* 1–2.

Ollendick, T. H., Allen, B., Benoit, K., & Cowart, M. J. (2011). The tripartite model of fear in children with specific phobia: Assessing concordance and discordance using the Behavioral Approach Test. *Behaviour Research and Therapy, 49,* 459–465.

Ollendick, T. H., & Cerny, J. A. (1981). *Clinical behavior therapy with children.* New York: Plenum Press.

Ollendick, T. H., & Hersen, M. (Eds.). (1984). *Child behavioral assessment: Principles and procedures.* New York: Pergamon Press.

Ollendick, T. H., & Hersen, M. (Eds.). (1993). *Handbook of child and adolescent assessment.* Boston: Allyn & Bacon.

Ollendick, T. H., & Mayer, J. A. (1984). School phobia. In S. M. Turner (Ed.), *Behavioral theories and treatment of anxiety* (pp. 367–411). New York: Plenum Press.

Ollendick, T. H., & Shirk, S. R. (2011). Clinical interventions with children and adolescents: Current status, future directions. In D. H. Barlow (Ed.), *Oxford handbook of clinical psychology* (pp. 762–788). Oxford, UK: Oxford University Press.

Olweus, D. (1979). Stability of aggressive reaction patterns in males: A review. *Psychological Bulletin, 86,* 852–875.

Patterson, G. R. (1976). The aggressive child: Victim and architect of a coercive system. In E. J. Mash, L. A. Hamerlynck, & L. C. Hardy (Eds.), *Behavior modification and families* (pp. 267–316). New York: Brunner/Mazel.

Prins, P. M. J., & Ollendick, T. H. (2003). Cognitive change and enhanced coping: Missing mediational links in cognitive behavior therapy with anxiety-disordered children. *Clinical Child and Family Psychology Review, 6,* 87–105.

Prinz, R. (Ed.). (1986). *Advances in behavioral assessment of children and families.* Greenwich, CT: JAI Press.

Rhodes, T. E., & Dadds, M. R. (2010). Assessment of conduct problems using an integrated, process-oriented approach. In R. C. Murrihy, A. D. Kidman, & T. H. Ollendick (Eds.), *Clinical handbook of assessing and treating conduct problems in youth* (pp. 77–116). New York: Springer.

Scotti, J. R., Mullen, K. B., & Hawkins, R. P. (1998). Child conduct and developmental disabilities: From theory to practice in the treatment of excess behaviors. In J. J. Plaud & G. H. Eifert (Eds.), *From behavior theory to behavior therapy* (pp. 172–202). Boston: Allyn & Bacon.

Silverman, W. K., & Albano, A. M. (1996). *Anxiety Disorders Interview Schedule for DSM-IV: Child and Parent Versions.* San Antonio, TX: Psychological Corporation.

Skinner, B. F. (1953). *Science and human behavior.* New York: Macmillan.

Skinner, B. F. (1957). The experimental analysis of behavior. *American Scientist, 45*(4), 343–371.

Staats, A. W. (1975). *Social behaviorism.* Homewood, IL: Dorsey Press.

Staats, A. W. (1986). Behaviorism with a personality. In R. O. Nelson & S. C. Hayes (Eds.), *Conceptual foundations of behavioral assessment* (pp. 244–296). New York: Guilford Press.

Ullmann, L. P., & Krasner, L. (Eds.). (1965). *Case studies in behavior modification.* New York: Holt, Rinehart & Winston.

Umbreit, J., Ferro, J. B., Liaupsin, C. J., & Lane, K. L. (2007). *Functional behavioral assessment and function-based intervention: An effective, practical approach.* Upper Saddle River, NJ: Pearson Education.

Wahler, R. G. (1976). Deviant child behavior in the family: Developmental speculations and behavior change strategies. In H. Leitenberg (Ed.), *Handbook of behavior modification and behavior therapy* (pp. 516–543). Englewood Cliffs, NJ: Prentice-Hall.

Wahler, R. G., House, A. E., & Stambaugh, E. E. (1976). *Ecological assessment of child problem behavior: A clinical package for home, school, and institutional settings.* New York: Pergamon Press.

Winett, R. A., Riley, A. W., King, A. C., & Altman, D. G. (1989). Preventive strategies with children and families. In T. H. Ollendick & M. Hersen (Eds.), *Handbook of child psychopathology* (2nd ed., pp. 499–521). New York: Plenum Press.

Yoman, J. (2008). A primer on functional analysis. *Cognitive and Behavioral Practice, 15,* 325–340.

4

Case Conceptualization, Treatment Planning, and Outcome Monitoring

Bryce D. McLeod, Amanda Jensen-Doss, and Thomas H. Ollendick

The primary goal of this chapter is to illustrate how diagnostic and behavioral assessment tools can be used together to develop a case conceptualization as a guide to the clinical assessment and treatment process. Chapter 1 has outlined general assessment principles; Chapters 2 and 3 have described the conceptual underpinnings of the diagnostic and behavioral assessment traditions, respectively. This integrative chapter illustrates how tools from both traditions can be used to develop and refine a case conceptualization, to plan for treatment, and to monitor the effects of treatment.

The ability to develop a case conceptualization is an important and fundamental psychotherapy skill. A case conceptualization provides a clinician with a roadmap that not only identifies the constructs for assessment and treatment, but also guides treatment planning and evaluation from intake through termination. It therefore is important for clinicians to understand how to use diagnostic and behavioral tools to develop an empirically based case conceptualization.

It can be a challenge to apply findings from the empirical treatment literature to particular clients. Such findings are primarily based upon nomothetic principles. Clinical trials provide general statements about how the average child responds to a given treatment, so it can be difficult to determine whether these findings apply to a particular child or family. Little research exists to indicate which child clients are more or less likely to respond to a particular treatment (Kazdin, 2007). Moreover, the demographic and clinical characteristics of the children treated in clinical trials do not always represent the youth seen across different practice settings (e.g., Baker-Ericzen, Hurlburt, Brookman-Frazee, Jenkins, & Hough, 2010; Ehrenreich-May et al., 2011). Clinicians therefore must determine the extent to which particular evidence-based treatments match the characteristics and background of each child client, and must then decide whether adaptations need to be made.

As noted earlier, similar problems can arise when clinicians are attempting to select assessment instruments. Few nomothetic tools have been normed on representative samples. Moreover, only a handful of diagnostic and behavioral tools have been validated for the diverse youth seen in practice settings, who come to treatment with a wide range of presenting problems. As a result, clinicians must select the best assessment tool available for a particular client and purpose, as the "perfect" assessment tool may not exist for any one youth seen in clinical practice.

A key skill for clinicians is to understand how to translate empirical findings from the assessment and treatment literatures for use in practice settings. Clinicians must know how to select the best-fitting evidence-based treatment and assessment tools. We suggest that the ability to develop a case conceptualization is critical to this process, because it allows clinicians to use scientific findings to inform the treatment of specific clients.

WHAT IS A CASE CONCEPTUALIZATION?

A "case conceptualization" is broadly defined as a set of hypotheses about the causes, antecedents, and maintaining factors of a client's emotional, interpersonal, and behavior problems (Eells, 2007; Haynes, O'Brien, & Kaholokula, 2011; Nezu, Nezu, Peacock, & Girdwood, 2004). Both diagnostic and behavioral assessment play a role in developing a case conceptualization. Baseline data generated early in the assessment process form the basis of the case conceptualization and are used to access the empirical literature. The literature is then used to identify the target behaviors, determine how the problems developed, and decide how the problems can be ameliorated.

As noted earlier, findings from a thorough assessment can generate a relatively complete picture of an individual child and her or his family. However, clinicians need a framework for interpreting the assessment data. A case conceptualization grounded in empirical findings provides this framework. Basically, a case conceptualization allows clinicians to synthesize assessment data into a comprehensive picture of an individual that describes how the target behaviors came about and how they can be alleviated (Eells & Lombart, 2004; Haynes et al., 2011). Once developed, the case conceptualization guides assessment and treatment by identifying treatment targets and markers for clinical change (Eells & Lombart, 2004).

Case conceptualization is an empirical process. Hypotheses are generated and then tested during treatment. We assert that the hypotheses should be driven by empirically supported developmental psychopathology theories regarding factors implicated in the development and maintenance of the target behaviors (Haynes et al., 2011; Hunsley & Mash, 2007; McFall, 2005). This information, in turn, should directly inform (1) treatment planning (i.e., the length and focus of treatment), (2) treatment selection (i.e., the interventions designed to alter the causal and maintaining factors), and (3) treatment monitoring/evaluation. In order to translate these theories into a case conceptualization, clinicians must understand when and how to use diagnostic and behavioral assessment tools. Below we outline how these different assessment approaches can be used to develop, evaluate, and refine a case conceptualization.

One final note should be offered regarding our approach to case conceptualization. Key to our assessment approach is a thorough understanding of behavioral theories and methods. A critical part of developing a case conceptualization is determining the extent to which a target behavior occurs across time and contexts. Not only is this information needed to generate a diagnosis; it also directly informs treatment planning and selection. Behavioral assessment is uniquely suited for this purpose. As a result, it is important for clinicians to understand behavioral theories and methods. That being said, in this book we do not advocate for a particular theoretical approach to therapy. Our focus here is on how to use diagnostic and behavioral assessment approaches to inform treatment, not on how to use a particular type of therapy with children and their families.

HISTORICAL CONSIDERATIONS

The roots of case conceptualization can be traced to the medical diagnostic tradition of ancient times (see Eells & Lombart, 2004). Associated with Hipprocrates and Galen, the medical diagnostic tradition emphasizes a rational, theory-driven approach to diagnosis guided by assessment. Developed in the 5th century B.C.E., the Hippocratic tradition emphasized a thorough assessment guided by reason, logic, and observation in order to arrive at the correct diagnosis of the underlying pathology. In the 2nd century C.E., Galen began to use empirical methods to understand disease and human anatomy so that he could test the accuracy of a diagnosis. The core diagnostic and empirical values underlying the medical diagnostic tradition are central to many of the case conceptualization approaches currently used in psychotherapy.

Case conceptualization has long been a critical part of psychotherapy. Each brand of psychotherapy takes a unique approach to case conceptualization that is based on the theory underlying its approach to treatment. Several books and chapters have been published on case conceptualization in the past decade (e.g., Haynes et al., 2011; Hersen & Porzelius, 2002;

Horowitz, 2005; McLeod, Jensen-Doss, Wheat, & Becker, in press; Nezu et al., 2004; Reitman, 2008). Despite these publications, little systematic research exists on the potential value of using different case conceptualizations to guide assessment and treatment (Eells & Lombart, 2004; Nelson-Gray, 2003). As a result, few empirically based guidelines exist to shape the process.

Despite the lack of research, case conceptualization is considered a critical component of assessment and treatment. The American Psychological Association Presidential Task Force on Evidence-Based Practice (2006) considers case conceptualization an important component of evidence-based practice: "The purpose of Evidence Based Practice in psychology is to promote effective psychological practice and enhance public health by applying empirically supported principles of psychological assessment, *case conceptualization*, therapeutic relationship, and intervention" (p. 273, emphasis added). In lieu of empirical findings to guide this process, we rely upon research on the correlates and contributors to child emotional and behavioral disorders to build an evidence-based approach to case conceptualization for the treatment of child emotional and behavioral problems. We now present a summary of this approach.

AN EVIDENCE-BASED APPROACH TO CASE CONCEPTUALIZATION

The primary goal of case conceptualization is to identify a set of testable hypotheses about the factors (independent variables) that serve to cause or maintain a target behavior (dependent variable). To test these hypotheses, a clinician introduces interventions designed to alter the causal and/or maintaining factors, and observes the resulting impact upon the target behavior. Collecting assessment data throughout treatment is a key part of testing the hypotheses. Indeed, regular outcome monitoring creates a feedback loop that allows a clinician to refine and reformulate the hypotheses. It is absolutely critical to test the hypotheses. Hypotheses that are generated early in treatment may not be specific enough, or may simply be wrong. Assessment data can help shed light upon the accuracy of the hypotheses, and thus can help identify when the hypotheses, and the treatment plan, may need to be altered.

Below we present the five steps involved in developing a case conceptualization: (1) Identify target behaviors and causal/maintaining factors; (2) arrive at a diagnosis; (3) form the initial case conceptualization; (4) proceed with treatment planning and selection; and (5) develop outcome-monitoring and evaluation strategies. Different assessment tools are used at each step. Information gathered at any one step will not provide a definitive understanding of a youth and her or his problems. Rather, the data collected at each step can be used to develop, evaluate, and reformulate the hypotheses. Table 4.1 summarizes the five steps.

TABLE 4.1. Steps in Building a Case Conceptualization

Number	Step and definition
Step 1:	*Identify target behaviors and causal/maintaining Factors.* Identify and define the relevant target behaviors. Map out the historical, causal, antecedent, and maintaining factors for each target behavior.
Step 2:	*Arrive at a diagnosis.* Determine whether the child meets diagnostic criteria for one or more *Diagnostic and Statistical Manual of Mental Disorders* (DSM) diagnoses.
Step 3:	*Form the initial case conceptualization.* Synthesize and interpret the assessment data within the context of the developmental psychopathology literature. Produce a comprehensive picture of the child, along with a set of hypotheses for how the target behaviors developed, are maintained, and can be ameliorated.
Step 4:	*Proceed with treatment planning and selection.* Use the case conceptualization to generate a treatment plan designed to target the key hypotheses. Search the treatment literature, and select an appropriate evidence-based treatment.
Step 5:	*Develop outcome-monitoring and evaluation strategies.* Develop a plan for ongoing outcome monitoring that focuses on target behaviors and causal/maintaining factors, and that will permit the hypotheses to be tested. At treatment termination, conduct a thorough assessment that evaluates treatment effectiveness, the child's functioning, and the need for further treatment.

STEPS IN BUILDING A CASE CONCEPTUALIZATION

The initial meetings with the child and his or her family generally focus upon defining the target behaviors and formulating a diagnosis. Depending upon setting constraints, this information may need to be gathered across a number of sessions.

Step 1: Identify Target Behaviors and Causal/Maintaining Factors

One important goal of the initial meetings is to identify the target behaviors, along with a preliminary sketch of the historical, causal, and maintaining factors that may be related to one or more of the target behaviors. Clearly defining the target behaviors establishes why the child and his or her family have presented for treatment and forms the basis for setting collaborative treatment goals. Next, we detail the information that can be gathered during the initial meetings to achieve these goals.

Target Behaviors

One of the first tasks of a therapist meeting a new client is to identify relevant target behaviors. An accurate description of the target behaviors is critical to treatment planning. If possible, each target behavior should be defined in terms of three response modes (i.e., behavior/motoric, affective/physiological, cognitive/verbal) as well as the target behavior's topography (i.e., frequency, intensity, and duration; see our discussion in Chapter 3 for more detail). Generating a precise definition of each target behavior facilitates treatment monitoring, because the target behaviors represent markers of treatment progress that should be closely aligned with what the child and family want to gain from treatment.

The next step is to rank the target behaviors in terms of treatment priority. Target behaviors should be ordered according to severity, desires of the child and his or her family, and the potential of the target behavior to cause future impairment. In some cases, the child, parents, and clinician may not agree on what precisely the target behaviors are or how to rank them. In such cases, collaborative goal setting can be used to ensure that the child and family can agree upon what target behaviors to address in treatment (see Hawes & Dadds, Chapter 12, this volume).

Historical Events and Causal Factors

The initial meetings should also be used to identify historical events and causal factors, in order to provide a context for understanding each target behavior. Understanding whether historical events (e.g., speech delays, medical complications/hospitalizations, temperament) have set the stage for current problems via specific causal factors (e.g., poor social skills, poor emotion regulation) is important for developing a case conceptualization (Freeman & Miller, 2002). Historical events (i.e., risk factors) cannot be altered; however, the historical factors produce changes in the child (causal factors) that do influence the target behaviors and can be targeted in treatment. For example, a traumatic event can influence a child's affective and cognitive functioning, and these factors can be addressed directly in treatment, even though the event itself cannot be retracted or altered. To identify potential historical and causal factors, the clinician should gather information in such areas as developmental history, medical history, school history, and family psychiatric history. This information helps a clinician formulate a prognosis and generate a complete picture of an individual child. See Table 4.2 for examples of areas that can be assessed.

Contextual Information

It is important to determine where (e.g., home, school, public settings) and when (i.e., at what times) each target behavior occurs. During the initial meetings, a functional interview can be used to identify whether particular variables reliably precede the target behavior (i.e., antecedent variables) and/or make a target behavior more likely to occur (i.e., establishing

TABLE 4.2. Factors That May Contribute to the Development and Maintenance of Childhood Emotional and Behavioral Problems

Factors	Sample questions
Developmental factors	Did the child experience any prenatal, perinatal, or postnatal complications? Did the child achieve all developmental milestones? What is the child's social history? Does the child have a history of any learning difficulties?
Trauma	Has the child been exposed to any traumatic events or witnessed violence?
Medical history	Does the child have a history of medical illnesses, hospitalizations, or significant injuries? Is the child taking any medications or other substances that could explain the presenting problems?
Genetic factors	Is there a family history of emotional and/or behavioral problems? Does the child have a history of behavioral inhibition?
Biological factors	To what extent do physical or somatic symptoms play a role in the presenting problem? Does the child have particular markers of physiological overreactivity, such as a strong startle response and strong gag reflex?
Behavioral skills	Has the child developed the appropriate behavioral skills? If not, what (if any) role do the skill deficits play in causing or maintaining the target behavior?
Cognitive processes	How does the child view his or her target behaviors? Does the child believe in his or her ability to deal effectively with the target behaviors? Are there any cognitive biases that might influence the child's perception of his or her environment? Are any cognitive processes missing that might aid the target behavior (e.g., problem-solving skills)?
Learning processes	Does a specific event and/or stressor predate the onset of the target behavior? Did a direct (conditioning) and/or indirect (operant, modeling) learning experience influence the development of the target behavior?
Parental influences	What opportunities do the parents provide for mastery experiences? Do the parents negatively influence the child's opportunities for behavioral practice? Do the parents routinely take tasks over for the child that she or he could reasonably do without help? Do the parents model certain behaviors?

operations) in particular contexts (see Chapter 3). As noted earlier, this type of information is important for generating a diagnosis. For example, inattention and hyperactivity that occur across contexts might indicate a diagnosis of attention-deficit/hyperactivity disorder (ADHD), whereas this diagnosis is not indicated if these target behaviors only occur at home. This information also assists the clinician in treatment planning. For example, behavior that only occurs in the home may indicate the need for parent-focused interventions.

Maintaining Factors

The initial assessment should also identify maintaining factors. These factors are the internal and/or external conditions that influence the occurrence of behavior via the operant mechanisms of reinforcement or punishment (see Chapter 3 for more detail). For example, negative reinforcement can serve to maintain anxiety when avoidance of specific situations reduces the unpleasant experience of fear and anxiety; as a result, avoidant behavior can become a habitual behavioral response to feared stimuli or situations, even when there is no real threat.

Step 2: Arrive at a Diagnosis

The next step is to determine whether a child meets criteria for one or more disorders. Assigning a diagnosis represents an important step in building a case conceptualization. This step provides access to the area of the developmental psychopathology literature that will help a clinician identify possible maintaining and/or controlling variables. Assigning a diagnosis also represents the best way to identify relevant assessment tools and evidence-based treatment options.

Gathering Data for Steps 1 and 2

The assessment data used to generate the initial case conceptualization are typically collected during the initial treatment meetings. As noted in previous chapters, and detailed in subsequent chapters, a variety of assessment tools can be used to gather the data. Standardized interviews represent the most psychometrically sound approach to gathering information. However, standardized interviews take time to administer and do not exist for all domains, so unstructured interviews may be needed. Whenever possible, data gathered via interviews should be supplemented with self-report questionnaires and/or idiographic measures (e.g., self-monitoring assignments). Nomothetic measures can help quantify the severity of a child's problems, provide data on functioning, and identify potential target behaviors. Idiographic measures can help define the target behaviors and identify potential causal and maintaining factors. The decision to use a particular assessment approach will be guided by the psychometric properties of the measures, as well as the constraints of the setting in which the assessment will occur.

Step 3: Form the Initial Case Conceptualization

The next step is to generate the initial case conceptualization. The initial case conceptualization should provide a comprehensive picture of the young client that tells how the problems developed, how the problems are maintained, and how the problems can be ameliorated (Eells & Lombart,

2004; Haynes et al., 2011). The key components of the case conceptualization are the hypotheses about the causes, antecedents, and maintaining factors of each target behavior (Eells, 2007; Nezu et al., 2004). These hypotheses constitute the roadmap that guides assessment, identifies targets for treatment, and highlights potential markers for clinical change (Eells & Lombart, 2004). Figure 4.1 is a worksheet that can be used to develop a case conceptualization.

Generating the initial case conceptualization begins with outlining the treatment goals. Each goal should focus upon one target behavior and the expected outcome of treatment for that behavior. For example, school refusal can represent a target behavior, and the expected outcome of treatment can be no missed school days for a month. As noted above, it is often helpful to generate the treatment goals in collaboration with the child and family.

The next step is to synthesize the available data for each target behavior. The clinician must rely upon the developmental psychopathology literature to interpret the data. Using the list of possible risk (historical) factors generated in the initial meetings, the clinician must determine whether one or more risk factors have contributed to the development and maintenance of the target behavior via specific causal factors. For example, a child with an inhibited temperament (historical factor) may not have learned appropriate social skills (causal factor), which serves to increase anxiety in social situations (target behavior). A primary goal of this step is to generate a coherent "story" that explains how specific historical and causal variables have contributed to each target behavior.

Once the causal variables are mapped out for each target behavior, the next step is to consider whether contextual issues influence the target behavior. If a target behavior varies across contexts, then it is important to pinpoint relevant antecedent and maintaining variables. It is possible that a functional interview during the intake may help identify relevant antecedent and maintaining variables. However, more information may need to be gathered following the intake to perform a functional analysis. This process should help explain the function of each target behavior within particular contexts.

The last part of this step is to synthesize the data and produce hypotheses about the relations among the causal, antecedent, and maintaining variables for each target behavior. For example, one hypothesis for school refusal might be that it is maintained by the positive attention provided by the parents during the school day. It can help to produce a figural drawing that depicts the relations among the variables (see Jensen-Doss, Ollendick, & McLeod, Chapter 15, this volume, for examples).

The initial case conceptualization produced by this process is used to guide treatment planning and selection. Data gathered from the initial meetings will probably not provide a complete picture of the child. Rather, the goal is to gather enough information to formulate tentative hypotheses

FIGURE 4.1. Worksheet for generating a case conceptualization.

Step 1: Operationalize the target behaviors.
What are the target behaviors? What are the cognitive, behavioral, and affective components of each target behavior? What are the frequency, intensity, and duration of each target behavior?

Target behavior	Cognitive	Behavioral	Affective	Intensity (1–10)	Frequency and duration

What historical factors may be linked to one or more target behaviors?

What causal factors may be linked to one or more target behaviors?

What antecedents appear to precede the occurrence of one or more target behaviors?

What factors appear to be maintaining one or more target behaviors?

Step 2: Arrive at a diagnosis.
Does the child meet diagnostic criteria for a DSM disorder?

Step 3: Form the initial case conceptualization
What are the treatment targets? What historical factors may be linked to the treatment targets? What causal factors are contributing to the treatment targets? What role do contextual factors (antecedents, maintaining variables) play in the target behavior?

Treatment targets	Historical factors	Causal factors	Antecedents	Maintaining factors

Step 4: Proceed with treatment planning and selection.

List the hypotheses to be addressed in treatment, in terms of treatment priority and interventions that target those hypotheses.

Hypothesis	Intervention
1.	
2.	
3.	
4.	
5.	
6.	

List evidence-based treatments designed to address the treatment targets.

Step 5: What measures will be used for ongoing assessment to monitor the target behavior and intervening variables?

Measure	Domain	Reporter	Frequency

What measures will be used for treatment evaluation?

Posttreatment Assessment Battery	Domain	Reporter

that can be tested and refined in subsequent therapy sessions. Filling out the Figure 4.1 worksheet and producing a figural drawing can help shed light on areas where further assessment is needed. As treatment progresses, data can be gathered that can be used to test the hypotheses and further refine the case conceptualization. Behavioral assessment tools, such as self-monitoring, are particularly useful for this purpose.

Step 4: Proceed with Treatment Planning and Selection

Next, the case conceptualization is used to guide treatment planning and selection. Treatment planning involves taking the hypotheses and translating them into a plan of action. As noted above, each hypothesis should identify causal, antecedent, and maintaining factors that represent potential treatment targets. The first step in treatment planning is to determine which hypotheses should be targeted and in what order.

Nezu et al. (2004) suggest using a cost–benefit analysis to develop the treatment plan. They recommend considering the following factors:

1. What is the probability that altering the causal, antecedent, or maintaining factor will produce meaningful change in the target behavior (e.g., is the factor modifiable, is the client motivated to change the factor)?
2. What is the probability that altering the causal, antecedent, or maintaining factor will impact multiple variables (e.g., multiple target behaviors)?
3. What is the feasibility of producing change in the causal, antecedent, or maintaining factors (e.g., would the cost be prohibitive, would the interventions take too much time, does the client have the requisite skills, does the therapist have the expertise)
4. What is the likelihood of changing the target behaviors (e.g., what is the probability that lasting change can be produced)?
5. What are the short- and long-term consequences of altering the causal, antecedent, or maintaining variables (e.g., will targeting specific variables lead to alliance ruptures)?

Each of these questions needs to be carefully considered in formulating the treatment plan. The clinician must weigh the need to produce change in a particular area with the likely impact the intervention will have upon the client's motivation and therapy engagement. The end product is a treatment plan that identifies which hypotheses will be tested and in what order.

The next step is treatment selection. Treatment selection should be guided by the treatment outcome literature. Numerous evidence-based treatments exist for a variety of diagnoses (e.g., depression, conduct disorder). Treatment planning begins with identifying the treatments that are designed to treat the disorder(s) a child is diagnosed with. We advocate a prescriptive approach to treatment, in which particular interventions within an evidence-based treatment are matched to the factors hypothesized to play a role in causing and maintaining a particular disorder. Empirical findings support this type of prescriptive approach for certain child problems. Research indicates that cognitive-behavioral treatment (CBT) for child anxiety is more effective when the therapeutic interventions are matched to the specific symptoms exhibited by individual youth (Eisen & Silverman, 1993, 1998; Ollendick, 1995; Ollendick, Hagopian, & Huntzinger, 1991). For example, Eisen and Silverman (1993) found that CBT was maximally effective when children presenting primarily with worry were provided with cognitive interventions and when children presenting primarily with somatic complaints were provided with relaxation training. These findings provide support for the utility of the prescriptive approach to treatment planning.

The first step is to identify therapeutic interventions that address the causal, antecedent, or maintaining variables found in each hypothesis. The clinician must then examine the literature to identify appropriate treatment options. Given the constraints of many clinical settings, it can be challenging to search the treatment literature efficiently. Several recent books identify specific evidence-based treatments for common childhood disorders (e.g., Kendall, 2011; Weisz & Kazdin, 2010). In addition, several online databases now allow clinicians to search for evidence-based treatment options for clients with various childhood disorders and with different demographic characteristics; these databases provide efficient access to the current literature (see *www.effectivechildtherapy.com*, or the California Evidence-Based Clearinghouse, *www.cebc4cw.org*).

Next, the clinician must select the appropriate treatment among the available options. In treatment selection, a number of issues need to be considered:

1. *The existence of several evidence-based treatments for some disorders.* For example, both group-based and individual-focused forms of CBT have demonstrated positive effects for anxious children. Similarly, both interpersonal psychotherapy and CBT have been found to be efficacious for adolescents with depressed mood. In these cases, clinicians must take into consideration how the characteristics of a particular treatment may, or may not, fit their clients and fit within their own clinical practice. Treatments that target the core processes and/or address particular client characteristics should be given preference.

2. *Comorbidity.* It is common for children to present with multiple disorders. In this case, a hierarchical list of target behaviors can help determine how to proceed. Target behaviors that are at the top of the list can be given treatment priority. It may be the case that different treatments are needed to address multiple target behaviors. If so, a modular approach to

treatment (see below) may be the most efficient approach, since it allows target behaviors to be addressed in order of treatment priority.

3. *The lack of an evidence-based treatment for a given disorder.* For example, evidence-based treatments have not yet been developed for adjustment disorders. In this case, the clinician must survey the literature and determine how best to modify existing evidence-based treatments for the child's target behaviors. A case conceptualization that clearly identifies the causal and maintaining factors can help the clinician identify interventions designed to target those processes.

Once a treatment is selected, issues of intervention sequence and intensity must be determined. Modular treatments have certain advantages, as this treatment approach allows for the flexible delivery of interventions based upon the case conceptualization (Chorpita, Daleiden, & Weisz, 2005). Modular treatments have free-standing modules for particular causal, antecedent, and maintaining factors. This allows clinicians to take a patient-centered approach to treatment that matches the sequence and duration of interventions to the needs of particular young clients. Modular treatments are also designed to address multiple disorders, which helps address some of the challenges noted above.

Step 5: Develop Outcome-Monitoring and Evaluation Strategies

The final step involves developing an outcome-monitoring and evaluation plan. The collection and evaluation of assessment data will allow a clinician to test the hypotheses embedded within a case conceptualization. Using the principles of functional assessment and single-case series designs, the clinician can determine whether changes in the independent variables (interventions) produce improvements in the target behaviors via alterations in the causal, antecedent, or maintaining processes. If treatment proceeds as predicted by the hypotheses, then alterations to the treatment plan may not be needed. However, the collection of assessment data allows the clinician to determine whether the hypotheses are accurate and to change the treatment plan if necessary.

Because lengthy assessment during treatment can become burdensome, targeted assessment of specific symptoms and contributing factors is suggested (Southam-Gerow & Chorpita, 2007). Ongoing assessment should include some measure of the target behaviors (dependent variables), along with assessment of the causal, antecedent, or maintaining factors (mediators) that are the target of intervention. A number of different tools exist for ongoing assessment. Brief checklists that assess specific symptoms or idiographic measures often represent the best fit. Idiographic measures can be used to monitor changes in causal, antecedent, or maintaining factors, as standardized measures often do not exist for these constructs (Weisz et al., 2011). It is important to select measures that are designed for repeated assessment and have demonstrated sensitivity to change (see our discussion in Chapter 1).

A more comprehensive assessment is conducted at the end of treatment, because it is important to understand the impact of treatment as well as to determine whether further intervention is needed. We recommend that the assessment include measures of the disorder or disorders (and target behaviors) that were the focus of treatment, if feasible. Such an assessment might include a structured interview, broad- and narrow-band self-report measures, and idiographic measures (Southam-Gerow & Chorpita, 2007). In selecting outcome measures for either form of outcome assessment, it is important to choose measures that have been demonstrated to be sensitive to change. Finally, it is recommended that this assessment answer the question of whether the client experienced clinically significant change.

SUMMARY

The five-step process described above is designed to provide clinicians with a structured approach to case conceptualization and assessment during treatment of children and adolescents. We have emphasized the importance of using assessment to develop testable hypotheses regarding the nature and causes of a young client's target behaviors. These hypotheses can then be used to guide treatment planning and selection. By relying upon empirically validated theories and findings throughout this process, clinicians can produce treatment plans tailored to each individual client and thus help maximize the beneficial effects of evidence-based treatments for youth emotional and behavioral disorders.

CLINICAL CASE EXAMPLES

Up to this point we have provided an overview of the fundamental issues that clinicians need to consider as they rely on diagnostic and behavioral assessment procedures to guide the clinical process from intake to termination. The ideas and concepts thus covered serve as the foundation for the remainder of this book. Part II of the book describes the core diagnostic and behavioral assessment strategies used with children and adolescents throughout the assessment and treatment process. First, however, we present two sample cases: one of a youth with an internalizing disorder, and the other of a youth with an externalizing disorder. The two sample cases provide general information about the presenting problem and the history of the presenting problem that would normally be collected at intake. These sample cases are then used throughout Part II to illustrate the application of diagnostic and behavioral assessment strategies.

INTERNALIZING DISORDERS CASE EXAMPLE: SOFIA

Sofia was a 15-year-old Hispanic female who presented for treatment after her school contacted her parents because she had not been attending classes. This occurred in May of her sophomore year at Central High School, a public high school. Sofia lived with her parents, Adriana (age 35) and Sergio (age 35), both immigrants from Guatemala; she had one older brother (age 19) who lived outside the home. At the time Sofia presented for the initial assessment, her school was considering placing her in an alternative education setting because of her truancy, as she had missed more than 100 days of school during the present academic year. She was accompanied to the intake appointment by her mother, Adriana.

Presenting Problem

Sofia and her mother came to treatment seeking help for Sofia's anxiety about attending school. Sofia indicated that she was not attending school because of embarrassment over experiencing panic attacks at school. Although her panic symptoms had remitted at the time of the intake, her avoidance related to these panic attacks had led her to fall behind academically, which was also a source of embarrassment and shame for her. Sofia's parents hoped that treatment would help Sofia begin attending school again, while Sofia hoped that treatment might help her identify academic alternatives to returning to her current school.

History of the Presenting Problem

Both Sofia and her mother attributed Sofia's school nonattendance to anxiety. Sofia's attendance problems had begun 8 months earlier, at the beginning of her sophomore year, when she was 14 years old. At that time, she experienced an "attack" during her physical education class. While running, Sofia began to experience shortness of breath, a racing heart, chest pains, and dizziness. Sofia became convinced that she was going to die of a heart attack and became quite agitated. Her parents subsequently sought medical help for her, but no medical cause for her symptoms was found. Her doctor advised the family that he believed Sofia had experienced a panic attack. Following this attack, Sofia began to avoid school. She told her parents that she was afraid to participate in physical education again, due to the possibility of another panic attack. She was also embarrassed because her classmates had seen her "freak out" and she feared everybody would be making fun of her. When she again attended school, she experienced additional panic attacks and stopped attending school altogether.

After Sofia had missed a month of school, her guidance counselor suggested to the family that they seek treatment for Sofia. The family followed through on that recommendation, and Sofia participated in 16 sessions of exposure-based CBT. The treatment focused on helping Sofia learn to recognize and manage her panic symptoms and on getting her to attend school again. The family reported that this treatment was helpful in decreasing Sofia's panic attacks, and that after 4 months of coping skills training and graduated exposure, Sofia had resumed attending school on a regular basis. In February, the family discontinued treatment.

Although Sofia's treatment was successful, she had missed a significant amount of school due to her avoidance and had fallen behind academically. Her therapist had worked with the school to come up with a plan to help Sofia catch up in school, but the amount of work proved insurmountable. In April, the school informed Sofia that it would not be possible for her to make up the work and that she would have to repeat her sophomore year. Sofia then stopped attending school completely, leading to the current treatment referral.

In the initial appointment, Sofia said she had stopped attending school because she did not "see the point." She reported feeling very embarrassed about being retained and concerned about everybody knowing about her problems when the next school year started. She said that she had been spending most of her time at home sleeping. In addition to not attending school, she had withdrawn from her friends. She said that she felt "weak" for not being able to get control of her panic symptoms sooner, and "stupid" for not being able to make up her work more quickly; she thus could not imagine why any of her friends would want to spend time with her. She reported feeling very demoralized and having a hard time envisioning any type of a future for herself.

Sofia's mother, Adriana, said she was at a loss as to how to deal with Sofia's problems. She said that she currently felt unable to force Sofia to face her fears and begin attending school. She reported that because of her own considerable difficulty tolerating her daughter's distress, she was allowing her to stay home rather than risking upsetting her daughter. She reported that she had experienced similar difficulties during Sofia's exposure-based CBT, but that the support of Sofia's therapist had helped her tolerate that distress. She also indicated that she was having difficulty working together with the school to address Sofia's problems, due to a language barrier. Adriana had moved to the United Stated from Guatemala when she was in her late teens and had a limited grasp of the English language. She said that she typically relied on Sofia to help her communicate with the school, but that Sofia was now refusing to help her in this capacity.

Psychosocial History

Sofia lived with her mother, Adriana, and father, Sergio; she had one older brother who was living outside the home and attending community college. Both of Sofia's parents were immigrants from Guatemala; her father worked in construction, and her mother worked part-time doing house-keeping at a hotel. Adriana reported that Sofia's current difficulties were placing strain on her marriage. Sergio, who worked very long hours and had limited involvement in child rearing, was impatient with her for not "taking control" of the situation and forcing Sofia to go to school. She said that Sergio was also fighting frequently with Sofia; in these fights, he typically pointed to her brother's hard work and academic achievements, and called Sofia "lazy" for not engaging in school. Sofia said that these fights often left her feeling guilty and depressed. Adriana said she thought it was unlikely that Sergio would be able to participate in treatment, due to his work schedule.

Prior to the onset of her first panic attack, Sofia had been reasonably popular at school. She reported having a good group of girlfriends who had been friends since middle school, including one best friend who still kept in touch with her despite her recent social withdrawal. During her freshman year, she had started dating a boy at her school. They dated for about 6 months before they broke up. She said that the breakup happened over the fact that he was "pushy" about having sex. When this was queried further, she said that she did not want to talk about what happened, but that "guys don't always know how to stop." She denied that this incident with her boyfriend had anything to do with her problems, although her panic attacks had begun around the time of this breakup.

Developmental, Educational, and Medical History

Adriana reported that her pregnancy with Sofia was unremarkable and that Sofia had reached all of her developmental milestones within normal limits. She did say that Sofia had always been a somewhat timid child. As a toddler, Sofia had been reluctant to separate from her mother, which Adriana felt was not a problem because it meant that she always knew that Sofia was nearby and safe. Although it was difficult to get Sofia to start going to kindergarten, Sofia soon grew to love school and had no more difficulties separating to go to school.

Prior to the onset of her panic attacks, Sofia had been primarily an A student and had been in several honors classes. She reported that she had enjoyed school before it became too "embarrassing" to attend school any more. She felt that her history of being a strong student would make the fact that she was being held back even more obvious to her classmates. Before she was told she was being retained, Sofia had planned on attending college like her brother; she said that this plan had been very important to her father, who had never been able to attend college.

Sofia's medical history was also unremarkable. When she had her first panic attack, her doctor had conducted a thorough battery of tests to rule out any physical sources for her symptoms. Prior to receiving the 16 sessions of CBT, Sofia had never received any psychological treatment.

Adriana said that before the CBT, no one in their family had ever attended therapy, although she said that she herself had experienced panic attacks occasionally during her life and described herself as a "worrier." She said that she had also experienced a period of feeling severely "homesick" after immigrating to the United States and had difficulty getting out of bed for a period of about 6 months. She reported no medical complications for her husband and denied any other family history of medical or mental health difficulties.

EXTERNALIZING DISORDERS CASE EXAMPLE: BILLY

Billy was a 10-year-old European American male referred by his family doctor for various problems related to his behavior at home, at school, and in the community. He and his family presented for treatment in October of his fourth-grade year at the local public elementary school. Billy lived with his mother, Mary (age 42), and his older sister, Meredith (age 13 years). He also had an older brother, Mike, who was 16 years of age and who had been adjudicated for breaking and entering and for assaulting a police officer upon his arrest. At the time of referral, Mike was detained in the local juvenile detention facility. Mary was divorced from Billy's father, James, who had not been very involved with the family for the past 8 years. James presently lived in another state and had infrequent contact with the family (a few times a year for the holidays and for the children's birthdays). He had remarried. At the time of referral, Billy's medical doctor inquired about placement outside the family home and in a residential school, due to increasing levels of negativistic and aggressive behavior. Billy also had been having behavioral difficulties at school, even though he was thought to be a bright student. He was described as argumentative and disrespectful to his teachers and as unable to get along with his classmates. Although he had not gotten into physical fights with his classmates, he was frequently bullied both physically and verbally by bigger boys in the school. He had not failed any grades and was achieving at an average level.

Presenting Problem

Billy was brought to treatment by his mother, who was seeking help for his oppositional, negativistic, and noncompliant behaviors both at home and at school. She also described him as a somewhat "anxious" child who was "deathly afraid" of sleeping in his own bed and who seemed to be afraid of the dark. Interestingly, Billy's mother indicated that he was at times a very "good" and caring child who seemed to need extra attention and affection, but who at the same time could be very mean and spiteful toward both her and his older sister. His mother was quite perplexed by his behavior, as it seemed to vary a lot; she stated, "I can never tell what he will be like—he is just so hard to predict." In addition, his mother wondered whether he had ADHD, "since he hardly ever listens to me and always seems to be on the go."

Billy did not want to attend the session, but did come upon the promise of a reward for doing so. Initially, he stated that nothing was wrong and that this was all "her problem." He stated further that "She is hardly ever home, and when she is home, she's reading a book or in her room. She never listens to me." Upon further discussion, he acknowledged problems at home and school, but said that they were not his fault. He attended the session reluctantly and offered little insight into the problems that were presented.

History of the Presenting Problem

According to his mother, Mary, Billy had "carried a chip on his shoulder" ever since his father left the home 8 years earlier. She noted that his behavioral problems had escalated following his brother's recent detention. Mary also indicated that Billy was just like his older brother, Mike, in many ways, and that both were hard-to-manage children. Meredith, on the other hand, was described as a model child: "How I wish I had two more girls like Meredith rather than those two boys. They are a handful."

His mother also reported that Billy had "always been afraid of sleeping in his own bed, even though he had a room of his own" in their suburban three-bedroom ranch-style home. She could not recall any precipitating event, but noted that he had always worried at nighttime and had longstanding trouble falling asleep. According to Mary, Billy would tell her that he was afraid of monsters and that someone might break into his room and beat him up. The family dreaded nighttime, as it could take up to 2 hours for Billy to fall asleep. Frequently he wandered into his mother's bedroom if he awakened during the night. He also did not like to be left alone at other times of the day, and he sought out his mother or his sister to be near them, even though he did not get along with them and argued with them most of the time. He would not go outside to play alone even during the daylight, but especially not at nighttime. He never enjoyed activities in the yard at night, such as playing hide and seek, catching fireflies, or even watching the stars.

In reference to his problems with paying attention and being overly active, Mary reported that she did not recall specifically when "all this" started, but that she recalled Billy's kindergarten teacher telling her that he was "a very active and energetic child who does not like to sit still . . . he is all boy." He also reportedly liked to play rough-and-tumble games and to get into shoving matches at school, and to "boss the other kids around" in his early years.

In the initial appointment, as noted above, Billy disclosed little about the history of his problems. He did, however, reluctantly indicate that he had "a little" trouble getting along with his family and his classmates at school. He stated, "I don't know why they don't like me or get along with me. It seems like everyone is picking on me and won't give me a fair chance. They just seem out to get me . . . my mom, my sister, and even my friends . . . they just want to get me in trouble." Initially, he denied problems with sleeping in his own bed and his nighttime fears. Upon further inquiry, however, he indicated that he had "some" problems falling asleep and playing alone at home, but that he could not figure out why he felt that way. He simply stated, "Yeah, I guess someone might come in my room or outside while I'm playing and take me away—there are lots of mean people out there, you know." He denied any difficulties with paying attention or being overly active.

Billy's mother, Mary, said that she was at a loss as to how to deal with him and his problems. She reported "trying everything" and added, "Besides, sometimes he is a really good kid and I guess I do love him . . . he is just so hard to figure out. I don't understand how he can be so nice and loving sometimes, but then be so mean and argue with me at other times. He is hard to figure out."

Psychosocial History

As noted, Billy lived with his mother and older sister in a suburban home in a small town. His older brother was in residential placement at a nearby delinquency facility, and his father lived in another state some 500 miles away. His mother was gainfully employed as an executive secretary, and she described the family as "lower middle class." Her ex-husband continued to provide child support, though the amount of money "does not begin to cover the expenses of raising three kids." Mary received some support from her parents (Billy's maternal grandparents), who lived nearby and had a good relationship with the family. Still, she reported that her father thought she was "not strict enough with the kids" and "let them get their way." Her mother, on the other hand, felt that Mary was doing a good job raising the kids; the grandmother especially liked Meredith and did a number of things with her whenever she could. In contrast, Mary's mother and father did very little with either of the boys. There were no other family members in the community.

Developmental, Educational, and Medical History

Mary reported that her pregnancy with Billy had been relatively uneventful, except that she and her husband had begun to have marital difficulties at about that time. The husband was reportedly having an affair with a coworker at that time, and she reported considerable stress in dealing with his infidelity. Billy weighed 7 pounds, 9 ounces at birth. Although he was jaundiced, no other problems were noted at birth. However, Billy was delayed in speech and wet the bed up to about 8 years of age. He also seemed to have some emotion regulation difficulties, as he was excessively shy with strangers, but overly aggressive in his play with his sister and preschool classmates. Surprisingly to his mother, he seemed to want to go to kindergarten so that he could be near his sister and brother (who went to the same small school, but with whom he frequently fought at home).

Billy was always a good student, earning grades of A's, B's, and C's, even though he hardly ever studied or did homework. According to his mother, this was quite a contrast to Meredith, who was a straight-A student and who studied a lot. Her mother reported that Meredith was a lot like her (she too had been a good student who earned a bachelor's degree in English) and that Billy was a lot like his dad (who was reportedly a mediocre student and who had obtained a trade school degree in automotive mechanics). She described her ex-husband as "bright enough, but just not motivated to do well."

Billy's medical history was unremarkable, with one exception: As an infant and toddler, he had numerous earaches. At about 3 years of age, he had his adenoids removed and seemed to get better. However, he subsequently developed more earaches and had trouble with these until he was about 7 years of age. Even though Billy's behavioral problems were long-standing, he had never received any psychological treatment. Mary reported that she had relied first on her pediatrician and then on her family doctor for advice. She reported that this advice was good for the most part, and that it had permitted her to do as well as she had for so many years. Mary reported a history of alcoholism and drug abuse in Billy's father's family and depression in her own family (her older sister and her maternal grandmother). She reported no psychiatric problems in her own parents, though her mother had diabetes. Finally, Mary herself reported feeling depressed at times, but stated that she had never been diagnosed with a depressive disorder. She also reported considerable distress associated with Billy's problems and her older son's detention. She remarked that she felt she had failed as a parent.

REFERENCES

American Psychological Association Presidential Task Force on Evidence-Based Practice. (2006). Evidence-based practice in psychology. *American Psychologist, 61,* 271–285.
Baker-Ericzén, M. J., Hurlburt, M. S., Brookman-Frazee, L., Jenkins, M. M., & Hough, R. L. (2010). Comparing child, parent, and family characteristics in usual care and empirically supported treatment research samples for children with disruptive behavior disorders. *Journal of Emotional and Behavioral Disorders, 18,* 82–99.
Chorpita, B. F., Daleiden, E. L., & Weisz, J. R. (2005). Identifying and selecting the common elements of evidence based interventions: A distillation and matching model. *Mental Health Services Research, 7,* 5–20.

Eells, T. D. (2007). *Handbook of psychotherapy case formulation* (2nd ed.). New York: Guilford Press.

Eells, T. D., & Lombart, K. G. (2004). Case formulation: Determining the focus in brief dynamic psychotherapy. In D. P. Charman (Ed.), *Core processes in brief psychodynamic psychotherapy: Advancing effective practice* (pp. 119–144). Mahwah, NJ: Erlbaum.

Ehrenreich-May, J., Southam-Gerow, M. A., Hourigan, S. E., Wright, L. R., Pincus, D. B., & Weisz, J. R. (2011). Characteristics of anxious and depressed youth seen in two different clinical contexts. *Administration and Policy in Mental Health and Mental Health Services Research, 38*, 398–411.

Eisen, A. R., & Silverman, W. K. (1993). Should I relax or change my thoughts?: A preliminary study of the treatment of overanxious disorder in children. *Journal of Cognitive Psychotherapy, 7*, 265–280.

Freeman, K. A., & Miller, C. A. (2002). Behavioral case conceptualization for children and adolescents. In M. Hersen (Ed.), *Clinical behavior therapy: Adults and children* (pp. 239–255). New York: Wiley.

Haynes, S. N., O'Brien, W. H., & Kaholokula, J. K. (2011). *Behavioral assessment and case formulation*. Baltimore, MD: Johns Hopkins University Press.

Hersen, M., & Porzelius, L. K. (2002). *Diagnosis, conceptualization, and treatment planning for adults: A step-by-step guide*. Mahwah, NJ: Erlbaum.

Horowitz, M. (2005). *Understanding psychotherapy change: A practical guide to continued analysis*. Washington, DC: American Psychological Association.

Hunsley, J., & Mash, E. J. (2007). Evidence-based assessment. *Annual Review of Clinical Psychology, 3*, 29–51.

Kazdin, A. E. (2007). Mediators and mechanisms of change in psychotherapy research. *Annual Review of Clinical Psychology, 3*, 1–27.

Kendall, P. C. (Ed.). (2011). *Child and adolescent therapy: Cognitive-behavioral procedures* (4th ed.). New York: Guilford Press.

McFall, R. M. (2005). Theory and utility: Key themes in evidence-based assessment: Comment on the special section. *Psychological Assessment, 17*, 312–323.

McLeod, B. D., Jensen-Doss, A., Wheat, E., & Becker, E. M. (in press). Evidence-based assessment and case formulation for child anxiety. In C. Essau & T. H. Ollendick (Eds.), *Treatment of childhood and adolescent anxiety*.

Nelson-Gray, R. O. (2003). Treatment utility of psychological assessment. *Psychological Assessment, 15*, 521–531.

Nezu, A. M., Nezu, C. M., Peacock, M. A., & Girdwood, C. P. (2004). Case formulation in cognitive-behavior therapy. In M. Hersen (Series Ed.) & S. N. Haynes & E. M. Heiby (Vol. Eds.), *Comprehensive handbook of psychological assessment: Vol. 3. Behavioral assessment* (pp. 402–426). Hoboken, NJ: Wiley.

Ollendick, T. H. (1995). Cognitive behavioral treatment of panic disorder with agoraphobia in adolescents: A multiple baseline study. *Behavior Therapy, 26*, 395–399.

Ollendick, T. H., Hagopian, L. P., & Huntzinger, R. M. (1991). Cognitive-behavior therapy with nighttime fearful children. *Journal of Behavior Therapy and Experimental Psychiatry, 22*, 113–121.

Reitman, D. (Vol. Ed.). (2008). *Vol. 2. Children and adolescents*. In M. Hersen (Series Ed.), *Handbook of psychological assessment, case conceptualization, and treatment*. Hoboken, NJ: Wiley.

Southam-Gerow, M. A., & Chorpita, B. F. (2007). Anxiety in children and adolescents. In E. J. Mash & R. A. Barkley (Eds.), *Assessment of childhood disorders* (4th ed., pp. 347–397). New York: Guilford Press.

Weisz, J. R., Chorpita, B. F., Frye, A., Ng, M. Y., Lau, N., Bearman, S. K., & Hoagwood, K. E. (2011). Youth top problems: Using idiographic, consumer-guided assessment to identify treatment needs and to track change during psychotherapy. *Journal of Consulting and Clinical Psychology, 79*, 369–380.

Weisz, J. R., & Kazdin, A. E. (Eds.). (2010). *Evidence-based psychotherapies for children and adolescents.* (2nd ed.). New York: Guilford Press.

Part II

ASSESSMENT TOOLS

5

Interviews

Carla E. Marin, Yasmin Rey, and Wendy K. Silverman

As evident in other chapters in this volume, the clinical assessment of children and adolescents may involve a myriad of assessment procedures—from checklists and rating scales completed by children, parents, and/or teachers; to behavior observation tasks, self-monitoring procedures, laboratory and physiologically based measures; and finally to unstructured and structured interviews. The primary role of interviews in the assessment process is to gather information about a youth's presenting problem for diagnosis, prognosis, case conceptualization, and treatment planning (Mash & Barkley, 2007). Interviews are used to assess both internalizing and externalizing problems in children and adolescents (from here on, we use the term "youth" unless we are referring to a specific developmental period).

In the first few sections of the chapter, we describe the different types of interview schedules available, discuss the theory underlying the use of the interviews, and summarize their psychometric support. The next part of the chapter details the application of interview schedules to the two clinical cases. This is followed by a discussion of the implications for treatment planning and evaluation of treatment outcomes. The chapter concludes with a discussion of the limits of interviews, as well as clinical and research recommendations.

DESCRIPTION OF THE ASSESSMENT METHOD

Before we proceed, a few comments are in order about developmental considerations when clinicians are administering interviews to youth. The most distinctive characteristic of youth relative to adults is ever-unfolding change (Mash & Barkley, 2007; Silverman & Ollendick, 2005). When a clinician is evaluating a youth with internalizing and/or externalizing problems, a common question arises: When is change in the youth in a particular context normative? To address this question, Ollendick and Hersen (1984) encourage the interviewer to employ "normative-developmental" principles. These principles highlight the importance of evaluating behavior in light of the context in which it occurs. The normative-developmental perspective underscores the importance of assessing changes in behaviors in relation to reference groups (Ollendick, Grills, & King, 2001). This typically involves comparing youth of the same age group on specific domains of functioning (e.g., cognitive, behavioral, emotional, and social functioning). For instance, certain externalizing behavior problems such as temper tantrums are deemed non-normative in older children (Mash & Barkley, 2007), but not in younger children. The developmental perspective underscores the importance of accounting for various quantitative and qualitative changes in a youth's behavior as due to the natural progression of development (Ollendick et al., 2001).

However, normative information on youth behavioral and emotional problems in the general population is generally scarce. Most of the available age-related information on youth problems is derived from either cross-sectional or single-birth-cohort longitudinal studies (Bongers, Koot, van der Ende, & Verhults, 2003). Unfortunately, youth age is a relatively crude index for determining developmentally appropriate behaviors (Silverman & Ollendick, 2005).

Another important age-related concern is that use of interviews with young children (i.e., younger than 9 years old) who present with externalizing behavior problems may lead to biased and unreliable diagnoses (McMahon & Frick, 2005). It is therefore recommended that interviews be conducted with other informants, especially parents. The use of multiple informants in the assessment of youth problems is relevant not only to young children who present with externalizing behavior problems, but to youth in general (Mash & Hunsley, 2005).

Contextual considerations are also significant. It is not uncommon for youth to display transient fears in everyday situations (e.g., giving a class presentation). It also is not uncommon for youth to experience sadness at the loss of a pet or losing contact with friends when families move to other cities. Level of impairment associated with behavioral and emotional problems is another important issue to consider relative to the contexts in which those problems occur. For instance, even though it is not uncommon for youth to experience sadness at the loss of a friendship, if a youth's sadness prevents him or her from making new friends or keeping up with schoolwork, then this level of sadness could be indicative of depressive symptomatology; the youth should thus be evaluated for such symptoms.

Unstructured Interviews

The unstructured interview, often referred to as the "clinical interview," has been the hallmark of assessment in most clinical settings (Cashel, 2002; Elliot, Miltenberger, Kaster-Bundgaard, & Lumley, 1996; O'Brien, McGrath, & Haynes, 2003). One of its main advantages is its flexibility across several aspects of the assessment process. Specifically, the unstructured interview allows a clinician the greatest flexibility in terms of assessing the presenting problem(s); it also allows the clinician to use his or her clinical judgment to probe further, such as when a response from a youth or parent is unclear or vague. Because of the flexible nature of the unstructured interview, the clinician can also use his or her judgment regarding the need to follow up with additional probes, such as those relating to the youth's psychiatric and family history, relevant stressors, and contextual factors associated with the presenting problem(s). Yet another advantage is increased flexibility with respect to administration time.

Clearly, however, a higher level of professional or clinical expertise and skill is needed to conduct an unstructured interview effectively, and to glean reliable and valid information relative to that obtained via structured and semistructured interviews. Indeed, among the main limitations of the unstructured interview are its reliability and validity (Lucas, 2003; Villa & Reitman, 2007). Reports in the youth assessment literature suggest that seasoned clinicians make up their minds regarding diagnostic status within the first few minutes of meeting and speaking with their clients (Lucas, 2003). Clinicians' tendency to "rush to judgment" (so to speak) can be problematic, because it may preclude them from considering alternative explanations for problem behaviors (e.g., are a child's difficulties in going to school due to social phobia [SOP], major depressive disorder [MDD], or both?). Given its insufficient psychometric support coupled with the high level of expertise and skill needed to conduct an effective interview, the clinical interview is generally not recommended for use in research settings. Still, it is a mainstay in ongoing clinical practice.

Structured and Semistructured Interviews

Structured interviews are considered respondent-based interviews, in that questions are standardized and are typically read verbatim to the youth (Shaffer, Lucas, & Richters, 1999). Responses to interview questions, for the most part, require either "yes" or "no" answers. Because respondent-based interviews are highly structured, they require little familiarity with diagnostic criteria. As such, these interviews may be administered by lay clinicians and are most often employed in epidemiological and other research settings. We refer to respondent-based interviews as "structured interviews" throughout the rest of the chapter.

Semistructured interviews are considered interviewer-based interviews;

questions are also standardized, but with room for flexibility of question delivery and responses. Although responses to many questions also require "yes" or "no" answers, interviewer-based interviews include several open-ended questions for additional probing and/or clarification as deemed necessary by the clinician. These interviews require deeper knowledge of diagnostic criteria and are most often employed in treatment research settings. We refer to interviewer-based interviews as "semistructured interviews" throughout the rest of the chapter.

Structured and semistructured interview schedules were designed in part to reduce the error variance associated with unstructured interviewing approaches. They cover the most prevalent psychiatric diagnoses found in youth (e.g., anxiety disorders, mood disorders, conduct disorder [CD], attention-deficit/hyperactivity disorder [ADHD]). The interview schedules reviewed in this chapter are all structured around the criteria of the *Diagnostic and Statistical Manual of Mental Disorder*, fourth edition (DSM-IV; American Psychiatric Association, 1994) and its text revision (DSM-IV-TR; American Psychiatric Association, 2000). Several of the interview schedules' diagnostic criteria are also based on the *International Statistical Classification of Diseases and Related Health Problems*, 10th revision (ICD-10; World Health Organization, 1993). Interview schedules will need to be revised around the new diagnostic criteria of the *Diagnostic and Statistical Manual of Mental Disorders, Fifth Edition* (DSM-5; American Psychiatric Association, 2013). However, as of the publication of this volume, no revised interview schedules have been released.

All of the interview schedules for youth psychopathology have respective youth and parent versions, and most can be administered to youth ages 6–18 years. All of them also require minimal verbal responses (i.e., "yes" or "no"), and most contain rating scales to assist the interviewer in prioritizing the diagnoses that may be assigned to the youth. Sections covering developmental history, medical history, and youth functioning in academic and social domains are also included in most of the schedules.

A semistructured interview schedule often has an introductory section, which includes questions requesting a brief description of the presenting problems, as well as questions about the youth's schooling, friendships, and extracurricular activities. These questions serve not only to gain information, but to build rapport with the youth and/or parent. Both structured and semistructured interviews then typically proceed with modules assessing specific disorders, which often begin with a small number of screening questions. If an informant responds "yes" to a screening question, the entire set of questions for that section is administered, which includes obtaining frequency, intensity, and interference ratings of endorsed symptoms. If an informant responds "no" to the screening questions, the diagnostic section may be skipped.

In research studies, the complete diagnostic section is typically administered, even if the screening items are not endorsed. The utility of the screening items in interview schedules remains a question for future research. Specifically, empirical research is needed to determine the relative utility of specific symptoms for diagnosing a given disorder. Pina, Silverman, Alfano, and Saavedra (2002), for example, evaluated the diagnostic efficiency of symptoms comprising Criteria A and B (uncontrollable and excessive worry), as well as Criterion C (physiological symptoms) of DSM-IV generalized anxiety disorder (GAD) in a sample of anxious youth and their parents. Findings showed that uncontrollable and excessive worry in the areas of "health of self" and "health of others," and four of six physiological symptoms associated with worry (e.g., irritability, trouble sleeping), were stronger predictors of GAD in youth than other worry areas and/or physiological symptoms were. Further research is needed to determine whether these findings can be replicated in independent samples. Accumulation of such data might then be used to assist in the development of empirically derived and clinically useful screening items (Pina et al., 2002; see also Lucas et al., 2001).

Diagnoses are yielded from interview schedules by administering parallel versions to the youth and parent, with the wording often simplified in the youth version. Diagnoses based on combined youth and parent interviews are most often determined through using rules derived by the interview developers. For the majority of interview schedules, if the required number of criteria is met for a particular diagnostic section within either the youth or parent interview schedule, then a diagnosis is warranted. For instance, if a child meets criteria for a primary diagnosis of separation anxiety disorder (SAD) and a secondary diagnosis of SOP on the Anxiety Disorders Interview Schedule for DSM-IV: Child Version (ADIS-IV: C; Silverman & Albano, 1996), and a primary diagnosis of only SAD on the Parent Version (ADIS-IV: P), then the combined diagnostic profile would be this: primary diagnosis of SAD, and secondary diagnosis of SOP. Some interview schedules use computerized algorithms to derive the diagnostic profile when multiple informants are interviewed (e.g., see Shaffer, Fisher, Lucas, Dulcan, & Schwab-Stone, 2000).

The interview schedules discussed in the following section were selected for review in this chapter because they are the most widely used and researched in the youth mental health field, and have the most psychometric support. We also wanted to provide readers with a wide selection of interview schedules to fit their specific needs, as well as the contexts in which the schedules will be used (i.e., research or clinical settings). Table 5.1 summarizes the characteristics of the interview schedules described below.

Review of Structured Interview Schedules

National Institute of Mental Health Diagnostic Interview Schedule for Children, Version IV

The National Institute of Mental Health Diagnostic Interview Schedule for Children, Version IV (NIMH DISC-IV; Shaffer et al., 2000) is in its fourth revision, and its diagnostic criteria are based on DSM-IV and ICD-10. The

TABLE 5.1. Characteristics of Structured and Semistructured Diagnostic Interview Schedules

Interview	Type (S or SS)	Age range (years)	Number of diagnoses covered	Informants	Administration time (per informant)	Computerized version (Y/N)	Translations
NIMH DISC-IV (Shaffer et al., 2000)	S	6–17	>30	Youth Parent	70 minutes	Y	Spanish (Bravo et al., 2001)
MINI-KID (Sheehan et al., 2010)	S	6–17	24	Youth Parent Youth/parent together	30 minutes	N	
ChIPS (Weller et al., 2000)	S	6–18	20	Youth Parent	40 minutes	N	Spanish (Moreno et al., 2006)
ADIS-IV: C/P (Silverman & Albano, 1996)	SS	6–18	15	Youth Parent	90 minutes	N	Spanish (Marin et al., 2012)
CAPA (Angold & Costello, 2000)	SS	9–17	>30	Youth Parent	60 minutes	N	Spanish (Angold & Costello, 2000)
DICA (Reich, 2000)	SS	6–17	26	Child Adolescent Parent	60 minutes	Y	
K-SADS (Ambrosini, 2000)	SS	6–18	>30	Youth Parent	75–90 minutes	N	

Note. NIMH DISC-IV, National Institute of Mental Health Diagnostic Interview Schedule for Children, Version IV; MINI-KID, Mini International Neuropsychiatric Interview for Children and Adolescents; ChIPS, Children's Interview for Psychiatric Syndromes; ADIS-IV: C/P, Anxiety Disorders Interview Schedule for DSM-IV: Child and Parent Versions; CAPA, Child and Adolescent Psychiatric Assessment; DICA, Diagnostic Interview for Children and Adolescents; K-SADS, Schedule for Affective Disorders and Schizophrenia for School-Age Children; S, structured; SS, semistructured; Y/N, yes or no.

original version of the DISC was developed primarily for epidemiological studies to examine prevalence rates of mental disorders in youth (Shaffer et al., 2000). It was designed to be administered by lay interviewers and has a computerized version available to assist in administration. The DISC-IV assesses current problems, as well as problems occurring over the past 12 months. The DISC-IV also includes an optional module for lifetime diagnoses. In community samples, the interview requires about 70 minutes for each informant to complete. To shorten administration time, the authors recommend skipping diagnostic modules that are not relevant to the study or particular setting (Shaffer et al., 2000). When an interviewer is using more than one diagnostic module, the authors further recommend employing the computer program to aid in the interview's administration (Shaffer et al., 2000).

The DISC-IV assesses more than 30 internalizing and externalizing disorders in youth ages 6–17 years. For the internalizing disorders modules, the DISC assesses all the anxiety disorders, as well as the most common mood disorders and associated mood episodes (e.g., MDD, dysthymia, manic episode). The externalizing disorders modules assess all the disruptive behaviors most commonly diagnosed in youth (e.g., ADHD, oppositional defiant disorder [ODD], and (CD). The DISC-IV is also available in Spanish (Bravo et al., 2001).

Mini International Neuropsychiatric Interview for Children and Adolescents

The Mini International Neuropsychiatric Interview for Children and Adolescents (MINI-KID; Sheehan et al., 2010) uses DSM-IV-TR or ICD-10 diagnostic criteria to asses 24 psychiatric disorders as well as suicidality in youth ages 6–17 years. For the internalizing disorders modules, the MINI-KID assesses all the anxiety disorders, as well as the most common mood disorders and associated mood episodes. The externalizing disorders modules assess all the disruptive behaviors most commonly diagnosed in youth, as well as substance abuse and dependence.

The MINI-KID was developed to answer increasing calls for a brief and reliable diagnostic instrument. Most currently available structured and semistructured interview schedules (e.g., the ADIS-IV: C/P, the DISC-IV, and the Schedule for Affective Disorders and Schizophrenia for School-Age Children, Present and Lifetime [K-SADS-P/L; Ambrosini, 2000]) can be time-consuming; as much as 2–3 hours may be required to administer the full interview to both the youth and parent. The majority of the semistructured interviews also require considerable training and at a minimum, a basic understanding of childhood and adolescent psychopathology, whereas structured interviews can often be administered by lay interviewers without such knowledge. The MINI-KID is brief, as it focuses only on identifying current diagnoses. Furthermore, it relies on the use of screening questions (so that if the informant responds negatively, the rest of the diagnostic module may be skipped, as described earlier). These questions were based on theory, rather than by a formal evaluation of the diagnostic efficiency of symptoms.

Sheehan et al. (2010) compared administration times between the MINI-KID and K-SADS-P/L and found that for youth diagnosed with any internalizing or externalizing disorder, the length of administration of the MINI-KID was between 35 and 40 minutes, versus 95 and 120 minutes for the K-SADS-P/L.

Children's Interview for Psychiatric Syndromes

The Children's Interview for Psychiatric Syndromes (ChIPS; Weller, Weller, Fristad, Rooney, & Schecter, 2000) uses DSM-IV diagnostic criteria to assess 20 disorders in youth ages 6–18 years. For the internalizing disorders modules, the ChIPS assesses all of the anxiety disorders, as well as the most common mood disorders and associated mood episodes. The externalizing disorders modules assess all the disruptive behaviors most commonly diagnosed in youth (e.g., ADHD, ODD, and CD) as well as substance abuse. The last two sections of the interview assess psychosocial stressors such as parental neglect and abuse.

The ChIPS was developed initially by assessing the adherence of extant interview schedules (i.e., DISC-IV and K-SADS) to DSM-III criteria and the degree to which the questions were child-friendly. The authors concluded that the interview schedules' language was not adequate for interviewing youth. To address this issue, the questions were rewritten to take sentence length, age-appropriate word selection, and comprehensibility into account. The ChIPS was subsequently revised to meet DSM-III-R and DSM-IV criteria. It takes about 40 minutes to administer.

The ChIPS offers a couple of advantages that are not offered by other interview schedules. The language has been adapted for better child understanding as well as increased child cooperation with the interviewer. A second advantage is that the results of the interview are presented in an easy-to-interpret one-page summary sheet. The parent version of the ChIPS is available in Spanish (Moreno, Basurto, Becerra, & San Pedro, 2006).

Review of Semistructured Interview Schedules

Anxiety Disorders Interview Schedule for DSM-IV: Child and Parent Versions

The Anxiety Disorders Interview Schedule for DSM-IV: Child and Parent Versions (ADIS-IV: C/P; Silverman & Albano, 1996) is the most widely used interview in the assessment of anxiety disorders in youth ages 6–18 years, due in part to its comprehensive coverage of these disorders. The ADIS-IV: C/P also includes modules for assessing MDD and dysthymia, as well as the most common externalizing problems in youth. In addition to items assessing diagnostic criteria, the ADIS-IV: C/P contains severity rating scales, which youth, parents, and clinicians use to rate the youth's level of distress and/or impairment in functioning specific to each disorder, using a scale from 0 ("none") to 8 ("very much") (Silverman & Albano, 1996). If either the youth or parent reports impairment ratings of 4 or higher, this may warrant a DSM-IV diagnosis. The most severe and interfering disorder, ascertained by the severity rating scale, is considered the primary diagnosis, followed by a ranking of the other severity ratings (secondary, tertiary). The severity ratings derived by the clinicians are based on the information obtained from both the youth and parent interviews, and their respective severity ratings. The ADIS-IV: C/P severity rating scales are also used to obtain ratings from youth and parents on the severity of the youth's fear and/or avoidance in specific situations for those DSM-IV anxiety disorders in which fear and/or avoidance occurs (e.g., SOP, specific phobia [SP], GAD). In this way, clinicians can ascertain which symptoms/situations are most severe and require targeting in treatment. The time required to administer the ADIS-IV: C/P to each informant is about 90 minutes. There is a Spanish version available, and its psychometric properties are currently being evaluated (Marin, Rey, & Silverman, 2012).

Although the ADIS-IV: C/P contains diagnostic modules on affective (mood) disorders as well as the externalizing disorders, it was initially designed to improve test–retest reliability estimates of the anxiety disorders (Silverman & Nelles, 1988). With previously available diagnostic instruments (e.g., the DISC), the anxiety disorders modules demonstrated the lowest reliability. Although subsequent revisions of other structured and semistructured interviews have resulted in improved reliability values, the ADIS: C/P remains the most detailed and heavily anxiety-focused interview schedule for use with young people and their parents. It has been used in the majority of randomized clinical trials for youth anxiety, including the Child/Adolescent Anxiety Multimodal Study (Walkup et al., 2008). Recently, Jarrett, Wolff, and Ollendick (2007) have demonstrated the reliability, validity, and clinical utility of the ADIS-IV: C/P in the diagnosis of ADHD, while Anderson and Ollendick (2012) have similarly demonstrated its psychometric properties and its equivalence to the DISC-IV in the diagnosis of ODD.

Child and Adolescent Psychiatric Assessment

The Child and Adolescent Psychiatric Assessment (CAPA; Angold & Costello, 2000) assesses the duration, frequency, and intensity of symptoms associated with over 30 psychiatric diagnoses in youth ages 9–17 years. The CAPA's diagnostic criteria are based on DSM-IV and ICD-10. It also includes diagnostic modules covering a number of disorders that were included in DSM-III-R but were removed in DSM-IV (e.g., overanxious disorder). For the internalizing disorders modules, the CAPA assesses all the anxiety disorders and most of the mood disorders commonly found in youth. The externalizing disorders modules assess all the disruptive behavior disorders. Due to concerns regarding reliability of recall beyond 3 months, the CAPA only assesses problems occurring during this time period, referred to as the "primary period" (Angold, Erkanli, Costello, & Rutter, 1996).

The CAPA employs a modular format, such that specific diagnostic modules may be administered independently from the entire interview. A unique feature of the CAPA is the inclusion of a glossary. The glossary is used by the interviewer to determine (based on the descriptions provided by the interviewee) presence or absence of symptoms, as well as coding instructions for different levels of symptom severity. The total administration time for the CAPA for each informant is about 60 minutes.

Diagnostic Interview for Children and Adolescents

The Diagnostic Interview for Children and Adolescents (DICA; Herjanic & Campbell, 1977; Reich, 2000) is available in three versions: a child (DICA-C), adolescent (DICA-A), and parent version (DICA-P). Similar to the DISC-IV, it was developed initially for use in epidemiological research, and early versions of the instruments were therefore highly structured and designed to be administered by lay interviewers. Over the years, however, it evolved into a semistructured interview (Reich, 2000). The DICA can be used to derive diagnoses based on DSM-III-R or DSM-IV criteria. It assesses 26 psychiatric disorders in youth ages 6–17 years. It evaluates current diagnoses as well as lifetime diagnoses. For the internalizing disorders modules, the DICA assesses all the anxiety disorders and most of the mood disorders commonly found in youth. The externalizing disorders modules assess all the disruptive behavior disorders. Unlike the other interview schedules, the DICA is unique in its assessment of risk and protective factors (e.g., interpersonal conflicts between parents at home, parental substance use, and incarceration). The DICA also includes a perinatal and psychosocial module. The total administration time for the DICA for each informant is about 60 minutes.

All three versions of the DICA are available in a computerized form, allowing for self-administration. However, studies on the psychometric properties of the computerized DICA have yielded less than optimal kappa coefficients relative to the clinician-administered DICA (Reich, Cottler, McCallum, Corwin, & VanEerdwegh, 1995). As such, Reich et al. (1995) have recommended that the computerized DICA be used a screening tool rather than a diagnostic interview.

Schedule for Affective Disorders and Schizophrenia for School-Age Children

The Schedule for Affective Disorders and Schizophrenia for School-Age Children (K-SADS; Ambrosini, 2000) is currently in its fourth revision;

DSM-III-R or DSM-IV diagnostic criteria may be used to derive diagnoses. Diagnoses may also be derived by using the Research Diagnostic Criteria (Spitzer, Endicott, & Robins, 1978). The K-SADS assesses over 30 psychiatric disorders in youth ages 6–18 years. It includes modules for assessing all of the internalizing and externalizing disorders most commonly found in youth. The authors of the current K-SADS also included the Clinical Global Impressions Scale to measure symptom severity and symptom improvement.

Currently, there are three versions available: the K-SADS-Present State (K-SADS-P) to assess current diagnoses, and two epidemiological versions, the K-SADS—Epidemiologic (K-SADS-E) and K-SADS—Present and Lifetime (K-SADS-P/L). Although the K-SADS-E assesses the most severe past episode of psychiatric problems, it also assesses for current problems at the administration of the interview. The K-SADS-P/L, unlike the K-SADS-P and K-SADS-E, includes an 82-symptom Screen Interview. It assesses past and current symptoms on 20 different diagnostic areas. Time to administer is between 75 and 90 minutes for each informant. As noted earlier, if an informant responds "no" to the screening sections, the specific diagnostic section is skipped, shortening the administration of the interview. The K-SADS-P/L is available in Spanish (Ulloa et al., 2006).

Psychometric Properties

The most commonly reported psychometric properties for structured and semistructured interviews are (1) "interrater reliability," defined as the level of diagnostic agreement between independent interviews; (2) "test–retest reliability," defined as the level of diagnostic agreement between two different time points; and (3) "concurrent validity," defined as the level of diagnostic agreement between the interview of interest and a criterion (e.g., another well-established interview). Kappa coefficients, which capture agreement between categorical decisions while correcting for chance agreement (Cohen, 1960), are most often used to evaluate these different levels of reliability and validity. According to Landis and Koch's (1977) criteria, kappa coefficients greater than .74 indicate excellent reliability; kappas between .60 and .74 indicate good reliability; kappas between .40 and .59 indicate fair reliability; and kappas less than .40 indicate poor reliability. These criteria are used to evaluate the reliability estimates of all the interview schedules we describe. Below we provide an overview of the psychometric properties of the interview schedules described earlier. Summaries of the interviews' reliabilities for internalizing and externalizing diagnoses are included in Tables 5.2 and 5.3 respectively. Test–retest reliability information is provided for all of the interview schedules; interrater reliability is provided for those schedules where such data are available. Below, in the text, concurrent validity information is provided for all summarized interview schedules.

TABLE 5.2. Reliability Estimates of Structured and Semistructured Diagnostic Interview Schedules—Internalizing Diagnoses

Interview	Internalizing diagnoses	Test–retest reliability (kappa)			Interrater reliability (kappa)		
		Youth	Parent	Combined	Youth	Parent	Combined
NIMH DISC-IV (Shaffer et al., 2000)	GAD		.65	.58			
	MDD	.92	.66	.65			
	SAD	.46	.58	.51			
	SOP	.25	.54	.48			
	SP	.68	.96	.86			
MINI-KID (Sheehan et al., 2010)	Dysthymia			.41			.79
	GAD			.64			1.00
	MDD			.75			1.00
	OCD			.75			.94
	PD			.42			.88
	PTSD			.71			1.00
	SAD			.70			.93
	SOP			.64			1.00
	SP			.65			1.00
ADIS-IV: C/P (Lyneham et al., 2007; Silverman et al., 2001)	GAD	.63	.72	.80	.82	.82	.80
	OCD						.91
	SAD	.78	.88	.84	.81	.83	.89
	SOP	.71	.86	.92	.87	.83	.82
	SP	.80	.65	.81	.85	.87	1.00

(continued)

Instrument	Disorder		
CAPA (Angold & Costello, 2000)	Dysthymia	.85	
	GAD	.79	
	MDD	.90	
DICA (Reich et al., 2000)	MDD	.55–.80	
	SAD	.60–.75	
	SP	.65	
K-SADS (Ambrosini, 2000)	Dysthymia	.70–.89	1.00
	Any AD	.24–.80	
	MDD	.54–1.00	1.00
	PTSD	.60–.67	
	GAD	.78	1.00
	SAD	.65	1.00

Note. NIMH DISC-IV, National Institute of Mental Health Diagnostic Interview Schedule for Children, Version IV; MINI-KID, Mini International Neuropsychiatric Interview for Children and Adolescents; ADIS-IV: C/P, Anxiety Disorders Interview Schedule for DSM-IV: Child and Parent Versions; CAPA, Child and Adolescent Psychiatric Assessment; DICA, Diagnostic Interview for Children and Adolescents; K-SADS, Schedule for Affective Disorders and Schizophrenia for School-Age Children; AD, anxiety disorder; GAD, generalized anxiety disorder; MDD, major depressive disorder; OCD, obsessive compulsive disorder; PTSD, posttraumatic stress disorder; SAD, separation anxiety disorder; SOP, social phobia; SP, specific phobia.

TABLE 5.3. Reliability Estimates of Structured and Semistructured Diagnostic Interview Schedules—Externalizing Diagnoses

Interview	Internalizing diagnoses	Test–retest reliability (kappa)			Interrater reliability (kappa)		
		Youth	Parent	Combined	Youth	Parent	Combined
NIMH DISC-IV (Shaffer et al., 2000)	ADHD-C	.42	.79	.62			
	ODD	.51	.54	.59			
	CD	.65	.43	.55			
MINI-KID (Sheehan et al., 2010)	ADHD-C			1.00			.90
	ADHD-I			.80			.93
	ADHD-H						.65
	ODD			.71			1.00
	CD			.85			1.00
ADIS-IV: C/P (Silverman et al., 2001)	ADHD-C	.61	1.00	1.00			
	ODD		.78	.62			
CAPA (Angold & Costello, 2000)	ADHD-C						
	ODD						
	CD	.55					
DICA (Reich et al., 2000)	ADHD-C	.32–.65					
	ODD	.46–.60					
	CD	.92					
K-SADS (Ambrosini, 2000)	ADHD-C			.55–.91			.80
	ODD			.46–.77			1.00
	CD			.83			

Note. NIMH DISC-IV, National Institute of Mental Health Diagnostic Interview Schedule for Children, Version IV; MINI-KID, Mini International Neuropsychiatric Interview for Children and Adolescents; ADIS-IV: C/P, Anxiety Disorders Interview Schedule for DSM-IV: Child and Parent Versions; CAPA, Child and Adolescent Psychiatric Assessment; DICA, Diagnostic Interview for Children and Adolescents; K-SADS, Schedule for Affective Disorders and Schizophrenia for School-Age Children; ADHD-C, attention-deficit/hyperactivity disorder—combined; ADHD-H, attention-deficit/hyperactivity disorder—hyperactive; ADHD-I, attention-deficit/hyperactivity disorder—inattentive; ODD, oppositional defiant disorder; CD, conduct disorder.

Reliability and Validity of the NIMH DISC-IV

Test–retest reliability estimates of the most common internalizing and externalizing disorders on the NIMH DISC-IV are generally in the acceptable range (with the exception of SOP; Shaffer et al., 2000). These rates are comparable to those for earlier versions of the DISC (Jensen et al., 1995; Schwab-Stone et al., 1996). Interrater reliability of the DISC-IV has been not evaluated. Studies on the validity of earlier versions of the DISC have found that agreement between the DISC 2.3 and clinician-generated ratings is generally in the moderate to good range (see Schwab-Stone et al., 1996). A later study conducted with a small sample of adolescents ($N = 25$) found a similar pattern of agreement between clinician-rated diagnoses and the DISC-IV (see Roberts, Parker, & Dagnone, 2005).

Reliability and Validity of the MINI-KID

Test–retest reliability estimates (1- to 5-day retest interval) for specific anxiety diagnoses made with the MINI-KID have been found to be in the good to excellent range (Sheehan et al., 2010), with the exception of panic disorder (PD), which is in the fair range (kappa = .42). Test–retest reliability estimates for depressive disorders are also in the good to excellent range (Sheehan et al.) with the exception of dysthymia, which is in the fair range (kappa = .41). Sheehan et al. note that the kappa value for dysthymia should be interpreted with caution, given the small number of cases meeting criteria for this disorder. Interrater reliability estimates for all internalizing disorders are in the excellent range. Test–retest and interrater reliability estimates for the externalizing disorders are in the good to excellent range.

Concurrent validity of the MINI-KID has been examined with the K-SADS-PL as the criterion. Kappa values at the syndromal level of diagnoses are in the fair to good range. Kappa values for most of the DSM-IV anxiety disorders are in the poor range, with the exception of obsessive–compulsive disorder (OCD; kappa = .47) and PD (kappa = .56). Kappa values for the mood disorders and episodes are also in the poor range, with the exception of mania and hypomania (kappa = .50). Concurrent validity for the externalizing disorders are in the fair to good range, with the exception of ODD (kappa = .34).

Reliability and Validity of the ChIPS

Test–retest or interrater reliability estimates are not yet available for the ChIPS; thus the ChIPS is not included in Tables 5.2 and 5.3. However, a study (Fristad et al., 1998) examining the concurrent validity of the ChIPS with the DICA as the criterion found kappa estimates for the internalizing disorders to be in the fair to excellent range; a similar pattern of findings were observed for the externalizing disorders. Studies on earlier versions of the ChIPS found validity estimates to be in the poor to good range for both the internalizing and externalizing disorders (e.g., Teare, Fristad, Weller, Weller, & Salmon, 1998).

Reliability and Validity of the ADIS-IV: C/P

Test–retest reliability estimates for specific anxiety diagnoses made with the ADIS-IV: C/P have been found to be good to excellent for most DSM-IV anxiety disorders (i.e., GAD, SAD, SOP, and SP) in youth, parent, and combined youth and parent reports (Silverman, Saavedra, & Pina, 2001). Lyneham, Abbott, and Rapee (2007) found good to excellent interrater reliability estimates for most DSM-IV anxiety diagnoses (i.e., GAD, OCD, SAD, SOP, and SP) when youth, parent, and combined youth and parent reports in an Australian sample of clinic-referred anxious youth were examined.

Wood, Piacentini, Bergman, McCracken, and Barrios (2002) examined the concurrent validity of the ADIS-IV: C/P with the Multidimensional Anxiety Scale for Children (MASC; March, 1998) and found strong convergence between the ADIS-IV: C/P DSM-IV anxiety diagnoses (except for GAD) and the MASC subscale scores corresponding to the respective disorders. Findings also supported divergent validity of the ADIS-IV: C/P in the predicted direction (e.g., MASC Social Anxiety subscale scores, but no other subscale scores, were significantly elevated for children meeting DSM-IV criteria for SOP).

Reliability and Validity of the CAPA

Test–retest reliability estimates of internalizing diagnoses made with the CAPA are in the good to excellent range; test–retest reliability estimates are only available for CD (Angold & Costello, 1995). Intraclass correlation coefficients using DSM-III-R criteria for symptom scale scores are also in the good to excellent range (Angold & Costello, 1995). The validity of the CAPA was evaluated along 10 criteria pertaining to youth psychiatric diagnoses (e.g., age, sex, functional impairment, parental psychopathology). Construct validity across these criteria was also good. For example, diagnoses based on parent and child interviews were positively correlated with parent and teacher reports on the Child Behavior Checklist (CBCL; Achenbach, 1991) and the Teacher's Report Form (Achenbach & Edelbrock, 1986), respectively (see Angold & Costello, 2000).

Reliability and Validity of the DICA

Test–retest reliability estimates for the DICA-C and DICA-A in clinical and community samples are generally in the acceptable range, with the exception of DSM-IV ADHD diagnoses (kappa = .32) on the DICA-C (Reich, 2000). No formal validity tests have been conducted on the current version of the DICA. Reich (2000) notes, however, that two studies of children with bipolar parents who were evaluated with the 1992 DICA demonstrated that it was able to discriminate children with differing levels of psychopathology.

Reliability and Validity of the K-SADS

Interrater and test–retest reliability estimates are only available for earlier versions of the K-SADS. Kappas for the most common youth internalizing and externalizing problems are in the acceptable range, with the exception of anxiety disorders (kappa = .24), on the second version of the K-SADS-P. Validity was demonstrated by showing that depression symptoms and severity were significantly related to symptom scores on several depression rating scales, such as the Beck Depression Inventory (Beck, Ward, Mendelson, Mock, & Erbaugh, 1961), the Children's Depression Inventory (Kovacs, 1992), and the Hamilton Depression Rating Scale (Hamilton, 1960). Validity of earlier versions of the K-SADS-P/L (Kaufman, Birmaher, Brent, & Rao, 1997) has also been demonstrated by showing that anxiety symptoms and severity are significantly related to symptom scores on the Screen for Child Anxiety Related Emotional Disorders (Birmaher et al., 1997) and the Internalizing broad-band scale of the CBCL (Achenbach, 1991).

THEORY UNDERLYING THE METHOD

The theory underlying the interviewing methodology conceptualizes mental illness from the perspective of the categorical medical model of diseases. The DSM (American Psychiatric Association, 2013) and ICD (World Health Organization, 2003) diagnostic systems stem from the medical model. This model assumes that psychiatric disorders are qualitatively different from each other. From this perspective, disorders are characterized by a specific set of criteria, represented in the form of cognitive, behavioral, and/or physiological symptoms. There are no laboratory tests yet available to diagnose psychiatric disorders, and thus clinicians rely on their clinical expertise, using a "present–absent" approach to symptoms to determine whether an individual meets criteria for a specific disorder. This determination is based largely on a youth's and/or parents' reports of the youth's cognitive, behavioral, and/or physiological experiences, as well as the clinician's observation of the youth's behavior.

DSM recently underwent a fifth revision (American Psychiatric Association, 2013). Decisions about earlier revisions were determined by clinical consensus among members of an expert committee. Revisions made thereafter also took into consideration the empirical literature that had accumulated on diagnosis, assessment, and treatment of the various disorders (American Psychiatric Association, 1994, 2000, 2013). The categorical perspective is useful because it provides the field with a common language to describe psychopathological conditions. In addition, having a specific set of symptoms that map onto a given psychiatric disorder (e.g., distress upon separation from major attachment figures is a hallmark symptom of SAD) allows the therapist to focus on the reduction of those specific symptoms associated with the disorder. The categorical system further affords the researcher the capability to make formal comparisons between different groups of youth. This allows for comparisons on diagnostic categories based on youth age, sex, and ethnicity.

FACTORS TO CONSIDER IN SELECTING A DIAGNOSTIC INTERVIEW

Given the different characteristics of structured, semistructured, and unstructured interviews, several factors should be considered in deciding which interview approach to utilize. One factor is the clinician's level of expertise. As noted, unstructured interviews require a high level of expertise (e.g., master's-level or doctoral-level), familiarity with diagnostic criteria, correlates of symptom presentation, and contextual factors associated with the presenting problem(s). Semistructured interviews (e.g., the ADIS-IV: C/P, the K-SADS) also require some level of expertise, but with training, these interviews can be administered by bachelor's level clinicians and graduate students. Structured interviews (e.g., the DISC-IV, the ChIPS) are the only interviews that may be administered by lay interviewers, after some training is completed.

A second factor to consider is the time available for the administration of the interview. Apparent from the above, several of the structured interviews (e.g., the DISC-IV) and semistructured interviews (e.g., the ADIS-IV: C/P) require some time to administer (about 1–2 hours per informant, or a total of 2–4 hours for both youth and parent). If time is of concern, the clinician may choose to administer the ChIPS or MINI-KID, both of which yield reliable and valid diagnoses comparable to those of other interview schedules (e.g., the K-SADS-P/L).

A third factor to consider is the purpose of the interview: Is it being administered in a clinical or research setting? If the interview is intended to evaluate the efficacy of an intervention for the purposes of research, for example, then interviews with strong psychometric support need to be utilized. That being said, however, the psychometric support of the interview should always be considered, regardless of setting. Finally, given the growing minority population in the United States (U.S. Census Bureau, 2007), the primary language of the informant may need to be considered. Some of the interview schedules summarized earlier have been translated into Spanish as well as other languages. Refer back to Table 5.1 for more information regarding the interviews' characteristics.

In the last couple of decades, much attention has been paid to developing evidence-based treatment approaches for internalizing and externalizing behavior problems in youth (Silverman, Pina, & Viswesvaran, 2008;

Pelham & Fabiano, 2008). Just as important as evidence-based treatment approaches are evidence-based assessment approaches. Such an approach is important to ensure that the disorder one is hoping to alleviate in a youth, such as anxiety, is *the* disorder associated with the youth's presenting problem and impairment (Silverman & Ollendick, 2005). In light of this, the final consideration in selecting an interview for use is the evidence that has accumulated regarding the interview's psychometric support.

APPLICATION TO THE CASE OF SOFIA

Sofia was a 15-year-old Hispanic girl who was referred by school personnel to treatment after difficulties staying in school. At the time of the initial referral, she had missed about 100 days of school. Her refusal to go to school had been attributed to panic attacks, as well as fear of re-experiencing the panic attacks. Sofia successfully completed a 16-week exposure-based cognitive-behavioral treatment (CBT). She was able to return to school, but shortly afterward, the school informed Sofia and her family that she was going to be retained and she would have to repeat sophomore year. Upon learning this information, Sofia became so distraught that she stopped attending school altogether, leading to a second treatment referral.

Interviewing Strategies

Given that Sofia's primary difficulties appeared to be panic attacks and possible depressive symptoms (refer to McLeod, Jensen-Doss, & Ollendick, Chapter 4, this volume, for the complete case description), the ADIS-IV: C was administered to her and the ADIS-IV: P to her mother. The ADIS-IV: P was deemed adequate for interviewing Sofia's mother because it was available in Spanish. As noted earlier, the ADIS-IV: C/P contains an introductory section with questions about the presenting problem. This section thus provided an opportunity for the interviewer to begin to establish rapport with Sofia. Given that Sofia was also presenting with depressive symptoms, it would be important for the interviewer to determine the primary problem for treatment planning. That is, was Sofia depressed as a result of her inability to stay in school (which would be related to panic symptoms), or should the focus of treatment be on reducing her depressive symptoms?

Below we present brief excerpts from the interview that was conducted with Sofia. The clinician used the PD module of the ADIS-IV: C. Because the ADIS-IV: C/P is a semistructured interview, the interview questions do not need to be read verbatim; they may be modified to reflect the interviewer's awareness of the information gathered at intake, the interviewee's developmental level, and other factors.

> INTERVIEWER: We know that sometimes people get scared because they are scared of a specific thing. But sometimes people feel

really scared for no reason at all! They are not in a scary place and there is nothing scary around, but all of a sudden, out of the blue, they feel really scared and they don't know why. Is that what happened to you in the past?

SOFIA: Yes, I think so. The first time I felt really panicky, I was very confused. I really thought there was something physically wrong with me. It felt like I was going to die.

At this juncture, the interviewer went on to obtain more information about the antecedents of Sofia's panic attack, as well as about the frequency, intensity, and duration of her panic symptoms. This was important, because the interviewer needed to determine whether Sofia's positive response to the main criterion question of the PD section of the ADIS-IV: C was not due to another anxiety disorder (fear of negative evaluation from others, fear in the presence of a certain situation or object, etc.). It was important to assess that the "unexpected" panic attack did not occur immediately before or upon exposure to a situation that almost always causes anxiety. One way to achieve this would be to ask, as the interviewer did:

INTERVIEWER: OK, Sofia. You just told me about getting scared when you were in P.E. Now, at that time, were you scared of what the other kids around you were thinking about you? Were you thinking about that? Or were you feeling panicky for no reason at all?

SOFIA: No, I don't remember thinking about what the other students were thinking. I was focused on the sensations in my body. It was really scary.

After completing the PD section of the ADIS-IV: C, the interviewer obtained an overall rating of interference, using the rating scale described earlier (i.e., a "Feelings Thermometer").

INTERVIEWER: OK, I want to know how much this problem has messed things up in your life. That is, how much has it messed things up for you with friends, in school, or at home? How much does it stop you from doing things you would like to do? Tell me how much by using the Feelings Thermometer we discussed earlier, OK?

After the interviewer obtained an interference rating for PD, she also administered the SOP module, given that Sofia also reported some concerns at intake, regarding fear of negative evaluation by others. Specifically, she reported that she was embarrassed to return to school because she was being retained. Finally, the interviewer proceeded to the affective disorders modules and assessed for dysthymia or MDD.

Interviews with Sofia's Parents

The ADIS-IV: P was conducted with Sofia's mother to obtain more information about Sofia's difficulties with attending school. The ADIS-IV: P follows the same format as the ADIS-IV: C and is available in Spanish. It was also recommended, if her father agreed, to conduct the ADIS-IV: P with him as well, to get a comprehensive picture of Sofia's functioning and any difficulties at home that might be maintaining or exacerbating her school refusal behavior.

Diagnostic Impression

The diagnostic impression was formulated after interviewing Sofia and her mother. The ADIS-IV: C indicated that Sofia met criteria for two primary diagnoses: SOP and MDD. Both diagnoses were primary because Sofia rated them as equally interfering, giving them both an interference rating of 7 on the Feelings Thermometer. She also met criteria for a secondary diagnosis of PD with agoraphobia. This was considered a secondary diagnosis because Sofia's interference rating was lower than SOP and MDD, since her panic attacks had decreased after her previous round of treatment.

The ADIS-IV: P indicated that Sofia only met criteria for a diagnosis of PD with agoraphobia, with an interference rating of 7 on the Feelings Thermometer. Thus the composite diagnostic profile generated by the ADIS-IV interviews was as follows: a primary diagnosis of SOP, a primary diagnosis of MDD, and a secondary diagnosis of PD with agoraphobia.

APPLICATION TO THE CASE OF BILLY

Billy was a 10-year-old European American boy who was referred to treatment by his family doctor for behavior problems at home, at school, and in his community. He lived with his older sister, Meredith, who was 13, and his mother, Mary, who was 42. He also had a 16-year-old brother, Mike, who was being detained at a juvenile detention facility at the time of referral. Mike had been adjudicated for breaking and entering and for assaulting a police officer upon his arrest. Billy's mother was divorced from his father, who had infrequent contact with the children. Mary wanted help in managing Billy's oppositional, negativistic, and noncompliant behaviors at home and school. She was also concerned about his nighttime fears and described him as a somewhat "anxious" child, although anxiety was not the chief complaint for his referral. Refer to Chapter 4 for the complete case description.

Interviewing Strategies

Billy was reluctant to participate in the intake process. It is not uncommon for youth with externalizing behavior problems to refuse to participate in the assessment process (Greene & Doyle, 1999; Handwerk, 2007; McMahon & Frick, 2005). Indeed, defiance and noncompliance are the defining characteristics of youth presenting with ODD, a possible problem for Billy. Thus obtaining an accurate, reliable, and valid interview with Billy proved challenging. Furthermore, it was Mary who initiated the referral because of *her* difficulties in managing Billy's behavior. It is rarely the case that youth with externalizing behavior problems are distressed by their noncompliance and defiant behaviors (McMahon & Frick, 2005). As such, conducting the interview with the mother was most critical in this case; however, information from Billy was also useful in determining the extent of his nighttime fears and his other worries.

Handwerk (2007) recommends that with youth who refuse to participate in the assessment process, establishing rapport with the youth is of upmost importance. This can be accomplished at the first session by suggesting playing a board game or a video game, instead of immediately beginning with the diagnostic interview. The use of a semistructured interview is better for establishing rapport than a structured interview, because most semistructured interviews start with open-ended questions about what brought the family to treatment. This allows the clinician to talk about the youth's interests and other nonthreatening subjects. Validating the youth's interests and establishing mutual respect are also important for the establishment of rapport (see Handwerk, 2007; see also Shirk, Reyes, & Crisostomo, Chapter 14, this volume). Furthermore, many semistructured interviews consist of standardized questions requiring mainly "yes" or "no" responses, and thus only requiring minimal verbal interaction.

If Billy had shown reluctance to respond to this interviewing strategy, it would have been worthwhile to consider switching to one of the more highly structured interview schedules, such as the DISC-IV. Some children may actually prefer the structure of such an interview, given the relative lack of structure and order they may feel in their daily lives. Unfortunately, there is no research to date that guides a clinician regarding which course to choose first (i.e., unstructured or structured) in cases such as Billy's, and this is why all options need to be placed on the table, tried, and adjusted accordingly.

Interviews with Billy and His Mother

As noted above, most of the information about Billy's oppositional and negativistic problems needed to be obtained from his mother. It was recommended that a semistructured interview like the ADIS-IV: P or the DICA-P be completed with Mary (the former was chosen). During the interview, it was critical for the clinician to obtain information regarding the frequency, intensity, and duration of Billy's negativistic and noncompliant behaviors. Specifically, it was most important to learn about the antecedents and consequences of Billy's outbursts. This helped the clinician determine which factors might have led to the development and maintenance of Billy's oppositional behavior (McMahon & Frick, 2005; Murrihy, Kidman, & Ollendick, 2010). Finally, it was important for the interviewer to obtain interference ratings of Billy's other difficulties (e.g., nighttime fears, difficulties with focusing and attention) for the purpose of developing treatment targets (detailed further below). So, too, it was important to interview Billy to get his report, especially about the nighttime fears and about the inattention and hyperactivity problems.

Diagnostic Impression

The diagnostic impression was formulated after interviewing Billy and his mother. On the ADIS-IV: C, Billy met diagnostic criteria for SP of dark/being alone, a subclinical diagnosis of ADHD—combined type (ADHD-C), and a subclinical diagnosis of GAD. On the ADIS-IV: P completed with his mother, he met criteria for a primary diagnosis of ODD and a secondary diagnosis of SP of dark/being alone. He also met subclinical criteria for ADHD-C. He did not meet subclinical criteria for GAD on the ADIS-IV: P. After reviewing all the interference ratings for the respective youth and parent derived diagnoses, the clinician determined that his primary diagnosis was ODD and that his secondary diagnosis was SP of dark/being alone. Hence it was determined that initial treatment would focus on helping Mary manage Billy's ODD and that a secondary goal of intervention would be to treat his SP. As Jensen-Doss, Ollendick, and McLeod describe in Chapter 15, other assessment information did not support the subclinical diagnosis of ADHD-C.

IMPLICATIONS FOR TREATMENT PLANNING AND OUTCOME EVALUATION

Diagnostic interviews can be utilized at various stages during the treatment process. At intake, they are used to determine presence or absence of diagnoses; to evaluate contextual factors that may be maintaining, contributing to, or exacerbating the presenting problem; and to establish a baseline of impairment level for treatment planning, and outcome evaluation.

Treatment Planning

After the interviews with the youth and her or his parents, the next step is to select the specific symptoms that will be targeted during the youth's treatment. Given the high level of comorbidity among youth with internalizing and externalizing behavior problems (e.g., Brady & Kendall, 1992; Last, Perrin, Hersen, & Kazdin, 1992; Zoccolillo, 1992), a key issue involves prioritizing the various difficulties reported by the youth and parents. In cases where a youth has been diagnosed with more than one disorder, as in the cases of Sofia and Billy, it is important to determine how much the symptoms related to each of the disorders interfere in the youth's functioning at school, at home, or with peers. One way to prioritize the youth's difficulties is by obtaining youth and parent ratings of interference. Many of the interviews described earlier contain rating scales for determining level of interference.

Evaluating Treatment Outcome

Interviews like the DISC-IV, ADIS-IV: C/P, and K-SADS-P/L have been widely used to evaluate treatment outcome for youth presenting with both internalizing and externalizing problems. Specifically, they have been used frequently in the treatment outcome evaluation process to determine the diagnostic recovery rates of various samples from pretreatment to posttreatment (e.g., Silverman et al., 2008; Pelham & Fabiano, 2008). Youth and/or parents are administered a diagnostic interview at pretreatment, to determine whether the youth meet the diagnostic criteria (which is the main requirement) for enrolling in a randomized clinical trial. To evaluate the efficacy of the treatment, it is important to know the percentage of youth who no longer meet diagnostic criteria at posttreatment relative to pretreatment. For example, such data may reveal that at posttreatment 80% of youth are recovered or are no longer meeting diagnostic criteria. Interviews that also contain severity ratings, such as the ADIS-IV: C/P, have also been used to evaluate outcome from a dimensional perspective. For example, if a mean severity rating for a particular diagnosis is 7.4 on a 9-point Likert scale at pretreatment, and that mean severity rating drops to 5.5 at posttreatment (and the mean difference is statistically significant), then the researcher may conclude that the treatment was efficacious.

The practice of systematically evaluating diagnostic recovery rates via diagnostic interviews is more often employed in research settings than in clinical settings. Indeed, the American Psychological Association Presidential Task Force on Evidence-Based Practice (2006) has placed a great emphasis on increasing the use of evidence based practices in clinical settings, which include employing assessment methods that also have a strong empirical basis. In the past, clinicians have been resistant to adopting evidence-based practices in their own work (Beutler, 2000). Nevertheless, the youth mental health field has witnessed a significant change in clinicians' willingness to adopt such practices (Silverman & Hinshaw, 2008). Increased efforts are still needed to continue promoting the use of evidence-based practices in clinical settings.

LIMITATIONS OF DIAGNOSTIC INTERVIEWS

Although semistructured and structured diagnostic interviews have strong psychometric support for deriving reliable and valid diagnoses, they also have limitations. First, the "yes–no" or "present–absent" approach, which underlies all interview approaches, implies that an individual either has a disorder or does not. It fails to consider the possibility that the individual not fully meet diagnostic criteria for a disorder, but still may display symptoms of that disorder, leading to significant impairment (Angold, Costello, Farmer, Burns, & Erkanli, 1999). Second, although clinical disorders are assumed within a categorical perspective to be qualitatively distinct from each other, the high levels of comorbidity among many of the DSM disorders call this assumption into question (Widiger & Clark, 2000). Finally, the categorical perspective pays insufficient attention to likely sex and age differences in the manifestation of clinical diagnoses.

SUMMARY AND RECOMMENDATIONS FOR FUTURE RESEARCH

This chapter presents a review of the most widely used and researched diagnostic interview schedules available for use with youth presenting with internalizing and externalizing behavior problems. The chapter also describes how a diagnostic interview was used in the assessment process for an adolescent presenting with anxiety and depressive symptomatology, as well as for a child presenting mainly with disruptive behavior problems that were leading to significant interference at home and school. It is important to note that a comprehensive assessment of youth problems involves the use of not only diagnostic interviews, but self-rating scales, direct behavioral observation systems, and self-monitoring forms. Those assessment modalities are reviewed in other chapters of this book.

   Although a great deal of evidence has accumulated on the use of diagnostic interviews, much remains to be explored. For instance, information about the reliability of such interviews when used in community clinics and when diagnosing disorders of varying base rates is still needed. Another concern relates to research findings in the anxiety disorders area that show high discordance among the tripartite features of anxiety. Thus more work is needed in understanding this discordance and in incorporating this understanding into the existing assessment armamentarium and treatment decisions. Discordance among systems in general might suggest, for example, behavioral versus cognitive interventions (see, e.g., Eisen & Silverman, 1998). Evidence regarding the incremental validity of using a multi-informant assessment and multiresponse assessment procedure is also needed.

   As noted earlier, another development that is likely to have implications for the use of diagnostic interview schedules is the inclusion of dimensional severity ratings in some of the diagnostic categories of the DSM-5 (see also Jensen-Doss, McLeod, & Ollendick, Chapter 2, this volume). Such ratings have the potential to address several disadvantages of a pure categorical approach to classifying psychopathology, such as the DSM-IV system's inability to capture individual differences in the severity of a given disorder, as well as other clinically significant features that are either subsumed by other diagnoses or fall below diagnostic thresholds (Brown & Barlow, 2005, 2009). Research on whether including dimensional severity ratings successfully addresses the disadvantages of a pure categorical approach will be needed. The current diagnostic interview schedules will need to be modified to reflect the changes made in DSM-5.

ACKNOWLEDGMENTS

Preparation of this chapter was supported in part by a grant from the National Institute of Mental Health (R01MH079943).

REFERENCES

Achenbach, T. M. (1991). *Manual for the Child Behavior Checklist and Revised Child Behavior Profile (Revised)*. Burlington: University of Vermont, Department of Psychiatry.

Achenbach, T. M., & Edelbrock, C. S. (1986). *Manual for the Teacher's Report Form and the Teacher Version of the Child Behavior Profile*. Burlington: University of Vermont, Department of Psychiatry.

Ambrosini, P. J. (2000). Historical development and present status of the Schedule for Affective Disorders and Schizophrenia for School-Age Children (K-SADS). *Journal of the American Academy of Child and Adolescent Psychiatry, 39*, 49–58.

American Psychiatric Association. (1994). *Diagnostic and statistical manual of mental disorders* (4th ed.). Washington, DC: Author.

American Psychiatric Association. (2000). *Diagnostic and statistical manual of mental disorders* (4th ed., text rev.). Washington, DC: Author.

American Psychiatric Association. (2013). *Diagnostic and statistical manual of mental disorders* (5th ed.). Arlington, VA: Author.

American Psychological Association Presidential Task Force on Evidence-Based Practice. (2006). Evidence-based practice in psychology. *American Psychologist, 61*, 271–285.

Anderson, S. R., & Ollendick, T. H. (2012). The reliability and validity of the Anxiety Disorders Interview Schedule for the diagnosis of oppositional defiant disorder. *Journal of Psychopathology and Behavioral Assessment*. Publishes online May 19, 2012.

Angold, A., & Costello, E. J. (1995). A test–retest reliability study of child-reported psychiatric symptoms and diagnoses using the Child and Adolescent Psychiatric Assessment (CAPA-C). *Psychological Medicine, 25*(4), 755–762.

Angold, A., & Costello, E. J. (2000). The Child and Adolescent Psychiatric Assessment. *Journal of the American Academy of Child and Adolescent Psychiatry, 39*, 39–48.

Angold A., Costello, E. J., Farmer, E. M. Z., Burns, B. J., & Erkanli, A. (1999).

Impaired but undiagnosed. *Journal of the American Academy of Child and Adolescent Psychiatry, 38*, 129–137.

Angold, A., Erkanli, A., Costello, E. J., & Rutter, M. (1996). Precision, reliability, and accuracy in the dating of symptom onset in child and adolescent psychopathology. *Journal of Child Psychology and Psychiatry, 37*, 657–664.

Beck, A. T., Ward, C. H., Mendelson, M., Mock, J., & Erbaugh, J. (1961). An inventory for measuring depression. *Archives of General Psychiatry, 4*(6), 561–571.

Beutler, L. E. (2000). Empirically based decision making in clinical practice. *Prevention and Treatment, 3*, no pagination specified.

Birmaher, B., Khetarpal, S., Brent, D. A., Cully, M., Balach, L., Kaufman, J., & McKenzie, N. (1997). The Screen for Child Anxiety Related Emotional Disorders (SCARED): Scale construction and psychometric characteristics. *Journal of the American Academy of Child and Adolescent Psychiatry, 36*, 545–553.

Bongers, I. L., Koot, H. M., van der Ende, J., & Verhulst, F. C. (2003). The normative development of child and adolescent problem behavior. *Journal of Abnormal Psychology, 112*, 179–192.

Brady, E. U., & Kendall, P. C. (1992). Comorbidity of anxiety and depression in children and adolescents. *Psychological Bulletin, 111*, 244–255.

Bravo, M., Ribera, J., Rubio-Stipec, M., Canino, G., Shrout, P., Ramírez, R., & Taboas, A. M. (2001). Test–retest reliability of the Spanish version of the Diagnostic Interview Schedule for Children (DISC-IV). *Journal of Abnormal Child Psychology, 29*, 433–444.

Brown, T. A., & Barlow, D. H. (2005). Dimensional versus categorical classification of mental disorders in the fifth edition of the Diagnostic and Statistical Manual of Mental Disorders and beyond: Comment on the special section. *Journal of Abnormal Psychology, 114*, 551–556.

Brown, T. A., & Barlow, D. H. (2009). A proposal for a dimensional classification system based on the shared features of the DSM-IV anxiety and mood disorders: Implications for assessment and treatment. *Psychological Assessment, 21*, 256–271.

Cashel, M. L. (2002). Child and adolescent psychological assessment: Current clinical practices and the impact of managed care. *Professional Psychology: Research and Practice, 33*, 446–453.

Cohen, J. (1960). A coefficient of agreement for nominal scales. *Educational and Psychological Measurement, 20*, 37–46.

Eisen, A. R., & Silverman, W. K. (1998). Prescriptive treatment for generalized anxiety disorder in children. *Behavior Therapy, 29*, 105–121.

Elliot, A. J., Miltenberger, R. G., Kaster-Bundgaard, J., & Lumley, V. (1996). A national survey of assessment and therapy techniques used by behavior therapists. *Cognitive and Behavior Practice, 3*, 107–125.

Fristad, M. A., Cummins, J., Verducci, J. S., Teare. M., Weller, E. B., & Weller, R. A. (1998). Study IV: Concurrent validity of the DSM-IV revised Children's Interview for Psychiatric Syndromes (ChIPS). *Journal of Child and Adolescent Psychopharmacology, 8*, 227–236.

Greene, R. W., & Doyle, A. E. (1999). Toward a transactional conceptualization of oppositional defiant disorder: Implications for assessment and treatment. *Clinical Child and Family Psychology Review, 2*, 129–148.

Hamilton, M. (1960). A rating scale for depression. *Journal of Neurology, Neurosurgery and Psychiatry, 23*(1), 56–62.

Handwerk, M. L. (2007). Oppositional defiant disorder and conduct disorder. In M. Hersen & J. C. Thomas (Eds.), *Handbook of clinical interviewing with children* (pp. 212–248). Thousand Oake, CA: Sage.

Herjanic, B., & Campbell, W. (1977). Differentiating psychiatrically disturbed children on the basis of a structured interview. *Journal of Abnormal Child Psychology, 5,* 127–134.

Jarrett, M. A., Wolff, J. C., & Ollendick, T. H. (2007). Concurrent validity and informant agreement of the ADHD module of the Anxiety Disorders Interview Schedule for DSM-IV. *Journal of Psychopathology and Behavioral Assessment, 29,* 159–168.

Jensen, P., Roper, M., Fisher, P., Piacentini, J., Canino, G., Richters, J., & Schwab-Stone, M. E. (1995). Test–retest reliability of the Diagnostic Interview Schedule for Children (DISC 2.1). *Archives of General Psychiatry, 52,* 61–71.

Kaufman, J., Birmaher, B., Brent, D., & Rao, U. (1997). Schedule for Affective Disorders and Schizophrenia for School-Age Children—Present and Lifetime Version [K-SADS-PL]: Initial reliability and validity data. *Journal of the American Academy of Child and Adolescent Psychiatry, 36*(7), 980–980.

Kovacs, M. (1992). *Children's Depression Inventory manual.* North Tonawanda, NY: Multi-Health Systems.

Landis, J. R., & Koch, G. G. (1977). The measurement of observer agreement for categorical data. *Biometrics, 33*(1), 159–174.

Last, C. G., Perrin, S., Hersen, M., & Kazdin, A. E. (1992). DSM-III-R anxiety disorders in children: Sociodemographic and clinical characteristics. *Journal of the American Academy of Child and Adolescent Psychiatry, 31,* 1070–1076.

Lucas, C. P. (2003). Use of structured diagnostic interviews in clinical child psychiatric practice. In M. B. First (Ed.), *Standardized evaluation in clinical practice* (pp. 75–101). Arlington, VA: American Psychiatric Publishing, Inc.

Lucas, C. P., Zhang, H., Fisher, P. W., Shaffer, D., Regier, D. A., Narrow, W. E., & Friman, P. (2001). The DISC Predictive Scales (DPS): Efficiently screening for diagnoses. *Journal of the American Academy of Child and Adolescent Psychiatry, 40,* 443–449.

Lyneham, H. J., Abbott, M., A., & Rapee, R. M. (2007). Interrater reliability of the Anxiety Disorders Interview Schedule for DSM-IV: Child and Parent Version. *Journal of the American Academy of Child and Adolescent Psychiatry, 46,* 731–736.

Marin, C. E., Rey, Y., & Silverman, W. K. (2012). *Test–retest reliability of the Spanish version of the Anxiety Disorders Interview Schedule for DSM-IV: Child and Parent Versions.* Manuscript in preparation.

March, J. (1998). *Manual for the Multidimensional Anxiety Scale for Children (MASC).* Toronto: Multi-Health Systems.

Mash, E. J., & Barkley, R. A. (2007). Assessment of child and family disturbance: A developmental–systems approach. In E. J. Mash & R. A. Barkley (Eds.), *Assessment of childhood disorders* (pp. 3–50). New York: Guilford Press.

Mash, E. J., & Hunsley, J. (2005). Evidence-based assessment of child and adolescent disorders: Issues and challenges. *Journal of Clinical Child and Adolescent Psychology, 34,* 362–379.

McMahon, R. J., & Frick, P. J. (2005). Evidence-based assessment of conduct problems in children and adolescents. *Journal of Clinical Child and Adolescent Psychology, 34,* 477–505.

Moreno, A. M. M., Basurto, F. Z., Becerra, I. G., & San Pedro, E. M. (2006). Discriminant and criterion validity of the Spanish version of the Children's Interview for Psychiatric Syndromes—Parents Version (P-ChIPS). *European Journal of Psychological Assessment, 22*, 109–115.

Murrihy, R. C., Kidman, A. D., & Ollendick, T. H. (Eds.). (2010). *Clinical handbook of assessing and treating conduct problems in youth.* New York: Springer.

O'Brien, W. H., McGrath, J. J., & Haynes, S. N. (2003). Assessment of psychopathology: Behavioral approaches. In J. Graham & J. Naglieri (Eds.), *Handbook of psychological assessment* (pp. 509–529). New York: Wiley.

Ollendick, T. H., & Hersen, M. (1984). An overview of child behavioral assessment. In T. H. Ollendick & M. Hersen (Eds.), *Child behavioral assessment: Principles and procedures* (pp. 3–19). New York: Pergamon Press.

Ollendick, T. H., Grills, A. E., & King, N. J. (2001). Applying developmental theory to the assessment and treatment of childhood disorders: Does it make a difference? *Clinical Psychology and Psychotherapy, 8*, 304–314.

Pelham, W. E., & Fabiano, G. A. (2008). Evidence-based psychosocial treatments for attention-deficit/hyperactivity disorder. *Journal of Clinical Child and Adolescent Psychology, 37*, 184–214.

Pina, A. A., Silverman, W. K., Alfano, C. A., & Saavedra, L. M. (2002). Diagnostic efficiency of symptoms in the diagnosis of DSM-IV generalized anxiety disorder in youth. *Journal of Child Psychology and Psychiatry, 43*, 959–967.

Reich, W. (2000). Diagnostic Interview for Children and Adolescents (DICA). *Journal of the American Academy of Child and Adolescent Psychiatry, 39*, 59–66.

Reich, W., Cottler, L., McCallum, K., Corwin, D., & VanEerdewegh, M. (1995). Computerized interviews as a method of assessing psychopathology in children. *Comprehensive Psychiatry, 36*, 40–45.

Roberts, N., Parker, K. C. H., & Dagnone, M. (2005). Comparison of clinical diagnoses, NIMH-DISC-IV diagnoses and SCL-90-R ratings in an adolescent psychiatric inpatient unit: A brief report. *Canadian Child and Adolescent Psychiatry Review, 14*(4), 103–105.

Schwab-Stone, M. E., Shaffer, D., Dulcan, M. K., Jensen, P. S., Fisher, P., Bird, H. R., & Rae, D. S. (1996). Criterion validity of the NIMH Diagnostic Interview Schedule for Children version 2.3 (DISC-2.3). *Journal of the American Academy of Child and Adolescent Psychiatry, 35*, 878–888.

Shaffer, D., Fisher, P., Lucas, C. P., Dulcan, M. K., & Schwab-Stone, M. E. (2000). NIMH Diagnostic Interview for Children Version IV (NIMH DISC-IV): Description, differences from previous versions, and reliability for some common diagnoses. *Journal of the American Academy of Child and Adolescent Psychiatry, 39*, 28–38.

Shaffer, D., Lucas, C. P., & Richters, J. E. (Eds.). (1999). *Diagnostic assessment in child and adolescent psychopathology.* New York: Guilford Press.

Sheehan, D. V., Sheehan, K. H., Shytle, R. D., Janavs, J., Bannon, Y., Rogers, J. E., & Wilkinson, B. (2010). Reliability and validity of the Mini International Neuropsychiatric Interview for Children and Adolescents (MINI-KID). *Journal of Clinical Psychiatry, 71*, 313–326.

Silverman, W. K., & Albano, A. M. (1996). *Anxiety Disorders Interview Schedule for DSM-IV: Child and Parent Versions.* San Antonio, TX: Psychological Corporation.

Silverman, W. K., & Hinshaw, S. T. (2008). The second special issue on evidence-based psychosocial treatments for children and adolescents: A 10-year update. *Journal of Clinical Child and Adolescent Psychology, 37,* 1–7.

Silverman, W. K., & Nelles, W. B. (1988). The Anxiety Disorders Interview Schedule for Children. *Journal of the American Academy of Child and Adolescent Psychiatry, 6,* 772–778.

Silverman, W. K., & Ollendick, T. H. (2005). Evidence-based assessment of anxiety and its disorders in children and adolescents. *Journal of Clinical Child and Adolescent Psychology, 34,* 380–411.

Silverman, W. K., Pina, A. A., & Viswesvaran, C. (2008). Evidence-based psychosocial treatments for phobic and anxiety disorders in youth and adolescents. *Journal of Clinical Child and Adolescent Psychology, 37,* 105–130.

Silverman, W. K., Saavedra, L. M., & Pina, A. A. (2001). Test–retest reliability of anxiety symptoms and diagnoses with the Anxiety Disorders Interview Schedule for DSM-IV: Child and Parent Versions. *Journal of the American Academy of Child and Adolescent Psychiatry, 40,* 937–944.

Spitzer, R. L., Endicott, J., & Robins, E. (1978). Research Diagnostic Criteria: Rationale and reliability. *Archives of General Psychiatry, 35,* 773–782.

Teare, M., Fristad, M. A., Weller, E. B., Weller, R. A., & Salmon, P. (1998). Study I: Development and criterion validity of the Children's Interview for Psychiatric Syndromes (ChIPS). *Journal of Child and Adolescent Psychopharmacology, 8,* 205–211.

Ulloa, R. E., Ortiz, S., Higuera, F., Nogales, I., Fresán, A., Apiquian R., & de la Peña, F. (2006). Interrater reliability of the Spanish version of the Schedule for Affective Disorders and Schizophrenia for School-Age Children—Present and Lifetime Version (K-SADS-P/L). *Actas Españolas de Psiquiatría, 34*(1), 36–40.

U.S. Census Bureau. (2007). Census 2000 redistricting data (Public Law 94-171). Retrieved from *www.census .gov/support/PLData .html*

Villa, M., & Reitman, D. (2007). Overview of interviewing strategies with children, parents, and teachers. In M. Hersen & J. C. Thomas (Eds.), *Handbook of clinical interviewing with children* (pp. 2–15). Thousand Oaks, CA: Sage.

Walkup, J. T., Albano, A. M., Piacentini, J., Birmaher, B., Compton, S. N., Sherrill, J. T., & Kendall, P. C. (2008). Cognitive behavioral therapy, sertraline, or a combination in childhood anxiety. *New England Journal of Medicine, 359,* 2753–2766.

Weller, E. B., Weller, R. A., Fristad, M. A., Rooney, M. T., & Schecter, J. (2000). Children's Interview for Psychiatric Syndromes (ChIPS). *Journal of the American Academy of Child and Adolescent Psychiatry, 39,* 76–84.

Widiger, T. A., & Clark, L. A. (2000). Toward DSM-V and the classification of psychopathology. *Psychological Bulletin, 126,* 946–963.

Wood, J., Piacentini, J. C., Bergman, R. L., McCracken, J., & Barrios, V. (2002). Concurrent validity of the anxiety disorders section of the Anxiety Disorders Interview Schedule for DSM-IV: Child and Parent Versions. *Journal of the American Academy of Child and Adolescent Psychiatry, 31,* 335–342.

World Health Organization. (1993). *International statistical classification of diseases and related health problems.* Geneva: Author.

Zoccolillo, M. (1992). Co-occurrence of conduct disorder and its adult outcomes with depressive and anxiety disorders: A review. *Journal of the American Academy of Child and Adolescent Psychiatry, 31,* 547–556.

6

Checklists and Rating Scales

Thomas M. Achenbach

Numerous checklists and rating scales have been constructed for assessing many aspects of human functioning.[1] On most rating instruments for assessing children's behavioral, emotional, and social problems, informants rate specific items on multistep Likert scales, although items on some instruments are rated dichotomously as "present–absent." Various instruments are designed to be completed by parents, teachers, clinicians, observers, and children themselves.

"Narrow-band" instruments are designed to assess a single, narrow class of problems, often defined in terms of a particular diagnostic category, such as attention-deficit/hyperactivity disorder (ADHD). An example is the ADHD Rating Scale–IV (DuPaul, Power, Anastopoulos, & Reid, 1998). "Broad-band" instruments, by contrast, are designed to assess a broad spectrum of problems. The problems assessed by some broad-band instruments are chosen to correspond to symptom criteria for multiple diagnostic categories and are scored in terms of those categories. An example is the Adolescent Symptom Inventory–4 (ASI-4; Gadow & Sprafkin, 1998). Other broad-band instruments tend to focus on symptoms of a particular diagnostic category but include problems that may fall outside that category. As an example, the Conners Rating Scales—Revised (Conners, 2001) focus mainly on ADHD problems, but non-ADHD items are also included.

Some broad-band instruments have been subjected to factor analysis as part of the development process, but items were ultimately assigned to

---

[1]For brevity, the term "rating instruments" is used from here on to include checklists and rating scales, and the term "children" is used to include ages from 1½ through 18 years.

scales on the basis of the authors' judgments, rather than directly reflecting statistically identified associations among items. Examples of such instruments are the Strengths and Difficulties Questionnaire (SDQ; Goodman, 1997), which is a brief broad-band screening instrument; the Devereux Scales of Mental Disorders (Naglieri & Pfeiffer, 2004), which is a longer instrument; and the Behavior Assessment System for Children (BASC; Reynolds & Kamphaus, 1992), which is a much longer instrument with numerous scales.

Rather than surveying the many existing instruments, this chapter illustrates the contributions of rating instruments as exemplified by the Achenbach System of Empirically Based Assessment (ASEBA; Achenbach, 2009). The ASEBA includes developmentally appropriate instruments for ages 1½–5, 6–18, 18–59, and 60–90+ years. Different versions of the instruments are designed for completion by untrained lay informants, including parents, daycare providers, teachers, children, adults assessing their own functioning, and collaterals of adults who are being assessed. Other versions are designed for completion by clinical interviewers, clinicians who administer individual ability or achievement tests, and nonparticipant observers of children in group settings such as schools. Consistent with the case studies presented in this book, the chapter focuses mainly on ages 6–18. However, because parents and other family members are often involved in the assessment and treatment of children, the chapter also illustrates how assessment of these important adults can contribute to helping children.

DESCRIPTION OF THE ASSESSMENT METHOD

The ASEBA instruments are designed to be used for many research, training, and clinical purposes. Instruments completed by lay respondents—such as parents, daycare providers, teachers, and children—can be self-administered by respondents with fifth-grade reading skills. If a respondent's ability to complete an instrument is questionable, a lay interviewer with no specialized training can read the instrument's items to the respondent and enter the respondent's answers. The instruments designed for lay informants include items describing a broad spectrum of problems that can be rated by the respondents with a minimum of inference. Each item is rated 0 ("not true"), 1 ("somewhat or sometimes true"), or 2 ("very true or often true"), based on a specified rating period—such as 2 months for ages 1½–5 and for teachers' ratings of 6 to 18-year-olds, and 6 months for parents' ratings of 6 to 18-year-olds, for self-ratings by 11 to 18-year-olds and adults, and for ratings by adult collaterals. Instruments designed for completion by clinicians and by observers in settings such as schools have four-step scales for rating behaviors observed during particular real-time periods. In addition to problem items, most instruments also have items for describing and rating competence and adaptive functioning, plus open-ended items for providing additional information, such as descriptions of specific problems and the "best" things about the person being rated. Table 6.1 summarizes the ASEBA instruments and respondents.

Brief Problem Monitor

Most of the instruments listed in Table 6.1 are designed to contribute to comprehensive initial assessments on which to base decisions about who needs help, for what, to what degree, and in what contexts (such as home and school). The instruments are also designed to aid in targeting interventions on particular problems and competencies, assessing the progress of interventions at intervals of ≥ 2 months, and evaluating outcomes and functioning during follow-up periods. To meet needs for brief assessments that can be repeatedly applied at shorter intervals, the Brief Problem Monitor (BPM) includes Internalizing, Attention, and Externalizing problem items for rating 6 to 18-year-olds at user-selected intervals of days, weeks, or months (Achenbach, McConaughy, Ivanova, & Rescorla, 2011). The Internalizing, Attention Problems, and Externalizing scale scores are summed to provide a Total Problems score. Users can also write in items for rating additional problems and strengths.

TABLE 6.1. ASEBA Forms for Ages 1½ to 90+ Years

Name of form	Filled out by …
Child Behavior Checklist for Ages 1½–5 (CBCL/1½–5)	Parents, surrogates
Caregiver–Teacher Report Form for Ages 1½–5 (C-TRF)	Daycare providers, preschool teachers
Child Behavior Checklist for Ages 6–18 (CBCL/6–18)	Parents, surrogates
Teacher's Report Form for Ages 6–18 (TRF)	Teachers, school counselors
Youth Self-Report for Ages 11–18 (YSR)	Youth
Brief Problem Monitor for Ages 6–18 (BPM)	Parents, teachers, youth
Semistructured Clinical Interview for Children and Adolescents (SCICA)	Clinical interviewers
Direct Observation Form (DOF)	Observers
Test Observation Form (TOF)	Psychological examiners
Adult Self-Report for Ages 18–59 (ASR)	Adults
Adult Behavior Checklist for Ages 18–59 (ABCL)	Adult collaterals
Older Adult Self-Report for Ages 60–90+ (OASR)	Older adults
Older Adult Behavior Checklist for Ages 60–90+ (OABCL)	Older adult collaterals

Completed in about 1–2 minutes, parallel BPM forms obtain ratings from parent figures and staff in residential facilities (BPM-P), teachers and other school staff (BPM-T), and youths who rate their own functioning (BPM-Y). The BPM can be completed repeatedly to monitor functioning and to assess a child's responses to interventions (RTIs), as well as for research comparisons of children receiving different intervention conditions. To link BPM scores with the more comprehensive instruments needed for initial and outcome assessments, the BPM items and scales have counterparts on the Child Behavior Checklist for Ages 6–18 (CBCL/6–18), Teacher's Report Form (TRF), and Youth Self-Report (YSR). Equally important, like the software for other ASEBA instruments (described later), the BPM software provides cross-informant comparisons of ratings by different informants, as well as comparisons with norms for the child's age and gender, the type of informant (parent, teacher, youth), and dozens of different societies, as explained later.

THEORY UNDERLYING THE METHOD

Numerous theories have been constructed to explain human behavior and emotions. Very broad psychoanalytic and behavioral theories for explaining most aspects of human functioning have given way to theoretical models for representing relations among particular measurable variables. Consistent with the shift from broad explanatory theories to more specific models, ASEBA research employs computerized multivariate methods to derive taxonomic models for behavioral, emotional, and social problems from ratings of large samples of individuals by various informants. Psychometric theory has guided the construction of the rating instruments and the derivation of taxonomic models from data obtained with the instruments.

Figure 6.1 illustrates the hierarchical model derived from CBCL/6–18, TRF, and YSR ratings of tens of thousands of clinically referred and nonreferred children, as detailed elsewhere (Achenbach & Rescorla, 2001). The base of the hierarchy in Figure 6.1 comprises problem items rated 0, 1, or 2 by parents, teachers, and children themselves. Exploratory factor analyses (EFAs) and confirmatory factor analyses (CFAs) were used to identify syndromes of covarying problems. These syndromes are embodied in the following eight scales, which are labeled in terms of summary descriptions of their constituent items: Anxious/Depressed, Withdrawn/Depressed, Somatic Complaints, Social Problems, Thought Problems, Attention Problems, Rule-Breaking Behavior, and Aggressive Behavior. Second-order factor analyses have yielded a broad grouping of the Anxious/Depressed, Withdrawn/Depressed, and Somatic Complaints syndromes that are collectively scored on a scale designated as Internalizing, plus a broad grouping of the Rule-Breaking Behavior and Aggressive Behavior syndromes that are

	Total Problems							
Broad Groupings	Internalizing						Externalizing	
Syndromes	Anxious/ Depressed	Withdrawn/ Depressed	Somatic Complaints	Social Problems	Thought Problems	Attention Problems	Rule-Breaking Behavior	Aggressive Behavior
Examples of Problem Items*	Cries	Enjoys little	Aches, pains	Clumsy	Can't get mind off thoughts	Acts young	Bad companions	Argues
	Fears	Lacks energy	Eye problems	Gets teased	Hears things	Can't concentrate	Breaks rules	Attacks people
	Feels Unloved	Rather be alone	Feels dizzy	Jealous	Repeats acts	Can't sit still	Lacks guilt	Disobedient
	Feels too guilty	Refuses to talk	Headaches	Lonely	Sees things	Confused	Lies, cheats	Fights
	Talks or thinks of suicide	Sad	Nausea	Not liked	Strange behavior	Daydrams	Sets fires	Loud
	Worries	Secretive	Overtired	Prefers younger kids	Strange ideas	Fails to finish	Steals	Mean
		Shy, timid	Stomachaches	Too dependent		Impulsive	Swearing	Screams
		Withdrawn	Tired			Inattentive	Truant	Temper
			Vomiting			Stares	Vandalism	Threatens

*Abbreviated versions of the CBCL/6–18, TRF, and YSR items.

FIGURE 6.1. Hierarchical model of ASEBA assessment levels exemplified with items and syndromes scored from the CBCL/6–18, TRF, and YSR. From Achenbach (2009, p. 82). Copyright 2009 by Thomas M. Achenbach. Reprinted by permission.

collectively scored on a scale designated as Externalizing. The syndrome scales and the broad Internalizing and Externalizing scales are scored by summing the 0–1–2 ratings of the items comprising each scale. The Total Problems scale shown at the top of the hierarchy in Figure 6.1 is scored by summing the 0–1–2 ratings of all problem items of the CBCL/6–18, TRF, or YSR, including items that are not on any of the eight syndrome scales. The Total Problems score serves as a general psychopathology measure analogous to Full Scale IQ scores on ability tests.

The model illustrated in Figure 6.1 is supported by thousands of studies of the reliability, validity, and utility of scores at each of the four levels of the hierarchy and of relations between the levels (see Achenbach, 2009; Bérubé & Achenbach, 2013). These studies include longitudinal and outcome tests of the long-term predictive power of ASEBA scores (e.g., Hofstra, van der Ende, & Verhulst, 2002; MacDonald & Achenbach, 1999); tests of genetic and environmental influences on ASEBA scales (e.g., Eley, Lichtenstein, & Moffitt, 2003); and tests of the replicability of ASEBA syndromes in many societies (Ivanova, Achenbach, Rescorla, Dumenci, Almqvist, Bathiche, et al., 2007; Ivanova, Achenbach, Rescorla, Dumenci, Almqvist, Bilenberg, et al., 2007; Ivanova, Dobrean, et al., 2007; Ivanova et al., 2010, 2011).

The eight syndrome scales, the Internalizing and Externalizing scales, and the Total Problems scale can be viewed as measuring hierarchically related taxonomic constructs; "constructs" are defined as "object(s) of thought constituted by the ordering or systematic uniting of experiential elements" (Gove, 1971, p. 489). Each construct comprises a set of covarying problems identified in ratings by parents, teachers, and children. In statistical terms, each construct can be viewed as a latent variable that is measured by the sum of 0–1–2 ratings of the CBCL/6–18, TRF, or YSR items constituting the scale that measures the construct. Profiles display CBCL/6–18, TRF, and YSR item ratings and scale scores in a hierarchical fashion, as illustrated in Figure 6.2.

The ASEBA model illustrated in Figure 6.1 was derived from empirical data, but it can be used to generate and aggregate new data, which in turn may be used to modify the model. The model in Figure 6.1 is, in fact, an outgrowth of earlier models that were revised on the basis of new data (Achenbach, 1991; Achenbach & Edelbrock, 1983). In addition to being scored in terms of scales for empirically derived constructs, ASEBA instruments are scored in terms of scales based on diagnostic categories of the American Psychiatric Association's (2000) *Diagnostic and Statistical Manual of Mental Disorders* (DSM) and other constructs. DSM-oriented scales were constructed by having expert psychiatrists and psychologists from many societies identify ASEBA items they judged to be very consistent with criteria for particular DSM diagnostic categories. Items identified by a large majority of the experts were used to construct the following DSM-oriented scales for ages 6–18: Affective Problems, Anxiety Problems,

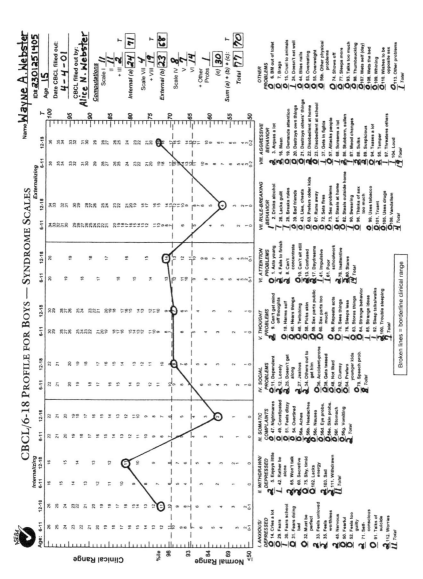

FIGURE 6.2. Hand-scored Syndrome Profile from CBCL/6–18 completed for 15-year-old Wayne Webster by his mother. Computer-scored profiles are also available. From Achenbach and Rescorla (2001, p. 23). Copyright 2001 by Thomas M. Achenbach. Reprinted by permission.

139

Somatic Problems, Attention Deficit Hyperactivity Problems, Oppositional Defiant Problems, and Conduct Problems (Achenbach & Rescorla, 2001). In addition, sets of ASEBA problems shown by research to be good measures of other clinical constructs have been used to construct scales for scoring the CBCL/6–18, TRF, and YSR. These include scales designated as Obsessive–Compulsive Problems, Posttraumatic Stress Problems, and Sluggish Cognitive Tempo (Achenbach & Rescorla, 2007a). Note that the empirically derived scales shown in Figure 6.1, the DSM-oriented scales, and the latter three scales are all scored from the same pool of CBCL/6–18, TRF, and YSR items. Some items are included in all three kinds of scales, whereas other items are included in only one or two kinds of scales. In effect, the three different kinds of scales provide different templates for aggregating the items rated by parents, teachers, and children.

PSYCHOMETRIC PROPERTIES

Psychometric theory provides a variety of criteria for evaluating assessment scales in terms of data obtained on samples of people (see McLeod, Jensen-Doss, & Ollendick, Chapter 1, this volume, for a discussion of psychometric qualities relevant to checklists and rating scales). Extensive psychometric data have been published for all ASEBA instruments (Bérubé & Achenbach, 2013). Table 6.2 summarizes Cronbach's (1951) alpha coefficients for internal consistency and Pearson correlations (r) for test–retest reliabilities of competence, adaptive functioning, and problem scales scored from ASEBA forms completed by lay informants for ages 6–18. For all the scales, criterion-related validity has been supported by findings that children referred for mental health services scored significantly *lower* on competence and adaptive functioning scales and significantly *higher* on problem scales than demographically similar non-referred children, after age, ethnicity, gender, and socioeconomic status (SES) were partialed out (Achenbach et al., 2011; Achenbach & Rescorla, 2001, 2007a).

The construct validity of the scales has been supported by hundreds of studies that have found significant associations with many other measures of psychopathology, including the Conners (2001) scales, the BASC (Reynolds & Kamphaus, 1992), the SDQ (Goodman, 1997), and DSM diagnoses obtained from standardized diagnostic interviews and from clinical evaluations (Achenbach & Rescorla, 2001; Bérubé & Achenbach, 2013; Ferdinand, 2008). Other studies have found significant associations with particular genetic and neurophysiological factors, as well as significant predictions of long-term outcomes for children receiving treatment and children in general population samples (Achenbach, 2009; Achenbach & Rescorla, 2007b; Hofstra et al., 2002; Visser, van der Ende, Koot, & Verhulst, 2003).

TABLE 6.2. Alphas and Test–Retest Reliabilities for CBCL/6–18, TRF, YSR, and BPM Scales

Scales	Alpha[a]	Test–retest reliability[b]
Competence and Adaptive Functioning		
CBCL/6–18 Narrow-Band Competence scales	.67	.88
CBCL/6–18 Total Competence	.79	.91
TRF Academic Performance	NA	.93
TRF Total Adaptive	.90	.93
YSR Narrow-Band Competence scales	.64	.87
YSR Total Competence	.75	.89
YSR Positive Qualities	.75[c]	.83
Empirically based syndromes		
CBCL/6–18	.83	.89
TRF	.85	.89
YSR	.79	.79
BPM[d] Attention Problems	.82	.84
DSM-oriented scales		
CBCL/6–18	.82	.88
TRF	.84	.85
YSR	.76	.79
Internalizing and Externalizing		
CBCL/6–18	.92	.92
TRF	.93	.88
YSR	.90	.85
BPM[d]	.82	.84
Total Problems		
CBCL/6–18	.97	.94
TRF	.97	.95
YSR	.95	.87
BPM[d]	.89	.89
Problem scales added in 2007		
CBCL/6–18	.61[e]	.84
TRF	.69[e]	.84
YSR	.70[e]	.80

Note. Samples included children referred for mental health services and nonreferred children, as detailed by Achenbach and Rescorla (2001). Except for Total Problems, coefficients are means computed by averaging coefficients for all the relevant scales. NA, not applicable.

[a]Mean alphas for N = 1,938–3,210.

[b]Mean test–retest intervals = 8–16 days. N = 44–89.

[c]Mean alpha for 27,206 alphas from multicultural samples, as detailed by Achenbach and Rescorla (2007a).

[d]BPM alphas and test–retest reliabilities are averaged over versions completed by parents, teachers, and youth (BPM-P, BPM-T, BPM-Y; Achenbach et al., 2011).

[e]Mean alphas for 55,508 CBCLs, 30,957 TRFs, and 27,206 YSRs from multicultural samples, as detailed by Achenbach and Rescorla (2007a).

Cross-Informant Comparisons

Meta-analyses of many studies using many different rating and interview instruments have yielded correlations in the .20s and .30s between ratings of children's problems by informants playing different roles with respect to the children who are rated, such as parents versus teachers versus mental health workers versus observers (Achenbach, McConaughy, & Howell, 1987; Duhig, Renk, Epstein, & Phares, 2000; Renk & Phares, 2004). Correlations between children's self-ratings and ratings by adults tend to be even lower. Correlations in the .60s are often found between ratings by adults who see children in similar contexts, such as mothers and fathers, or pairs of teachers in the same school setting. However, even these correlations are not high enough to ensure that a particular adult's ratings of a child will yield the same information as ratings by another adult who sees the child in the same general context, much less ratings by adults who see the child in other contexts or self-ratings by the child.

Because discrepancies between informants' ratings of children's problems are regarded as being "among the most robust findings in clinical child research" (De Los Reyes & Kazdin, 2005, p. 483), most professionals who work with children now recognize the need to obtain data from multiple informants. Unfortunately, when discrepancies are found between different informants, some professionals ask, "Which one should I believe?" Because the reliability, validity, and utility of parent, teacher, and self-ratings have been supported in numerous studies, ratings by all these kinds of informants can be valuable, even when they disagree. It is therefore important to glean information from discrepancies as well as from agreements between informants, rather than to try choosing which informant to believe.

Informant discrepancies may reflect important differences between children's behaviors in different contexts (such as home vs. school) and with different interaction partners even in the same general context (such as a child's mother vs. the child's father, or a teacher in math class vs. a teacher in history class). Discrepancies may also stem from differences between informants' mindsets, sensitivity to the occurrence of particular behaviors, memories of particular behaviors, and thresholds for reporting particular observations of a child for purposes of clinical assessments. For example, behaviors of concern to a teacher who is trying to teach and maintain discipline in a class of many students may not be observed or reported by a parent who sees a child in family contexts.

Documentation of informant discrepancies is essential for comprehensive clinical assessment in order to identify differences between a child's functioning in different contexts, as perceived and rated by different informants. By obtaining data from multiple informants, practitioners can also identify "outlier" informants who differ from all the other informants in reporting more, fewer, or different problems than other informants report. When cross-informant comparisons reveal an outlier informant, practitioners can investigate to determine whether something about the context in which this informant sees the child, or the informant's characteristics, or both might help explain the differences from other informants' ratings.

Methods for Using Cross-Informant Data

To make it easy for practitioners to obtain parallel data for comparison among multiple informants, most problem items on the CBCL/6–18, TRF, and YSR have counterparts on all three forms, although a few items are specific to one or two forms. The items that are specific to one or two forms assess problems that are unlikely to be ratable by all three kinds of informants. For example, an item for rating nightmares is on the CBCL/6–18 and YSR but not on the TRF, whereas an item for rating disruption of class discipline is on the TRF but not on the CBCL/6–18 or YSR.

To enable practitioners to identify agreements and disagreements between informants' ratings of parallel items, the ASEBA software provides side-by-side displays of 0–1–2 ratings of the parallel problem items by up to eight informants, as illustrated in Figure 6.3. The cross-informant comparisons can include any combination of parent, teacher, and self-ratings. As Figure 6.3 shows, practitioners can quickly identify problems that are rated 0 by all informants (e.g., item 21 on the Anxious/Depressed syndrome), items that are endorsed (i.e., are rated 1 or 2) by all informants (e.g., item 5 on the Withdrawn/Depressed syndrome), and items that are endorsed by some informants but not others (e.g., item 75 on the Withdrawn/Depressed syndrome). The fact that item 75 ("Too shy or timid"), was endorsed only by two teachers suggests that this characteristic may have been evident only in those teachers' classes.

In addition to the side-by-side displays of item ratings, the ASEBA software also displays standardized scale scores in terms of bar graphs, as illustrated in Figure 6.4. Each bar represents the T score for a scale scored from a particular informant's ratings. The T scores are standardized on the basis of norms for the child's age and gender, the type of informant (parent, teacher, self), and the user-selected multicultural norm group (explained in the following section). T scores below 65 (i.e., below the bottom broken line in Figure 6.4) are in the normal range (< 93rd percentile for the child's age and gender, the type of informant, and the multicultural norm group). T scores of 65–69 (i.e., in the interval demarcated by the two broken lines in Figure 6.4) are in the borderline clinical range (93rd–97th percentile). And T scores above 69 (i.e., above the top broken line in Figure 6.4) are in the clinical range (> 97th percentile). Similar bar graphs display children's scores on the six DSM-oriented scales, as well as on the Internalizing, Externalizing, and Total Problems scales.

As an additional aid to using data from multiple informants, the ASEBA software displays a Q correlation between the 0–1–2 ratings of

Cross-Informant Comparison - Problem Items Common to the CBCL/TRF/YSR

ID: 23012511405 Name: Wayne Webster Gender: Male Birth Date: 03/03/1986 Comparison Date: 04/13/2001

Form	Eval ID	Age	Informant Name	Relationship	Date
CBC1	001	15	Alice N. Webster	Biological Mother	04/04/2001
CBC2	002	15	Ralph F. Webster	Biological Father	04/05/2001
YSR3	003	15	Self	Self	04/08/2001
TRF4	004	15	George Jackson	Classroom Teacher [M]	04/10/2001

Form	Eval ID	Age	Informant Name	Relationship	Date
TRF5	005	15	Carmen Hernandez	Classroom Teacher (F)	04/11/2001
TRF6	006	15	Charles Dwyer	Classroom Teacher (M)	04/12/2001

Columns 1–8: CBC · CBC · YSR · TRF · TRF · TRF · (7) · (8)

Anxious/Depressed

Item	1	2	3	4	5	6
14.Cries	0	0	0	0	0	0
29.Fears	0	1	0	0	0	0
30.FearSchool	1	0	0	0	0	0
31.FearDoBad	0	0	0	0	0	0
32.Perfect	2	1	2	0	0	1
33.Unloved	2	2	2	0	0	0
35.Worthless	2	2	2	1	0	0
45.Nervous	2	2	2	2	1	0
50.Fearful	0	0	0	0	0	0
52.Guilty	0	0	0	0	0	0
71.SelfConc	2	2	1	1	2	0
91.Suicide	0	0	2	0	0	0
112.Worries	2	2	2	2	0	0

Withdrawn/Depressed

Item	1	2	3	4	5	6
5.EnjoysLittle	2	1	2	2	2	1
42.PreferAlone	1	1	2	2	1	2
65.Won'tTalk	2	1	2	2	1	2
69.Secretive	2	1	2	2	1	2
75.Shy	0	0	0	2	0	0
102.LacksEnergy	2	2	0	0	1	0
103.Sad	2	2	2	2	1	0
111.Withdrawn	2	1	2	2	2	2

Somatic Complaints

Item	1	2	3	4	5	6
51.Dizzy	0	1	1	0	0	0
54.Tired	0	2	1	0	0	0
56a.Aches	0	2	0	0	0	0
56b.Headaches	2	0	0	0	0	0
56c.Nausea	0	0	0	0	0	0
56d.EyeProb	0	0	0	0	0	0
56e.SkinProb	0	0	1	0	0	0
56f.Stomach	0	0	0	0	0	0
56g.Vomit	0	0	0	0	0	0

Social Problems

Item	1	2	3	4	5	6
11.Dependent	0	2	2	0	1	2
12.Lonely	2	0	2	1	0	0
25.NotGetAlong	2	1	1	0	1	0
27.Jealous	2	1	0	0	0	0
34.OutToGet	2	2	2	2	1	0
36.GetsHurt	0	2	2	0	1	0
38.Teased	0	0	1	1	0	2
48.NotLiked	0	1	2	0	1	2
62.Clumsy	0	0	0	0	1	0
64.PreferYoung	1	0	0	1	0	1
79.SpeechProb	0	0	0	0	0	0

Thought Problems

Item	1	2	3	4	5	6
9.MindOff	2	1	2	2	1	2
18.HarmSelf	0	0	0	0	0	0
40.HearsThings	0	0	1	0	0	0
46.Twitch	0	0	2	0	0	0
58.PicksSkin	0	0	0	0	0	0
66.RepeatsActs	2	2	1	1	0	0
70.SeesThings	0	0	0	0	0	0
83.StoresUp	0	1	0	0	2	0
84.StrangeBehav	0	0	1	1	0	2
85.StrangeIdeas	1	0	2	2	0	1

Attention Problems

Item	1	2	3	4	5	6
1.ActsYoung	0	2	0	0	2	2
4.FailsToFinish	2	2	2	2	1	0
8.Concentrate	2	2	2	2	1	1
10.SitStill	0	2	2	0	1	0
13.Confused	2	2	2	2	1	2
17.Daydream	2	1	1	2	1	2
41.Impulsive	1	2	2	2	2	0
61.PoorSchool	1	1	2	1	2	0
78.Inattentive	2	2	2	2	1	1

Columns 1–8: CBC · CBC · YSR · TRF · TRF · TRF · TRF · (8)

Rule-Breaking Behavior

Item	1	2	3	4	5	6	7
26.NoGuilt	1	2	0	2	1	1	
28.BreaksRules	1	2	0	2	0	1	
39.BadFriends	2	1	2	0	0	0	
43.LieCheat	0	0	0	0	0	0	
63.PreferOlder	0	0	0	0	0	0	
82.StealsOther	0	0	0	0	0	0	
90.Swears	1	2	1	2	0	0	
96.ThinksSex	0	0	0	1	0	0	
99.Tobacco	0	0	0	0	0	0	
101.Truant	0	0	1	0	0	0	
105.UsedDrugs	0	0	0	0	0	0	

Aggressive Behavior

Item	1	2	3	4	5	6	7
3.Argues	2	1	2	2	1	2	
16.Mean	0	1	1	0	1	0	
19.DemAtten	0	1	0	1	0	2	
20.DestroyOwn	0	0	0	0	0	0	
21.DestroyOther	0	0	0	0	0	0	
23.DisobeySchl	1	2	1	2	1	0	
37.Fights	0	1	0	1	0	0	
57.Attacks	0	2	0	1	0	0	
68.Screams	1	2	0	2	0	2	
86.Stubborn	2	1	2	1	2	2	
87.MoodChang	2	1	2	2	2	2	
89.Suspicious	2	1	2	2	0	2	
94.Teases	0	2	0	2	0	0	
95.Temper	2	2	2	2	1	1	
97.Threaten	2	0	0	2	0	0	
104.Loud	1	0	1	0	0	0	

Other Problems

Item	1	2	3	4	5	6	7
44.BiteNail	0	0	0	0	0	0	
55.Overweight	0	2	0	2	0	0	
56h.OtherPhys	0	0	0	0	0	0	

{F}=Female {M}=Male

FIGURE 6.3. Cross-informant comparisons of item scores for Wayne Webster. From Achenbach and Rescorla (2001, p. 36). Copyright 2001 by Thomas M. Achenbach. Reprinted by permission.

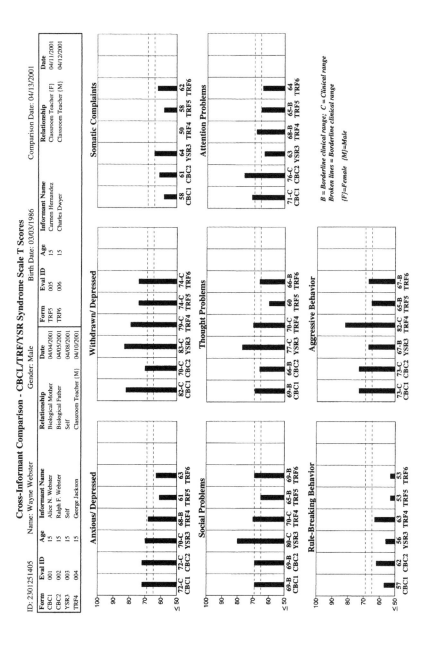

FIGURE 6.4. Cross-informant comparisons of syndrome scores for Wayne Webster. From Achenbach and Rescorla (2001, p. 39). Copyright 2001 by Thomas M. Achenbach. Reprinted by permission.

problem items by each pair of informants. Each Q correlation is computed by applying the formula for Pearson r to the two sets of item ratings from a pair of informants. In other words, the Q correlations (ranging from −1.00 to +1.00) indicate the degree of agreement between the two informants' ratings of one child, unlike R correlations, which indicate the degree of agreement between scores for two variables across many cases. To help practitioners evaluate the magnitude of the Q correlation between each pair of informants, the software also displays the 25th percentile, mean, and 75th percentile correlations obtained in large reference samples of pairs of informants like those whose Q correlation is being evaluated. If the correlation between a pair of informants for a particular child is below the 25th percentile, it is labeled as "below average"; if the correlation is between the 25th and 75th percentile, it is labeled as "average"; and if the correlation is above the 75th percentile, it is labeled as "above average". If the Q correlation between particular informants is below average for those kinds of informants, this could prompt the practitioner to investigate why agreement between the informants is so low. For example, if the Q correlation between a child's mother and father is below average, the practitioner could discuss with the parents why one parent reported more problems in general or more problems of a particular kind than the other parent did.

To provide practitioners with text that can be exported into reports and used for other purposes, the ASEBA software generates narrative reports of the findings. To alert practitioners to problems that may be especially critical, the narrative reports display each informant's ratings of critical items that clinicians have identified as raising particular challenges for management. Examples include "Deliberately harms self or attempts suicide," "Hears sounds or voices that aren't there", "Physically attacks people," and "Sets fires."

Norms

In order to evaluate scores on measures of behavioral, emotional, and social problems, practitioners need to compare scale scores obtained by a particular child with normative distributions of scores. Some measures have no norms, whereas "norms" for other measures are based on samples of convenience that are not representative of any relevant populations. To be valid, norms should be based on distributions of scores obtained by large samples of children who are like the child being assessed with respect to such important characteristics as age and gender, and who are representative of the population relevant to the child with respect to variations in such characteristics as ethnicity, SES, urban–suburban–rural residence, and geographical area. To obtain the representative samples needed for valid norms, it is necessary to assess children who are selected from the relevant population by systematic procedures, such as stratified random sampling. It is also necessary to have assessments completed for high percentages of the children selected for the samples. Otherwise, even if samples are well selected to be representative of relevant populations, low completion rates are apt to yield biased results because the noncompleters may differ from the completers in important ways.

Because the distributions of scores obtained from different kinds of informants may also differ, it should not be assumed that norms obtained from parent ratings can be used to evaluate teacher or self-ratings, or vice versa. Consequently, it is necessary to obtain different informants' ratings of normative samples of children and to construct separate norms for the different kinds of informants. Based on stratified random sampling procedures, the first normative data for CBCL/6–18 ratings were obtained by interviewers who visited randomly selected homes in Washington, D.C., Maryland, and Virginia in the 1970s (Achenbach & Edelbrock, 1981). The 1991 and 2001 norms for the CBCL/6–18, TRF, and YSR were obtained from ratings of national probability samples of children residing throughout the United States in randomly selected homes visited by interviewers, who asked parents to complete the CBCL/6–18 and asked 11- to 18-year-olds to complete the YSR (Achenbach, 1991; Achenbach & Rescorla, 2001). For the national sample on which the 2001 CBCL/6–18 was normed ($N = 1,753$), the completion rate was 93%. Of the 11- to 18-year-olds whose parents completed the CBCL/6–18, 96.5% completed the YSR ($N = 1,057$). With parents' consent, the TRF was mailed to the children's teachers for completion. Gender distributions were approximately 50–50 female–male. Ethnicity was approximately 60% European American, 20% African American, 9% Hispanic/Latino, and 12% mixed or other.

Constructing Multicultural Norms

The distributions of scale scores found for the U.S. national sample were used to construct gender-specific norms for CBCL/6–18 and TRF ratings separately for ages 6–11 and 12–18, as well as YSR ratings for ages 11–18. Because ASEBA instruments have been translated into 90 languages, and there are published reports of findings from 80 societies (Bérubé & Achenbach, 2013), ASEBA instruments are widely used to assess children from many societies and cultural groups. In order to provide norms for evaluating children outside the United States, as well as children whose families immigrate to the United States and other host societies, norms have been constructed from ASEBA ratings of population samples of children from many societies, as listed in Table 6.3. Most of the societies are countries, but some are not, such as Puerto Rico, Hong Kong, and Flanders (the Flemish-speaking region of Belgium). CFAs have supported the fit of the CBCL/6–18, TRF, and YSR eight-syndrome model to ratings of children in all societies in which population samples were assessed with one or more of these forms (Ivanova, Achenbach, Rescorla, Dumenci, Almqvist, Bathiche,

TABLE 6.3. Group 1, 2, and 3 Societies for CBCL, C-TRF, TRF, and YSR Scales

Society	CBCL/1½–5	C-TRF	CBCL/6–18	TRF	YSR	YSR-PQ[a]
ASEBA Standard[b]	2	2	2	2	2	2
Algeria	NA	NA	3	NA	NA	NA
Australia	2	NA	2	2	2	3
Austria	NA	2	NA	NA	NA	NA
Bangladesh	NA	NA	NA	NA	3	NA
Belgium (Flanders)	2	NA	2	NA	NA	NA
Brazil	NA	NA	3	NA	3	3
Chile	3	2	NA	NA	NA	NA
China	2	2	1	1	2	NA
Colombia	NA	NA	3	NA	NA	NA
Croatia	NA	NA	2	2	2	3
Denmark	1	1	2	2	2	2
Ethiopia	NA	NA	3	NA	2	1
Finland	2	NA	2	1	1	2
France	2	NA	2	2	3	2
Germany	2	2	1	NA	1	2
Greece	NA	NA	2	2	3	3
Hong Kong	NA	NA	2	2	3	1
Iceland	1	1	1	NA	2	2
India (Telegu)	NA	NA	NA	NA	3	2
Iran	2	3	2	2	2	2
Israel	NA	NA	2	NA	2	2
Italy	2	2	2	2	3	2
Jamaica	NA	NA	2	3	2	2
Japan	NA	NA	1	1	2	1
Korea (South)	2	NA	2	NA	2	1
Kosovo	2	NA	2	2	3	2
Lebanon	NA	NA	NA	2	NA	NA
Lithuania	3	3	2	2	3	2
Netherlands	2	2	2	2	2	2
Norway	NA	NA	1	2	1	3
Pakistan	NA	NA	3	NA	NA	NA
Peru	2	NA	2	NA	NA	NA
Poland	NA	NA	2	2	2	2
Portugal	2	2	3	2	NA	NA
Puerto Rico	NA	NA	3	3	2	2
Romania	2	3	2	2	2	2
Russia	NA	NA	2	NA	NA	NA
Serbia	1	2	1	2	NA	NA
Singapore	2	NA	2	1	NA	NA
Spain	1	NA	NA	NA	3	2
Sweden	NA	NA	1	2	2	2
Switzerland (German)	NA	NA	2	NA	2	2

TABLE 6.3. *(continued)*

Society	CBCL/1½–5	C-TRF	CBCL/6–18	TRF	YSR	YSR-PQ[a]
Taiwan	3	NA	2	2	NA	NA
Thailand	NA	NA	2	3	NA	NA
Tunisia	NA	NA	3	NA	3	2
Turkey	2	NA	2	3	2	2
United Arab Emirates	2	NA	NA	NA	NA	NA
United States	2	2	2	2	2	3
Uruguay	NA	NA	2	NA	NA	NA

Note. NA, normative sample not available at this writing. Group 1, societies with mean Total Problems scores more than 1 *SD* below the omnicultural mean; Group 2, societies with mean Total Problems scores between –1 and +1 *SD* from the omnicultural mean; and Group 3, societies with mean Total Problems scores more than 1 *SD* above the omnicultural mean.

[a]PQ, Positive Qualities scale (from Achenbach & Rescorla, 2007a, p. 2).

[b]ASEBA Standard, default (Group 2) norms if norms are not available for the user-selected society.

et al., 2007; Ivanova, Achenbach, Rescorla, Dumenci, Almqvist, Bilenberg, et al., 2007; Ivanova, Dobrean, et al., 2007).

We (Achenbach & Rescorla, 2007a, 2010) provide details elsewhere of how multicultural norms were constructed for ages 6–18 and 1½–5, respectively. The procedures can be summarized as follows:

1. For each instrument, the mean Total Problems score was computed for the population sample from each society.
2. The "omnicultural mean" (Ellis & Kimmel, 1992) Total Problems score was computed by summing the mean Total Problems scores from all the societies and dividing by the number of societies.
3. For each instrument, the mean Total Problems scores from all the available societies formed a normal distribution around the omnicultural mean.
4. Because the mean Total Problems scores from all the available societies spanned a relatively small range with no extreme outliers, the societies were divided into the following groups: Group 1 (societies with mean Total Problems scores more than 1 *SD* below the omnicultural mean); Group 2 (societies with mean Total Problems scores between –1 and +1 *SD* from the omnicultural mean); and Group 3 (societies with mean Total Problems scores more than 1 *SD* above the omnicultural mean).
5. Multicultural norms for Group 1 societies were constructed by averaging the cumulative frequency distributions of scores from all Group 1 societies on each problem scale of an instrument to form a single cumulative frequency distribution of scale scores. This was done separately for scores obtained by each age group and gender on the CBCL, TRF, and YSR. Normalized *T* scores were then

assigned to each raw scale score, based on the score's percentile in the cumulative frequency distribution. The same procedure was followed for constructing multicultural norms for the Group 3 societies. Because the mean Total Problems score for the U.S. national sample was close to the omnicultural mean for each instrument, and because the U.S. norms have been used in so many clinical and research applications, the U.S. norms are used for Group 2 societies' problem scale scores.

Using Multicultural Norms

The Group 1, Group 2, and Group 3 norms are programmed into the software for scoring the CBCL/6–18, TRF, and YSR. The software lists the societies for which normative data are available for each instrument, and indicates whether they are included in Group 1, 2, or 3 for that instrument. When practitioners select a particular society for scoring a particular instrument, such as a Chinese translation of the CBCL/6–18 completed by a father from mainland China, the software will display the scale scores in relation to norms for that society. If a form is completed by an informant from a society that is not listed, the practitioner can select norms for a society that is thought to be similar to the informant's society. If the practitioner does not select a particular society, Group 2 norms serve as the default.

When scale scores from multiple informants are displayed in bar graphs like those illustrated in Figure 6.4, the T score represented by each bar is standardized for Group 1, 2, or 3 norms, depending on the society selected by the user as being appropriate for each informant. As explained earlier, each bar is also standardized for the age and gender of the child being assessed and for the type of informant (parent, teacher, self). For some children, it may be appropriate to display scale scores from instruments completed by different informants in relation to different sets of multicultural norms. For example, if a boy's father came from mainland China, scale scores from the father's CBCL/6–18 would be displayed in relation to Group 1 CBCL/6–18 norms. If the boy's mother came from Hong Kong, scale scores from the mother's CBCL/6–18 would be displayed in relation to Group 2 CBCL/6–18 norms appropriate for Hong Kong. If the boy attended a U.S. school, scale scores from the TRFs completed by his teachers would be displayed in relation to Group 2 norms appropriate for the United States. If the boy was moderately acculturated to the United States, his YSR scale scores could be displayed in relation to Group 2 YSR norms, which are appropriate for both mainland China and the United States, as illustrated by the profile in Figure 6.5 for the YSR DSM-oriented scales.

If the boy had lived in Hong Kong or if his Hong Kong mother was thought to be especially influential, his YSR scores could also be displayed in relation to Group 3 YSR norms appropriate for Hong Kong, as illustrated by the profile in Figure 6.6. A practitioner evaluating the boy could

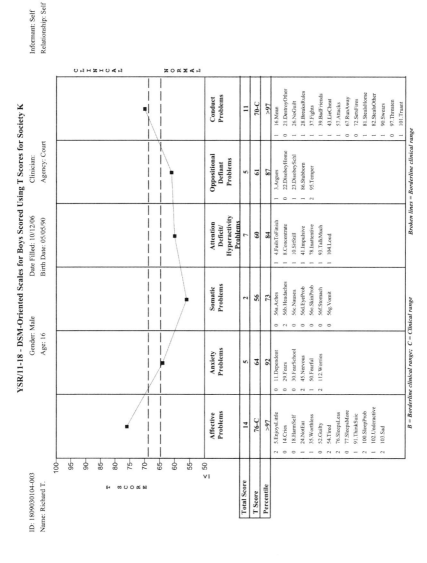

FIGURE 6.5. Profile of DSM-oriented YSR scales in relation to Group 2 norms. From Achenbach and Rescorla (2007a, p. 12). Copyright 2001 by Thomas M. Achenbach. Reprinted by permission.

151

look at all his scores displayed in relation to the appropriate multicultural norms and determine which scales were in the borderline or clinical ranges according to any of the norms and which scales did not reach even the borderline range according to any of the norms. If there were major discrepancies between the elevations of scales scored from instruments completed by different informants and/or the boy's YSR scores in relation to Group 2 versus Group 3 norms, the practitioner could consider possible cultural variations in whether particular problem levels were deviant in relation to mainland Chinese, Hong Kong, or U.S. norms. For example, by comparing the profiles shown in Figures 6.5 and 6.6, the practitioner would see that the boy's score for the DSM-oriented Affective Problems scale was in the clinical range, according to both Group 2 and Group 3 norms. However, the boy's score for the DSM-oriented Conduct Problems scale was in the clinical range according to Group 2 norms but not Group 3 norms.

APPLICATION TO THE CASE OF SOFIA

The editors of this volume have provided the case of Sofia in Chapter 4 as an example of "internalizing disorders." Several of Sofia's problems were consistent with the second-order factor-analytically derived grouping of problems for which I (Achenbach, 1966) coined the term "internalizing." Comprising problems such as depression, anxiety, social withdrawal, and somatic complaints without known medical cause, internalizing groupings of problems have been found in many other studies, using many samples, assessment instruments, and analytic methods (Achenbach & Edelbrock, 1978, 1984; Achenbach, Conners, Quay, Verhulst, & Howell, 1989; Krueger & Piasecki, 2002).

Internalizing groupings consist of diverse problems having varying degrees of association with one another. Very few children manifest either all or none of the problems that might be labeled as internalizing. Furthermore, although the term "externalizing" was coined for another second-order factor-analytically derived grouping of problems (aggressive and rule-breaking behavior; Achenbach, 1966), children may have both internalizing and externalizing problems in various degrees, as well as problems that are associated with both groupings or are not strongly associated with either grouping (e.g., attention problems, social problems, thought problems; Achenbach & Rescorla, 2001). Even among those whose problems are mainly associated with the internalizing grouping, children vary in the degree to which they manifest problems of depression or anxiety, social withdrawal, somatic complaints, or various combinations of these problems. A particular child may also manifest different patterns and degrees of problems in different contexts, with different interaction partners (e.g., mother vs. father, math teacher vs. history teacher), at different points in time, and during different developmental periods.

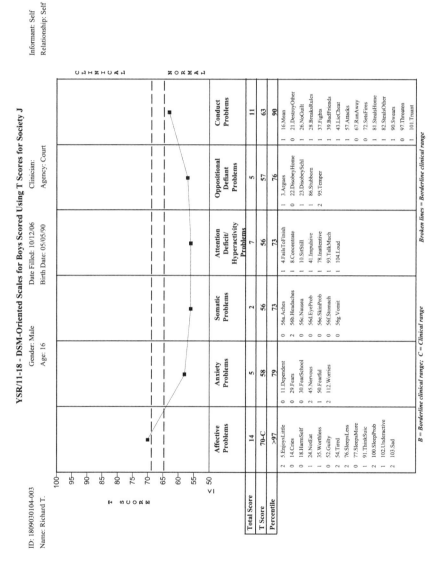

FIGURE 6.6. Profile of DSM-oriented YSR scales in relation to Group 3 norms. From Achenbach and Rescorla (2007a, p. 11). Copyright 2001 by Thomas M. Achenbach. Reprinted by permission.

153

For all the foregoing reasons, it is essential that even children for whom referral complaints specify certain disorders (e.g., internalizing, externalizing, ADHD) receive assessments that are sufficiently comprehensive to take account of a broad spectrum of problems, competence, adaptive functioning, and family variables. In other words, referral complaints should not be allowed to cause premature closure on assumed disorders. It is especially important to avoid assessing children only with procedures targeted on the referral complaints. For example, if we use only ADHD instruments to assess children who are referred for ADHD, we may fail to find that they have problems such as depression, anxiety, aggression, and so on, instead of or in addition to attention problems.

The cases provided by the editors richly illustrate the multiple facets of child and family functioning that can and should be assessed. The following discussion outlines applications of ASEBA instruments to Sofia's case. It would, of course, also be important to consider the history of Sofia's development and problems, as well as medical and psychoeducational evaluations. To communicate effectively with Sofia's parents, the practitioner would need to be able to speak Spanish.

Initial Assessment of Sofia's Competence, Adaptive Functioning, and Problems

Completion of the CBCL/6–18 would be requested as a routine part of the intake process. Parents who have at least fifth-grade reading skills can typically complete the CBCL/6–18 in 15–20 minutes, either in paper-and-pencil or online format, at home or in the practitioner's office. The Latin American Spanish CBCL/6–18 would be provided for Adriana and Sergio. If there was any doubt about their ability to complete the CBCL/6–18 alone, it could be read to them, and their answers could be entered on a paper copy or online by a staff member (such as a receptionist). If the CBCL/6–18 was completed in paper-and-pencil format, a clerical worker could subsequently enter the responses into the scoring software in about 3–5 minutes or could complete a hand-scored profile in about 5–10 minutes. Sofia would be asked to complete the YSR in English or Latin American Spanish, whichever she preferred. With parental consent, the TRF would be sent to one or more of Sofia's teachers, either in paper-and-pencil format or online, whichever they preferred.

As part of the initial assessment, a practitioner would typically conduct a clinical interview with Sofia. The Semistructured Clinical Interview for Children and Adolescents (SCICA; McConaughy & Achenbach, 2001) provides a protocol of semistructured open-ended questions that can be flexibly tailored to the interviewee. The questions cover various areas of functioning, such as school, relations with family and peers, interests, fantasies, and emotions. It also includes exploration of the interviewee's attitudes toward six problems that have been rated as "very true" or "often true" on the CBCL/6–18 and/or TRF completed for the interviewee. Interviewees are encouraged to express their feelings and to describe events and their own reactions. The interviewer makes brief notes about what the interviewee reports and also about how the interviewee looks and behaves. The interview can be audio- or video-recorded.

Unlike many standardized interviews, the SCICA is designed to document interviewees' appearance and behavior, as well as what they report. Also unlike other interviews, the SCICA provides sets of items on which the interviewer rates the interviewee's self-reports, plus the interviewee's observed behaviors. The ratings are entered into scoring software or on hand-scored profiles that display the interviewee's scores on factor-analytically derived syndromes, DSM-oriented scales, Internalizing, Externalizing, and Total Problems. T scores and percentiles are based on large samples of clinically referred children. The SCICA can make especially important contributions to diagnostic decisions, because it provides a standardized framework within which the practitioner can test diagnostic hypotheses about the child's problems, and can document the child's verbal and other responses. The practitioner can also compare scores on the SCICA's DSM-oriented scales with scores on the DSM-oriented scales for the other ASEBA forms completed for the child.

The SCICA blends well with most practitioners' customary assessment interviews. However, to hone practitioners' skills for administering and rating the SCICA, a training video available in videotape and DVD formats enables practitioners to rate segments of interviews with six children manifesting various patterns of problems. When entered into the SCICA software, the trainees' ratings are compared with the mean of ratings by experienced interviewers. The software displays Q correlations that measure agreement between scale scores for ratings by the trainees and the experienced raters. Displays of ratings for each item and scale, plus profiles based on ratings by the trainee and the experienced raters, reveal specific agreements and discrepancies between the trainee and experienced raters. The trainee can then view and rate the interview segments again as many times as necessary to reach good agreement with the experienced raters.

Initial Assessment of Sofia's Parents

As Table 6.1 shows, ASEBA instruments include self-report and collateral-report forms for ages 18–59 and 60–90+ years. Whenever possible, assessment of children for mental health services should include assessment of adult family members whose functioning is apt to be relevant to the child's functioning and whose participation is important for helping the child. When parents have routinely completed self-report instruments as part of mental health services for their children, significant associations have been found between parent and child scores for particular kinds of psychopathology (Vidair, et al., 2011). Multicultural norms for the ASEBA adult forms are scheduled for release in 2013.

ASEBA adult forms can be self-administered in 15–20 minutes at home or in the practitioner's office, in paper-and-pencil or online format. The forms cover a wide range of adaptive functioning; personal strengths; substance use; and behavioral, emotional, social, and thought problems. Furthermore, the parallel self-report and collateral-report forms provide cross-informant comparisons of item ratings and scale scores like those described earlier for the CBCL/6–18, TRF, and YSR. At no cost in a practitioner's time, parents can routinely complete the adult self-report and collateral-report forms to describe themselves and the other parent. The practitioner can then view the item ratings and profiles to identify issues that may be related to the child's needs for help. For example, if a parent's scores are elevated in areas such as depression, attention problems, or aggressive behavior, these problems may affect the child's functioning, as well as the parent's ability to collaborate in interventions for the child. In some cases, a parent's high problem scores and/or low adaptive functioning or personal strength scores may indicate that the parent needs help separately from or in conjunction with services for the child.

If more than one parent completes the self-report and collateral-report forms, cross-informant comparisons can be used to pinpoint discrepancies and consistencies between how parents see themselves and how each is seen by the other parent. For example, if a mother rates the father much higher on aggressive behavior than he rates himself and he rates the mother much higher on attention problems than she rates herself, these discrepancies would need to be considered in working with the parents in regard to their own functioning as well as the child's.

If the practitioner deems it appropriate and the parents consent, the profiles scored from the self-report and collateral-report forms can be shown to both parents. The profiles make it easy to document concretely how parents see themselves and each other, and to point out discrepancies between their views. This can facilitate parents' understanding of how personal perspectives differ and how one parent may be seen by the other parent as needing help. If the parents are also shown profiles scored from the CBCL/6–18 and from other forms completed for their child, insights gained from seeing their own self-report and collateral-report profiles can help them understand how their child's functioning may be seen differently by different informants. This, in turn, can facilitate more sophisticated and proactive involvement by parents in interventions for helping their child.

In Sofia's case, Adriana's feelings about being unable to cope with Sofia's distress and Sergio's criticisms of Adriana and Sofia would certainly argue for having Adriana and Sergio complete the Adult Self-Report (ASR) to describe themselves, as well as the Adult Behavior Checklist (ABCL) to describe the other parent. Both forms are available in Latin American Spanish translations. Although Adriana said that Sergio was unlikely to participate in treatment, his obvious concerns about Sofia might at least motivate him to complete the ASR and ABCL at home. If necessary, the forms could be administered by phone or by a lay interviewer (e.g., the practitioner's receptionist).

Whether or not the practitioner deemed it appropriate to show the ASR and ABCL profiles to Adriana (and to Sergio if he could be persuaded to attend), the practitioner could use the information to help one or both parents collaborate more effectively in interventions for Sofia. If the ASR and/or ABCL profiles revealed high levels of problems, interventions for one or both parents might also be considered. The limited success of Sofia's previous exposure-based cognitive-behavioral therapy indicated that the behavior of one or both parents might need to change in order to help. Cross-informant comparisons of the CBCL/6–18, TRF, and YSR data could also reveal variations in Sofia's functioning as seen by her parents, her teachers, and herself, which would provide targets for a more differentiated approach than was used previously. A more differentiated approach could be designed to overcome deficits in competencies and adaptive functioning revealed by the CBCL/6–18, TRF, and YSR, as well as to reduce problems. Equally important, the SCICA could indicate the degree to which Sofia could express important issues in one-to-one interviews with the practitioner, and thus whether Sofia was a good candidate for talking therapies versus other approaches.

Assessing Responses to Interventions (RTIs)

If the practitioner recommended interventions and if the family accepted the recommendation, the practitioner could use the BPM to monitor RTIs. Sofia could complete the BPM-Y and one or both parents could complete the BPM-P at intervals selected by the practitioner, such as weekly or every 2 weeks. If Sofia attended school again, teachers could be asked to complete the BPM-T. Because Sofia's school avoidance was intertwined with social withdrawal, inferiority feelings, self-consciousness, anxiety, depression, and worrying, as well as arguments with her father, the BPM's repeated assessments of these problems (as well as additional user-specified problems and strengths) would be important. In fact, alleviation of the problems was apt to be necessary to help Sofia resume normal developmental progress. The practitioner could use the BPM scoring software to make cross-informant comparisons and to track changes in item and scale scores during the course of work with Sofia and her parents. Because Sofia had previously been a good student, was now 15, and could quit school at 16, options such as attending a community college or an alternative school program might be considered.

Assessing Outcomes for Sofia and her Parents

Brief assessments with the BPM can track changes in a child's functioning during the course of interventions and under other conditions where repeated evidence-based assessments are needed, such as after placement in inpatient and residential facilities. However, evaluations of outcomes require more comprehensive assessments that enable practitioners to make rigorous comparisons with comprehensive initial assessments.

At the conclusion of interventions for Sofia, completion of the CBCL/6–18 by one or both parents, the YSR by Sofia, and the TRF by Sofia's teacher(s) (if Sofia was attending school by then) would provide scale scores that could be precisely compared with Sofia's initial scale scores. By comparing the preintervention and postintervention profiles, the practitioner could quickly identify scale scores that had moved from the borderline or clinical range to the normal range and vice versa. To test the statistical significance of changes in scale scores, the practitioner could follow the instructions on page 195 of the *Manual for the ASEBA School-Age Forms & Profiles* (Achenbach & Rescorla, 2001) for applying the standard error of measurement, which is listed for CBCL/6–18, TRF, and YSR scales in Appendix D of the *Manual*. Because Sofia's functioning might change after termination of the intervention, a thorough outcome evaluation would include completion of the ASEBA forms again for at least one follow-up assessment at 6 or more months after termination. If any scale scores were in the borderline or clinical range at that point, the practitioner could consider possible needs for further help. Adriana and Sergio could also be asked to complete the ASR and ABCL for outcome and follow-up assessments of their functioning. Page 179 of the *Manual for the ASEBA Adult Forms & Profiles* (Achenbach & Rescorla, 2003) provides instructions for applying the standard error of measurement data displayed in Appendix D of the *Manual* to test the significance of changes in ASR and ABCL scale scores.

APPLICATION TO THE CASE OF BILLY

As pointed out in the case of Sofia, it is important to assess a broad spectrum of functioning in every case, rather than allowing referral complaints to cause premature closure and to limit assessment only to the referral complaints. Although Billy is described in Chapter 4 as a case example of externalizing disorders, the need to assess nonexternalizing as well as externalizing problems was indicated by his mother's report that he was anxious, feared the dark and sleeping in his own bed, and might have ADHD.

Initial Assessment of Billy's Competencies, Adaptive Functioning, and Problems

As described for Sofia, completion of the CBCL/6–18 would be requested as a routine part of the intake procedure. Because Billy's mother, Mary, was evidently the only adult in the home and Billy's father had little contact with the family, Mary might be the only informant available to complete the CBCL/6–18. However, as Billy was attending school, the practitioner could request Mary's consent to send the TRF to Billy's main teacher for completion. If more than one teacher had regular contact with Billy, a TRF could be sent to each teacher. Although Billy was slightly younger than the 11- to 18-year norm group for the YSR, he could be asked to complete the YSR after his 11th birthday, if the clinical contacts continued that long.

Because of the kinds of problems that were of greatest concern at home and school, and because of Billy's tendency to blame others, the SCICA could be especially useful for assessing Billy's self-reports and behavior in a one-to-one interview with the practitioner. In addition to providing scores for self-reported problems and for observations of Billy, the SCICA would enable the practitioner to judge whether a therapeutic approach that included one-to-one talking sessions might be effective with Billy.

Initial Assessment of Billy's Mother

As part of the routine assessment procedure, Mary would be asked to complete the ASR to describe her own functioning. Mary could also be asked to complete the ABCL to describe Billy's father. Although Billy's father had left the family and was unlikely to be involved in interventions, the practitioner could consider the ABCL profile in relation to Mary's ASR profile and Billy's CBCL/6–18 and TRF profiles. If the ABCL profile revealed high scores on scales that were also elevated for Billy, this might shed light on the development of Billy's problems, Mary's views of similarities between Billy and his father, and the like. The ASR profile could indicate areas in which Mary might need help, either in conjunction with the practitioner's work with Billy or via referral to another practitioner. If the practitioner deemed it appropriate, the CBCL/6–18, ASR, ABCL, and (with the teacher's consent) TRF profiles could be shown to Mary for discussion of similarities and differences among the profiles. The practitioner could also use the SCICA findings and interactions with Mary to judge whether family meetings with Mary, Billy, and possibly Meredith (Billy's sister) would be worthwhile. If Mary expressed concerns about Meredith and/or if the practitioner decided to involve Meredith, Mary could be asked to complete the CBCL/6–18 for Meredith, and Meredith could be asked to complete the YSR.

Assessing Responses to Interventions

Because Billy's problems were reported to occur at school as well as at home, the practitioner would probably include Billy's teachers in intervention plans, such as contingency management and behavioral report cards to keep Mary and the practitioner informed of problems and adaptive functioning in school. If a teacher or teachers were involved, the practitioner could send copies of the BPM-T to Billy's teacher(s), as well as giving copies of the BPM-P to Billy's mother, for completion at intervals such as weekly.

As many children younger than 11 are able to complete the BPM-Y, the practitioner could also ask Billy to complete it. After entry into the BPM software, the data could be used to make cross-informant comparisons of BPM-P, BPM-T, and BPM-Y scores and to track changes in item and scale scores. If sufficient improvements were not found, home and school interventions could be modified as needed.

Assessing Outcomes for Billy and His Mother

The BPM would provide repeated short-term assessments of subsets of Billy's Internalizing, Attention, and Externalizing problems, plus strengths and problems added by the practitioner. After the interventions ended, the practitioner would ask Mary to complete the CBCL and Billy's teacher(s) to complete the TRF. The item and scale scores obtained at this point would be compared with the initial item and scale scores to identify improvements, as well as possible worsening or failure to change. If important problems, competencies, or adaptive functioning failed to show sufficient improvement, further interventions could be targeted on these areas. If interventions had been implemented to help Mary and/or Meredith, the ASR, CBCL/6–18, and YSR could also be completed to evaluate their outcomes. To identify possible subsequent changes for the better or worse, the forms would also need to be completed 6 or more months later.

SUMMARY

Many rating instruments have been constructed for assessing children and adolescents. Examples include the ADHD Rating Scale–IV, the ASI-4, the Conners Rating Scales—Revised, the SDQ, the Devereux Scales, and the BASC. This chapter has illustrated contributions of rating instruments as exemplified by the ASEBA, which includes instruments completed by lay informants (parents, other adults, adult collaterals, teachers, children), by clinicians, and by observers.

Psychometric theory has guided the construction of the ASEBA instruments and the derivation of taxonomic models from data obtained with these instruments. Psychometric data on the test–retest reliability and internal consistency of ASEBA scales are summarized in Table 6.2. Thousands of publications report validity data for ASEBA instruments, including their criterion-related and construct validity.

To enable users to identify both discrepancies and agreements between ratings by different informants, the ASEBA includes parallel forms for parent and teacher ratings, youth self-ratings, adult self-ratings, and adult collateral ratings. The ASEBA software displays side-by-side comparisons of item ratings and scale scores obtained from up to eight informants, plus Q correlations between item ratings by each pair of informants.

Because practitioners need valid norms with which to compare scale scores obtained by individual children, ASEBA scores are displayed in relation to percentiles and *T* scores based on normative population samples for the child's gender and age, the type of informant, and the user-selected multicultural norm group.

Applications of ASEBA parent-, teacher-, self-, and practitioner-completed instruments have been illustrated for the cases of Sofia and Billy. These applications included use of comprehensive ASEBA instruments for initial, outcome, and follow-up assessments, plus repeated assessments at brief intervals with the BPM. The applications also included use of the ASR and ABCL for initial and outcome assessments of the parents of children referred for mental health services. Because translations of ASEBA instruments are available in 90 languages and there are published reports of their use in 80 societies, they can be applied to people from many cultural backgrounds.

REFERENCES

Achenbach, T. M. (1991). *Manual for the Child Behavior Checklist/4-18 and 1991 Profile*. Burlington: University of Vermont, Department of Psychiatry.

Achenbach, T. M. (2009). *The Achenbach System of Empirically Based Assessment (ASEBA): Development, findings, theory, and applications*. Burlington: University of Vermont, Research Center for Children, Youth, and Families.

Achenbach, T. M., Conners, C. K., Quay, H. C., Verhulst, F. C., & Howell, C. T. (1989). Replication of empirically derived syndromes as a basis for taxonomy of child/adolescent psychopathology. *Journal of Abnormal Child Psychology, 17*, 299–323.

Achenbach, T. M., & Edelbrock, C. (1978). The classification of child psychopathology: A review and analysis of empirical efforts. *Psychological Bulletin, 85*, 1275–1301.

Achenbach, T. M., & Edelbrock, C. (1981). Behavioral problems and competencies reported by parents of normal and disturbed children aged four to sixteen. *Monographs of the Society for Research in Child Development, 46*(1, Serial No. 188).

Achenbach, T. M., & Edelbrock, C. (1983). *Manual for the Child Behavior Checklist and Revised Child Behavior Profile*. Burlington: University of Vermont, Department of Psychiatry.

Achenbach, T. M., & Edelbrock, C. (1984). Psychopathology of childhood. *Annual Review of Psychology, 35*, 227–256.

Achenbach, T. M., McConaughy, S. H., & Howell, C. T. (1987). Child/adolescent behavioral and emotional problems: Implications of cross-informant correlations for situational specificity. *Psychological Bulletin, 101*, 213–232.

Achenbach, T. M., McConaughy, S. H., Ivanova, M. Y., & Rescorla, L. A. (2011). *Manual for the ASEBA Brief Problem Monitor (BPM)*. Burlington: University of Vermont, Research Center for Children, Youth, and Families.

Achenbach, T. M., & Rescorla, L. A. (2001). *Manual for the ASEBA School-Age Forms & Profiles*. Burlington: University of Vermont, Research Center for Children, Youth, and Families.

Achenbach, T. M., & Rescorla, L. A. (2003). *Manual for the ASEBA Adult Forms & Profiles*. Burlington: University of Vermont, Research Center for Children, Youth, and Families.

Achenbach, T. M., & Rescorla, L. A. (2007a). *Multicultural supplement to the Manual for the ASEBA School-Age Forms & Profiles*. Burlington: University of Vermont, Research Center for Children, Youth, and Families.

Achenbach, T. M., & Rescorla, L. A. (2007b). *Multicultural understanding of child and adolescent psychopathology: Implications for mental health assessment*. New York: Guilford Press.

Achenbach, T. M., & Rescorla, L. A. (2010). *Multicultural supplement to the Manual for the ASEBA Preschool Forms & Profiles*. Burlington: University of Vermont, Research Center for Children, Youth, and Families.

American Psychiatric Association. (2000). *Diagnostic and statistical manual of mental disorders* (4th ed., text rev.). Washington, DC: Author.

Bérubé, R. L., & Achenbach, T. M. (2013). *Bibliography of published studies using the Achenbach System of Empirically Based Assessment (ASEBA)*. Burlington: University of Vermont, Research Center for Children, Youth, and Families.

Conners, C. K. (2001). *Conners' Rating Scales—Revised technical manual*. North Tonawanda, NY: Multi-Health Systems.

Cronbach, L. J. (1951). Coefficient alpha and the internal structure of tests. *Psychometrika, 16,* 297–334.

De Los Reyes, A., & Kazdin, A. E. (2005). Informant discrepancies in the assessment of childhood psychopathology: A critical review, theoretical framework, and recommendations for further study. *Psychological Bulletin, 131,* 483–509.

Duhig, A. M., Renk, K., Epstein, M. K., & Phares, V. (2000). Interparental agreement on internalizing, externalizing, and total behavior problems: A meta-analysis. *Clinical Psychology: Science and Practice, 7,* 435–453.

DuPaul, G. J., Power, T. J., Anastopoulos, A. D., & Reid, R. (1998). *ADHD Rating Scale–IV: Checklists, norms, and clinical interpretation*. New York: Guilford Press.

Eley, T. C., Lichtenstein, P., & Moffitt, T. E. (2003). A longitudinal behavioral genetic analysis of the etiology of aggressive and nonaggressive antisocial behavior. *Development and Psychopathology, 15,* 383–402.

Ellis, B. B., & Kimmel, H. D. (1992). Identification of unique cultural response patterns by means of item response theory. *Journal of Applied Psychology, 77,* 177–184.

Ferdinand, R. F. (2008). Validity of the CBCL/YSR DSM-IV scales Anxiety Problems and Affective Problems. *Journal of Anxiety Disorders, 22,* 126–134.

Gadow, K. D., & Sprafkin, J. (1998). *Adolescent Symptom Inventory–4 norms manual*. Stony Brook, NY: Checkmate Plus.

Goodman, R. (1997). The Strengths and Difficulties Questionnaire: A research note. *Journal of Child Psychology and Psychiatry, 38,* 581–586.

Gove, P. (Ed.). (1971). *Webster's third new international dictionary of the English language*. Springfield, MA: Merriam.

Hofstra, M. B., van der Ende, J., & Verhulst, F. C. (2002). Child and adolescent problems predict DSM-IV disorders in adulthood: A 14-year follow-up of a

Dutch epidemiological sample. *Journal of the American Academy of Child and Adolescent Psychiatry, 41*, 182–189.

Ivanova, M. Y., Achenbach, T. M., Rescorla, L. A., Bilenberg, N., Kristensen, S., Bjarnadottir, G., Dias, P., et al. (2011). Syndromes of preschool psychopathology reported by teachers and caregivers in 14 societies. *Journal of Early Childhood and Infant Psychology, 7*, 88–103.

Ivanova, M. Y., Achenbach, T. M., Rescorla, L. A., Dumenci, L. Almqvist, F., Bathiche, M., et al. (2007). Testing the Teacher's Report Form syndromes in 20 societies. *School Psychology Review, 36*, 468–483.

Ivanova, M. Y., Achenbach, T. M., Rescorla, L.A., Dumenci, L., Almqvist, F., Bilenberg, N., Verhulst, F. C., et al. (2007). The generalizability of the Youth Self-Report syndrome structure in 23 societies. *Journal of Consulting and Clinical Psychology, 75*, 729–738.

Ivanova, M. Y., Achenbach, T. M., Rescorla, L. A., Harder, V. S., Ang, R. P., Bilenberg, N., & Verhulst, F. C. (2010). Preschool psychopathology reported by parents in 23 societies: Testing the seven-syndrome model of the Child Behavior Checklist for Ages 1.5–5. *Journal of the American Academy of Child and Adolescent Psychiatry, 49*, 1215–1224.

Ivanova, M. Y., Dobrean, A., Dopfner, M., Erol, N., Fombonne, E., Fonseca, A. C., Chen, W. J., et al. (2007). Testing the 8-syndrome structure of the CBCL in 30 societies. *Journal of Clinical Child and Adolescent Psychology, 36*, 405–417.

Krueger, R. F., & Piasecki, T. M. (2002). Toward a dimensional and psychometrically-informed approach to conceptualizing psychopathology. *Behaviour Research and Therapy, 40*, 485–499.

MacDonald, V. M., & Achenbach, T. M. (1999). Attention problems versus conduct problems as six-year predictors of signs of disturbance in a national sample. *Journal of the American Academy of Child and Adolescent Psychiatry, 38*, 1254–1261.

McConaughy, S. H., & Achenbach, T. M. (2001). *Manual for the Semistructured Clinical Interview for Children and Adolescents* (2nd ed.). Burlington: University of Vermont, Research Center for Children, Youth, and Families.

Naglieri, J. A., & Pfeiffer, S. I. (2004). Use of the Devereux Scales of Mental Disorders for dignosis, treatment, planning, and outcome assessment. In M. E. Maruish (Ed.), *The use of psychological testing for treatment planning and outcomes assessment* (Vol. 2, pp. 305–330). Mahwah, NJ: Erlbaum.

Renk, K., & Phares, V. (2004). Cross-informant ratings of social competence in children and adolescents. *Clinical Psychology Review, 24*, 239–254.

Reynolds, C. R., & Kamphaus, R. W. (1992). *Behavior Assessment System for Children (BASC)*. Circle Pines, MN: American Guidance Service.

Vidair, H. B., Reyes, J. A., Shen, S., Parrilla-Escobar, M. A., Heleniak, C. M., Hollin, I. L., & Rynn, M. A. (2011). Screening parents during child evaluations: Exploring parent and child psychopathology in the same clinic. *Journal of the American Academy of Child and Adolescent Psychiatry, 50*, 441–450.

Visser, J. H., van der Ende, J., Koot, H. M., & Verhulst, F. C. (2003). Predicting change in psychopathology in youth referred to mental health services in childhood or adolescence. *Journal of Child Psychology and Psychiatry, 44*, 509–519.

7

Direct Observation

David Reitman, Stacey McGregor, and Alexis Resnick

Reason, observation, and experience—the holy trinity of science.
—ROBERT GREEN INGERSOLL

As suggested by the quotation above, few human actions are more closely aligned with scientific activity than direct observation. That being said, recent trends in psychological science generally and in clinical practice specifically seem to be moving away from this time-honored tradition. Within the psychological tradition, the historical record is replete with observation. Freud's clinical insights, though unstructured and unsystematic by today's standards, were the bedrock of his theorizing (Freud, 1909/1953). Pavlov's accidental movement into the study of "psychic secretions" were inspired by observations of preexperimental behavior among the canines involved in his Nobel-Prize-winning research on the digestive reflex (Pavlov, 1927). Landmark studies in social psychology—the Robber's Cave experiment (Sherif, 1966), Zimbardo's prison experiments (Haney, Banks, & Zimbardo, 1973), and Milgram's studies of obedience to authority (Milgram, 1963)—all involved direct observation of human behavior, albeit under experimental conditions. More recently, the American Psychological Association's "Decade of Behavior" (2000–2010) campaign would seem to imply that observational activity would be at the center of such an enterprise.

Given the prominent role of direct observation in laying the foundation of contemporary psychology, the abandonment of studies involving direct observation within social psychology over the past few decades is all the more striking (Baumeister, Vohs, & Funder, 2007). From 1976 to 2006, the percentage of studies that included direct assessment of behavior in the *Journal of Personality and Social Psychology* dropped from 80% to 20%. By way of explanation, Baumeister et al. (2007) argue that funding priorities, publication pressures, and the current intellectual/theoretical emphasis on cognitive science have combined to diminish the likelihood of social and behavioral scientists' observing "actual" human behavior. Rhetorically questioning whether the abandonment of direct inquiry matters, Baumeister et al. (2007) illustrate with a particularly relevant study of helping behavior. Participants were first asked about the likelihood of providing assistance and financial support to a hypothetical accident victim, and attractiveness of the victim was found to have played no role in hypothetical giving. However, when the event was *actually staged*, attractiveness had a significant impact on both the level of giving and who was helped (West & Brown, 1975). Drawing on this study and many more, Baumeister et al. offer a frank assessment of the state of social psychology and its transformation into a science of self-report and "keystrokes and reaction times":

> Surely some important behavior involves a person standing up? Or actually talking to another live person, even beyond getting instructions to sign a consent form and activate a computer program? Whatever happened to helping, hurting, playing, working, talking, eating, risking, waiting, flirting, goofing off, showing off, giving up, screwing up, compromising, selling, persevering, pleading, tricking, outhustling, sandbagging, refusing, and the rest? Can't psychology find ways to observe and explain these acts, at least once in a while? (p. 399)

Not that clinical psychology has been immune to such trends. Indeed, as early as 1990, Gross asserted that trends in behavior therapy research and practice suggested a move away from careful observation of individuals in favor of group research designs that relied more heavily on paper-and-pencil measures (as stand-ins for behavior). Gross (1990) specifically identified the direct measurement of behavior change as a hallmark of behavior therapy, and lamented the drift from direct observation in research and clinical practice. Given the pivotal contributions of direct observation to psychological science, abandonment of direct observation in clinical practice would be a striking development.

In recent years, numerous texts, book chapters, and reviews have extolled the merits of evidence-based assessment and weighing the relative benefits of various assessment practices (Frick, Barry, & Kamphaus, 2010). Among children and families, core evidence-based practices include interviews, checklists and rating scales, self-monitoring, sociometric ratings, physiological assessment, laboratory measures, and of course direct observation of behavior (Frick et al., 2010). A central theme explored in the present chapter is whether or not behavioral observation should continue to occupy an important place in contemporary child behavioral assessment or more specifically, whether direct observations of behavior can in any way be shown to be functionally related to better treatment outcomes (Gresham, 2003; Nelson-Gray, 2003, Pelham, Fabiano, & Massetti, 2005).

DESCRIPTION OF THE ASSESSMENT METHOD

There is broad consensus among child behavior therapists and researchers that behavioral assessments should consist of multiple measures/methods (e.g., interviews, rating scales, and direct observation) and informants/ sources (e.g., parents, child/adolescent, and teachers) (Pelham et al., 2005). However, for child therapists trained in the behavioral tradition, behavioral observation occupies a special place among these measurement options (Baer, Harrison, Fradenburg, Petersen, & Milla, 2005). Chief among the salutary qualities of behavioral or "direct" observation is the oft-cited notion that direct observation yields estimates of child behavior problems that are less prone to bias and error than self- and behavior ratings (Patterson & Forgatch, 1995). Direct observation involves careful selection of operationally well-defined behaviors that require the assessor to be in direct contact with the behaving participant (Cone & Foster, 1982). When behavioral observation occurs in the context of a functional assessment or experimental functional analysis (Alberto & Troutman, 2006), the observation will also involve describing the conditions under which a behavior is most or least likely to occur, via study of its associated antecedents and consequences. Finally, to ensure reliability and maximize the validity of the behavioral observation, the protocol must be used in a consistent manner across place and time, and the data must be interpreted in a systematic fashion that is logically related to the initial research or clinical question (Chafouleas, Riley-Tillman, & Sugai, 2007).

Before settling on behavioral observation as a measurement strategy, a clinician needs to consider several factors, including whether the response properties of the behavior lend themselves to the method. Specifically, is the behavior readily observable (accessible), and does it occur with sufficient frequency to permit reliable sampling? For example, stealing may not be directly observable, and fighting may be insufficiently frequent to capture via direct observation methods (Foster & Cone, 1986). Moreover, high-frequency behaviors lend themselves to different methods of observation than low-base-rate behaviors, and the observer must decide whether event recording or time-based recording will best suit the behavior of interest. As recommended by Mash and Hunsley (2005), the assessor should also consider the purpose of data collection (i.e., description/diagnosis, determination of functional relationships, intervention monitoring, or program evaluation) because some methods, such as antecedent–behavior–consequence (A-B-C) analysis, may be useful for describing functional relationships but insensitive to change (Alberto & Troutman, 2006; Cone & Foster, 1982; Foster & Cone, 1986).

An evaluator should also consider the number of behaviors and individuals he or she plans to observe. As a practical matter, the observation will be constrained by available resources (e.g., number of observers, equipment limitations, and time needed to train observers), as well as by whether or not the behavior observation is practical—or even permitted—in the setting of interest. For example, in our experience, schools may sometimes limit or even attempt to bar classroom observations of children. Under these circumstances, parents occasionally must assert their rights under the Individuals with Disabilities Education Improvement Act (IDEA) and apply pressure until school personnel allow an observation to take place.

Steps in Conducting Behavioral Observations

Having determined the appropriateness of direct observation, one begins by defining the target behavior(s). Depending on the level of analysis (i.e., molar or molecular), the target behavior(s) may be defined at the level of distinct behaviors, behavioral constellations, or interactions (Cone & Foster, 1982; Frick et al., 2010). Definitions should be as specific, clear, and objective as possible, with the ultimate "goodness" of a definition defined as the extent to which two independent observers using this definition agree on the presence or absence of a given behavior (see Foster & Cone's 1995 discussion of "accuracy" for additional considerations). Next, the setting of the behavioral observation must be determined. A vital decision involves whether the observation takes place in a naturalistic environment (e.g., at school), an analogue setting (e.g., a clinic room that "simulates" a classroom), or both. Naturalistic observations produce data that are putatively more ecologically valid (Frick et al., 2010). However, naturalistic observations can be viewed as time-consuming and impractical, especially among private practitioners (Pelham et al., 2005). Indeed, such considerations apply even for school-based psychologists (Hintze, 2005). On the other hand, if greater control is desired, or if one hopes to elicit the problem behavior (i.e., by presenting a feared stimulus or difficult academic assignment), it may be desirable or even essential to conduct observations in analogue settings. Analogue behavioral observations may not only help observers estimate behavioral frequency in a natural environment, but may also help observers identify the factors maintaining the behavior(s) in question, as in functional analysis manipulations (Haynes, 2001). Despite their promise, concerns about analogue observations include difficulties with ensuring uniformity in administration, limited information about their psychometric properties, and uncertainty about the extent to which they generalize to other settings (Haynes, 2001; Mash & Foster, 2001).

After deciding what, when, and where to observe, clinicians and researchers must turn their attention to the collection and coding of data.

Users of direct observation may choose from narrative, event-based, or time-based recording strategies (Chafouleas et al., 2007; Cone & Foster, 1982). For more exhaustive accounts of the strengths and weaknesses of the data collection methods introduced below, readers are encouraged to consult the excellent texts by Miltenberger (2008) and Alberto and Troutman (2006) for child clinical or school-based resources, respectively.

Narrative Recording

Narrative recording consists of an observer's oral or written account of behavior (Cone & Foster, 1982). When employing narrative recording procedures, observers should describe rather than infer (Reitman & Hupp, 2003). For instance, rather than recording that a child was "aggressive," an observer should describe the events that led the observer to label the act "aggressive" (e.g., the child was observed hitting and kicking a peer on the playground). Concerns about narrative recording include observers' failing to record occurrences, or using different identifiers to document the same occurrence (Cone & Foster, 1982). Narrative records may be difficult to quantify and time-consuming to transcribe, code, and summarize, yet may still be quite useful if the observer is unfamiliar with the population or behavior under investigation. Thus narrative accounts may serve as sources of preliminary information for "pinpointing" behaviors and improving the quality of the operational definitions (Alberto & Troutman, 2006).

The form of narrative recording that appears to have the greatest clinical utility is A-B-C analysis or "functional assessment" (Gresham, 2003; O'Neill et al., 1997). When researchers formally manipulate the antecedent and consequent conditions in an experimental analogue, the result is functional analysis (Alberto & Troutman, 2006). Developed in the early days of child behavior therapy and strongly associated with contingency-based accounts of problem behavior (Baer et al., 2005), the narrative requires the observer to document "everything the participant says and does and everything said and done to the participant child" (Alberto & Troutman, 2006, p. 61). Observers then record the type and relative frequency of antecedent stimuli (e.g., requests, reprimands) as well as carefully describing the consequences of the problem or "target" behavior (e.g., peers laugh, teacher ignores, child is removed from classroom, etc.). The free-form narrative is sometimes called an "anecdotal observation," and is usually organized post hoc and subdivided into A-B-C categories for review by a treatment team or therapist (Alberto & Troutman, 2006). From such data, it is often possible to develop plausible hypotheses concerning the possible functions (utility) of problem behavior that can be used to develop interventions. Although some support exists for functional assessment in classroom settings (see Ervin, DuPaul, Kern, & Friman, 1998), the strongest support for this approach is presently found in the developmental disabilities literature (Nelson-Gray, 2003). Gresham (2003) has raised many concerns about the support for functional assessment and has called for more studies of its treatment utility.

Event-Based Recording

Event-based recording may determine "frequency" (how often the behavior occurs) or "rate" (how often the behavior occurs per unit of time). Less commonly, behavioral events may be described in terms of "duration" (how long the behavioral event lasts) or "latency" (how much time elapses between a signal and the initiation of a response). Under certain circumstances, the behavior may not be directly observed, but the action results in "products" that may be observed, evaluated, and counted (i.e., permanent products) (Chafouleas et al., 2007). In contrast to narrative recording, event-based recording requires the observer to document specific response properties for operationally defined behavior(s) chosen in advance (Cone & Foster, 1982). Event-based recording is often used to monitor the effects of treatment, but it may not be useful for documenting time-related behavior patterns, for observing low-frequency behaviors, or for determining the onset and termination of behaviors (Cone & Foster, 1982). In addition, if the target behavior occurs at high rates, it may be difficult to record the behavior accurately and challenging to record multiple behaviors. If the observer wishes to record several behaviors simultaneously, or the behaviors of a group of students, then time-based techniques may be more suitable than event-based strategies (Chafouleas et al., 2007).

Time-Based Recording

Time-based recording requires an observer to subdivide an observation interval into equal subintervals. For example, if the observer wishes to obtain a 10-minute sample of behavior, subdividing the period into 10-second intervals would result in 60 equal intervals. When the behavior of interest is observed, an occurrence is scored. Two time-based strategies are common: "interval recording" and "momentary time sampling" (Chafouleas et al., 2007). In momentary time sampling or simply "time sampling," observers record whether a behavior occurs, but score an occurrence only if the behavior is observed at the *end* of a given interval. Time sampling generally involves intervals of 1–60 minutes, though shorter or longer intervals are possible. For example, an observer using a 5-minute time sampling strategy over the course of 30-minute recess period could note whether a socially withdrawn child was engaged in social interaction. Such a strategy would yield a total of six observations during the recess period. Assuming that a fixed as opposed to a variable time-sampling strategy was used, samples would be obtained at 5, 10, 15, 20, 25, and 30 minutes.

If whole-interval recording is selected, observers score an occurrence only if the behavior is observed for the entirety of the interval. By contrast, partial-interval recording requires the observer to note only whether the behavior occurred at any time during the interval. According to Cone and Foster (1982), "interval systems have the potential for greater data yield than does event recording, and are better suited to theoretical or practical research questions that require analyses of fine-grained data" (p. 321). However, time-based recording is rarely feasible for participant-observers (e.g., teachers, parents), and may result in fatigue because observers must remain vigilant during all or most of the interval. In addition, time-based recording may not be sensitive to variation in low-base-rate behaviors (Cone & Foster, 1982). Finally, in communications about time-based recording, data should not be interpreted as frequency estimates. A child who is scored as out of seat during 15 of 30 intervals should not be described as having been out of seat 15 times, but rather should be described as being out of seat during 50% of the observed intervals.

Formal Observational Systems

An issue frequently raised about the viability of direct observation as a practical aid to clinical assessment concerns the resources that must be allocated for the development of new observational systems (Volpe, DiPerna, Hintze, & Shapiro, 2005). At the top of any list of resources would be the time and effort needed to develop the observational system itself, including the time needed to create and refine operational definitions, choose methods, develop data-recording forms, and graph or otherwise consolidate data so that clinical decisions can be made about treatment progress or classification. Historically, clinicians and researchers, primarily those trained within the operant tradition, have developed observational systems and codes idiosyncratically. This has the advantage of better capturing the unique facets of a given participant's or client's behavioral repertoire (Foster & Cone, 1995); on the other hand, such an approach limits the use of direct observation to those trained in the method or with access to such individuals. As alternatives, several observational systems have been created to reduce the effort needed to employ direct observation, promote greater measurement consistency, and enhance the reliability and validity of observation. To date, most standardized behavioral observation systems have been designed for use in classroom settings and are geared toward the assessment of putatively externalizing behaviors, such as out-of-seat, off-task, or other forms of disruptive behavior.

Two examples of classroom-based behavioral observation tools that employ the aforementioned recording techniques are the Classroom Observation Code (COC; Abikoff & Gittelman, 1985) and the Revised Edition of the School Observation Coding System (REDSOCS; Jacobs et al., 2000). The COC, which has mainly been used with hyperactive, inattentive, and disruptive children, utilizes a time-sampling approach to record child behavior across 14 observational categories. The tool has adequate interobserver reliability and discriminates hyperactive from control children. The REDSOCS employs an interval coding system, assessing inappropriate, noncompliant, and off-task behaviors. REDSOCS reliability coefficients are high; scores correlate with the Sutter–Eyberg Student Behavior Inventory—Revised and the Conners Teacher Rating Scale—Revised; and the measure discriminates referred children from controls (Jacobs et al., 2000).

Two other measurement systems have been developed in concert with comprehensive multidimensional rating systems. The first, the Direct Observation Form (DOF), is part of the Achenbach System of Empirically Based Assessment (ASEBA; Achenbach, 2009), which includes the well-known Child Behavior Checklist as well as the Youth Self-Report and Teacher's Report Form. The Student Observation System is the direct observation scheme employed as part of the school-based Behavior Assessment System for Children, Second Edition (BASC-2; Reynolds & Kamphaus, 2004). These simple and brief observation systems incorporate both time-sampling methods and narrative descriptions of behavior, and sample a wide range of child behaviors in the classroom. Norm-referenced data are not available for these behavioral observation systems; however, the data gathered on the rating scales can be compared to the data gathered from the observations to provide a more comprehensive picture of the problem behavior(s) (Achenbach, 2009). Recently the DOF has been the subject of extensive study, and we review some of the psychometric data produced by these efforts in the next section (Volpe, McConaughy, & Hintze, 2009).

Limitations of the Approach

Direct observation has a number of strengths, including the assessment of targets that generally have high face validity and often have high social validity (Wolf, 1978). Direct observation also facilitates the development of measures that may be more sensitive to change and thus more useful in promoting ongoing progress assessment and treatment planning (Chafouleas et al., 2007). Nevertheless, some limitations are apparent. First, the act of targeting specific behaviors for observation and change can result in the selection of well-defined but trivial treatment targets that lack social validity (Hawkins, 1986; Wolf, 1978). Moreover, since significant resource allocation is associated with the use of direct observation, the benefits of direct observation could be outweighed by its costs. Alternatively, behaviors that are too broadly defined (i.e., when response classes with similar topographies but different functions are combined) make it difficult or impossible to establish functional relations and may render the observational measure insensitive to change.

Notwithstanding concerns about the resources needed to obtain reliable observations of behavior (see "Psychometric Properties," below), one of the chief concerns about direct observation has involved reactivity to the observer's presence (especially for naturalistic observations). The best data on this phenomenon have been obtained by Patterson, Reid, and Dishion

(1992), with the consensus being that concerns about reactivity may be somewhat exaggerated. In general, when efforts are made to minimize the intrusiveness of the observation, and a child is given an opportunity to habituate to an observer's presence, the validity of the observations do not appear to be seriously compromised (at least not by reactivity effects). Beyond obvious problems, such as biases introduced by observer expectancy, other sources of error such as "observer drift" may be corrected by periodic feedback from another observer and by reliability checks, which can be scheduled to prevent such problems from developing (Baer et al., 2005; Patterson et al., 1992). As noted previously, the effort that must be expended to maintain the integrity of the observations may constitute one of the largest perceived impediments to conducting observations. As such, efforts should be made to minimize complexity and reduce "informant load" as much as possible (Chafouleas et al., 2007; Volpe et al., 2009). Other problems that may arise during the course of conducting behavioral observations and may compromise the reliability and validity of the observations have been well documented elsewhere (see Cooper, Heron, & Heward, 2007, for a comprehensive list).

THEORY UNDERLYING THE METHOD

Observations always involve theory.
            —EDWIN HUBBLE

Direct observation is so closely identified with behaviorism and its associated clinical traditions that the theoretical and practical arguments offered in favor of the practice can be challenging to elucidate. Indeed, many of the arguments made by the early developers of behavioral research and therapy in favor of direct observation flow directly from the limitations associated with "indirect" measures (i.e., data collection methods that do not place the scientist or practitioner in direct contact with the behaving individual) (Gresham, 2003; Skinner, 1953). The most prominent concerns about indirect measurement involve the tendency of respondents to misrepresent or perhaps to "misremember" events, as well as participants' difficulties in making important discriminations or detecting change when it is present (Cooper et al., 2007).

Classical Test Theory and Generalizability Theory

Early behavior therapists were notably pragmatic in their clinical approach, and it took some time for behavior therapists to examine seriously the theoretical models underlying clinical practice (Cone, 1992). Early proponents of direct observation rejected traditional assessment and classical psychometric or "test" theory on several grounds (Nelson, Hay, & Hay, 1977). First, behaviorists rejected the characterization of direct observation data as providing an "estimate of an underlying construct." In contrast to indirect measures, no such appeal to underlying constructs was thought necessary. Secondly, the classical test theory (CTT) model was resisted due to its association with the study of individual differences (i.e., efforts to establish the meaning of an individual score in relation to norms and deviations from normal for similar individuals) (see Hintze, 2005). Instead, the study of the individual's behavior in context, and in relation to "one's own control" or baseline, was preferred over normative comparisons (Sidman, 1960). Finally, the conceptualization of true score and error variance in CTT was considered inconsistent with a behavioral theory that viewed "true score variance" as reflecting behavior in context. Mischel's (1968) seminal work illustrated that cross-situational variability was a core assumption in behavioral theory. Variability in performance, rather than being relegated to "error," was viewed as a phenomenon important to understand in its own right (and preferably through experimental manipulation) (Sidman, 1960).

Despite arguments to the contrary, a consensus that traditional psychometric considerations were applicable to behavioral assessment began to emerge (Cone, 1977). Although traditional psychometric concepts such as reliability and validity require modification, with some effort they (and their many subcategories) were in fact relevant and potentially important for demonstrating the effectiveness of behavior therapy (Foster & Cone, 1995; Haynes, Richard, & Kubany, 1995; Johnston & Pennypacker, 1993). In an effort to address the conceptual and technical limitations of CTT, generalizability (G) theory (Cronbach, Gleser, Nanda, & Rajaratnam, 1972) was proposed as an alternative method of evaluating the psychometric adequacy of behavioral observation (see Hinzte & Matthews, 2004).

With respect to direct observation, the most appealing aspect of G theory is that rather than viewing measurement "error" as random and thus unknowable, the theory explicitly addresses sources of variability (i.e., "facets") that contribute to observed scores. Importantly, G theory also reminds assessors that reliability and validity are properties of the uses to which test scores are put, rather than properties of the measures themselves (Suen & Ary, 1988). According to Shavelson, Webb, and Rowley (1989), "A score's usefulness then, largely depends on the extent to which it allows us to generalize accurately to behavior in some wider set of situations, a *universe of generalization*" (p. 922; emphasis in original). Cone and Foster (1982) identify five such universes of generalization that are relevant to direct observation: (1) observers, (2) time, (3) settings, (4) behavior, and (5) methods. The concept of reliability in CTT is addressed in G theory via the universes of observers and time, while traditional notions of validity can typically be addressed via studies examining the characteristics of scores across settings, behavior, methods, and other universes as dictated by the nature of the research question. Due to space limitations, we focus our discussion of the psychometric adequacy of direct observation on the four most commonly explored universes: observers, time, settings, and method.

PSYCHOMETRIC PROPERTIES

Reliability of Behavioral Observation

Traditional psychometric theory as applied to indirect measures such as self-report and rating scales emphasizes internal consistency and test–retest reliability, whereas direct observation has generally relied on intraobserver reliability and interobserver agreement to establish consistency of measurement (Hintze, 2005). Strong interobserver agreement is often touted as the signature strength of systematic direct observation (Briesch, Chafouleas, & Riley-Tillman, 2010) and is by far the most frequently reported form of reliability information for direct observation (Gresham, 2003). According to this logic, assessors feel more confident in the reliability of direct observation when multiple (at least two) independent individuals observing the same behavior during the same period (interobserver agreement) see that same thing, or when the consistency of a single person's observations of the same participant(s) over multiple sessions (intraobserver reliability) remains high (Suen & Ary, 1989). Because in most instances it is impossible for a rater to rate the same behavior multiple times without video records, "for better or worse" the most frequently obtained and studied form of agreement is interobserver agreement (Cone & Foster, 1982).

The choice of an agreement index should be suited to the method of behavioral observation and the frequency of the behavior being observed. For instance, if only the frequency of a target behavior (e.g., the number of times a child was out of seat during an entire class period) was recorded, a "smaller/larger" index (the quotient of the smaller number of observed behaviors divided by the larger number) would be the only method by which to calculate agreement for two independent observers. However, other methods of behavioral observation call for different agreement indices. Examples include the "percentage agreement" index (the average percentage of occasions when two independent raters agree that a behavior did or did not occur); "occurrence" or "nonoccurrence" agreement indices (separate calculations of the agreement indices for occurrences and nonoccurrences); coefficient kappa (an estimate of agreement between observers, corrected for chance); and coefficient phi (the correlation between the two sets of scores). (See Hintze, 2005, for a more complete discussion of the types of agreement indices).

In general, recommendations for a threshold of interobserver agreement tend to fall around .80 (Cooper et al., 2007). Higher thresholds tend to be recommended for less rigorous measures of agreement (i.e., .90 or greater), such as smaller/larger or percentage agreement indices. Less rigorous methods of agreement tend to capitalize on chance agreement and are sensitive to the base rate of the behavior of interest. By contrast, for more rigorous indices such as the kappa coefficient, estimates as low as

.40–.60 may be considered "fair" and .60–.80 may be regarded as "substantial" (Hintze, 2005). Practically speaking, if used in isolation, high reliabilities found for occurrence or nonoccurrence agreement can be highly misleading, but when *both* occurrence and nonoccurrence agreement are calculated, high values for both do a more than adequate job of ruling out chance agreement as a threat to reliability estimation (Baer et al., 2005).

Generalizability over Observers

In the context of G theory, interobserver reliability is deemed a form of "scorer generalizability," and studies evaluating this facet address the question "To what extent do data obtained from this observation depend on the person doing the observing?" (Cone & Foster, 1982, p. 325). In short, one hopes that the answer to this question is "no." That is, one wishes to view observers as essentially interchangeable and, statistically speaking, as accounting for little or no variability in the analysis of variance. Interobserver agreement in direct observation depends upon a variety of factors, including the expertise of the coders, the behaviors being observed, the number of indicators of the construct being observed, and the complexity of the coding system. Though interobserver agreement is a form of scorer generalizability, the two concepts are not interchangeable. Indeed, in a study of off-task behavior in a classroom setting that utilized momentary time sampling, Hintze and Matthews (2004) found high levels of interobserver agreement as estimated by using point-by-point percentage agreement (range = .88–.92), and acceptable kappa coefficients (average = .65), but lower levels of reliability as estimated using G theory (range = .62–.63). The meaning and significance of this distinction are addressed in the section below.

Generalizability over Time

Generalizability over time or occasions deals with the extent to which data collected at a specific time are comparable to data collected at other times that are not observed. Such data are important in clinical practice when professionals need to know how representative their direct observation data is of a child's behavior at other times, or how accurately they can predict future behavior from their data. The critical clinical assessment question arising from these data is this: How many observations of a given behavior are necessary to establish reliability or consistency of measurement (Hintze, 2005; Hintze & Matthews, 2004)?

A series of primarily classroom-based studies will illustrate some of the differences between interobserver agreement and consistency of measurement across time (generalizability), as well as highlight some of the clinical insights that seem to be produced by the approach. For example, Hintze and Matthews (2004) conducted systematic direct observations of on-task behavior for 14 boys across time (10 days) and "setting" (actually, time of day confounded with setting; math [A.M.] and reading [P.M.] activities), while simultaneously holding scorer, item, method, and dimension constant. The authors concluded that in order to obtain adequate levels of reliability (.80), some children (the children displaying the least stable patterns) would need to be observed as frequently as four times per day over a 4-week (20-day) period. If however, a child displayed greater initial stability, reliability could be achieved with a single observation per day for seven days.

To illustrate how variance is partitioned in G theory, consider that in the "standard model" (essentially, the experimental conditions), the majority of the variance was due to variation in the actual behavior of the persons (62%), whereas about 13% of the variability was explained by an interaction between the persons' behavior and the "setting." Time (days) contributed little variance by itself, though a sizable 24% of the variance was attributed to "unexplained error." A more recent study of the part of the ASEBA's DOF that samples on-task behavior (using a form of time sampling in which a child had to be on task for the majority of the last 5 seconds of each minute, for 10 minutes) resulted in high interobserver reliability (.97), yet rather low test–restest (.47, 12-day interval) and adequate generalizability and dependability coefficients (.70) (Volpe et al., 2009). In addition, while estimates of the number of days needed to achieve generalizability and dependability may vary as a function of type of behavior observed, Briesch et al. (2010) found that three to five observations either across or within days to could result in dependable estimates of "academic engagement." Interestingly, similar recommendations appear in the behavior-analytic literature (Miltenberger, 2008).

Accuracy

Accuracy has been described as a psychometric property uniquely associated with behavioral assessment (Foster & Cone, 1995). When data subjected to assessment for interobserver reliability show a high level of correlation, results are sometimes presented as if accuracy of measurement has been achieved. Accuracy has also been defined as what is "true" about a given behavior (Foster & Cone, 1995; Johnston & Pennypacker, 1993). Cone and Foster (1982) have argued that accuracy could be established by comparing observations of the behavior to video recordings—an "unimpeachable source of information about the phenomenon of interest" (p. 336). Other standards for establishing accuracy have been discussed by Baer et al. (2005). Unfortunately, where direct observations are concerned, attempting to establish a "gold standard" is exceptionally challenging. Interestingly, when attempts are made to establish a gold standard for other measurement methods, most often it is behavioral observation that serves as the incontrovertible index (Foster & Cone, 1995)!

Validity of Behavioral Observations

In asserting the importance of establishing the reliability and validity of tests independently, Foster and Cone (1995) note that confusing reliability and validity can result in problematic interpretations, especially when negative results are obtained. Indeed, the problem may be even more acute in clinical settings. Consider the observation that child behavior as directly observed changed in a favorable direction, but teacher ratings, for example, did not. "Is it the test, the theory, or the study that is bad?" (Foster & Cone, 1995, p. 249). Suffice it to say that while reliability of observation may be high, questions about the validity of the observation may still remain.

Generalizability over Settings

For the purposes of the present discussion, the most pertinent form of setting generalizability for direct observations occurs when practitioners or researchers attempt to elicit clinically relevant behaviors under controlled (analogue) conditions and seek to generalize the results to other settings (typically, home or school). A special series on clinical analogues published in *Psychological Assessment* in 2001 summarized much of what is presently known and made numerous recommendations concerning future directions in research. In general, these studies suggested that clinical analogues (e.g., playroom observation tasks for attention-deficit/hyperactivity disorder [ADHD] assessment, parent–child interaction, etc.) of naturalistic observations were lacking in psychometric development (Haynes, 2001). Notably, depending on the behavior and type of analogue system used, there was conflicting evidence for cross-setting generalization. For example, some studies examining aggression and noncompliance have demonstrated generalizability (e.g., Hinshaw, Zupan, Simmel, Nigg, & Melnick, 1997), whereas observations of children's social behavior have not been shown to generalize to the school setting (Mori & Armendariz, 2001). Finally, studies concerned with the generalizabilty of clinic analogues of parenting were reviewed by Roberts (2001), who concluded that parent-directed-chore analogues were the most psychometrically sound (i.e., provided evidence of content and criterion validity) and yielded the highest utility for assessment (e.g., facilitated diagnostic decisions) and treatment (e.g., provided goals for treatment).

Generalizability over Methods

Research examining the generalizability of direct observation across methods has generally asked this question: To what extent do parent self-reports or other ratings of child behavior correspond with naturalistic or clinic analogues? The driving force in this sort of comparison has to do with reducing the costs of assessment, treatment, and/outcome monitoring. Indeed, if data supported this kind of generalization, the implications of these findings would be profound. Methodologically, these studies are carried out by comparing data obtained via direct observation to several (usually indirect) assessment methods that measure the *same* behavior (Foster & Cone, 1995). In this regard, it is helpful to think of the indirect measures as establishing the convergent validity of the behavioral observation. Demonstrating high correlations for the same behavior when "maximally different" assessment methods are used provides the best evidence of validity or, in G theory terms, "generalizability" (Foster & Cone, 1995, p. 250).

Research examining the convergent validity of behavioral observations has been examined widely in child and family settings. In an early example of such work, Risley and Hart (1968) found a weak correspondence between child self-reports and observed play until child "accuracy" was reinforced (as cited in Cone & Foster, 1982). Hawes and Dadds (2006) found that parent discipline, as measured by the Alabama Parenting Questionnaire, was related to observations of both "parental praise" and "harsh/aversive parenting" for parents of children with conduct problems. Collectively, the magnitude of the relations observed between self- or other-ratings and direct observation has been modest at best. We explore a few possible explanations for these findings in our discussion.

APPLICATION TO THE CASE OF SOFIA

Having addressed the theoretical and technical aspects of direct observation, we turn now to application, drawing on the vignettes presented by McLeod, Jensen-Doss, and Ollendick in Chapter 4 of this volume. Recall that Sofia, the adolescent in the first Chapter 4 study, missed many days of school, presumably in an effort to minimize panic symptoms. Sofia subsequently fell behind academically, and her family sought treatment. Following treatment, Sofia temporarily returned to school, but ceased attending after being informed that she would be retained due to her previous absences. Sofia expressed embarrassment over her academic failure. Upon presenting to the clinic, Sofia's parents asserted their desire for her to return to school and earn her diploma.

Though there are many "purposes" of assessment (Mash & Hunsley, 2005), our efforts to inform the evaluation of change would begin in Sofia's case with operationalizing "school refusal behaviors." Indirect assessments such as the Functional Assessment Interview (O'Neill et al., 1997) could be used to help define "school refusal," as well as to obtain information about antecedents and consequences that could be useful in treatment planning. Operationalization requires a target behavior to be named, described, and elaborated with examples and nonexamples (Miltenberger, 2008).

To illustrate a systematic direct observation in Sofia's case, consider that a descriptive assessment of Sofia's school refusal might reveal that if she could be induced to get out of bed, she was more likely to attend school. Direct assessment of her school refusal behaviors might therefore allow for a more sensitive assessment of treatment progress. Since the observation would be likely to involve the home setting, it might make more sense to train the parents to observe than to deploy evaluators to the home each morning (Hawkins & Mathews, 1999). At baseline, the parents could prompt Sofia at 6:30 A.M., saying, "It is time to wake up, Sofia. Please get out of bed now," and then use a digital stopwatch or smart phone to record the length of time it took for Sofia to get out of bed. One could thus obtain an approximation of baseline latency to compliance (recording in this way would also preserve the natural ecology of repeated requests for Sofia to get up). Subsequent antecedent (e.g., preparing a delicious breakfast) or consequent (e.g., providing highly salient rewards such as a family outing contingent on prompt waking) interventions could then be evaluated by comparing pre- and postintervention latencies.

In the present example, "refusal to get out of bed" would be defined in a manner similar to noncompliance. Specifically, refusal would be scored if, 10 seconds after an instruction to get out of bed, any part of Sofia's body remained in contact with the bed. Examples of refusal behaviors would include such behaviors as "complaining that it was too early," "throwing the pillows," "pulling the covers over her head," or "lying quietly with her eyes closed in the bed" after 10 seconds had elapsed. Nonexamples of refusal to get out of bed would include any behaviors that resulted in her no longer being in contact with the bed prior to 10 seconds' elapsing (e.g., "getting out of bed," "putting on a robe," "cursing her father while brushing her teeth," "getting materials prepared for the day," etc.). Refusal could be measured as the latency (in seconds) between the initial command to get out of bed and actually getting up (after allowing 10 seconds for her to respond to the request).

A behavioral observation technique that requires the same kind of operationalization as described above, but that requires more formal control of the setting, is a "behavioral avoidance test" (BAT; Lang & Lazovik, 1963). BATs are presently considered a standard of care in much anxiety treatment for children (see Velting, Setzer, & Albano, 2004). A BAT in this case would involve observing Sofia's response to intentionally presented anxiety-provoking stimuli (e.g., requests to go to school, the school bus, etc.) and then observing her movements relative to the feared stimulus in graduated steps. Objective criteria for evaluating her reaction (e.g., how closely she approached the stimulus, the number of steps taken, and/or the time spent in the anxiety-provoking situation) would be customized for Sofia. BATs provide observable measures of avoidance, and have been regarded as easy to use, efficient, and psychometrically sound (i.e., they yield high interobserver agreement, are sensitive to treatment, and require minimal observer training) (Frick et al., 2010). Nevertheless, there is no standardized way to perform BATs; demand characteristics may influence behavior during the simulation; and the results of a BAT may not generalize. Of course, BATs can be considered both assessment and intervention—an important point that we return to later in the chapter.

With respect to treatment planning, functional assessment has been shown to play an important role in facilitating reductions in school refusal behavior (Kearney, 2001). As a form of narrative direct observation, functional assessment (known earlier in the history of behavior therapy as A-B-C analysis) facilitates an understanding of the factors presumed to explain (influence or cause) the display of the problem behavior. In general, the functional assessment of antecedents and consequences would be expected to reveal that problem behaviors are related to the contingent presentation of social reinforcers (e.g., attention), material reinforcers (i.e., tangibles, access to activities, etc.), or escape or avoidance of stimuli (Reitman & Hupp, 2003). On some occasions, problem behaviors may produce their own reinforcers (automatic or sensory reinforcement). In Sofia's case, functional assessment would be expected to produce meaningful information about the settings and times most strongly associated with Sofia's avoidance behavior. Regarding settings, her school refusal behavior tended to occur at home, as Sofia generally successfully avoided attending school altogether. Avoidance behaviors might start and intensify in the morning before school started and might persist throughout school hours (if Sofia was unsuccessful in avoiding school). School refusal behaviors might be least likely to be observed on weekends or evenings, as no demands to attend school were made at these times.

In Sofia's case, functional assessment could reveal several possible avenues for treatment planning. First, Sofia's initial panic attacks at school, and the associated distress she experienced, would likely have produced a strong response from others ("Are you OK?", etc.). In addition, the initial panic attacks seemed to have resulted in removal from the situation (escape). Consequences that might be contributing to *maintenance* of school refusal behaviors would include her being allowed to remain at home, which could have had a variety of other important consequences. For example, avoidance of school would have eliminated contact with stimuli associated with her declining academic performance (e.g., reducing or eliminating thoughts about being "stupid" or thoughts about the likelihood of having to repeat a grade), as well as eliminating the need for her to confront peers whom she perceived as evaluating her negatively.

APPLICATION TO THE CASE OF BILLY

The study of externalizing behaviors has frequently employed direct observation, most likely because of the overtness of most behaviors that fall under the externalizing umbrella (exceptions for very-low-base-rate behaviors, or explicitly covert behaviors such as theft). In Billy's case, his mother sought help for his oppositional, negativistic, and noncompliant behaviors at home and school. He also presented with some symptoms of anxiety and attention difficulties. Functionally, he appeared to be having significant social difficulties as well as peer conflict at school.

Given the range of potential behavioral targets in such a case, it becomes clear that one the most important tasks in behavior therapy, and hence behavior assessment, is the selection of the problem target. In Billy's case, concerns about his social interactions were high on both his teacher's and his mother's list of concerns, and problems in these interactions were evident both at home and at school. Peer or sibling conflict would be recorded if Billy was observed to be either the instigator or the victim of physical (e.g., hitting with hand, fist, or an object) or verbal (calling names, criticizing, tattling) aggression or conflict. Physical aggression would need to be forceful enough to be heard at a distance of 5 feet, or to cause the victim's body to be displaced by 6 inches. Verbal aggression such as name calling would be defined based on Billy's verbal repertoire (he tended to call others "jerk" or "stupid"), while definitions of critical statements or tattling would be based on whether a statement constituted a negative evaluation (e.g., saying that a picture "looks like it was drawn by a 2-year-old" to a peer) or had the effect of causing a peer to be immediately punished or reprimanded (e.g., a peer was told to "stop" or "cut it out" by a teacher). Note too that Billy need not always be the initiator of the physical or verbal aggression, as the purpose here would be to document "conflict" rather than assign blame. As always, the adequacy of the definition would ultimately be determined by the extent to which it was possible to achieve interobserver reliability. If accuracy was sought as well, a video recording could be constructed by expert raters (i.e., the "creators" of the code) and could be used to establish the criterion or gold standard against which the accuracy of the assessment could be determined (see Baer et al., 2005)

Having defined the code, the observer would need to select the best recording method or technique. In Figure 7.1, we present a partial-interval recording form similar to one we use for academic behavior, as well as for recess or home (living room) behavior. If the form were to be used during recess at Billy's school, for example, the observer could record Billy's behavior in relation to same-sex peers. This form provides six 10-second intervals per row, for a total of 6 minutes of observation. Billy's recess behavior could be recorded in the first minute, and the observer could record a different student's behavior during the next minute. The physical aggression (PA) and verbal aggression (VA) categories represent "examples" (nonexamples would be considered any behaviors inconsistent with the PA or VA code). The "Look" category may be used if an observer wishes to approximate a reactivity effect (i.e., a child spent over 50% of an interval looking at the observer). In partial-interval recording, a behavior is scored if it occurs "at any point" within a 10-second interval. At the end of the observation of Billy at recess the percentages of intervals in which Billy and his "composite" peer displayed physical and verbal aggression and reactivity could be calculated. Such data would likely be of value in establishing the baseline level of conflict Billy experienced during free play at school, and would permit some assessment of

FIGURE 7.1. Partial-interval recording form. PA, physical aggression; VA, verbal aggression; Look, looking at observer.

Setting/activity: _____ Observer: _____

Date: _____ Time began: _____ Target child: _____

	0–10 (sec)	11–20 (sec)	21–30 (sec)	31–40 (sec)	41–50 (sec)	51–60 (sec)
0 minutes (Target)	PA VA Look	PA VA Look	PA VA Look	PA VA Look	PA VA Look	PA VA Look
1 minute (Composite 1)	PA VA Look	PA VA Look	PA VA Look	PA VA Look	PA VA Look	PA VA Look
2 minutes (Target)	PA VA Look	PA VA Look	PA VA Look	PA VA Look	PA VA Look	PA VA Look
3 minutes (Composite 2)	PA VA Look	PA VA Look	PA VA Look	PA VA Look	PA VA Look	PA VA Look
4 minutes (Target)	PA VA Look	PA VA Look	PA VA Look	PA VA Look	PA VA Look	PA VA Look
5 minutes (Composite 3)	PA VA Look	PA VA Look	PA VA Look	PA VA Look	PA VA Look	PA VA Look

Observation Results						

Code	# Intervals (n/30)	%	Comments:
PA			
VA			
LOOK			

the effectiveness of any treatment directed at this very important form of functional impairment.

Functional assessment of Billy's behavior at home and school might also be attempted, to elucidate the factors involved in eliciting and maintaining peer conflict. Several antecedent factors might be identified as contributing to Billy's peer conflict, most notably unskilled (e.g., taking a ball, pulling a girl's hair, or calling someone names) or poorly timed (e.g., interrupting a game in progress) efforts to join his peers in play. Interestingly, such efforts to engage peers, though unsuccessful in maintaining or establishing cooperative, collaborative play bouts, could be very effective in generating immediate attention, albeit usually in the form of "counterattacks." As such, Billy's efforts to engage peers, however unskilled, would be effective (or functional), at least in the short term. Billy's "acting up" or "anxious behavior" and the adult attention it produced could also play a role in maintaining the problem behavior. Finally, ineffective consequences for noncompliance and socially inappropriate behavior (e.g., providing attention for inappropriate behavior and allowing inappropriate behaviors to occur without punishment, as his mother "let him get his way") might contribute further to maintenance of the problem behavior. Many treatments based on the Hanf (1968) model (Reitman & McMahon, 2012) utilize direct observation of dyadic interactions to facilitate the assessment of child behavior problems and guide parent training efforts.

In summary, clinical applications of direct observation may be used during any assessment phase to aid in documenting the existence of a behavior problem (in a relative or an absolute sense), or even as part of the treatment protocol to help determine whether or not mastery criteria for skill acquisition have been met. If functional assessment is employed, direct observation of the child in the setting(s) of interest can play an important role in facilitating successful outcomes. Finally, our examination of these case studies has also identified opportunities for using direct observation to monitor progress. At present, the data suggest that direct observation will continue to be used in concert with assessment tools described in other chapters (e.g., behavior ratings and interviews), to the benefit of children like Sofia and Billy.

IMPLICATIONS FOR TREATMENT PLANNING AND OUTCOMES EVALUATION

In the present chapter, we have sought to examine the role that direct observation should play in the larger enterprise of multimodal assessment. We now turn our attention to the implications of direct observation for treatment planning and outcome evaluation. Specifically, can it be said that direct observation contributes to better outcomes? And should direct observation continue to play a role in short-term treatment monitoring and/ or the assessment of long-term outcomes in clinical practice?

Diagnosis (as Treatment Planning)

In recent reviews of empirically based assessment and intervention for ADHD, Pelham and colleagues (Pelham et al., 2005; Pelham & Fabiano, 2008) have argued that rating scales obtained from parents and teachers can produce accurate, efficient diagnosis. Indeed, failure to observe an externalizing problem behavior on a given day would not be considered sufficient to challenge the accuracy of data obtained from rating scales (Hintze & Matthews, 2004).

Potentially more profitable uses of direct observation for diagnostic purposes may obtain when diagnostic taxa are less closely aligned with rating scales—specifically, when the diagnostic taxonomy is evolving, and/or where assessments are less well developed. For example, diagnosis of autism spectrum disorder (ASD) is challenging and made more so by the frequent inability of the individuals being assessed to contribute data via other assessment methods (because they are young, because their cognitive development is limited, or both) (Malloy, Murray, Akers, Mitchell, & Manning-Courtney, 2011). The cost of making a diagnostic error in the treatment of a child with ASD may also render direct observation more cost-effective. Specifically, a diagnosis of ASD would be likely to suggest a very different course of treatment than would a diagnosis of ADHD with a predominantly inattentive presentation, comorbid with language disorder. In the former case, intensive, in-home, costly behavior-analytic intervention might be called for, whereas outpatient therapy and in-school consultation and/or enhanced school-based services might be the treatment of choice in the latter instance. By contrast, behavioral observations to establish a differential diagnosis of, say, oppositional defiant disorder (ODD) and ADHD with a combined presentation might not be cost-effective, in the sense that empirically based interventions for both tend to call for behavior management training as a first-line course of treatment (Pelham & Fabiano, 2008). Of course, it may well be possible to distinguish children diagnosed with ODD and ADHD— combined via home- or school-based observations (McConaughy et al., 2010), but would it truly be cost-effective to do so? Put differently, does a differential diagnosis of ODD and ADHD—combined have treatment utility? If not, then using direct observation or any other assessment method to improve diagnostic accuracy cannot have treatment utility!

Treatment Planning

Of all the purposes of assessment noted by Mash and Hunsley (2005), treatment planning appears to be the one in which direct observation may be of greatest utility, especially when the focus is on identification of behavioral antecedents (whether proximal or distal). Adherents of the school-based behavior management system known as "positive behavioral support" emphasize the modification of behavioral antecedents over the manipulation of consequences, especially aversive consequences (Horner, 1994). Indeed, the use of direct observation in the context of severe behavior disorders such as self-injurious behavior and feeding disorders can be considered a standard of care (Piazza et al., 1998). In the field of applied behavior analysis, experimental procedures collectively referred to as "functional analysis" (distinguished from "functional assessment" by the emphasis on experimental manipulation of the assessment conditions) have been employed to facilitate improvements in treatment outcome for children with and without disabilities (Gresham, 2003; Sasso, Conroy, Peck-Stichter, & Fox, 2001). For internalizing problems such as phobias and school refusal, exposure to feared stimuli—through role plays or virtual-reality exposures, *in vivo*, or in clinical analogues—constitutes a core feature of treatment. As a result, at some stage of treatment, it is a near-certainty that a child's response to treatment—using (or failing to use) skills learned in the context of therapy—will be subject to direct observation (Kearney, 2001; Velting et al., 2004). When direct observation is utilized in this way, it is difficult to disentangle its treatment planning function from its role in formative (ongoing) or summative outcome evaluation.

Behavior therapists pioneered the entry of paraprofessionals and laypersons into treatment roles (Reitman & McMahon, 2012); thus it should come as no surprise that such individuals have also been engaged in assessment roles, including the use of direct observation. Training parents, for example, to observe and record their own and their children's behavior has also been shown to facilitate positive treatment response (Reitman & Drabman, 1999). Called "Level 1 research" by Hawkins and Mathews (1999), this approach calls for parents (or other laypersons or paraprofessionals) to observe and record clinically relevant child behaviors. The approach is described as "freewheeling" and is devoid of many, if not most, of the requirements for assuring the technical adequacy of direct observations. In Level 1 research, the goal is simply to ask the parent (or other person) to directly observe the child, record the child's activity, and work collaboratively with the therapist to evaluate and make decisions about treatment based on the child's response. Indeed, when parents observe and record child behavior in this way, they have reported changes in child behavior that they were not otherwise aware of; anecdotally, parents sometimes report surprise at the magnitude and frequency of their children's positive behavior in cases where their preexisting biases may have been negative (see Reitman & Drabman, 1999, for an example). Conversely, when parents view their child's behavior in an unrealistically positive light, direct observation through a one-way mirror or via a video recording is sometimes sufficient to alter the parents' perspective. When used in this fashion, direct observation may indeed be exceptionally important to facilitating clinically meaningful change and could significantly affect such important treatment mediators as attendance and/or homework/treatment adherence (Nock & Kurtz, 2005; Pelham et al., 2005; Reitman & Hupp, 2003). Feedback on direct observation may benefit treatment in much the same way that other forms of "feedback" have done (Lambert & Hawkins, 2004). However, we are unaware of any systematic program of research that has sought to evaluate the benefits of direct observation in this way.

In school settings, it has long been customary for teachers, school psychologists, and other interventionists to conduct classroom observations (Alberto & Troutman, 2006). However, many such observations are not functional in the sense that they add to an understanding of the factors that contribute to maintaining such problems, and thus they may not be useful for intervention planning. For example, observational measures derived from child assessment systems such as the ASEBA and the BASC-2 are theoretically agnostic and allow a clinician only to document the existence of a problem (relative to the appropriate normative group) or to document behavior change (e.g., to note pre–post changes after implementation of an intervention). Interestingly, federally mandated functional behavioral assessments typically call for direct observation as part of a larger set of assessment activities including interviews, rating scales, and the examination of records (i.e., the cumulative file, as well as permanent products such as grades or referrals). As to whether such observations add incremental validity to classroom-based interventions (as opposed to incremental validity with respect to diagnostic accuracy, or "pseudotreatment" utility), much remains to be learned. Indeed, Nelson-Gray (2003) has asserted that although there is fairly strong evidence of incremental validity for functional assessment for children with disabilities (and thus, at least indirectly, evidence supporting the use of behavioral observation), more evidence is needed to assert this more generally. A review by Gresham (2003) suggests an absence of clear evidence demonstrating the treatment utility of functional assessment in school-based settings with typically functioning children.

Generalization of behavior from observations obtained via analogues such as functional analysis and via BATs should also be viewed cautiously, as there is no guarantee of generalization—and ample evidence to suggest that there may not be any (Mash & Foster, 2001). Thus, although a child may demonstrate use of skills learned to combat anxiety under the supervision of a parent or therapist, the child may or may not be able to utilize such skills effectively when unaccompanied or outside of the training environment.

Outcome Evaluation

Few would dispute the ultimate value of establishing change in the setting(s) of interest. However, as noted here and elsewhere (see Cone & Foster,

1982), a level of abstraction exists between any given instance of observed behavior and the clinical constructs we attempt to influence (e.g., "being on-task" or "playing cooperatively," or even more abstractly, "developing or maintaining friendships"). Indeed, though empirically based assessment almost reflexively invokes the phrase "multimodal assessment," in practice most clinical assessment (and the vast majority of empirically based clinical research) relies to a surprisingly strong degree on client self-ratings and/or ratings of others (Patterson & Forgatch, 1995). As noted by Patterson and Forgatch (1995), such problems may affect our understanding of the treatment outcome literature:

> Most researchers who study treatment use parent ratings because they are easy to obtain and intrinsically appealing. Who would know better than parents whether a child had changed? However, the findings here ... suggest that mothers' ratings of child behavior reflect improvement even when there is no treatment. Based on maternal reports everything works. (p. 283)

As such, probably the strongest case for collecting direct observation data arises from concerns about whether we can "trust" treatment outcome data that rely (too) heavily on self-reports. Indeed, self-reported reductions in speaking anxiety lack social validity when clinical analogues and direct observation reveal no change in a client's willingness to give a speech or no change in others' ratings of a speaker's level of comfort and persuasiveness. In this respect, the validity of direct observations, when these are conducted with a sufficient level of rigor to be considered accurate and generalizable, is virtually unassailable. In the context of behavioral or cognitive-behavioral treatment, direct observation data *are* incontrovertible indices. If such a measure can be considered reliable and accurate, the most damning critique that can be offered is that the behavior as measured does not capture the larger clinical construct of interest (e.g., reduced aggressive behavior is not equivalent to improved social functioning), or in essence, is not socially valid (Hawkins, 1986; Wolf, 1978).

SUMMARY AND RECOMMENDATIONS

In recent years, clinical applications of direct observation have generally been regarded as important and valuable, but impractical (see Pelham et al., 2005). However, when viewed through the prism of recent developments in our conceptualization of child clinical assessment in general and empirically based assessment in particular, a more nuanced assessment of behavioral observation seems warranted. When it is utilized to facilitate diagnostic assessment, and especially when the diagnostic criteria are closely aligned with behavioral rating scales, direct observation is probably unnecessary (i.e., has no incremental validity). When it is used for treatment planning, however, direct observation appears to have more convincing evidence of clinical utility. As noted by Nelson-Gray (2003), functional analysis, which requires direct observation, is considered "best practice" in the treatment of children with developmental disabilities and severe behavioral disorders. Indeed, as Mash and Foster (2001) hoped, increasingly inventive researchers appear to be revolutionizing analogue behavioral assessments, broadening contexts in which they may be employed, and utilizing research to improve the analogues so that they better capture important behavioral dimensions (treatment mediators) that can more readily be assessed in clinical settings. For example, though the data are not exclusively derived from direct observation, Dishion's Family Check-Up (Lunkenheimer et al., 2008), is an example of a clinical analogue that generates meaningful data on parent–child interaction and communication patterns while serving as a proximal indicator of clinical improvement/treatment outcome.

It is hard to imagine contemporary behavioral and cognitive-behavioral interventions without behavioral observation (Velting et al., 2004). Indeed, Velting et al. (2004) assert that direct observation outside the office, though difficult, is vital. They suggest that the use of visual media and telecommunications could be an important way to reduce costs and eliminate logistical problems associated with the treatment of separation anxiety, social phobia, and generalized anxiety disorder. With the advent of smart phones, obtaining and sharing such information would seem more feasible than ever, although ethical and legal barriers to sharing such information may present themselves as this practice evolves. Velting et al. (2004) also note that while families may exhibit resistance to the additional effort and planning that may go into arranging for BATs, or family BAT, it may be worthwhile to expend extra clinical effort to gaining the families' support for such exercises.

Correspondence of Direct Observation to Self-Reports and Rating Scales: Artifacts and Alternatives

Informant ratings and direct observation have traditionally shown only low to modest relationships—a finding that has been vexing to both researchers and clinicians (Achenbach, McConaughy, & Howell, 1987). However, Lorenz, Melby, Conger, and Xu (2007) suggest that relations between direct observation and ratings could be attenuated by a "context-by-measurement confound." This type of confound is produced by the mismatch between direct observations, which tend to be specific and context-dependent, and questionnaires and rating scales, which typically ask respondents to recall their behavior or the behavior of others under "more heterogeneous or amorphous conditions" (p. 499). Extrapolating from data on ratings of couples' hostility during discussions, Lorenz et al. (2007) found that correlations between direct observations of hostility and ratings of hostility for the observation were nearly twice the magnitude of correlations between the observations and questionnaires that asked them to report about hostility over the past month. Similarly, in a study seeking to validate the Parenting Scale (PS), Arnold, O'Leary, Wolff, and Acker (1993) found unusually large correspondence between videotaped direct observations of parent–child interaction and parents' self-ratings of their parenting style on the PS (i.e., r range = .38–.79). Interestingly, observers in this study utilized an observational rating system that closely resembled the PS as completed by the parents themselves (in fact, it appeared simply to have been reworded). As a result, not only did Arnold et al. (1993) address the context-by-measurement confound; they also held constant the item content and format used to respond. Given the widespread extent to which such artifacts might exist in studies examining the correspondence of analogue behavioral observations and ratings by others, Lorenz et al. (2007) assert that analogue assessments may relate more strongly to questionnaire reports than was previously believed.

Notwithstanding the arguments in favor of obtaining direct observations of behavior, there will undoubtedly still be circumstances where such observations will be cost-prohibitive or impractical. Under such circumstances, alternative sources of data, which share at least some of the positive characteristics of observational data (perhaps by virtue of being "direct"), may be still be preferable to rating scales and self-reports. Among such alternatives may be "direct behavior ratings" (DBRs), which have been used to assess the construct of student engagement in classroom-based studies (Briesch et al., 2010; Riley-Tillman, Chafouleas, Sassu, Chanese, & Glazer, 2008). DBRs place observers in direct contact with the behavior(s) in question, but rather than being concerned with moment-to-moment changes in the behavior in question, respondents provide global assessments of more molar behavioral units. Although a preliminary study appeared to support the use of DBRs (Riley-Tillman et al., 2008), a more recent evaluation was decidedly less supportive of the notion that DBRs could be used in lieu of direct observation (Briesch et al., 2010).

Efforts to assess more molar behavioral categories may turn out to be far less intensive in terms of training and more reliable, which would significantly reduce many of the costs associated with direct observation (Mash & Foster, 2001). Indeed, Patterson et al. (1992) have utilized more molar behavioral observation schemes to good effect in building latent models of important constructs related to antisocial behavior. Another innovation associated with Patterson's Oregon Social Learning Center, the telephone checklist (e.g., the Parent Daily Report), provides outcome data based on short-term client recall that is more closely tied to the behavioral events than is typically possible with rating scales and self-reports. Such measures have the added benefit of being able to be "customized" to address only a client's presenting concerns.

A final form of behavioral assessment, "individualized target behavior evaluation" (ITBE), is a hybrid behavioral assessment that utilizes a form of direct observation, but the observations are greatly simplified so that teachers and parents can provide the necessary data. Examples of ITBEs that are already in common use are daily report cards. Such approaches relate directly to observed behavior in that these forms of data are produced directly by behavioral actions professionals might hope to observe, but lack the resources to obtain. Copies of completed assignments or school behavior logs, also known as "permanent products" in the school psychology literature (see Atkins, Pelham, & Licht, 1985), can likewise be reviewed. Permanent products should be highly correlated with direct observations of on-task behavior, but come at greatly reduced cost. Similarly, one might wish to determine whether a child has or has not utilized a set of organizational skills, which might prove quite daunting to observe via naturalistic observation. Using an ITBE, a teacher or parent can rate the condition of a child's desk or book bag for organizational quality. Importantly, ITBEs may address many of the criticisms previously leveled at direct observations in clinical settings, especially those aimed at the high level of effort and cost associated with obtaining such data.

Recommendations

The most central lesson emerging from the past four decades of research on assessment is the recognition that tests (assessment) are not "valid" in and of themselves, but rather are validated for specific purposes (Cone & Foster, 1982; Mash & Hunsley, 2005). Moreover, our evaluation of the utility of any given form of assessment is likely to depend upon the nature of the task and the purposes of assessment. Ultimately, behavioral observations, like functional behavioral assessment itself, may not be called for until less labor-intensive assessment and protocols have been tried—which is consistent with the "least restrictive intervention" principle (Cooper et al., 2007).

In the early days of behavioral assessment, ongoing measurement of progress was considered a core feature of behavioral interventions. Thus the distinctions among assessment, treatment planning, and treatment outcome were not as clear as in other clinical traditions (Hayes, Nelson, & Jarrett, 1987). Indeed, sharing and incorporating the results of ongoing assessment appear to have a positive impact on treatment outcome (Lambert & Hawkins, 2004). Hawkins and Mathews (1999) have also argued that feedback regarding treatment progress is beneficial, especially when clients participate in the assessment. Though direct observation does not seem crucial for informing diagnostic decision making, it does seem likely to facilitate the achievement of better outcomes, though the mechanism for this is unknown and data supporting this contention are limited. Technology may hold the key and shift the balance from pencil-and-paper methods to a blend of assessment approaches that maximizes the benefits of clinical assessment.

One of the most important developments affecting the clinical usage of direct observation, and one that has undoubtedly fueled a renewed interest in this assessment method, is the inclusion of direct observation in recent legislation concerned with the requirements of IDEA and functional assessment (Gresham, 2003; Nock & Kurtz, 2005). Indeed, although systematic or formal observations may be rare in clinical settings (Pelham et al., 2005), the use of direct observation in schools appears well established, despite its questionable fidelity (Sasso et al., 2001). Current legislation *requires* a commitment of resources to facilitate compliance with the law, which ultimately supports the practice. Thus, while behavioral observations may be "expensive," legal requirements to comply with IDEA necessitate that school systems provide the resources needed to conduct them. By contrast, no such contingencies appear to operate in clinical practice, so the use of systematic behavioral observation languishes. Research settings are the only other contexts in which direct observation appears common, and this occurs because editors require it and funding agencies are willing to pay for it (Baer et al., 2005). Finally, recent advances in theory, specifically G theory, appear to be driving a resurgence of research on direct observation and behavioral assessment (Brennan, 2010). Although it may be too early to make any predictions, our knowledge and understanding of the purposes of assessment and the role that various assessment practices may play in promoting advances in child interventions seem certain to increase over the next decade.

REFERENCES

Abikoff, H., & Gittelman, R. (1985). Classroom Observation Code: A modification of the Stony Brook code. *Psychopharmacology Bulletin, 21,* 901–909.

Achenbach, T. M. (2009). *The Achenbach System of Empirically Based Assessment (ASEBA): Development, findings, theory, and applications.* Burlington: University of Vermont Research Center for Children, Youth, and Families.

Achenbach, T. M., McConaughy, S. H., & Howell, C. T. (1987). Child/adolescent behavioral and emotional problems: Implications of cross-informant correlations for situational specificity. *Psychological Bulletin, 101,* 213–232.

Alberto, P., & Troutman, A. (2006). *Applied behavior analysis for teachers* (7th ed.). Columbus, OH: Pearson.

Arnold, D. S., O'Leary, S. G., Wolff, L., & Acker, M. (1993). The Parenting Scale: A measure of dysfunctional parenting in discipline situations. *Psychological Assessment, 5,* 137–144.

Atkins, M., Pelham, W. E., & Licht, M. (1985). A comparison of objective classroom measures and teacher ratings of attention deficit disorder. *Journal of Abnormal Child Psychology, 13,* 155–167.

Baer, D. M., Harrison, R., Fradenburg, L., Petersen, D., & Milla, S. (2005). Some pragmatics in the valid and reliable recording of directly observed behavior. *Research on Social Work Practice, 15,* 440–451.

Baumeister, R. F., Vohs, K. D., & Funder, D. C. (2007). Psychology as the science of self-reports and finger movements: Whatever happened to actual behavior? *Perspectives on Psychological Science, 2*(4), 396–403.

Brennan, R. L. (2010). Generalizability theory and classical test theory, *Applied Measurement in Education, 24,* 1–21.

Briesch, A. M., Chafouleas, S. M., & Riley-Tillman, T. C. (2010). Generalizability and dependability of behavior assessment methods to estimate academic engagement: A comparison of systematic direct observation. *School Psychology Review, 39,* 408–421.

Chafouleas, S. M., Riley-Tillman, T. C., & Sugai, G. (2007). *School-based behavioral assessment: Informing intervention and instruction.* New York: Guilford Press.

Cone, J. D. (1977). The relevance of reliability and validity for behavioral assessment. *Behavior Therapy, 8,* 411–426.

Cone, J. D. (1992). That was then! This is now! *Behavioral Assessment, 14,* 219–228.

Cone, J. D., & Foster, S. L. (1982). Direct observation in clinical psychology. In P. Kendall & J. Butcher (Eds.), *Handbook of research methods in clinical psychology* (pp. 311–354). New York: Wiley.

Cooper, J. O., Heron, T. E., & Heward, W. L. (2007). *Applied behavior analysis* (2nd ed.). Columbus, OH: Pearson.

Cronbach, L. J., Gleser, G. C., Nanda, H., & Rajaratnam, N. (1972). *The dependability of behavioral measurements.* New York: Wiley.

Ervin, R. A., DuPaul, G. J., Kern, L., & Friman, P. C. (1998). Classroom-based functional and adjunctive assessments: Proactive approaches to intervention selection for adolescents with attention deficit hyperactivity disorder. *Journal of Applied Behavior Analysis, 31,* 65–78.

Foster, S. L., & Cone, J. D. (1986). Design and use of direct observation procedures. In A. Ciminero, K. Calhoun, & H. Adams (Eds.), *Handbook of behavioral assessment* (2nd ed., pp. 253–234). New York: Wiley.

Foster, S. L., & Cone, J. D. (1995). Validity issues in clinical assessment. *Psychological Assessment, 7*(3), 248–260.

Freud, S. (1953). Analysis of a phobia in a five-year-old boy. In J. Strachey (Ed. & Trans.), *The standard edition of the complete psychological works of Sigmund Freud* (Vol. 10, pp. 3–149). London: Hogarth Press. (Original work published 1909)

Frick, P. J., Barry, C. T., & Kamphaus, R. W. (2010). *Clinical assessment of child and adolescent personality and behavior* (3rd ed.). New York: Springer.

Gresham, F. M. (2003). Establishing the technical adequacy of functional behavioral assessment: Conceptual and measurement challenges. *Behavioral Disorders, 28,* 282–298.

Gross, A. M. (1990). An analysis of measures and design strategies in research in behavior therapy: Is it still behavioral? *The Behavior Therapist, 13,* 203–209.

Haney, C., Banks, W., & Zimbardo, P. (1973). Interpersonal dynamics in a simulated prison. *International Journal of Criminology and Penology, 1,* 69–97.

Hanf, C. (1968). *Modifying problem behaviors in mother–child interactions: Standardized laboratory situations.* Paper presented at the conference of the Association for Advancement of Behavior Therapy, Olympia, WA.

Hawes, D., & Dadds, M. R. (2006). Assessing parenting practices through parent-report and direct observation during parent-training. *Journal of Child and Family Studies, 15,* 555–568.

Hawkins, R. P. (1986). Selection of target behaviors. In R. O. Nelson & S. C. Hayes (Eds.), *Conceptual foundations of behavioral assessment* (pp. 331–385). New York: Guilford Press

Hawkins, R. P., & Mathews, J. R. (1999). Frequent monitoring of clinical outcomes: Research and accountability for clinical practice. *Education and Treatment of Children, 22,* 117–135.

Hayes, S. C., Nelson, R. O., & Jarrett, R. B. (1987). The treatment utility of assessment. *American Psychologist, 42*(11), 963–974.

Haynes, S. N. (2001). Clinical applications of analogue behavioral observation: Dimensions of psychometric evaluation. *Psychological Assessment, 13,* 73–85.

Haynes, S. N., Richard, D. C. S., & Kubany, E. S. (1995). Content validity in psychological assessment: A functional approach to concepts and methods. *Psychological Assessment, 7*(3), 238–247.

Hinshaw, S. P., Zupan, B. A., Simmel, C., Nigg, J. T., & Melnick, S. (1997). Peer status in boys with and without attention deficit disorder: Predictions from overt and covert antisocial behavior, social isolation, and authoritative parenting beliefs.. *Child Development, 68,* 880–896.

Hintze, J. M. (2005). Psychometrics of direct observation. *School Psychology Review, 34*(4), 507–519.

Hintze, J. M., & Matthews, W. J. (2004). The generalizability of systemic direct observations across time and setting: A preliminary investigation of the psychometrics of behavioral observation. *School Psychology Review, 33*(2), 258–270.

Horner, R. H. (1994). Functional assessment: Contributions and future directions. *Journal of Applied Behavior Analysis, 27*(2), 401–404.

Jacobs, J. R., Boggs, S. R., Eyberg, S. M., Edwards, D., Durning, P., Querido, J. G., & Funderburk, B. W. (2000). Psychometric properties and reference point data for the Revised Edition of the School Observation Coding System. *Behavior Therapy, 31,* 695–712.

Johnston, J. M., & Pennypacker, H. S. (1993). *Strategies and tactics of behavioral research* (2nd ed.). Hillsdale, NJ: Erlbaum.

Kearney, C. A. (2001). *School refusal behavior in youth: A functional approach to assessment and treatment.* Washington, DC: American Psychological Association.

Lambert, M. J., & Hawkins, E. J. (2004). Measuring outcome in professional practice: Considerations in selecting and using brief outcome instruments. *Professional Psychology: Research and Practice, 35,* 492–499.

Lang, P. J., & Lazovik, A. D. (1963). Experimental desensitization of a phobia. *Journal of Abnormal and Social Psychology, 66,* 519–525.

Lorenz, F. O., Melby, J. N., Conger, R. D., & Xu, X. (2007). The effects of context on the correspondence between observation ratings and questionnaire reports of hostile behavior: A multitrait, multimethod approach. *Journal of Family Psychology, 21,* 498–509.

Lunkenheimer, E. S., Dishion, T. J., Shaw, D. S., Connell, A. M., Gardner, F., Wilson, M. N., & Skuban, E. M. (2008). Collateral benefits of the Family Check-Up on early childhood school readiness: Indirect effects of parents' positive behavior. *Developmental Psychology, 44,* 1737–1752.

Malloy, C. A., Murray, D. S., Akers, R., Mitchell, T., & Manning-Courtney, P. (2011). Use of the Autism Diagnostic Observation Schedule (ADOS) in a clinical setting. *Autism, 15,* 143–162.

Mash, E. J., & Foster, S. L. (2001). Exporting analogue behavioral observation from research to clinical practice: Useful or cost-defective? *Psychological Assessment, 13*, 86–98.

Mash, E. J., & Hunsley, J. (2005). Evidence-based assessment of child and adolescent disorders: Issues and challenges. *Journal of Clinical Child and Adolescent Psychology, 34*(3), 362–379.

McConaughy, S. H., Harder, V. S., Antshel, K. M., Gordon, M., Eiraldi, R., & Dumenci, L. (2010). Incremental validity of test session and classroom observations in a multimethod assessment of attention deficit/hyperactivity disorder. *Journal of Clinical Child and Adolescent Psychology, 39*(5), 650–666.

Milgram, S. (1963). Behavioral study of obedience. *Journal of Abnormal and Social Psychology, 67*, 371–378.

Miltenberger, R. G. (2008). *Behavior modification: Principles and procedures* (4th ed.). Belmont, CA: Wadsworth/Thomson Learning.

Mischel, W. (1968). *Personality and assessment.* New York: Wiley.

Mori, L. T., & Armendariz, G. M. (2001). Analogue assessment of child behavior problems. *Psychological Assessment, 13*, 36–45.

Nelson, R. O., Hay, L. R., & Hay, W. M. (1977). Comments on Cone's "The relevance of reliability and validity for behavioral assessment." *Behavior Therapy, 8*, 427–430.

Nelson-Gray, R. O. (2003). Treatment utility of psychological assessment. *Psychological Assessment, 15*, 521–531.

Nock, M. K., & Kurtz, S. M. (2005). Direct behavioral observation in school settings: Bringing science to practice. *Cognitive and Behavioral Practice, 12*, 359–370.

O'Neill, R. E., Horner, R. H., Albin, R. W., Sprague, J. R., Storey, K., & Newton, J. S. (1997). *Functional assessment and program development for problem behavior: A practical handbook* (2nd ed.). Pacific Grove, CA: Brooks/Cole.

Patterson, G. R., & Forgatch, M. (1995). Predicting future clinical adjustment from treatment outcome and process variables. *Psychological Assessment, 7*, 275–285.

Patterson, G. R., Reid, J. B., & Dishion, T. R. (1992). *Antisocial boys.* Eugene, OR: Castalia.

Pavlov, I. P. (1927). *Conditioned reflexes* (G. V. Anrep, Ed. & Trans.). London: Oxford University Press.

Pelham, W. E., & Fabiano, G. A. (2008). Evidence-based psychosocial treatments for attention-deficit/hyperactivity disorder. *Journal of Clinical Child and Adolescent Psychology, 37*, 184–214.

Pelham, W. E., Fabiano, G. A., & Massetti, G. M. (2005). Evidence-based assessment of attention deficit hyperactivity disorder in children and adolescents. *Journal of Clinical Child and Adolescent Psychology, 34*, 449–476.

Piazza, C. C., Fischer, W. W., Hanley, G. P., LeBlanc, L. A., Wordsell, A. S., Lindauer, S. E., & Keeney, K. M. (1998). Treatment of pica through multiple analyses of its reinforcing functions. *Journal of Applied Behavior Analysis, 33*, 13–27.

Reitman, D., & Drabman, R. S. (1999). Multi-faceted uses of a simple time-out record in the treatment of a noncompliant 8-year-old boy. *Education and Treatment of Children, 22*, 194–203.

Reitman, D., & Hupp, S. D. A. (2003). Behavior problems in the school setting: Synthesizing structural and functional assessment. In M. L. Kelley, D.

Reitman, & G. Noell (Eds.), *Practitioner's guide to empirically based measures of school behavior* (pp. 23–36). New York: Kluwer Academic/Plenum.

Reitman, D., & McMahon, R. C. (2012). Constance "Connie" Hanf (1917–2002): The mentor and the model. *Cognitive and Behavioral Practice.*

Reynolds, C. R., & Kamphaus, R. W. (2004). *Behavior Assessment System for Children, Second Edition: Manual.* Circle Pines, MN: American Guidance Service.

Riley-Tillman, T. C., Chafouleas, S. M., Sassu, K. A., Chanese, J. A., & Glazer, A D. (2008). Examining the agreement of direct behavior ratings and systematic direct observation data for on-task and disruptive behavior. *Journal of Positive Behavior Interventions, 10*(2), 136–143.

Risley, T. R., & Hart, B. (1968). Developing correspondence between the nonverbal and verbal behavior of preschool children. *Journal of Applied Behavior Analysis, 1,* 267–281.

Roberts, M. W. (2001). Clinic observations of structured parent–child interaction designed to evaluate externalizing disorders. *Psychological Assessment, 13,* 46–58.

Sasso, G. M., Conroy, M. A., Peck-Stichter, J., & Fox, J. J. (2001). Slowing down the bandwagon: The misapplication of functional assessment for students with emotional or behavioral disorders. *Behavioral Disorders, 26,* 282–296.

Shavelson, R. J., Webb, N. M., & Rowley, G. L. (1989). Generalizabiity theory. *American Psychologist, 44,* 922–932.

Sherif, M. (1966). *In common predicament: Social psychology of intergroup conflict and cooperation.* Boston: Houghton Mifflin.

Sidman, M. (1960). *Tactics of scientific research.* New York: Basic Books.

Skinner, B. F. (1953). *Science and human behavior.* New York: Macmillan.

Suen, H. K., & Ary, D. (1989). *Analyzing quantitative behavioral observation data.* Hillsdale, NJ: Erlbaum.

Velting, O. N., Setzer, N. J., & Albano, A. M. (2004). Update on advances in assessment and cognitive-behavioral treatment of anxiety disorders in children and adolescents. *Professional Psychology: Research and Practice, 35,* 42–54.

Volpe, R. J., DiPerna, J. C., Hintze, J. M., & Shapiro, E. S. (2005). Observing students in classroom settings: A review of seven coding schemes. *School Psychology Review, 34*(4), 454–474.

Volpe, R. J., McConaughy, S. H., & Hintze, J. M. (2009). Generalizability of classroom behavior problem and on-task scores from the Direct Observation Form. *School Psychology Review, 38*(3), 382–401.

West, S. G., & Brown, T. J. (1975). Physical attractiveness, the severity of the emergency and helping: A field experiment and interpersonal simulation. *Journal of Experimental Social Psychology, 11,* 531–538.

Wolf, M. M. (1978). Social validity: The case for subjective measurement or how applied behavior analysis is finding its heart. *Journal of Applied Behavior Analysis, 11,* 203–214.

8

Self-Monitoring

Christine L. Cole and Catherine A. Kunsch

Self-monitoring is an evidence-based strategy that has been used success-fully with children and adolescents in clinical settings for several decades (Broden, Hall, & Mitts, 1971; Nelson, 1977; Shapiro & Cole, 1994). In self-monitoring, children and adolescents with emotional and behav-ioral problems are taught to observe and record specific aspects of their behavior. Because the technique involves the youth in assessing their own behavior, it conceptually allows therapists or other behavior change agents to monitor the youth's difficulties without involving other independent observers (Reid, 1996; Shapiro & Cole, 1994). In addition, self-monitoring potentially provides information about private events, such as thoughts and feelings, that are not accessible in any other way. Self-monitoring is gener-ally conceptualized as including the two activities of self-observation and self-recording. "Self-observation" involves being aware of one's actions and knowing whether or not the behavior of interest has occurred. "Self-record-ing" refers to the activity of noting the occurrence of the observed behavior by using either paper and pencil or some other recording method. Self-monitoring strategies such as journaling, self-reporting, and self-graphing are included in the broad framework of self-monitoring processes (Shapiro & Cole, 1999).

Self-monitoring is considered both an assessment and an intervention technique. When self-monitoring is used for assessment purposes, children and adolescents may be asked to monitor or assess their own behavior, independently of the intervention procedure used. This may be part of the initial assessment process that attempts to understand a behavior's func-tion or obtain an initial behavior level. Self-monitoring can also be used for more extended periods as an outcome measure to determine the effects of intervention procedures or other therapeutic activities over time. The most obvious benefit of using a self-monitoring approach for assessment is that the information gathered may only be accessible to the child or adolescent. In addition, child-collected data are more convenient to obtain than data collected by adult observers. A self-monitoring approach that shifts responsibility for data collection from the adult to the child or adolescent typically reduces time demands on adults.

In addition to being a potentially valuable assessment tool, self-monitoring may also be used as an intervention strategy to encourage behavior change. In fact, self-monitoring has strong empirical support for its use with children and adolescents in the behavior change process (Briesch & Chafouleas, 2009; Mooney, Ryan, Uhing, Reid, & Epstein, 2005; Reid, 1996). Numerous studies have demonstrated that the activities of observing and recording one's own behavior often result in "reactive effects," or positive changes in the behavior being self-monitored (Reid, 1996; Shapiro & Cole, 1994). Although reactivity does not always result from self-monitoring, it does occur frequently enough to support its usefulness as an intervention. In fact, self-monitoring is a well-established intervention for children and adolescents with a variety of problem behaviors (Briesch & Chafouleas, 2009; Mooney et al., 2005).

Although self-monitoring as an assessment tool is conceptually sensible, using self-monitoring for purposes of assessment with children introduces significant problems (Shapiro & Cole, 1999). The questionable accuracy of data collected through self-report when children are the sole reporters is an obvious difficulty. The accuracy of child or adolescent self-reports may vary widely, depending on their developmental level and on the nature of the behavior being reported (La Greca, 1990; Ollendick, Grills, & King, 2001; Stone & Lemanek, 1990). Furthermore, there is evidence that young children in particular can be greatly influenced by suggestions to report events that never actually occurred (Bruck, Ceci, & Hembrooke, 1998). Clearly, there are numerous potential biases in the data recorded by youth without independent verification, and this issue is explored more fully later in the chapter.

It is also important to note that the developmental literature has conceptualized self-monitoring in somewhat different ways. Whereas the clinical and behavior change literature has focused on the "monitoring" process within self-monitoring, the developmental literature has focused more on the "self." From the developmental perspective, self-monitoring is viewed as a cognitive construct or personality trait that reflects the extent to which individuals monitor their expressive behavior and self-presentation through the processes of self-observation and self-control (Snyder, 1979). Efforts within the social cognition and personality literature have been devoted to understanding the impact of the construct of self-monitoring.

Although examining the nature of the self-monitoring construct presents some interesting opportunities for predicting the effectiveness of the self-monitoring process, the purpose of this chapter is to describe evidence-based self-monitoring strategies used with children and adolescents throughout the assessment and treatment process. In addition, the emphasis of the chapter is on explaining the methodology of self-monitoring, rather than on comprehensively reviewing the outcomes of studies in which these techniques were used. Readers interested in comprehensive reviews of outcome studies are referred to Briesch and Chafouleas (2009), Mooney et al. (2005), Reid (1996), and Webber, Scheuermann, McCall, and Coleman (1993). In our examination of the use of self-monitoring in clinical work with children and adolescents, the methodology is described, and use of self-monitoring is explored for both internalizing and externalizing disorders. Specifically, we first examine the use of self-monitoring for internalizing disorders such as anxiety and depression in youth. The cognitive and personal nature of these disorders requires children and adolescents to engage in the monitoring of private events, and self-monitoring can serve as a potential vehicle to assess these internal emotional states. Next, the self-monitoring of externalizing problems in youth, including symptoms of attention-deficit/hyperactivity disorder (ADHD), is discussed. The final section summarizes and offers future directions for self-monitoring research and practice in clinical work with children and adolescents.

DESCRIPTION OF THE ASSESSMENT METHOD

Child and Adolescent Characteristics

The empirical literature has demonstrated the feasibility of self-monitoring techniques for children and adolescents with numerous individual differences. Children and adolescents who have a range of behavioral and emotional difficulties have successfully used self-monitoring to assess their behavior in various clinical, residential, school, and community settings. Included are individuals with diagnoses of developmental disabilities (Hughes et al., 2002), learning disabilities (Snyder & Bambara, 1997), autism (Loftin, Odom, & Lantz, 2007), and a variety of emotional/behavioral disorders (Barry & Messer, 2003), as well as those with no specific diagnosis (e.g., Wood, Murdock, & Cronin, 2002). Children of all ages, from preschool to high school, have learned to use self-monitoring. Empirical evidence suggests that this strategy can be useful for the entire range of children served in a variety of settings. The only exceptions may be very young children, or those who are unable to self-monitor because of severe cognitive or emotional limitations. In these instances, parents are often asked to monitor instead, as long as the targets to be monitored are overt behaviors. Although technically this is not self-monitoring, several studies reviewed later have demonstrated the successful use of parent monitoring in addition to child self-monitoring.

Self-monitoring typically has been used by an individual child or adolescent to observe and record target behaviors that occur in one or more settings (e.g., Kern, Marder, Boyajian, Elliot, & McElhattan, 1997). The types of behaviors that can be self-monitored by children and adolescents range from concrete behaviors that are readily observable by the youth and others (e.g., disruptive behaviors, cigarettes smoked) to more subjective behaviors that are observable only to the youth (e.g., negative thoughts, anxious feelings). As long as the behavior to be monitored can be clearly communicated to a child or adolescent, almost any behavior can be self-monitored.

Self-Monitoring Procedures

In selecting a procedure for self-monitoring, a clinician or evaluator should consider several factors to ensure that a child or adolescent will in fact self-record behavior and that this recording will be accurate. Initially, a procedure should be selected that is relatively easy to use and is appropriate for the behavior being recorded. For example, a procedure that requires a child to self-monitor at specified time intervals would be appropriate for high-rate or ongoing behaviors (e.g., attending behavior in a classroom setting). To be feasible for use, the procedure should be inexpensive and relatively unobtrusive. Although, as discussed later in this chapter, an obtrusive recording device may serve as a cue for self-monitoring and therefore potentially enhance the accuracy of self-monitoring, a balance is needed between the obtrusiveness of the recording device and its feasibility and acceptability to the child or adolescent and those in the setting in which it is being used.

Types of Information Collected

A commonly used procedure involves having a child or adolescent self-monitor each occurrence of a target behavior, usually at the time of occurrence. This procedure is most useful when the frequency of the behavior is relatively low, when the occurrence is of short duration, and when the behavior is discrete. Examples include self-monitoring of negative statements by an adolescent with mild intellectual and developmental disabilities (Martella, Leonard, Marchand-Martella, & Agran, 1993) or self-monitoring homework completion by adolescents with learning disabilities (Trammel, Schloss, & Alper, 1994). These types of data are typically summarized as "total frequency" or, if self-monitoring sessions vary in length, as "rate of occurrence" (i.e., total frequency divided by total observation time).

Most often, self-monitoring in school settings involves data collected via "time sampling." With time sampling, a target behavior is self-monitored at the end of each specified time interval. Sugai and Rowe (1984) used a time-sampling procedure to obtain self-monitoring data from a 15-year-old male with mild developmental disabilities. At the end of each 10-minute interval, the adolescent was signaled by a kitchen timer to assess whether he had remained in his seat for the entire 10-minute period and to record an "I" (in seat) or "O" (out of seat) as appropriate.

A popular procedure used with self-monitoring on-task behavior is that of spot-checking, called "momentary time sampling" (e.g., Prater, Hogan, & Miller, 1992). In using this procedure, children are signaled (usually by an auditory tone) to self-monitor several times throughout a class period following short intervals of time, such as every 5 minutes. At the tone, children are instructed to decide whether they were attending or not attending, and mark a + or – on their recording sheet. These self-monitored data are typically summarized as "percentage on task," calculated by dividing the number of on-task occurrences by the total number of times the signal was given, multiplied by 100.

Self-monitoring may also be useful in the initial stages of a functional behavioral assessment to select a target behavior and/or develop hypotheses about possible factors involved in its occurrence. This type of preliminary data may be provided by a child or adolescent in the form of narrative descriptions in a behavioral log or diary, and may be structured or unstructured. For example, the child or adolescent could be asked to record occurrences of a specified behavior and the circumstances involved, such as the setting or situation in which the behavior occurred (e.g., school cafeteria, friend's home, etc.), or antecedents and consequences of the action. Also, child functional behavioral assessment interviews such as the Student-Assisted Functional Assessment Interview (Kern, Dunlap, Clarke, & Childs, 1995) may be useful for gathering functional assessment data.

Recording Devices

Various types of recording devices are available for use in self-monitoring. Historically, the most popular recording devices have been paper-and-pencil procedures (e.g., Harris, Graham, Reid, McElroy, & Hamby, 1994). Paper-and-pencil recording forms may vary from a simple journal in which a child makes entries, to an index card or a slip of paper on which the child makes a tally mark at each cue, to a more detailed individualized form. Examples of the use of mechanical devices, such as hand-held, belt-worn, or wrist counters for self-monitoring, also appear in the literature (e.g., Ollendick, 1981).

More recently, electronic devices such as cell phones and electronic diaries have been used by children and adolescents for self-monitoring (e.g., Henker, Whalen, Jamner, & Delfino, 2002; Tan et al., 2012; Whalen, Henker, King, Jamner, & Levine, 2004). Other, less conventional strategies have been used for "recording" children's self-monitoring. In one example, preschoolers used a thumbs-up or thumbs-down signal when teachers asked them to monitor their behavior following transition, free-play, and small-group instruction times (Miller, Strain, Boyd, Jarzynka, & McFetridge, 1993). In another example, teenagers with autism removed a token from a back pocket and placed it in a front pocket to self-monitor each transition to a new activity (Newman et al., 1995).

A number of factors should be considered in selecting a recording device. First, to increase the accuracy of self-monitoring, the device should be available for recording the target behavior as it occurs. If it is to be used in more than one setting, obviously the recording device must be portable. Second, the recording device should be easy to use and not distracting. If the child continues to manipulate or attend to the device after self-monitoring, the child may not attend to the ongoing activities, and the goal of self-monitoring may not be met. Third, the device should be sufficiently obtrusive that the child is aware of it and will use it for recording, but should not be excessively conspicuous to attract attention from others. This is a particular concern in inclusive school-based and community settings. A final consideration in selecting a recording device is its cost. For example, although an iPhone or iPod may be ideal to use with a child or adolescent because the device is portable, is unobtrusive, and serves as a reminder for self-monitoring, the cost may be prohibitive.

Prompts to Self-Monitor

Many different types of prompts may be used to signal children or adolescents to self-monitor their behavior. In school settings, external prompts have most often been used. External prompts can be either verbal or nonverbal, and can be delivered by another person (e.g., teacher, aide, support person) or by a mechanical device (e.g., tone on a prerecorded tape, kitchen timer). Verbal prompts may be useful when an entire class is self-monitoring and can involve a simple reminder from the teacher to self-monitor at the end of each class period. In other cases in which only one or a few students are self-monitoring, it may be more feasible to use nonverbal prompts, such as having the teacher periodically signal or tap the individual student(s) on the shoulder when it is time for self-monitoring. One of the most commonly used prompts is a prerecorded tone, since it requires limited teacher time and can be used with an individual or an entire class.

In others settings, self-prompting may be used successfully. With self-prompting or noncued self-monitoring, children or adolescents are typically instructed to note on their own, from time to time during the designated self-monitoring period, whether or not they were engaging in the target behavior. No external prompting is provided. This type of self-prompting procedure has been used most often for self-monitoring internalizing behavior; it is described in more detail in an upcoming section.

Self-Monitoring Training

The methods used in instructing children and adolescents to self-monitor their behavior are related to the complexity of the information requested and of the self-monitoring procedure itself, as well as to individual characteristics such as age, cognitive level, and presence of competing behaviors. The training procedures may range from simple verbal instructions to detailed training programs involving instruction, modeling, behavior rehearsal, performance feedback, and reinforcement. Direct instruction combined with behavior rehearsal of simulated situations, or video-recorded scenes of actual behaviors and situations, may be used. Training may occur in the natural setting or in a separate training location.

The specific training procedures selected should ensure that the child or adolescent understands what is expected and has the skills to implement the self-monitoring procedure. To increase the probability of accurate self-monitoring, training programs should include: (1) explicit definition of the target behavior; (2) simplified behavior counting and recording procedures; (3) specific and relatively short time periods in which self-monitoring occurs; (4) accuracy checks and corrective feedback, if necessary; and (5) sufficient practice to ensure that fluency in self-monitoring is attained (Frith & Armstrong, 1985).

ISSUES OF ACCURACY AND REACTIVITY IN SELF-MONITORING FOR ASSESSMENT

Accuracy of Self-Monitoring

The usefulness of self-monitoring as an assessment strategy during target behavior selection, functional behavioral assessment, and/or outcome evaluation activities depends to a great extent on the accuracy with which children and adolescents are able to monitor their behavior. In most self-monitoring studies, accuracy of self-monitored data has been determined by comparing self-recordings made by a child with those made simultaneously by another observer, usually an adult (e.g., Dunlap & Dunlap, 1989). The extent to which the child is able to match an adult's recordings of a particular behavior will determine the accuracy of self-monitoring. Although logic would suggest that adult observers' recordings are more accurate than children's self-recordings and therefore should be used as the standard of comparison, there currently are insufficient data to support this assumption.

Many studies have demonstrated that children and adolescents varying widely in cognitive, social, emotional, and behavioral characteristics are capable of accurately self-monitoring a variety of target behaviors (e.g., Carr & Punzo, 1993; Kern et al., 1997; Wood et al., 2002). A majority of these studies have reported child–observer agreement levels of at least 80%, the generally established minimum for acceptable levels of agreement (e.g., Wood et al., 2002).

Although children's and adolescents' accuracy have been found to be acceptable in most instances, some studies have reported low or inconsistent accuracy. For example, in a study using self-monitoring with preschoolers during independent readiness tasks, De Haas-Warner (1992) found a wide range of accuracy levels, from 61% (minimally acceptable) to 100% (excellent). McDougall and Brady (1995) also found large variations between individual participants in their study of self-monitoring with individuals with severe behavior disorders; the accuracy levels ranged from an average of 30% to 83%. In addition, there were large day-to-day discrepancies in individuals' accuracy levels, ranging from 0% to 100%.

A large number of early studies in self-monitoring investigated factors that may influence the accuracy of self-monitoring. Specific variables found to influence self-monitoring accuracy of children and adolescents include their awareness of accuracy assessment (e.g., Nelson, Lipinski, & Black, 1975), reinforcement for accurate self-monitoring (e.g., Lloyd & Hilliard, 1989), training in accurate self-monitoring (e.g., Shapiro, McGonigle, & Ollendick, 1981), the valence of the target behavior (e.g., Nelson, Hay, Devany, & Koslow-Green, 1980), and the nature of the recording device (e.g., Nelson, Lipinski, & Boykin, 1978). Generally, this literature would advise targeting desired appropriate behaviors for self-monitoring and using a simple, but relatively obtrusive, recording device to enhance high levels of accuracy. In addition, children and adolescents should be provided with initial training in accurate self-monitoring, should be aware their accuracy will be checked, and should be reinforced whenever they are found to be accurately self-monitoring their behavior. Each of these issues should be considered whenever self-monitoring procedures are used for assessment purposes, to increase the likelihood of accurate assessment by children and adolescents.

Reactivity of Self-Monitoring

Although positive outcomes are usually welcomed by practitioners, behavior change is a consideration when self-monitoring is used primarily for assessment purposes. For example, because of potential reactivity it may be impossible to obtain a clear picture of initial behavioral levels, as self-monitoring is serving simultaneously as an assessment and an intervention procedure. The reactive effects could potentially begin with the initiation of self-monitoring, and as a result would confound interpretation of the information being gathered. Undoubtedly, this causes greatest concern when self-monitoring is used in research investigations. For example, a study evaluating the effects of a social skills intervention on the depressive symptoms of adolescents could use self-monitoring as the data collection procedure. However, any changes in the target symptoms following the implementation of social skills training might reflect the joint or interactive effects of self-monitoring and the intervention, which would cloud interpretation of the results. Reactivity may be of less concern when the goal is simply to effect positive behavior change.

APPLICATIONS OF SELF-MONITORING

Self-Monitoring of Internalizing Behaviors

Self-monitoring has been used for assessment of internalizing disorders such as childhood anxiety and depression (Beidel, Neal, & Lederer, 1991; King, Ollendick, & Murphy, 1997), and it offers some distinct advantages over the more traditional assessment methods, such as interview schedules, self-report inventories, and behavioral interviews. With self-monitoring, specific information concerning covert thoughts and feelings, levels of anxious or depressed feelings, and conditions surrounding the problem situations can be self-reported at the time they occur. This information is critical to accurate assessment of an internalizing disorder, yet inaccessible through more traditional assessment methods. In addition, self-monitoring procedures have often been viewed as providing a more efficient way to accomplish the same goals as direct observations of behavior, such as identifying and counting symptoms, antecedents, and consequences of behaviors (Silverman & Ollendick, 2005).

As might be expected, self-monitoring for assessment of internalizing disorders has typically been used with older children and adolescents, since very young children may not be able to accurately identify and report anxious or depressed thoughts, feelings, or situational events (King et al., 1997). Obviously, whenever self-monitoring is selected as an assessment strategy for use with children or adolescents, the behaviors should be well defined and the recording procedures should be uncomplicated (Shapiro, 1984).

When self-monitoring is used to assess internalizing disorders, children or adolescents are typically instructed to record specific behaviors that occur before, during, or immediately after problem situations. For example, commonly self-monitored responses for assessment of social anxiety include frequency and duration of contacts, number of social interactions, and rate of speech dysfluencies (Donohue, Van Hasselt, & Hersen, 1994). Historically, methods used for self-monitoring childhood anxiety and depression have included behavioral diaries and counting devices (e.g., wrist counters). However, more recently, electronic forms of behavioral diaries have emerged as a promising alternative assessment method. These are often described in the literature as "electronic diaries," "ecological momentary assessment," (EMA), or "experience sampling" (Piesecki, Hufford, Solhan, & Trull, 2007; Shiffman, Stone, & Hufford, 2008). For example, EMA has been described by Shiffman et al. (2008) as a range of assessment methods and traditions using repeated collection of real-time data on individuals' behavior and experience in their natural environment; it includes paper-and pencil methods, as well as electronic forms of data collection. Another possible electronic method for self-monitoring is the use of smart phones by children or adolescents to communicate daily anxious or depressed symptoms, or other information, to their therapists. In a recent example, text messaging was used in the assessment and treatment of childhood overweight (Bauer, de Niet, Timman, & Kordy, 2010). Forty children (mean age 10.05 years) were asked to text-message weekly self-monitoring data on eating behavior, exercise behavior, and emotions. Results showed that the children submitted 67% of the weekly data they were expected to send in, suggesting the usefulness of this method.

Self-monitoring has also been used to assess several different types of anxiety in children. In one investigation (Beidel et al., 1991), test-anxious elementary school children were selected for study based on prior research demonstrating that such children actually express a broad range of fears, particularly in the social-evaluative realm. The authors examined the use of a daily diary to assess the range and frequency of anxious events in children. A total of 57 children (32 with test anxiety and 25 without it) in third through sixth grade participated in the study. Children were given a diary that consisted of 50 formatted pages (printed version or picture version) bound in a spiral notebook, and were instructed to complete one diary page each time something happened that made them feel anxious. Children were also provided with a sample of a correctly completed diary page, and each step in the entry was reviewed verbally as well as illustrated in the sample. The diary itself assessed, in checklist format, situational parameters related to the occurrence of anxious events (including time of day, location, specific anxiety-producing event, and behavioral responses to the event). The specific items included on the checklist were based on prior research and were intended to present a range of potentially anxiety-producing situations across classrooms, school cafeteria, home, outside, or with friends.

Results indicated that in general, children complied with the self-monitoring instructions at an acceptable level, and the self-monitored data appeared to be reliable. Although the specific format appeared to make no difference in compliance or mean number of events recorded for fifth- and sixth-grade children, the third- and fourth-grade children who completed the written version of the diary were less likely to adhere to the diary format than the other groups. An additional finding was that children who met *Diagnostic and Statistical Manual of Mental Disorders* (DSM) criteria for overanxious disorder or social phobia reported significantly more emotional distress and more negative behaviors (e.g., crying, somatic complaints, or behavioral avoidance) surrounding the occurrence of self-monitored events than the matched normal control participants. This provided some initial validity for the use of self-monitoring as a tool for the assessment of specific anxious behaviors in children with anxiety disorders.

In a more recent study using a daily diary, Allen, Blatter-Meunier, Ursprung, and Schneider (2010) evaluated the feasibility and convergent validity of the Child Version of the Separation Anxiety Daily Diary (SADD-C). Participants were 125 children (ages 7–14 years) from German-speaking areas of Switzerland. Children with separation anxiety disorder

(SAD; $n=58$), "other" anxiety disorders ($n=36$), and healthy controls ($n=31$) recorded the frequency of parent–child separations, along with associated anxiety, thoughts, reactions, and subsequent parental responses. Both mothers and children completed the SADD separately, at home, each day for an 8-day period. The investigators found modest compliance rates for the completion of the daily diary (i.e., 26% of the child participants did not complete any part of the SADD-C). Convergent validity was demonstrated through moderate to strong associations between the SADD-C and measures of anxiety symptoms and perceived child quality of life. Strong associations were present between the SADD-C and a specific measure of separation anxiety (the Separation Anxiety Inventory), and moderate associations with a general measure of anxiety symptoms (the Revised Child Manifest Anxiety Scale). The SADD-C was found to differentiate children with SAD from healthy controls, but not from children with "other" anxiety disorders. Only ratings of anxiety intensity differentiated children with SAD from children with "other" anxiety disorders.

A daily diary was also used in another study (Beidel, Turner, & Morris, 2000) with children (ages 8–12 years) with social phobia, to assess the effects of a behavioral treatment program designed to increase social skills and decrease social anxiety. In addition to other forms of assessment, a daily diary was completed by the children for 2 weeks at pretreatment, posttreatment, and 6-month follow-up. The daily diary consisted of the children's recording their engagement in various social activities, recording their response to each event (i.e., positive or negative coping skills used), and rating their level of distress in each social encounter. Because use of the diary was not the central focus of the study, data regarding the participants' compliance with use of the diary, or the consistency of self-reported information in the diary as compared to other assessment measures, were not reported.

Two other studies (Henker et al., 2002; Whalen et al., 2004) used electronic diaries for self-monitoring of anxiety levels in adolescents. Henker et al. (2002) utilized electronic diaries in a community sample of 155 ninth graders, who completed an electronic diary every 30 minutes for two 4-day intervals, in addition to completing an anxiety questionnaire. Using handheld computers, the adolescents reported upon their mood, social context, activity, and what they had consumed (e.g., food, alcohol, cigarettes). The results indicated that electronic diary reporting was able to distinguish symptom levels between high-anxiety and low-anxiety participants.

Whalen et al. (2004) utilized electronic diary reporting in a longitudinal study of teenager stress and health. High school students ($n=171$) who were already participating in a longitudinal study were invited to complete additional reports concerning the events of September 11, 2001. Electronic diary measures of anxiety were found to predict students' posttraumatic stress related to that event. These findings, combined with those of Beidel et al. (1991) and Allen et al. (2010), support the use of daily diaries in the assessment of childhood anxiety; more specifically, they lend initial support to the use of electronic diaries by children and adolescents.

In a slightly different example, Tan et al. (2012) used self-monitoring to assess emotional regulation and reactivity in anxious youth and healthy controls; a cell phone EMA protocol was employed. Older children and adolescents (ages 9–13) with generalized anxiety disorder, social anxiety disorder, social phobia, and healthy controls participated in the study. Each participant was given a modified answer-only cell phone, and all received training on what questions they would be asked during the study. Participants received 14 calls from Thursday afternoon through Monday evening. Each call consisted of a brief structured interview approximately 5 minutes in duration, followed by participants' rating their current emotion, describing and rating a peak emotional event that happened within the past hour, and choosing which emotional regulation strategy they used for the event from a list of cognitive-behavioral strategies (distraction, cognitive restructuring, problem solving, acceptance, avoidance, and rumination). Compliance rates for phone call completion were high for both the participants with anxiety disorders (93%) and the participants in the control condition (91.3%), and did not significantly differ. The investigators found that, as expected, anxious youth reported more intense peak negative emotions than age-matched controls. However, surprisingly, anxious and nonanxious youth did not differ in their reports of momentary negative emotions. This latter finding is in contrast to findings from questionnaire or laboratory-based studies (e.g., Carthy, Horesh, Apter, & Gross, 2010).

Ollendick (1995) used self-monitoring successfully in the assessment and treatment of four adolescents diagnosed with panic disorder with agoraphobia. These adolescents were instructed to monitor the date, time, duration, location, circumstance, and symptoms experienced (the 13 DSM symptoms were used) during their panic attacks. They were asked to record this information on a daily basis for the upcoming week, and the information was reviewed at the beginning of each subsequent session. In addition to ongoing self-monitoring, participants were asked during each session to provide self-efficacy ratings for coping with panic, as well as ratings of the extent to which they had actually avoided each of three problematic agoraphobic situations. Results indicated that panic attacks were eliminated, agoraphobic avoidance was reduced, and self-efficacy for coping with attacks was enhanced as a function of cognitive-behavioral treatment. In addition, heightened levels of anxiety sensitivity, trait anxiety, fear, and depression were reduced to normative levels for these adolescents.

On occasion, self-monitoring has also been used by children and adolescents with more severe obsessive–compulsive disorder (OCD). Although common with adults, self-monitoring by children and adolescents with OCD is rare. This may be due to children's concealing their symptoms, being less motivated, or being less able to self-monitor OCD behaviors (Wolff & Wolff, 1991), or to their inability to adequately describe or give sufficient detail regarding their symptoms (Lewin & Piacentini, 2010). In some cases, children have been instructed to self-monitor the frequency of OCD behaviors (e.g., Ownby, 1983; Phillips & Wolpe, 1981). In others, children have been asked to provide global daily reports (e.g., Harbin, 1979; Wilmuth, 1988). There is some evidence to suggest that self-monitoring may be most useful in assessing children's ruminative cognitions (Wolff & Wolff, 1991). However, not all children are compliant or accurate. In fact, Apter, Bernhout, and Tyano (1984) found that adolescents' lack of cooperation with a treatment program that included self-monitoring resulted in a 100% failure rate.

In treatment of childhood and adolescent depression, self-monitoring has been employed as both an assessment and an intervention procedure (Lewinsohn & Clarke, 1999). With depression, self-monitoring typically involves recording the occurrence of a targeted response in either an unstructured journal format or a checklist of predetermined behaviors. As depressed children and adolescents, like depressed adults, tend to focus on negative rather than positive events (Kaslow, Rehm, & Siegel, 1984), they may need to be taught to self-monitor pleasant events. Reynolds and Stark (1985) developed a school-based procedure for creating a pleasant events schedule for children that ensures an up-to-date representation of pleasant activities. The procedure involves initial schoolwide administration of a short questionnaire to identify positive and current age-appropriate activities. From this, a list of the most frequently identified activities can be constructed and placed into each child's self-monitoring diary. Children can then be asked to self-monitor with a check mark every time they participate in an enjoyable activity or have a pleasant thought. This way, students are likely to pay more attention to, and perhaps participate more in, the positive activities in their lives (Reynolds & Stark, 1987).

Evidence suggests that child and adolescent depression may be related to a disruption in the experience and regulations of emotions in social contexts (Sheeber, Hops, & Davis, 2001). There are limitations to retrospective reporting of emotions, especially in children (Stone et al., 1998). However, self-monitoring of emotions in the natural setting may help to address these limitations, as children and adolescents can track their emotions in real time. An example is a recent study by Silk et al. (2011), who used a cell phone EMA methodology in a group of youth with current major depressive disorder (MDD) to examine the daily emotional dynamics of child and adolescent depression. The investigators developed the cell phone EMA protocol study to make EMA methods more feasible for studies including younger children with mental health problems. Participants were 48 girls and 31 boys ranging in age from 7 to 17 years, and either were in a current episode of MDD ($n = 47$) or were no-psychopathology controls ($n = 32$) considered to be at low risk for depression based on family history.

Participants were given a modified answer-only cell phone and received calls from Friday through Monday at five different times during the study. Each participant received 12 calls from trained interviewers, starting after school on a Friday and ending on the following Monday. The 4-day blocks occurred during baseline, at the end of the first week of treatment, and during weeks 3, 5, and 7, for a total of 60 calls. During each call, the participant was asked to rate his or her current emotion on a 5-point scale adapted from the Positive and Negative Affect Scale for Children (Laurent et al., 1999). Four negative and four positive emotions were assessed. In addition, participants were asked about their current social context, including activity, location, and companions. The investigators found the cell phone EMA methodology to be feasible across all age groups. The rate of call completion was 92%, and the average call time was 3.78 minutes. In addition, participants with MDD reported significantly more intense negative emotions and more lability in negative emotions than did participants in the control group. Using technology such as cell phones to aid in self-monitoring is an emerging area of assessment research for children and adolescents.

In general, self-monitoring has been used as an effective mechanism for identifying and monitoring the private events of children and adolescents with various types of internalizing disorders. Studies have typically used diaries, data recording devices, or electronic technology such as cell phones and electronic diaries that simplify the procedures to successfully assess and monitor various symptoms of anxiety and depression.

Application to the Case of Sofia

In the case of Sofia, self-monitoring could play a central role in the assessment and treatment of her anxiety about attending school. Considering her age, the therapist might ask Sofia to participate in the functional assessment process by collecting information about her specific fears or apprehensions about attending school, and the events surrounding the anxiety. Specifically, Sofia might be asked to keep a daily diary for the first week in which she would log her feelings of anxiety and the environmental events surrounding them, including events that preceded or led up to these feelings and the consequences of the anxious episodes. The diary might use a simple paper-and-pencil or computer format. This information would then be shared and used by the therapist and Sofia to identify specific triggers and maintaining factors (e.g., reinforcement, escape) that could become targets of a behavior intervention plan.

Sofia might also be asked to begin daily self-monitoring of her level of distress related to each social encounter or time of day. If she had access to a smart phone and could use text messaging, the self-monitored ratings could be texted to the therapist daily, as described by Bauer et al. (2010); if not, this information could be recorded in a notebook and either emailed regularly or shared with the therapist during face-to-face meetings. Sofia's self-monitoring would continue throughout the intervention phase until a satisfactory reduction in her level of anxiety had been achieved.

Although self-monitoring alone could have some positive effects on Sofia's anxiety, the intense and long-term nature of her symptoms would suggest that additional cognitive-behavioral intervention strategies for treatment of anxiety and panic attacks would probably be needed. However, in this case, self-monitoring could serve as a useful tool for helping to understand the source and function of Sofia's anxiety symptoms, for collecting ongoing data to determine the effectiveness of the intervention, and as a supplementary intervention strategy itself.

Self-Monitoring of Externalizing Behaviors

Self-monitoring of externalizing problems has frequently been used as an intervention strategy, rather than solely for assessment purposes (Cole & Bambara, 2000; Shapiro & Cole, 1999). For example, one study evaluated the use of a cell phone to prompt a kindergarten student to self-record his on- or off-task behavior, in an effort to decrease his off-task/disruptive behavior (Quillivan, Skinner, Hawthorn, Whited, & Ballard, 2011). However, several recent studies have evaluated the use of electronic diaries by children to self-monitor their symptoms of ADHD. In one study examining the daily lives of mothers and children in their natural environments and everyday tasks over a 1-week period, Whalen, Henker, Jamner, et al. (2006) used electronic diaries for both mothers and children to collect information on the primary dependent measures. Participants were 27 mother–child dyads in the ADHD group and 25 mother–child dyads in the comparison group. The study served as an initial test of whether an electronic diary approach would elicit meaningful information from children with ADHD, including moods and self-perceptions, as well as overt behaviors. For 7 consecutive days during nonschool hours, the electronic diary (a Palm Pilot Personal Digital Assistant) beeped every 30 minutes (+/– 5 minutes) to signal time for completion of the daily diary. The mothers and children completed their own electronic diaries independently. Participants answered brief questions regarding their current activity and social context (companions), and current mood; they also indicated whether the current activity was something they chose and perceived to be difficult. Mothers rated both their mood and their children's mood.

Despite receiving an average of 95 (mothers) or 91 (children) signals per week, completion rates were high. Mothers' average completion rates were 91% (ADHD group) and 92% (comparison group), and the comparable rates for the children were 89% (ADHD) and 90% (comparison). All participants completed at least 71% of prompted diaries, and some even completed 100%. The children with ADHD were more often sad, angry, and disappointed than the comparison group. They also reported more discord between themselves and their mothers than the comparison group.

As expected, mothers were more likely to report problem behaviors than their children, but this study does lend support to the feasibility of using electronic devices for self-monitoring by children with ADHD and their parents.

In a similar study, Whalen, Henker, Ishikawa, et al. (2006) used the same methodology to assess levels of ADHD symptoms during times of day when "getting-ready" activities would be occurring—activities that are typically difficult for individuals with ADHD. Again, participants were 27 mother–child dyads in the ADHD group and 25 mother–child dyads in the comparison group (all children were 7–12 years old). The same procedures were used as in the study just described; however, the focus was on the comparison of natural getting-ready activities and other activities during the day. In contrast to the comparison group, mothers of children with ADHD spent more time in getting-ready activities, reported more symptomatic behaviors during these times, and felt more stressed and angry. Children's self-ratings also revealed situational effects, indicating that school-age children with ADHD can use carefully structured electronic diaries to give meaningful self-reports. Additional research is needed to investigate the validity of maternal report and child report against other forms of measurement.

Recent research has also begun to involve children and adolescents more directly in the functional behavior assessment process for externalizing problems. Students can potentially provide valuable firsthand information regarding their externalizing behavior, typical antecedents of their behavior, and possible behavior support strategies. Including a student directly in the assessment process may help adults to better understand the child or adolescent's thoughts and feelings regarding the behavior of concern, as well as to clarify the functional value of the behavior for the individual. Although studies have used child and adolescent interviews to help predict what might serve as a successful intervention or reveal idiosyncratic aspects of the context that only the youth would be able to identify (e.g., Nippe, Lewis-Palmer, & Sprague, 1998; Reed, Thomas, Sprague, & Horner, 1997), future research should investigate the effects of having children or adolescents self-record aspects of their behavior as part of the functional behavior assessment process.

Application to the Case of Billy

As a first step for dealing with Billy's oppositional, negativistic, and noncompliant behaviors at home and school, the therapist would collect information regarding possible functions of these behaviors. Although adults would be the sources for most of this information, Billy might also be asked to help self-monitor events surrounding the problem behavior. To simplify this task for Billy, the therapist might explain that during 1 week he should write down things that "triggered" his outbursts and things that happened after the problem behavior occurred. It probably would be necessary to operationalize the problem behaviors, antecedents, and consequences for him, and to role-play some examples with him. Billy would be asked to record this information and bring it to the next meeting with the therapist, where it would be discussed and used in developing his behavior intervention plan. The intervention plan might focus on particularly difficult time periods (e.g., getting ready for bed, dinnertime) and might involve providing Billy with praise and token reinforcement for specific appropriate behaviors. In addition, the therapist might choose to ask both Billy and his mother to use electronic diaries, as in the Whalen, Henker, Jamner, et al. (2006) study, to collect information on Billy's appropriate and disruptive behaviors during these difficult time periods. The self-monitoring strategy could be a modified version of the one described previously, in which an electronic diary (e.g., an iPhone) would beep every 60 minutes (+/– 5 minutes) to signal time for completion of the daily diary. Billy and his mother would each complete an electronic diary independently. As in the Whalen, Henker, Jamner, et al. (2006) procedure, both would answer brief questions about their current activity, social context, and current mood, and would indicate whether the current activity was something they chose and perceived to be difficult. In addition, Billy's mother would rate both her mood and Billy's mood. This evidence-based strategy utilizing self-monitoring of behavior and mood could be used to supplement other assessment and intervention strategies for remediation of Billy's oppositional, negativistic, and noncompliant behaviors at home and school.

SUMMARY AND FUTURE DIRECTIONS

Self-monitoring is a behavioral assessment strategy that can be used in clinical work with children and adolescents for activities such as functional behavior assessment, intervention selection/planning, and treatment outcome monitoring. The literature on self-monitoring has provided several demonstrations of its successful use for assessment of internalizing disorders such as anxiety and depression, and more recently for assessment of externalizing behaviors related to ADHD. Although issues of accuracy and reactivity must be considered when self-monitoring is used as an assessment tool, from a practical standpoint a therapist desires to obtain maximum behavior change for minimal effort. If having young clients simply monitor their own behavior can result in positive outcomes, then use of self-monitoring for assessment and intervention may be an ideal strategy.

One exciting and relatively unexplored area is the use of technology for self-monitoring purposes. With increased access to technology, many potential applications to self-monitoring are becoming apparent. For example, in recent years cell phone technology has been rapidly embraced by the medical community, and has been used for assessment, treatment, and information exchange in medical conditions such as hypertension, asthma, chronic obstructive pulmonary disease, and diabetes (Boschen, 2009; Wei, Hollin, & Kachnowski, 2010). A recent illustration with adults examined the use of text messaging by a group of women to self-monitor symptoms of bulimia nervosa (Shapiro et al., 2010). Interestingly, use of technologies such as text messaging for self-monitoring has not been similarly embraced by cognitive-behavioral therapists and researchers (Boschen, 2009), particularly those working with children and adolescents. Despite this limited use, early studies suggest that electronic technologies may be promising tools for self-monitoring by children and adolescents with behavioral and emotional problems. The specific advantages of many electronic methods such as text messaging (e.g., widespread use, low cost, flexibility, convenience, interactivity, familiarity), especially for adolescents, are clear. Let us hope that they will lead to more creative and frequent use of self-monitoring in assessment and treatment of a broader range of child and adolescent problems.

REFERENCES

Allen, J. L., Blatter-Meunier, J., Ursprung, A., & Schneider, S. (2010). The Separation Anxiety Daily Diary: Child Version: Feasibility and psychometric properties. *Child Psychiatry and Human Development, 41*, 649–662.

Apter, A., Bernhout, E., & Tyano, S. (1984). Severe OCD in adolescence: A report of eight cases. *Journal of Adolescence, 7*, 349–358.

Barry, L. M., & Messer, J. J. (2003). A practical application of self-management for students diagnosed with attention-deficit/hyperactivity disorder. *Journal of Positive Behavior Interventions, 5*, 238–248.

Bauer, S., de Niet, J., Timman, R., & Kordy, H. (2010). Enhancement of care through self-monitoring and tailored feedback via text messaging and their use in the treatment of childhood overweight. *Patient Education and Counseling, 79*, 315–319.

Beidel, D. C., Neal, A. M., & Lederer, A. S. (1991). The feasibility and validity of a daily diary for the assessment of anxiety in children. *Behavior Therapy, 22*, 505–517.

Beidel, D. C., Turner, S. M., & Morris, T. L. (2000). Behavioral treatment of childhood social phobia. *Journal of Consulting and Clinical Psychology, 68*, 1072–1080.

Boschen, M. J. (2009). Mobile telephones and psychotherapy: II. A review of empirical research. *The Behavior Therapist, 32*, 175–181.

Briesch, A. M., & Chafouleas, S. M. (2009). Review and analysis of literature on self-management interventions to promote appropriate classroom behaviors (1988–2008). *School Psychology Quarterly, 24*, 106–118.

Broden, M., Hall, R. V., & Mitts, B. (1971). The effects of self-recording on the classroom behavior of two eighth-grade students. *Journal of Applied Behavior Analysis, 4*, 191–199.

Bruck, M., Ceci, S. J., & Hembrooke, H. (1998). Reliability and credibility of young children's reports: From research to policy to practice. *American Psychologist, 53*, 136–151.

Carr, S. C., & Punzo, R. P. (1993). The effects of self-monitoring of academic accuracy and productivity on the performance of students with behavior disorders. *Behavioral Disorders, 18*, 241–250.

Carthy, T., Horesh, N., Apter, A., & Gross, J. J. (2010). Patterns of emotional reactivity and regulation in children with anxiety disorders. *Journal of Psychopathology and Behavioral Assessment, 32*, 23–36.

Cole, C. L., & Bambara, L. M. (2000). Self-monitoring: Theory and practice. In E. S. Shapiro & T. R. Kratochwill (Eds.), *Behavioral assessment in schools: Theory, research, and clinical foundations* (2nd. ed., pp. 202–232). New York: Guilford Press.

De Haas-Warner, S. (1992). The utility of self-monitoring for preschool on-task behavior. *Topics in Early Childhood Special Education, 12*, 478–495.

Donohue, B. C., Van Hasselt, V. B., & Hersen, M. (1994). Behavioral assessment and treatment of social phobia. *Behavior Modification, 18*, 262–288.

Dunlap, L. K., & Dunlap, G. (1989). A self-monitoring package for teaching subtraction with regrouping to students with learning disabilities. *Journal of Applied Behavior Analysis, 22*, 309–314.

Frith, G. H., & Armstrong, S. W. (1985). Self-monitoring for behavior disordered students. *Teaching Exceptional Children, 18*, 144–148.

Harbin, H. T. (1979). Cure by ordeal: Treatment of an obsessive–compulsive neurotic. *International Journal of Family Therapy, 4*, 324–332.

Harris, K. R., Graham, S., Reid, R., McElroy, K., & Hamby, R. S. (1994). Self-monitoring of attention versus self-monitoring of performance: Replication and cross-task comparison studies. *Learning Disability Quarterly, 17*, 121–139.

Henker, B., Whalen, C. K., Jamner, L. D., & Delfino, R. J. (2002). Anxiety, affect, and activity in teenagers: Monitoring daily life with electronic diaries. *Journal of the American Academy of Child and Adolescent Psychiatry, 41*, 660–670.

Hughes, C. H., Copeland, S. R., Agran, M., Wehmeyer, M. L., Rodi, M. S., & Presley, J. A. (2002). Using self-monitoring to improve performance in general education high school classes. *Education and Training in Mental Retardation and Developmental Disabilities, 37*, 262–272.

Kaslow, N. J., Rehm, L. P., & Siegel, A. W. (1984). Social-cognitive and cognitive correlates of depression in children. *Journal of Abnormal Child Psychology, 12*, 605–620.

Kern, L., Dunlap, G., Clarke, S., & Childs, K. E. (1995). Student-Assisted Functional Assessment Interview. *Diagnostique, 19*, 29–39.

Kern, L., Marder, T. J., Boyajian, A. E., Elliot, C. M., & McElhattan, D. (1997). Augmenting the independence of self-management procedures by teaching self-initiation across settings and activities. *School Psychology Quarterly, 12*, 23–32.

King, N. J., Ollendick, T. H., & Murphy, G. C. (1997). Assessment of childhood phobias. *Clinical Psychology Review, 17*, 667–687.

La Greca, A. M. (1990). Issues and perspective on the child assessment process. In A. M. La Grecca (Ed.), *Through the eyes of the child: Obtaining self-reports from children and adolescents* (pp. 3–17). Boston: Allyn & Bacon.

Laurent, J., Catanzaro, S., Joiner, T., Rudolf, K., Potter, K., & Lambert, S. (1999).

A measure of positive and negative affect for children: Scale development and preliminary validation. *Psychological Assessment, 11*, 326–338.

Lewin, A. B., & Piacentini, J. (2010). Evidence-based assessment of child obsessive compulsive disorder: Recommendations for clinical practice and treatment research. *Child Youth Care Forum, 39*, 73–89.

Lewinsohn, P. M., & Clarke, G. N. (1999). Psychosocial treatment for adolescent depression. *Clinical Psychology Review, 19*, 329–342.

Lloyd, M. E., & Hilliard, A. M. (1989). Accuracy of self-recording as a function of repeated experience with different self-control contingencies. *Child and Family Behavior Therapy, 11*(2), 1–14.

Loftin, R. L., Odom, S. L., & Lantz, J. F. (2007). Social interaction and repetitive motor behaviors. *Journal of Autism and Developmental Disorders, 38*, 1124–1135.

Martella, R. C., Leonard, I. J., Marchand-Martella, N. E., & Agran, M. (1993). Self-monitoring negative statements. *Journal of Behavioral Education, 3*, 77–86.

McDougall, D., & Brady, M. P. (1995). Using audio-cued self-monitoring for students with severe behavior disorders. *Journal of Educational Research, 88*, 309–317.

Miller, L. J., Strain, P. S., Boyd, K., Jarzynka, J., & McFetridge, M. (1993). The effects of classwide self-assessment on preschool children's engagement in transition, free play, and small group instruction. *Early Education and Development, 4*, 162–181.

Mooney, P., Ryan, J. B., Uhing, B. M., Reid, R., & Epstein, M. H. (2005). A review of self-management interventions targeting academic outcomes for students with emotional and behavioral disorders. *Journal of Behavioral Education, 14*, 203–221.

Nelson, R. O. (1977). Assessment and therapeutic functions of self-monitoring. In J. D. Cone & R. P. Hawkins (Eds.), *Progress in behavior modification* (Vol. 5, pp. 263–308). New York: Academic Press.

Nelson, R. O., Hay, L. R., Devany, J., & Koslow-Green, L. (1980). The reactivity and accuracy of children's self-monitoring: Three experiments. *Child Behavior Therapy, 2*(3), 1–24.

Nelson, R. O., Lipinski, D. P., & Black, J. L. (1975). The effects of expectancy on the reactivity of self-recording. *Behavior Therapy, 6*, 337–349.

Nelson, R. O., Lipinski, D. P., & Boykin, R. A. (1978). The effects of self-recorders' training and the obtrusiveness of the self-monitoring device on the accuracy and reactivity of self-monitoring. *Behavior Therapy, 9*, 200–208.

Newman, B., Buffington, D. M., O'Grady, M. A., McDonald, M. E., Poulson, C. L., & Hemmes, N. S. (1995). Self-management of schedule following in three teenagers with autism. *Behavioral Disorders, 20*, 190–196.

Nippe, G. E., Lewis-Palmer, T., & Sprague, J. (1998). *The student-directed functional assessment: II. An analysis of congruence between self-report, teacher report, and direct observation.* Unpublished manuscript, University of Oregon.

Ollendick, T. H. (1981). Self-monitoring and self-administered overcorrection: The modification of nervous tics in children. *Behavior Modification, 5*, 75–84.

Ollendick, T. H. (1995). Cognitive behavioral treatment of panic disorder with agoraphobia in adolescents: A multiple baseline design analysis. *Behavior Therapy, 26*, 517–531.

Ollendick, T. H., Grills, A. E., & King, N. J. (2001). Applying developmental theory to the assessment and treatment of childhood disorders: Does it make a difference? *Clinical Psychology and Psychotherapy, 8*, 304–314.

Ownby, R. L. (1983). A cognitive behavioral intervention for compulsive handwashing with a thirteen-year-old boy. *Psychology in the Schools, 20*, 219–222.

Phillips, D., & Wolpe, S. (1981). Multiple behavioral techniques in severe separation anxiety of a twelve-year-old. *Journal of Behavior Therapy and Experimental Psychiatry, 12*, 329–332.

Piesecki, T. M., Hufford, M. R., Solhan, M., & Trull, T. J. (2007). Assessing clients in their natural environments with electronic diaries: Rationale, benefits, limitations, and barriers. *Psychological Assessment, 19*, 25–43.

Prater, M. A., Hogan, S., & Miller, S. R. (1992). Using self-monitoring to improve on-task behavior and academic skills of an adolescent with mild handicaps across special and regular education settings. *Education and Treatment of Children, 15*, 43–55.

Quillivan, C. C., Skinner, C. H., Hawthorn, M. L., White, D., & Ballard, D. (2011). Using a cell phone to prompt a kindergarten student to self-monitor off-task/disruptive behavior. *Journal of Evidence-Based Practices for Schools, 12*, 131–146.

Reed, H., Thomas, E., Sprague, J., & Horner, R. H. (1997). The student guided functional assessment interview: An analysis of student and teacher agreement. *Journal of Behavioral Education, 7*, 33–49.

Reid, R. (1996). Research in self-monitoring with students with learning disabilities: The present, the prospects, the pitfalls. *Journal of Learning Disabilities, 29*, 317–331.

Reynolds, W. M., & Stark, K. D. (1985). *Procedures for the development of pleasant activity schedules for children*. Unpublished manuscript.

Reynolds, W. M., & Stark, K. D. (1987). School-based intervention strategies for the treatment of depression in children and adolescents. *Special Services in the Schools, 3*(3–4), 69–88.

Shapiro, E. S. (1984). Self-monitoring procedures. In T. H. Ollendick & M. Hersen (Eds.), *Child behavioral assessment: Principles and procedures* (pp. 148–165). New York: Pergamon Press.

Shapiro, E. S., & Cole, C. L. (1994). *Behavior change in the classroom: Self-management interventions*. New York: Guilford Press.

Shapiro, E. S., & Cole, C. L. (1999). Self-monitoring in assessing children's problems. *Psychological Assessment, 11*, 448–457.

Shapiro, E. S., McGonigle, J. J., & Ollendick, T. H. (1981). An analysis of self-assessment and self-reinforcement in a self-managed token economy with mentally retarded children. *Applied Research in Mental Retardation, 1*, 227–240.

Shapiro, J. R., Bauer, S, Andrews, E., Pisetsky, E., Bulik-Sullivan, B., Hamer, R. M., & Bulik, C. M. (2010). Mobile therapy: Use of text-messaging in the treatment of bulimia nervosa. *International Journal of Eating Disorders, 43*, 513–519.

Sheeber, L., Hops, H., & Davis, B. (2001). Family processes in adolescent depression. *Clinical Child and Family Psychology Review, 4*, 19–35.

Shiffman, S., Stone, A. A., & Hufford, M. R. (2008). Ecological momentary assessment. *Annual Review of Clinical Psychology, 4*, 1–32.

Silk, J. S., Forbes, E. E., Whalen, D. J., Jakubcak, J. L., Thompson, W. K., Ryan, N. D., & Dahl, R. E. (2011). Daily emotional dynamics in depressed youth: A cell phone ecological momentary assessment study. *Journal of Experimental Child Psychology, 110,* 241–257.

Silverman, W. K., & Ollendick, T. H. (2005). Evidence-based assessment of anxiety and its disorders in children and adolescents. *Journal of Clinical Child and Adolescent Psychology, 34,* 380–411.

Snyder, M. (1979). Self-monitoring processes. In L. Berkowitz (Ed.), *Advances in experimental social psychology* (Vol. 12, pp. 85–128). New York: Academic Press.

Snyder, M. C., & Bambara, L. M. (1997). Teaching secondary students with learning disabilities to self-manage classroom survival skills. *Journal of Learning Disabilities, 30,* 534–543.

Stone, A. A., Schwartz, J. E., Neale, J. M., Shiffman, S., Marco, C. A., Hickcox, M., & Cruise, L. J. (1998). A comparison of coping assessed by ecological momentary assessment and retrospective recall. *Journal of Personality and Social Psychology, 74,* 1670–1680.

Stone, W. L., & Lemanek, K. L. (1990). Developmental issues in children's self-reports. In A. M. La Greca (Ed.), *Through the eyes of the child: Obtaining self-reports from children and adolescents* (pp. 18–56). Boston: Allyn & Bacon.

Sugai, G., & Rowe, P. (1984). The effect of self-recording on out-of-seat behavior of an EMR student. *Education and Training of the Mentally Retarded, 19,* 23–28.

Tan, P. Z., Forbes, E. E., Dahl, R. E., Ryan, N. D., Siegle, G. J., Ladouceur, C. D., & Silk, J. S. (2012). Emotional reactivity and regulation in anxious and non-anxious youth: A cell-phone ecological momentary assessment study. *Journal of Child Psychology and Psychiatry, 53,* 197–206.

Trammel, D. L., Schloss, P. J., & Alper, S. (1994). Using self-recording, evaluation, and graphing to increase completion of homework assignments. *Journal of Learning Disabilities, 27,* 75–81.

Webber, J., Scheuermann, B., McCall, C., & Coleman, M. (1993). Research on self-monitoring as a behavior management technique in special education classrooms: A descriptive review. *Remedial and Special Education, 14*(2), 38–56.

Wei, J., Hollin, I., & Kachnowski, S. (2010). A review of the use of mobile phone text messaging in clinical and healthy behavior interventions. *Journal of Telemedicine and Telecare, 17,* 41–48.

Whalen, C. K., Henker, B., King, P. S., Jamner, L. D., & Levine, L. (2004). Adolescents react to the events of September 11, 2001: Focused versus ambient impact. *Journal of Abnormal Child Psychology, 32,* 1–11.

Whalen, C. K., Henker, B., Ishikawa, S. S., Jamner, L. D., Floro, J. N., Johnston, J. A., & Swindle, R. (2006). An electronic diary study of contextual triggers and ADHD: Get ready, get set, get mad. *Journal of the American Academy of Child and Adolescent Psychiatry, 45,* 166–174.

Whalen, C. K., Henker, B., Jamner, L. D., Ishikawa, S. S., Floro, J. N., Swindle, R., & Johnston, J. A. (2006). Toward mapping daily challenges of living with ADHD: Maternal and child perspectives using electronic diaries. *Journal of Abnormal Child Psychology, 34,* 115–130.

Wilmuth, M. (1988). Cognitive-behavioral and insight-oriented psychotherapy of an eleven-year-old boy with obsessive–compulsive disorder. *American Journal of Psychotherapy, 42,* 472–278.

Wolff, R. P., & Wolff, L. S. (1991). Assessment and treatment of obsessive–compulsive disorder children. *Behavior Modification, 15,* 372–393.

Wood, S. J., Murdock, J. Y., & Cronin, M. E. (2002). Self-monitoring and at-risk middle school students: Academic performance improves, maintains, and generalizes. *Behavior Modification, 26,* 605–626.

9

Physiological Assessment

Michelle A. Patriquin, Angela Scarpa, and Bruce H. Friedman

As indicated by William James (1884), human behavior is the product of environment, emotions, *and* physiological responses. People do not just "meet a bear, are frightened, and run." Rather, when people meet a bear, a distinct physiological state is activated, they feel frightened, and they run. To understand behavior and response to the environment, "bodily manifestation must first be interposed between" (James, 1884, pp. 190). Psychophysiology provides a unique link between behavior and biology by providing a methodology to assess physiological states associated with environmental changes and psychological differences. In child and adolescent populations, psychophysiology can grant insight into processes (e.g., threat responses shown through increased heart rate) that would otherwise go unnoticed. Clinically, understanding the psychophysiological underpinnings of behavior in children may help to understand the function of a behavior. For example, assessing heart rate before, during, and after hand flapping in a child with an autism spectrum disorder (ASD) may suggest that the behavior serves a de-arousing function. Here, psychophysiological assessment informs the intervention strategy to decrease symptomatic behaviors by replacing hand flapping with another behavior (e.g., using a weighted vest) that serves the same calming function.

Unlike language-based measures in child assessment, psychophysiological assessment does not require language, reading, or writing ability; therefore, it broadens the range of functioning that may be assessed. For children who may show limited insight into their behaviors, psychophysiological reactivity can provide a window into their physical and psychological state. Yet psychophysiological assessment in children has its limitations. In particular, psychophysiological measurement may be difficult for children, depending on their age, cognitive ability, and ability to tolerate the procedures. Some common difficulties are described later in the chapter.

If accurate data can be collected, findings may elucidate biological processes that parallel psychiatric difficulties. Differences in psychophysiological responses have been found across various child and adolescent psychiatric populations, including those with ASD, specific phobia, conduct disorder, and oppositional defiant disorder (Ollendick, Allen, Benoit, & Cowart, 2011; Patriquin, Scarpa, Friedman, & Porges, 2011; Scarpa, Raine, Venables, & Mednick, 1997). These differences in psychophysiological activity reflect biological processes related to emotions and attention to stimuli that may be involved in shaping child behaviors, including those that may be maladaptive (e.g., stereotypic, aggressive). In addition, the inclusion of psychophysiological measures widens the perspective for understanding development in child and adolescent behavior not only by assessing behavioral and physiological responses separately, but also by examining the interaction of these biobehavioral processes.

This chapter gives a broad overview of psychophysiological measures and their use in child and adolescent assessment. If the reader is interested in learning more about the methodological and procedural aspects of psychophysiological assessment, we suggest the following texts: *Handbook of Psychophysiology*, third edition (Cacioppo, Tassinary, & Berntson, 2007), *Psychophysiology* (Andreassi, 2000), and *Psychophysiological Recording* (Stern, Ray, & Quigley, 2000). We also suggest a book chapter titled "Psychophysiological Assessment" (Wilhelm, Schneider, & Friedman, 2006) that reviews psychophysiological assessment in children; it is similar in scope to the present chapter. Lastly, for the most recent psychophysiological literature, the journals *Biological Psychology* and *Psychophysiology* often include articles on psychophysiological recording in children. Methodological papers can be found on the Society for Psychophysiological Research (SPR) website (*www.sprweb.org*).

Throughout this chapter, the term "children" is used to include all school-age children and adolescents (6–18 years old).

DESCRIPTION OF ASSESSMENT METHOD

Properties of Psychophysiological Measures

Psychophysiology quantifies nervous system activity through the noninvasive assessment of physiological activity such as muscle action potentials, sweat gland activity, movement of the blood through the heart, action potentials in the eye, and hemodynamic response in the brain, among others. (See Table 9.1 for a listing of commonly used measures and abbreviations.) The nervous system can be broken down into the central and peripheral nervous systems. The central nervous system contains the brain, spinal cord, and retina. The peripheral nervous system is made up of the

TABLE 9.1 Common Psychophysiological Measures in Children/Adolescents

Measure	Index/indices
Electrocardiogram (ECG)	Heart rate (HR) HR variability (HRV), high- or low-frequency Respiratory sinus arrhythmia (RSA)
Electrodermal activity (EDA)	Tonic: Skin conductance level (SCL) Phasic: Skin conductance response (SCR)
Respiration	Respiration rate
Blood pressure (BP)	Systolic BP (SBP) Diastolic BP (DBP) Mean arterial pressure (MAP)
Electrooculography (EOG)	Saccade latency Saccade amplitude Direction of movement Velocity Fixation pause time Blink amplitude Blink closure Blink frequency
Electromyography (EMG)	EMG amplitude
Cortisol (hydrocortisone)	Salivary cortisol level
Electroencephalography (EEG)	Alpha waves Beta waves Delta waves Theta waves Kappa waves Lambda waves Mu waves Gamma waves
Functional magnetic resonance imaging (fMRI)	Blood-oxygen-level-dependent (BOLD) method

somatic nervous system and the autonomic nervous system. The somatic nervous system is part of the peripheral nervous system that is related to the voluntary control of body movements through skeletal muscles; it can be measured via indices such as electrooculography or electromyography. Conversely, the autonomic nervous system controls visceral functions that are largely nonconscious, including heart rate, salivation, perspiration, respiration rate, and dilation of the pupils, and can be measured via indices such as electrocardiography and electrodermal activity. The autonomic nervous system is traditionally viewed as having two branches that are primarily distinguished anatomically. The sympathetic branch emerges from the thoracic and lumbar regions of the spinal cord; the parasympathetic system includes cranial nerves and nerves that emerge from the sacral spinal region. Functionally, the parasympathetic system is often portrayed as being restoring and calming, and the sympathetic as being activating, as in "fight–flight"; however, there are many exceptions to these generalizations (Wolf, 1995). Most organs, such as the heart, have dual parasympathetic and sympathetic innervation, but a few, such as the eccrine sweat glands, have only sympathetic innervation. The origins of physiological responses, including innervation patterns, are important for the accurate measurement, interpretation, and conceptualization of psychophysiological measures (Cacioppo et al., 2007). More recently, psychophysiological literature has been extended to include neuroendocrine (cortisol) responses as well.

Central Nervous System

Electroencephalography

Electroencephalography (EEG) measures the gross electrical activity of the brain and has been used to reflect how neural activation (e.g., frontal asymmetry) is associated with the development of fear, anxiety, and emotion regulation in children (Hannesdóttir, Doxie, Bell, Ollendick, & Wolfe, 2010). Unlike other central nervous system measures (e.g., functional magnetic resonance imaging; see below) EEG has a high temporal resolution that allows clinicians to examine millisecond changes within the electrical activity of the brain. More recent techniques, such as high-density EEG (128 or 256 channels), have allowed higher spatial resolution to be captured in child populations (Kurth et al., 2010). Recording EEG in psychiatric populations (e.g., children with ASD or attention-deficit/hyperactivity disorder [ADHD]) can be difficult due to the use of the electrode cap; a child can often pull on the cap and disrupt data collection. The use of dense arrays (128 or 256 channels), however, requires less stringent impedance requirements and less preparation of the electrode site. For less dense arrays, the impedance requirement is <5 KΩ, which is achieved by preparing a clear recording area on the head—clear of hair, oils, and dead skin. The skin is prepared with alcohol, acetone, and electrode paste. A blunted needle is used to clean and prepare the electrode site. These preparation procedures can be time-consuming, and a child's attention can be quickly lost while a clinician is completing them. Distracting techniques (e.g., watching a movie, playing a game with a parent) can be helpful to prevent the child from becoming bored and agitated during the electrode preparation.

Functional Magnetic Resonance Imaging

One of the most frequent uses of functional magnetic resonance imaging (fMRI) is to measure the metabolic and vascular changes that parallel neural activity (Cacioppo et al., 2007). It has been used to assess various neural underpinnings, including brain structures underlying psychopathologies (Kleinhans et al., 2008), face processing (Fitzgerald, Angstadt, Jelsone, Nathan, & Phan, 2006), and threat responses (Dalton et al., 2005). The blood-oxygen level-dependent (BOLD) method measures the oxygenated-to-deoxygenated hemoglobin ratio in the blood across the brain. As metabolic demands increase in particular brain regions, the supply of oxygenated blood to that region increases. Thus, areas on an fMRI image will be "brighter" when there are higher amounts of oxygenated blood in that brain region. The oxygenated blood supports neural activity by providing a source of energy. FMRI captures brain activation by repeated scanning of the brain. Unlike positron emission tomography, fMRI has a higher spatial and temporal resolution; single-subject analyses are possible; it costs less; and it allows the measurement of connectivity (correlations) between brain regions. As such, fMRI has been increasingly used in child populations to examine neural activation patterns associated with psychopathologies, as well as examining the connectivity between brain regions.

Connectivity analyses in children with ASD have revealed significant relationship between abnormal connectivity and severity of ASD symptoms (Kleinhans et al., 2008). Of importance is that even lower-functioning children with ASD seem able to acclimate to the MRI scanner. In one study, amygdala reactivity was examined successfully with fMRI in a lower-functioning child with autism (IQ standard score = 69) (Kleinhans et al., 2008). Despite the tendency for lower-functioning children with autism to move and create unusable images, the experimental protocol included presentation of the animated character Digimon to hold a child's interest. This tactic captured the child's attention and thus minimized movement artifact. This strategy stresses the importance of including attention-capturing tasks, particularly for children who have difficulty remaining still (e.g., those with ASD or ADHD).

Peripheral Nervous System

Electrocardiography and Impedance Cardiography

Electrocardiography (ECG) and impedance cardiography (ICG) provide cardiac indices that are related to parasympathetic and/or sympathetic functioning, and that help to elucidate physiological processes associated with various disorders. Within the child literature, cardiovascular measures have been related to cognitive ability (Patriquin et al., 2011; Staton, El-Sheikh, & Buckhalt, 2008), emotion recognition (Bal et al., 2010), attention (Suess, Porges, & Plude, 1994), and social stimuli (Van Hecke et al., 2009). The most common cardiac index is heart rate (HR), in beats per minute. Cardiac rate can also be quantified as "heart period," which refers to the average duration of the cardiac cycle expressed in milliseconds (Stern et al., 2000). Unfortunately, when one is attempting to elucidate the autonomic branches influencing HR, the influences of sympathetic and parasympathetic activity are inextricable. This dilemma stresses the importance of using HR variability (HRV) indices such as respiratory sinus arrhythmia

(RSA) and ICG indices such as pre-ejection period (PEP). RSA is a measure of the vagal (i.e., parasympathetic) deceleratory influence on HR (Demeersman & Stein, 2007), whereas PEP is a measure of the sympathetic influence on cardiac contractility (Sherwood et al., 1990). Important methodological papers regarding these two measures and other psychophysiological responses can be found in a section of the SPR website (*www.sprweb.org/journal/index.cfm#guidelines*).

In assessing child physiology, it is important to differentiate between parasympathetic and sympathetic systems in order to understand the underlying biological processes. Fortunately, ambulatory monitors have made psychophysiological assessment much more accessible to researchers and clinicians than prior equipment setups. For example, if a clinician is interested in examining HR and HRV measures, a comfortable apparatus that can be used is the Polar Heart Rate Monitor (*www.polarusa.com/us-en*). The Polar Heart Rate Monitor allows a child to move freely about the room without being restricted by ECG leads attached to a stationary machine. This allows for real-time measurement of physiological processes that may have otherwise been impeded by the use of stationary equipment. If a clinician is interested in collecting ECG and ICG simultaneously, the Ambulatory Monitoring System (AMS; Vrije Universiteit, Department of Psychophysiology, Amsterdam, the Netherlands) is an ambulatory monitor that is able to collect both ECG and ICG. The AMS, unlike the Polar Heart Rate Monitor, requires that the child wear multiple adhesive electrodes; however, it has been used with children (e.g., Gilissen, Bakermans Kranenburg, van IJzendoorn, & Linting, 2008).

For accurate assessment of cardiovascular response in children, multiple measures can be used. For example, in children with conduct problems and aggressive tendencies, both PEP and RSA can be examined in order to extract the autonomic branches that may/may not be activated in these children to a reward task (Beauchaine, Hong, & Marsh, 2008). Moreover, in assessing these children with conduct disorder, measures of electrodermal activity can be included.

Electrodermal Activity

Electrodermal activity (EDA) measures the activity of the eccrine sweat glands that are innervated by cholinergic fibers from the sympathetic nervous system (Andreassi, 2000). EDA has been used to examine stress responses (Gilissen et al., 2008) and response to reward (Beauchaine et al., 2008). Typically, EDA measurement is taken from the fingers or palm of the nondominant hand. The palms of the hands and soles of the feet contain the highest number of eccrine sweat glands on the body. EDA can be measured both tonically and phasically. Tonic measurements include skin conductance level (SCL) and skin potential level. Phasic measurement includes skin conductance response (SCR) and skin potential response.

Furthermore, there are other ways to quantify EDA: (1) SCL, (2) change in SCL, (3) frequency of nonspecific SCRs, (4) phasic SCRs, and (5) number of trials to SCR habituation. When a stimulus is presented, there is a latency period for the phasic response. The phasic response rises in amplitude (i.e., rise time), reaches the apex (highest point on the curve), and then drops back to half of the amplitude (i.e., half recovery time). This curve represents the phasic EDA response when an individual is presented with a discrete stimulus.

EDA has been used to assess stress in children. In particular, EDA was used with the Trier Social Stress Test for Children to examine childrens' reactivity during a public speaking task (Gilissen et al., 2008). The study used the AMS, version 36 (see above). The AMS allowed the experimenters to note when various events happened in the data by using an event marker button. The ability to insert event markers in the psychophysiological data record is important if a clinician is presenting specific stimuli to which a child's physiological response is of interest. The event marker will indicate where in the data record each stimulus was presented.

A more recent development in EDA ambulatory monitoring is the Affectiva Q Sensor (*www.affectiva.com/q-sensor*), developed by researcher Rosalind Picard and her team at the Massachusetts Institute of Technology Media Lab. The Affectiva Q Sensor is a wrist monitor that does not require electrodes, electrode gel, or wires. It is worn on the wrist, as one would wear a sweatband. When clinicians are measuring EDA in children who may have tactile sensitivities (e.g., children with ASD), the Affectiva Q Sensor provides accurate measurement of EDA while ensuring the children's comfort (Picard, 2009).

Blood Pressure

Blood pressure (BP) is a cardiovascular measure (specifically, it refers to the pressure of blood on the walls of the blood vessels) that has been related to various psychological constructs, including cognitive load, problem solving, stress, frustration, hostility, and anger (Andreassi, 2000). BP is measured via a pressure cuff to derive systolic BP (SBP) and diastolic BP (DBP). SBP is measured when the heart contracts to push blood into the arteries, whereas DBP is measured when the heart relaxes between beats. Another common psychophysiological index of BP is mean arterial pressure (MAP). MAP is the average pressure that pushes blood throughout the circulatory system and is calculated as follows: $MAP = 1/3(SBP - DBP) + DBP$ (Andreassi, 2000). Within the child literature, BP has been assessed with both ambulatory and stationary monitors.

In particular, one intervention study examined the effect of breathing awareness meditation, life skills training, and health education interventions on 24-hour ambulatory BP in African American ninth graders (Brown Wright, Gregoski, Tingen, Barnes, & Treiber, 2011). This study examined ambulatory BP before and after the interventions. Spacelab 90207 monitors (Spacelab, Inc., Issaquah, WA) were used to record the 24-hour measurements. An experimental study used BP to examine the physiological underpinnings of classroom effort in children ages 7–11 years (Carapetian, Siedlarz, Jackson, & Perlmuter, 2008). Notably, this study collected BP measurements within the same time period (3:00–4:30 P.M.), using a sphygmomanometer. This instrument consists of a pressure cuff, a rubber bulb, a mercury manometer, and a stethoscope (Andreassi, 2000). Although both of these studies collected BP measurements in school settings, the studies used different measurement methods, highlighting the flexibility of context in collecting BP.

Salivary Cortisol

Salivary cortisol is measured through the saliva in the mouth and is generally excepted to be a measure of stress responses (Cacioppo et al., 2007). Cortisol is a glucocorticoid or steroid hormone secreted by the adrenal glands (located above the kidneys) as part of the hypothalamic–pituitary–adrenal axis. Saliva samples can be collected by placing plain cotton dental rolls in the mouth or by having a child passively drool through a short drinking straw into a vial. At times, children may need stimulants (e.g., Trident sugarless gum; Cicchetti, Rogosch, Gunnar, & Toth, 2010) in order to increase saliva production. However, it is recommended that any stimulants used should be minimal and that the volume of saliva should be kept as consistent as possible across samples and between participants (Schwartz, Granger, Susman, Gunnar, & Laird, 1998).

Recent child studies have examined the relationship between salivary cortisol and childhood maltreatment, depression, and ADHD and comorbid disorders (Cicchetti et al., 2010; Freitag et al., 2009; Hankin, Badanes, Abela, & Watamura, 2010; Scarpa, 2004). Similar to the measurement of BP, the collection of cortisol is flexible in that it can be performed in various contexts. Specifically, studies have collected cortisol during home visits, and even during summer camp (Cicchetti et al., 2010; Hankin et al., 2010). As stated earlier, however, salivary cortisol needs to be collected at the same time of the day across participants and samples, due to the diurnal fluctuation of cortisol levels. Moreover, if measured in response to a stressor, saliva samples should be taken at least 10–20 minutes after the stressor onset in order to assure enough time for cortisol to appear in the saliva. In order to extract cortisol levels from the saliva, the samples must be placed in a centrifuge and then assayed using chemicals (e.g., competitive sold-phase, time-resolved fluorescence immunoassay; DELFIA; Wallac, Gaithersburg, MD). The easiest way to assess cortisol levels is to have the samples sent to companies who will complete this processes (e.g., Salimetric Laboratories, State College, PA). Conversely, if there is access to a centrifuge, immunoassay kits that allow individuals to complete their own cortisol assays can be purchased online (e.g., *www.oxfordbiomed.com*). It is important for saliva samples to be frozen and stored at −40°C.

Multimodal Measures

As described above, psychophysiological measurement can include indices of the autonomic nervous system (e.g., heart rate, digestion, respiration rate, salivation), central nervous system (e.g., brain, spinal cord), and peripheral/somatic activity (e.g., eye movement, muscle movement; Cacioppo et al., 2007; Stern et al., 2000). Often, too, multimodal forms of assessment are used that combine multiple measures from Table 9.1. For example, a clinician may both measure autonomic nervous system activity through HR and use a peripheral/somatic index of eye movement in examining a child's physiological reaction to a phobic stimulus. A new trend in physiological measurement is the combination of imaging and peripheral nervous system measures, as including peripheral measures with imaging will enrich the understanding of the mind–body relationship (Gray et al., 2009). Yet few studies have used the combination of imaging techniques (e.g., fMRI) and autonomic nervous system measures. Although such arrangements entail additional recording constraints, combinations of various physiological measurement modalities have untapped potential for examining biobehavioral patterns in all populations, including children and adolescents.

Psychophysiological Measurement in Children

Psychophysiological measurement in children presents unique difficulties that are not found in work with adults. Various adaptations need to be made to assessment procedures and to the equipment being used. We also discuss ways to make psychophysiological assessment fun for children, ways to include parents in the assessment, and other issues that need to be considered (e.g., medications a child is taking, the time of day the assessment is conducted).

Adapting Equipment and Assessment Procedures to Children

Often psychophysiological equipment is designed to measure physiological response in adults. For example, large electrodes with strong adhesive may not be suitable for children, who have sensitive skin and do not require a large surface area to be covered for physiological responses (e.g., ECG) to be accurately measured. One must also take special care when using psychophysiological measures with a child to make sure that the equipment fits the child. If, for example, a BP cuff is too large for the child, it will be difficult to collect accurate readings.

In addition to equipment adaptations, some psychophysiological data analyses will require changes to the frequency bands from which data are collected. For example, for extracting RSA or high-frequency HRV from the interbeat intervals collected through the ECG signal, the frequency band typically used for adults (i.e., 0.15–0.40 Hz) will unnecessarily limit the data extracted. To assess these measures accurately in children, a frequency band of 0.24–1.04 should be used. This bandwidth effectively captures the range of spontaneous breathing in children (Bal et al., 2010; Ollendick et al., 2011), who have both faster HR and respiration rates than adults because their nervous systems are less developed (Bal et al., 2010). In all psychophysiological measures, clinicians and researchers should be aware of developmental considerations and should keep in mind that data analysis techniques for adults may not be appropriate for the assessment of psychophysiological data in children.

Once psychophysiological data have been collected, clinicians may need to assess differences in physiological reactivity between or within subjects. Special considerations may be needed, depending on the type of comparisons a clinician will make. In particular, for between-subjects analysis, data must be compared/matched to those for typically developing age- and IQ-matched individuals, in order to get an assessment of "normality." Both age (e.g., adolescents, on average, will have lower HR than infants) and IQ will affect physiological variables. For example, greater reductions in RSA amplitude to an attention-demanding stimulus (e.g., a working memory task) are associated with better cognitive performance (Beauchaine, 2001; Morgan, Aikins, Steffian, Coric, & Southwick, 2007; Staton et al., 2008; Watson, Baranek, Roberts, David, & Perryman, 2010). Therefore, it is important to consider age and IQ in comparing data between individuals.

Within individuals, such as when a clinician is conducting an exposure, controlling for age and IQ is not as essential. For example, if a clinician is using EDA as a measure of autonomic activation to a feared stimulus (e.g., a snake) before and after treatment, the control is built into the situation. The child's pretreatment EDA measurement is the variable to which the clinician will compare the posttreatment EDA measurement.

Making Psychophysiological Assessment Fun

A drawback to using psychophysiological measures for assessment is that the recording equipment can seem daunting to children. If the equipment is explained simply yet accurately, children are more likely to be comfortable in the situation; this will increase the chances of valid measurement. The clinician should always answer children's questions simply and thoroughly. Creating a story surrounding the equipment (e.g., going into space, exploring a jungle) can help to relieve a child's fear and anxiety about the psychophysiological measurement. Also, a reward system or schedule for the steps that need to be completed can help a child stay on track.

One example, Daniel Klein's laboratory at Stony Brook University (*www.psychology.sunysb.edu/sbutmntstudy*) is decorated with space and jungle themes. When a child comes for an assessment, the experimenters talk about the EEG equipment within the context of either the space or the jungle theme. For example, when putting on the EEG cap, they may enthusiastically state, "This is your space cap! We are getting you all ready to go up in space! Are you excited?" If a child is particularly hesitant about the psychophysiology equipment, telling a story can divert the child's attention to the story and away from the application of the equipment—in this case, the electrode cap for the EEG.

Other distracting or comforting techniques can include having the child watch an age-appropriate movie, play with age-appropriate toys that do not require much movement, and/or have a parent in the room. The clinician can also create a poster listing the steps of the assessment and place a sticker next to each assessment step once it is completed. Once the child has completed all of the steps, he or she can receive a reward (e.g., picking out a pencil from a prize box). For an older child, a large schedule on a poster board can be created that allows the child to move a placeholder (e.g., arrow, flower, football, star) from one task to the next. Upon completion of each step of the procedures, the clinician needs to respond enthusiastically (e.g., clapping and praise) when a child, particularly a child under 6 years old, completes a task/step. This helps the child remain interested in the assessment.

Including Parents in the Assessment

Parents can be a helpful resource when a clinician is trying to attach psychophysiological equipment to a child. Parents need to be given explicit directions on their role in the assessment, and these directions should be standardized across assessments. Parents can help with attaching electrodes or other sensors (e.g., a BP cuff). Including parents can also help children have a positive experience in the testing room. In some cases, however, parents may become more distracting to children than helpful. If this is the case, having a one-way mirror or camera where parents can view the assessment may help to relieve any anxiety/fear in either the child or the parents.

Other Issues to Consider with Psychophysiological Assessment in Children

Psychophysiological assessment can often require children to sit completely still for accurate data collection. Movement artifact can make data completely uninterpretable and meaningless. Most sensitive to movement artifact are imaging techniques, such as fMRI, where millimeters of movement render data unusable. Peripheral measures, such as ECG, EDA, and respiratory activity, are more robust to movement artifact. Several companies now manufacture ambulatory monitors that allow for individuals to be monitored while walking. In addition, some companies have developed wireless central nervous system measures that allow children to move around a room while EEG measurements are taken. If ambulatory monitors are used, accelerometers should be attached to the child in order to assess the rate and position of the child's movement, which can be later examined as potential confounds.

Additional confounding variables include medications and the time of day the physiological assessment is conducted. Medications should be stopped during the day if possible, or recorded (i.e., name of medication, dosage, frequency, last taken) if they cannot be suspended. In some cases, medications may best be suspended for up to 2 weeks in advance of the measurement, if permitted by the child's physician. For many physiological measures, there is diurnal variation; for instance, cortisol levels are highest in the early morning and decline throughout the day (Klimes-Dougan, Hastings, Granger, Usher, & Zahn-Waxler, 2001). If a clinician is comparing pre- and post-treatment measures of cortisol to assess stress, or differences between subjects, the time of day should be recorded to control for any diurnal variation that may affect the result. Optimally, experimental sessions should be run at approximately the same time of day within a specific study to control for diurnal rhythms.

Paradigms for Eliciting Physiological Reactivity in Children

Physiological measurement helps clarify how external stimuli may be affecting internal biological processes. To assess physiology, paradigms typically elicit reactivity (i.e., change in physiological state) either from baseline (i.e., neutral physiological state) or from a prior elicited state. In this section, we review various stimuli and tasks that can be used to assess physiological reactivity with children.

Baseline

In order to assess differences in physiological reactivity during or after a task, baseline physiological state must be assessed in the child. Methodologies for assessing baseline reactivity include watching non-stress-inducing videos (e.g., *Sesame Street*; Hannesdóttir et al., 2010), sitting quietly (Bal et al., 2010), and reading children's magazines (Roemmich, Lambiase, Salvy, & Horvath, 2009). A truly "neutral" recording condition is an idealized state that cannot realistically be attained, and so many researchers use a "vanilla" baseline in which mild, nonarousing stimuli are presented (Jennings, Kamarck, Stewart, Eddy, & Johnson, 1992). This strategy may be particularly appropriate for children, who frequently find it difficult to sit still without stimulation for extended periods. For cardiovascular measures, a 5-minute baseline recording is recommended for the analysis of high- and low-frequency HRV (Task Force of the European Society of

Cardiology and the North American Society of Pacing and Electrophysiology, 1996). Other measures may not require as lengthy baseline epochs. For example, EEG baseline measurement can be taken from a 60-second epoch (Hannesdóttir et al., 2010). Type of stimulus presentation and the length of baseline epoch are important in ensuring that a relatively neutral physiological state is captured. The reader is referred to the appropriate section of the SPR website (*www.sprweb.org/journal/index.cfm#guidelines*) for guideline papers that describe important considerations, by physiological measure, for the collection of baseline data.

Behavioral Challenge Stressors

Behavioral challenge stressors include physiological stressors (e.g., the cold-pressor paradigm), anxiety-provoking tasks, and mental stressors. In the child psychophysiological literature, for example, the cold-pressor paradigm has been used to assess pain thresholds during distraction manipulations (e.g., video games; Dahlquist et al., 2009). The cold-pressor task uses a refrigerated bath circulator to keep the water temperature at 5°C (±0.1°C). Children are instructed to keep their nondominant hand in the cold water until it starts to feel uncomfortable or hurt. Once their hand hurts, they are instructed to tell the examiner. The task is used to measure pain thresholds (measured by the number of seconds the hand was in the cold water). Behavioral challenges have also been used within clinical interventions. For example, in a study of treatment for specific phobia, cardiac activity has been used to assess efficacy of exposures based on the behavioral approach test (BAT; Ollendick et al., 2011). In this study, the BAT was tailored to each child's specific phobia and was realistic (e.g., the child had to approach a live animal). The BAT consisted of multiple steps that increased in difficulty, and the number of steps toward the feared stimulus that the child completed was the primary behavioral measure of performance.

Interestingly, reactivity to reward has been assessed in middle schoolers with depression in order to examine PEP, a cardiac sympathetic index derived from ICG (Sherwood et al., 1990), as a biomarker for substance use (Brenner & Beauchaine, 2011). In this study, physiological signals were collected while large single-digit numbers were presented in random order on a computer screen. Participants had to press the corresponding number on a keyboard and were sometimes rewarded $.06 or sometimes were not rewarded $.06. Other paradigms used with EEG, ECG, and HP evoke anxiety by having children give a speech to a video camera or to "friends" (Hannesdóttir et al., 2010; Roemmich et al., 2009). Lastly, cognitive challenges, such as the Children's Stroop Test, have been used to look at the effects of mental stressors on psychophysiological response in children (Marcovitch et al., 2010).

Emotional Stimuli

To assess physiological reactivity to faces and emotional stimuli, discrete stimuli are often used (i.e., pictures). In particular, EEG studies have examined physiological response (i.e., early posterior negativity and late positive potential and modulation of event-related potentials) to emotional stimuli by presenting developmentally appropriate pictures from the International Affective Picture System to children (Hajcak & Dennis, 2009). Pictures of faces have also been used to assess physiological response to social stimuli in children. For example, children and adolescents with ASD were shown pictures from the Dynamic Affect Recognition Evaluation (Porges, Cohn, Bal, & Lamb, 2007) as stimuli, in order to assess their cardiovascular response to six basic emotions (anger, disgust, fear, happiness, sadness, and surprise; Bal et al., 2010).

Although emotional stimuli can be discrete stimuli, continuous assessment of emotions is possible through the use of standardized music and film clips (Gross & Levenson, 1995; Stephens, Christie, & Friedman, 2010). Videos have been used successfully to examine emotional responses in children with ASD (Balconi, Amenta, & Ferrari, 2012) and psychophysiological responses to emotions in children and adolescents with ASD (Bal et al., 2010; Van Hecke et al., 2009).

THEORY UNDERLYING THE METHOD

Psychophysiological theories provide important conceptual links from physiological measurement to psychological constructs. In both research and clinical practice, it is critical to understand theory in order to draw accurate inferences and conceptualizations (Friedman, 2007; Kazdin, 1999, 2001). Although there are many theories linking physiological measures to psychological constructs, this section provides examples of two developmental psychophysiological theories. Our discussion is by no means an exhaustive review of relevant theories, and the reader is referred to the *Handbook of Psychophysiology* (Cacioppo et al., 2007) for a more complete review.

Polyvagal Theory

The "polyvagal theory" (Porges, 1995, 1998, 2001, 2003, 2007, 2009; Porges & Lewis, 2009) describes psychophysiological response from a developmental perspective. In particular, this theory connects central nervous system and peripheral nervous system structures to behavioral responses. Within the polyvagal theory, three broad and phylogenetically organized physiological responses are described (from oldest to most recently developed): (1) immobilization (feigning death), (2) mobilization (fight–flight), and (3) social communication (self-soothing, calming). Relevant to the physiological assessment of child behavior, the social communication circuit consists of the vagus nerve (measured through RSA; peripheral nervous system component) and the nucleus ambiguus (central nervous system component). The polyvagal theory hypothesizes that a self-soothed/calmed state promotes social communication and social behavior (Porges, 2001). Due to the developmental and social difficulties of children with ASD, the polyvagal theory is particularly relevant in studying and assessing these children. Recent studies have found that children with ASDs demonstrate more cardiac mobilization than typically developing children (Bal et al., 2010; Ming, Julu, Brimacombe, Connor, & Daniels, 2005; Van Hecke et al., 2009), and that decreased RSA is significantly related to measures of social behavior (Van Hecke et al., 2009). Thus, the polyvagal theory provides a conceptual link between physiological responses and psychopathologies related to social and developmental issues.

Polyvagal Theory and BIS–BAS Theory

The polyvagal theory has been extended by Theodore Beauchaine to include Gray's theory of motivation (e.g., Gray & McNaughton, 2000). Beauchaine's extension combines Gray's hypothesized behavioral approach system (BAS) and behavioral inhibition system (BIS) with tenets from the polyvagal theory (Beauchaine, Gatzke-Kopp, & Mead, 2007). Beauchaine uses this integrative theory to conceptualize the biobehavioral processes underlying externalizing disorders in children and adolescents. Specifically, he suggests that dysregulation of the BAS (appetitive behaviors in response to reward) is problematic when combined with inappropriate vagal regulation to negative emotion. Moreover, he proposes that fight–flight responding (or the activation of the mobilization circuit in the polyvagal theory) is characterized by individual differences in BAS and BIS functioning (i.e., approach vs. avoidance), and that BAS-predominant responding may be a marker for sensation seeking and aggressive behavior (Beauchaine et al., 2007). To investigate this motivational approach to the polyvagal theory, multiple psychophysiological studies have been conducted in children and adolescents with externalizing disorders, measuring RSA, PEP, EDA, and HR responses to reward tasks (e.g., Beauchaine et al., 2008).

APPLICATION TO THE CASE OF SOFIA

In the internalizing disorders case example presented by McLeod, Jensen-Doss, and Ollendick in Chapter 4 of this volume, Sofia was a 15-year-old Hispanic female who had difficulty with anxiety in school. She had a history of panic attacks at school, which led her to avoid school as a situation where she might have another panic attack. This caused her to fall behind academically. After Sofia missed a month of school, she attended exposure-based cognitive-behavioral therapy (CBT) for 16 sessions. The CBT helped alleviate some of Sofia's problems, but 2 months after termination she was told that she would have to repeat a grade because of her prior absences, and she stopped attending school completely.

Notably, Sofia's panic symptoms were indicative of physiological activation (i.e., racing heart, chest pains, dizziness). These panic symptoms are similar to how individuals may respond when they feel threatened (i.e., "fight or flight" for protection from threat). These physiological symptoms seemed quite severe for Sofia and were significant enough for her to believe she was having a heart attack. Instead of finding tools to cope with her physiological reactions, however, she began to avoid the situation where she experienced them. The exposure-based CBT most likely targeted her avoidance behaviors and her thoughts regarding situations that elicited her physiological reactions. Yet Sofia's primary symptoms were physiological. As such, including psychophysiological measures in the next round of her treatment could have been beneficial in order for Sofia to gain control of her physiological state, in addition to her thoughts and behaviors.

In particular, Sofia's physiological state could be assessed during exposures to stimuli that elicited significant physiological reactions (i.e., stimuli related to school). The Polar Heart Rate Monitor, as discussed earlier in this chapter, is an easy-to-use ambulatory measure of HR and HRV. This monitor could be worn as Sofia approached the school or was exposed to school-based activities (e.g., homework). If the clinician identified Sofia's physiological state as activating or becoming more aroused (e.g., increased HR), biofeedback protocols could be implemented to help Sofia gain conscious control of her physiological state.

One method involving biofeedback could be to have Sofia use deep breathing techniques while approaching the school. With the Polar Heart Rate Monitor or another ambulatory system attached to her, Sofia would be able to watch her HR change in real time and thus see objectively how the deep breathing was affecting her physiological state. It could also be used to demonstrate the physiological need for, and impact of, coping techniques: When Sofia was placed in anxiety-provoking situations at school, it might become easier for her to identify when her HR was increasing and she should use coping skills (e.g., deep breathing) to gain control of her HR. Overall, the primary goal of including psychophysiological measures in further exposure-based CBT would be to give Sofia greater self-efficacy in controlling her physiological state. Using psychophysiological measures to provide objective and real-time accounts of her physiological state would help Sofia to avoid misperceiving this state and would give her more accurate and rapid control over the biological processes underlying her panic symptoms.

APPLICATION TO THE CASE OF BILLY

In the externalizing case presented in Chapter 4, Billy was a 10-year-old European American male who struggled with significant emotional regulation issues pertaining to stress and anger management. Both at home and at school, he displayed oppositional, negativistic, and noncompliant behaviors. By his report, his mother did not pay attention to him when he was at home. Thus some of his behaviors (e.g., not being able to sleep due to nightmares, acting out at school and home) might have the function of seeking attention or obtaining comfort.

Billy did not seem to have effective strategies for gaining attention from others in appropriate ways. Moreover, he did not seem to have developed any "tools" for stress and anger management. As such, psychophysiological measures could be used in this case to teach Billy appropriate methods of dealing with his frustration and subsequent aggression. The clinician could teach Billy progressive muscle relaxation techniques designed for children (e.g., see Ollendick & Cerny, 1981) or an imagery-based procedure (e.g., see Koeppen, 1974), and simultaneously collect psychophysiological data. For ease of assessment, the Affectiva Q Sensor or another ambulatory system could be used for this data collection. The quantitative assessment would provide Billy and the clinician with a visualization of how Billy's physiological state (EDA or sympathetic response) mirrored his emotional state (i.e., what his physiological state "looked" like when he was angry vs. calm). With successful use of relaxation, not only would he feel calm by self-report, but he and the clinician would also be able to validate how he was subjectively feeling with objective physiological output.

SUMMARY AND RECOMMENDATIONS

In sum, psychophysiological measures can provide objective insight into biobehavioral processes that might otherwise go unnoticed in children and adolescents. Throughout this chapter, multiple physiological assessment measures have been described, but we have not provided extensive coverage of the psychophysiological measures available. We highly recommend reading papers that present methodological guidelines (e.g., those on the SPR website, *www.sprweb.org*) or the textbooks cited in the chapter. Carefully considered and collected psychophysiological measures can add important insights to the assessment of child psychopathology, and thereby can advance clinical theory, research, and practice.

REFERENCES

Andreassi, J. L. (2000). *Psychophysiology: Human behavior and physiological response*. Mahwah, NJ: Erlbaum.

Bal, E., Harden, E., Lamb, D., Van Hecke, A. V., Denver, J. W., & Porges, S. W. (2010). Emotion recognition in children with autism spectrum disorders: Relations to eye gaze and autonomic state. *Journal of Autism and Developmental Disorders, 40*(3), 358–370.

Balconi, M., Amenta, S., & Ferrari, C. (2012). Emotional decoding in facial expression, scripts and videos: A comparison between normal, autistic and Asperger children. *Research in Autism Spectrum Disorders, 6*(1), 193–203.

Beauchaine, T. (2001). Vagal tone, development, and Gray's motivational theory: Toward an integrated model of autonomic nervous system functioning in psychopathology. *Development and Psychopathology, 13*(2), 183–214.

Beauchaine, T., Gatzke-Kopp, L., & Mead, H. (2007). Polyvagal theory and developmental psychopathology: Emotion dysregulation and conduct problems from preschool to adolescence. *Biological Psychology, 74*(2), 174–184.

Beauchaine, T. P., Hong, J., & Marsh, P. (2008). Sex differences in autonomic correlates of conduct problems and aggression. *Journal of the American Academy of Child and Adolescent Psychiatry, 47*(7), 788–796.

Brenner, S. L., & Beauchaine, T. P. (2011). Pre-ejection period reactivity and psychiatric comorbidity prospectively predict substance use initiation among middle schoolers: A pilot study. *Psychophysiology,* 1–9.

Brown Wright, L., Gregoski, M. J., Tingen, M. S., Barnes, V. A., & Treiber, F. A. (2011). Impact of stress reduction interventions on hostility and ambulatory systolic blood pressure in African American adolescents. *Journal of Black Psychology, 37*(2), 210.

Cacioppo, J. T., Tassinary, L. G., & Berntson, G. G. (2007). *Handbook of psychophysiology* (3rd ed.). Cambridge, UK: Cambridge University Press.

Carapetian, S., Siedlarz, M., Jackson, S., & Perlmuter, L. C. (2008). Orthostatic blood pressure regulation predicts classroom effort in children. *International Journal of Psychophysiology, 68*(1), 70–74.

Cicchetti, D., Rogosch, F. A., Gunnar, M. R., & Toth, S. L. (2010). The differential impacts of early physical and sexual abuse and internalizing problems on daytime cortisol rhythm in school aged children. *Child Development, 81*(1), 252–269.

Dahlquist, L. M., Weiss, K. E., Dillinger Clendaniel, L., Law, E. F., Ackerman, C. S., & McKenna, K. D. (2009). Effects of videogame distraction using a virtual reality type head-mounted display helmet on cold pressor pain in children. *Journal of Pediatric Psychology, 34*(5), 574–584.

Dalton, K. M., Nacewicz, B. M., Johnstone, T., Schaefer, H. S., Gernsbacher, M. A., Goldsmith, H. H., & Davidson, R. J. (2005). Gaze fixation and the neural circuitry of face processing in autism. *Nature Neuroscience, 8*(4), 519–526.

Demeersman, R., & Stein, P. (2007). Vagal modulation and aging. *Biological Psychology, 74*(2), 165–173.

Fitzgerald, D. A., Angstadt, M., Jelsone, L. M., Nathan, P. J., & Phan, K. L. (2006). Beyond threat: Amygdala reactivity across multiple expressions of facial affect. *NeuroImage, 30*(4), 1441–1448.

Freitag, C. M., Hanig, S., Palmason, H., Meyer, J., Wust, S., & Seitz, C. (2009).

Cortisol awakening response in healthy children and children with ADHD: Impact of comorbid disorders and psychosocial risk factors. *Psychoneuroendocrinology, 34*(7), 1019–1028.

Friedman, B. (2007). An autonomic flexibility–neurovisceral integration model of anxiety and cardiac vagal tone. *Biological Psychology, 74*(2), 185–199.

Gilissen, R., Bakermans Kranenburg, M. J., van IJzendoorn, M. H., & Linting, M. (2008). Electrodermal reactivity during the Trier Social Stress Test for Children: Interaction between the serotonin transporter polymorphism and children's attachment representation. *Developmental Psychobiology, 50*(6), 615–625.

Gray, J. A., & McNaughton, N. (2000). *The neuropsychology of anxiety* (2nd ed.). New York: Oxford University Press.

Gray, M. A., Minati, L., Harrison, N. A., Gianaros, P. J., Napadow, V., & Critchley, H. D. (2009). Physiological recordings: Basic concepts and implementation during functional magnetic resonance imaging. *NeuroImage, 47*(3), 1105–1115.

Gross, J. J., & Levenson, R. W. (1995). Emotion elicitation using films. *Cognition and Emotion, 9*(1), 87–108.

Hajcak, G., & Dennis, T. A. (2009). Brain potentials during affective picture processing in children. *Biological Psychology, 80*(3), 333–338.

Hankin, B. L., Badanes, L. S., Abela, J. R. Z., & Watamura, S. E. (2010). Hypothalamic–pituitary–adrenal axis dysregulation in dysphoric children and adolescents: Cortisol reactivity to psychosocial stress from preschool through middle adolescence. *Biological Psychiatry, 68*(5), 484–490.

Hannesdóttir, D. K., Doxie, J., Bell, M. A., Ollendick, T. H., & Wolfe, C. D. (2010). A longitudinal study of emotion regulation and anxiety in middle childhood: Associations with frontal EEG asymmetry in early childhood. *Developmental Psychobiology, 52*(2), 197–204.

James, W. (1884). What is an emotion? *Mind, 9*(34), 188–205.

Jennings, Y. R,., Kamarck, T., Steward, C., Eddy, M., & Johnson, P. (1992). Alternate cardiovascular baseline assessment techniques: Vanilla or resting baseline. *Psychophysiology, 29*(6), 742–750.

Kazdin, A. E. (1999). Current (lack of) status of theory in child and adolescent psychotherapy research. *Journal of Clinical Child Psychology, 28*(4), 533–543.

Kazdin, A. E. (2001). Bridging the enormous gaps of theory with therapy research and practice. *Journal of Clinical Child Psychology, 30*, 59–66.

Kleinhans, N. M., Richards, T., Sterling, L., Stegbauer, K. C., Mahurin, R., Johnson, L. C., & Aylward, E. (2008). Abnormal functional connectivity in autism spectrum disorders during face processing. *Brain, 131*(4), 1000–1012.

Klimes-Dougan, B., Hastings, P. D., Granger, D. A., Usher, B. A., & Zahn-Waxler, C. (2001). Adrenocortical activity in at-risk and normally developing adolescents: Individual differences in salivary cortisol basal levels, diurnal variation, and responses to social challenges. *Development and Psychopathology, 13*(3), 695–719.

Koeppen, A. S. (1974). Relaxation training for children. *Elementary School Guidance and Counseling, 9*(1), 14–21.

Kurth, S., Ringli, M., Geiger, A., LeBourgeois, M., Jenni, O. G., & Huber, R. (2010). Mapping of cortical activity in the first two decades of life: A high-density sleep electroencephalogram study. *Journal of Neuroscience, 30*(40), 13211–13219.

Marcovitch, S., Leigh, J., Calkins, S. D., Leerks, E. M., O'Brien, M., & Blankson, A. N. (2010). Moderate vagal withdrawal in 3.5 year old children is associated with optimal performance on executive function tasks. *Developmental Psychobiology, 52*(6), 603–608.

Ming, X., Julu, P., Brimacombe, M., Connor, S., & Daniels, M. (2005). Reduced cardiac parasympathetic activity in children with autism. *Brain and Development, 27*(7), 509–516.

Morgan, C. A., Aikins, D. E., Steffian, G., Coric, V., & Southwick, S. (2007). Relation between cardiac vagal tone and performance in male military personnel exposed to high stress: Three prospective studies. *Psychophysiology, 44*(1), 120–127.

Ollendick, T., Allen, B., Benoit, K., & Cowart, M. (2011). The tripartite model of fear in children with specific phobias: Assessing concordance and discordance using the behavioral approach test. *Behaviour Research and Therapy, 49*, 459–465.

Ollendick, T. H., & Cerny, J. A. (1981). *Clinical behavior therapy with children.* New York: Plenum Press.

Patriquin, M. A., Scarpa, A., Friedman, B. H., & Porges, S. W. (2011). *Respiratory sinus arrhythmia: A marker for positive social functioning and receptive language skills in children with autism spectrum disorders.* Poster presented at the International Meeting for Autism Research, San Diego, CA.

Picard, R. W. (2009). Future affective technology for autism and emotion communication. *Philosophical Transactions of the Royal Society of London: Series B. Biological Sciences, 364*(1535), 3575–3584.

Porges, S. W. (1995). Orienting in a defensive world: Mammalian modifications of our evolutionary heritage. A polyvagal theory. *Psychophysiology, 32*(4), 301–318.

Porges, S. W. (1998). Love: An emergent property of the mammalian autonomic nervous system. *Psychoneuroendocrinology, 23*(8), 837–861.

Porges, S. W. (2001). The polyvagal theory: Phylogenetic substrates of a social nervous system. *International Journal of Psychophysiology, 42*(2), 123–146.

Porges, S. W. (2003). Social engagement and attachment. *Annals of the New York Academy of Sciences, 1008*, 31–47.

Porges, S. W. (2007). The polyvagal perspective. *Biological Psychology, 74*(2), 116–143.

Porges, S. W. (2009). The polyvagal theory: New insights into adaptive reactions of the autonomic nervous system. *Cleveland Clinic Journal of Medicine, 76*(Suppl. 2), S86–S90.

Porges, S. W., Cohn, J. F., Bal, E., & Lamb, D. (2007). *The Dynamic Affect Recognition Evaluation [Computer software].* Chicago: Brain–Body Center, University of Illinois at Chicago.

Porges, S. W., & Lewis, G. F. (2009). The polyvagal hypothesis: Common mechanisms mediating autonomic regulation, vocalizations and listening. In S. M. Brudzynski (Ed.), *Handbook of mammalian vocalization: An integrative neuroscience approach* (pp. 255–264). Amsterdam: Academic Press.

Roemmich, J. N., Lambiase, M., Salvy, S. J., & Horvath, P. J. (2009). Protective effect of interval exercise on psychophysiological stress reactivity in children. *Psychophysiology, 46*(4), 852–861.

Scarpa, A. (2004). The effects of child maltreatment on the hypothalamic–pituitary–adrenal axis. *Trauma, Violence, and Abuse, 5*(4), 333–352.

Scarpa, A., Raine, A., Venables, P. H., & Mednick, S. A. (1997). Heart rate and skin conductance in behaviorally inhibited Mauritian children. *Journal of Abnormal Psychology, 106*(2), 182–190.

Schwartz, E. B., Granger, D. A., Susman, E. J., Gunnar, M. R., & Laird, B. (1998). Assessing salivary cortisol in studies of child development. *Child Development, 69*(6), 1503–1513.

Sherwood, A., Allen, M., Fahrenberg, J., Kelsey, R., Lovallo, W., & Van Doornen, L. (1990). Methodological guidelines for impedance cardiography. *Psychophysiology, 27*(1), 1–23.

Staton, L., El-Sheikh, M., & Buckhalt, J. A. (2008). Respiratory sinus arrhythmia and cognitive functioning in children. *Developmental Psychobiology, 51*(3), 249–258.

Stephens, C. L., Christie, I. C., & Friedman, B. H. (2010). Autonomic specificity of basic emotions: Evidence from pattern classification and cluster analysis. *Biological Psychology, 84*(3), 463–473.

Stern, R. M., Ray, W. J., & Quigley, K. S. (2000). *Psychophysiological recording* (2nd ed.). Oxford, UK: Oxford University Press.

Suess, P. E., Porges, S. W., & Plude, D. J. (1994). Cardiac vagal tone and sustained attention in school age children. *Psychophysiology, 31*(1), 17–22.

Task Force of the European Society of Cardiology and the North American Society of Pacing and Elecgtrophysiology. (1996). Heart rate variability: Standards of measurement, physiological interpretation and clinical use. *Circulation, 93*(5), 1043–1065.

Van Hecke, A. V., Lebow, J., Bal, E., Lamb, D., Harden, E., Kramer, A., & Porges, S. W. (2009). Electroencephalogram and heart rate regulation to familiar and unfamiliar people in children with autism spectrum disorders. *Child Development, 80*(4), 1118–1133.

Watson, L. R., Baranek, G. T., Roberts, J. E., David, F. J., & Perryman, T. Y. (2010). Behavioral and physiological responses to child-directed speech as predictors of communication outcomes in children with autism spectrum disorders. *Journal of Speech, Language, and Hearing Research, 53*(4), 1052–1064.

Wilhelm, F. H., Schneider, S., & Friedman, B. H. (2006). Psychophysiological assessment. In M. Hersen (Ed.), *Clinician's handbook of child behavioral assessment* (pp. 201–231). Burlington, MA: Elsevier.

Wolf, S. (1995). Dogmas that have hindered understanding. *Integrative Physiological and Behavioral Science, 30*(1), 3–4.

10

Laboratory-Based
Cognitive Methodologies

Kathryn J. Lester and Andy P. Field

This chapter provides an overview of laboratory-based methodologies used to study aspects of cognitive processing implicated in child and adolescent internalizing and externalizing disorders. By its nature, this chapter is highly selective. Rather than attempting to provide a review of the multitude of laboratory-based cognitive methodologies available, we highlight classic experimental measures used to assess facets of cognition at different stages of information processing: attention, automatic associations, inhibitory processes, and interpretation and reasoning. In choosing the measures to review, we have selected those that we believe have the greatest potential for application in pediatric populations to study both experimental and clinical phenomena. We highlight methodological, technical, and psychometric issues relevant to using these tasks with child and adolescent samples. We also use recent research to illustrate the potential of these measures for bettering our understanding of childhood disorders. Finally, we consider whether and how these different measures might be utilized in clinical practice to help inform case conceptualization, treatment planning, and outcome evaluation, using the case examples presented by McLeod, Jensen-Doss, and Ollendick in Chapter 4 as a basis for discussion.

DESCRIPTION OF THE ASSESSMENT METHOD

Deficits and biases in aspects of cognitive functioning are increasingly recognized in developmental models of internalizing and externalizing disorders as playing a causal role in the development of these disorders and in contributing to the maintenance of these disorders over time. A vast array of cognitive tasks, often stemming from experimental paradigms employed in adult psychopathology, exist and have been utilized to study diverse aspects of cognitive functioning in typically developing and disordered children and adolescents. Cognitive methodologies provide a window on information-processing abilities, granting insights into aspects of perception, learning, memory, judgment, and problem solving. In this section, we briefly describe a limited selection of these measures, focusing on established tasks that measure selective attention, automatic evaluations, inhibitory processes, and reasoning, as these cognitive functions have been consistently implicated as both causal and maintaining factors in a range of childhood psychological disorders.

Methods for Measuring Attentional Processes

Tasks measuring attentional processes are widely used in the anxiety literature. We focus on the two most prevalent tasks: the dot-probe task and visual-search tasks. In the dot-probe task, a valenced and a neutral cue (e.g., words or faces) are presented simultaneously on a screen. For internalizing disorders such as anxiety, the valenced cue would be a threat cue (e.g., an angry face might be used in a socially anxious sample); for depression, the valenced cue might be related to self-worth (e.g., the word "useless"). These cues disappear, and a probe appears in the location either of the valenced or neutral cue. The participant has to respond to the probe; the question is how reaction time and accuracy of responses are affected by whether the probe appears in the spatial location previously occupied by the valenced or neutral cue. Individuals with elevated or clinical levels of anxiety or depression (relative to controls) typically respond faster to probes appearing in the location of valenced rather than neutral cues. This pattern of responding implies one of two things: The individuals' attention was oriented toward the valenced cues, or they had difficulty disengaging their attention from the valenced cues.

In the anxiety literature, many studies have used the dot-probe paradigm for assessing attention bias to threat words or pictures in children and adolescents. For example, children diagnosed with anxiety disorders in general (Vasey, Daleiden, Williams, & Brown, 1995); children with generalized anxiety disorder (GAD) and posttraumatic stress disorder (PTSD) (Dalgleish, Moradi, Taghavi, Neshat-Doost, & Yule, 2001; Dalgleish et al., 2003; Taghavi, Neshat-Doost, Moradi, Yule, & Dalgleish, 1999); children with elevated anxiety sensitivity (Hunt, Keogh, & French, 2007); and nonclinical children and adolescents with high anxiety levels (Vasey, El Hag, & Daleiden, 1996) have all shown the prototypic response pattern: They had faster responses to probes preceded by a threatening rather than a neutral word/picture. Attentional biases may also have a degree of content specificity. Adolescents ages 10–13 years reporting high levels of social stress showed vigilance to social threat words, but not physical threat words. In contrast, adolescents who reported low social stress showed no bias at all (Helzer, Connor-Smith, & Reed, 2009).

In nonanxious children, the dot-probe task has been used to show that children selectively attend to novel stimuli after they have been given threatening verbal information about them (Field, 2006a, 2006b). There is also some evidence that all children (not just anxious ones) show an attentional bias for emotionally valenced images. Waters, Lipp, and Spence (2004) demonstrated that both nonselected and clinically anxious children ages 9–12 years showed an attentional bias for emotionally valenced stimuli. Clinically anxious and nonanxious control children showed vigilance for happy emotional faces compared to neutral ones, but only clinically anxious children diagnosed with GAD showed an attentional bias for angry faces compared to neutral ones (Waters, Henry, Mogg, Bradley, & Pine, 2010; Waters, Mogg, Bradley, & Pine, 2008). Interestingly, the magnitude of the bias for angry faces was equivalent to that of the bias for happy faces; this finding suggests that clinically anxious children may have a bias for emotional faces in general, whereas nonanxious children may have a bias only for happy faces.

We (Field, Hadwin, & Lester, 2011) have recently reviewed the literature on attentional biases in child and adolescent anxiety, and noted that the mechanism underlying the experimental effects was not clear-cut in youth samples: Some studies in clinical samples showed vigilance to threat stimuli (e.g., Roy et al., 2008), whereas others showed *avoidance* of threat faces (e.g., Pine et al., 2005). However, a meta-analysis suggests that on balance, high trait and clinical anxiety in child samples is associated with *vigilance* to threat stimuli (Bar-Haim, Lamy, Pergamin, Bakermans-Kranenburg, & van IJzendoorn, 2007). These conflicting results do, however, highlight an important limitation of the dot-probe task: To understand the temporal allocation of attention, one needs to vary stimulus presentation times within the task. However, this is particularly difficult in child samples, who rarely tolerate large numbers of trials. An alternative strategy is to employ eye tracking (which we discuss in due course) to obtain online measures of spatial and temporal attention allocation.

Dot-probe-type tasks have also been used to study children with conduct problems (Adalio, White, & Blair, 2011), aggression and callous–unemotional (CU) traits (Kimonis, Frick, Fazekas, & Loney, 2006; Kimonis, Frick, Munoz, & Aucoin, 2007), and attention-deficit/hyperactivity disorder (ADHD) (Sonuga-Barke, De Houwer, De Ruiter, Ajzenstzen, & Holland, 2004). In a sample of adolescent boys ages 13–17 years and detained in a juvenile detention center, those boys scoring high on CU traits who also showed reduced vigilance for distressing picture stimuli reported the highest levels of aggression and violent delinquency. Kimonis et al. (2007) argue that in these individuals, a reduced attentional bias toward distressing negative stimuli may serve to reduce the extent to which cues (e.g., angry parental response, victim's distress) that would typically provoke a negative internal affective experience act to inhibit aggressive behavior and violence.

With regard to ADHD, Sonuga-Barke (2002) has proposed a pathway to ADHD involving aversion to delay, underpinned by heightened delay–reward discounting. Delay aversion in ADHD has been shown primarily in choice tasks, where children with ADHD choose small immediate rewards over large delayed rewards when compared to their peers (e.g., Kuntsi, Oosterlaan, & Stevenson, 2001). This tendency appears strongest when selection of the smaller immediate reward reduces overall delay (e.g., via reduced trial and session length; see Sonuga-Barke, Taylor, Sembi, & Smith, 1992). The dot-probe task has been used to investigate selective attention to cues associated with delay in children with ADHD and control children ages 8–12 years. Participants were asked to indicate on which side of the screen the probe was presented. First, participants completed a conditioning phase in which they learned to associate specific colors with delay-related cues. The dot probe was presented surrounded by a patch of color: One color indicated that a response should be made immediately (no-delay cue); a second color indicated that they should wait for 3 seconds before responding (short-delay cue); and a third color indicated that they should wait for 9 seconds (long-delay cue) before responding. During a subsequent test phase, a fourth color was introduced as a neutral stimulus and was paired with a color previously associated with either an immediate, short-delay, or long delay response. Children with ADHD demonstrated an attentional bias for color cues previously associated with delay-related experiences compared to neutral color cues. No significant difference in attentional bias was observed for cues that signaled delay and the avoidance of delay (i.e., immediate response); the participants with ADHD showed an attentional bias for all delay-related stimuli. The results were also not explained by differences in the ability to condition delay-related cues in children with ADHD and controls. In interpreting their findings, Sonuga-Clarke et al. (2004) suggest that children with ADHD may find the experience of delay and the avoidance of delay as of equal motivational significance. They argue that vigilance toward delay-related cues may represent an initial stage in an ADHD-specific delay avoidance mechanism. Through the early identification of delay-related cues, children with ADHD can act in ways to reduce the experience of delay by choosing immediacy over delay where available or by attending to nontemporal cues within their environment.

A second method used to assess selective attention is a visual-search task. In general, participants in visual-search tasks make decisions about the presence or absence of a prespecified target set among distracters (top-down search) or decide whether all stimuli within a visual array are the same or different (bottom-up search). Various parameters can be manipulated within this general framework to increase task difficulty: for example, increasing the similarity of targets and distracters, or the set size (the number of targets or distracters within a visual array). Donnelly, Hadwin, Menneer, and Richards (2010) argue that visual-search paradigms are an effective way to explore engagement or disengagement to threat in anxiety, and to demonstrate the moderating effect of anxiety on individuals' decisions about when to terminate search. A typical finding for anxious individuals would be that they find threat stimuli more quickly.

Visual-search tasks are still a relatively new methodology in child and adolescent samples. Nevertheless, trait-anxious (and nondepressed) children showed increased search efficiency when making decisions about when to terminate search trials in which a target was absent (Hadwin et al., 2003), and increased search efficiency when detecting threat stimuli such as emotional faces (Waters & Lipp, 2008), fear-relevant animals (Waters, Lipp, & Spence, 2008), and angry faces (Perez-Olivas, Stevenson, & Hadwin, 2008). This later effect was moderated by age, in that self-report separation anxiety was negatively correlated with search efficiency, but only for those ages 10 years and above. This study also found that the vigilance for angry faces in older children acted as a potential mediator of the relationship between maternal overprotection and separation anxiety. This study highlights how these attentional tasks can be used to delineate the cognitive mechanisms that underpin known predictors of different childhood psychopathologies. Visual-search tasks have also been used to investigate whether search efficiency varies for phylogenetic threat-relevant items (e.g., snakes, spiders), ontogenetic threat-relevant items (e.g., guns, knives, syringes) and non-threat-relevant items (e.g., mushrooms, flowers). Studies in both adults and children suggest that search for phylogenetically relevant stimuli is efficient relative to search for non-threat-relevant items (LoBue, 2010; LoBue & DeLoache, 2008; Öhman, Flykt, & Esteves, 2001; Waters, Lipp, et al., 2008), and this search advantage could have an evolutionary basis. However, recent evidence has also shown a search advantage for ontogenetic threat-related object categories such as guns, knives, and syringes (Blanchette, 2006; Brosch & Sharma, 2005; Fox, Griggs, & Mouchlianitis, 2007; LoBue, 2010); for nonthreatening stimuli (Tipples, Young, Quinlan, Broks, & Ellis, 2002); and for stimuli with which participants have expertise and that are therefore highly relevant stimuli (Purkis, Lester, & Field, 2011).

Despite the relative lack of research, we (Field et al., 2011) have concluded that the results of studies using visual-search paradigms to explore internalizing problems in children and adolescents are consistent with research using paradigms such as the dot-probe task and with adult research generally. In research on externalizing problems, these paradigms are much less frequently used (probably because of the difficulties inherent in, for example, asking a child with ADHD to attend to tens or hundreds of visual trials). However, a small number of studies have used visual-search tasks to assess attentional deficits in children with ADHD (see Mullane &

Klein, 2007, for a review). A review of these studies has shown that compared to control children, children with ADHD show less efficient search at both the lowest and highest levels of search complexity (with search complexity defined according to set size and target–distracter similarity). These findings could be accounted for by deficits in self-regulation, with attentional impairments in ADHD most commonly occurring under complex or boring task conditions. Very simple search tasks may fail to provide sufficient stimulation for children with ADHD to reach an optimal level of arousal for efficient search performance to occur. Complex search tasks may exceed these children's ability to allocate effort and attention so as to complete the search task efficiently. A study by Mehta, Goodyer, and Sahakian (2004) also demonstrated that performance on a matching-to-sample visual-search task can be affected by the administration of an acute single dose of a stimulant medication, methylphenidate, relative to a placebo control. Participants were a sample of boys ages 9–13 years with an ADHD diagnosis. In the visual-search task, participants were presented with a complex visual pattern (target); then, when they pressed a button, one, two, four, or eight distracter patterns surrounding the target were presented, one of which was identical to the target pattern. Participants were asked to keep the button pressed while searching for the matching stimulus and then to release the button to touch it. When given the stimulant medication, children made fewer incorrect responses relative to when they were given a placebo control, but there was no difference in latency of search responses. Mehta et al. (2004) suggest that this may reflect an improvement in distractibility as a result of receiving the stimulant medication.

Eye-tracking methods have also been used in conjunction with visual-search and dot-probe tasks to study attentional allocation in youth samples. Eye-tracking methods overcome one of the greatest limitations of reaction time and accuracy-based measures (e.g., dot-probe tasks, Stroop task), in that they provide a continuous rather than a snapshot view of attentional deployment; moreover, they are not influenced by motor responses. Eye movements are divided into "saccades" (rapid movements of the eye to fixate the fovea on a new location in the visual field) and "fixations" (periods between saccades when the eye pauses in a certain position). Eye-tracking devices measure eye positions, eye movements, and pupil dilation, with the direction of gaze being highly correlated (albeit not perfectly) with the uptake of visual information (In-Albon & Schneider, 2010). Thus, by tracking someone's eye movements, researchers can measure what captured and held the individual's attention and how that stimulus was perceived over time. Caseras, Garner, Bradley, and Mogg (2007) argue that eye movements possess ecological validity because people look at the stimuli they attend to. Using eye movements also allows researchers to investigate temporal components of attention, as it is possible to extract measures of biases in orienting as indexed by the direction and latency of the first shift in gaze, while duration of gaze is informative about the maintenance of attention.

Several different types of eye trackers are available. However, the most common and practical for use with children are video-based eye trackers, because these are unobtrusive. Video-based trackers work by capturing video images of the eye and then calculating the eye's x and y coordinates relative to the screen being viewed. Various eye-tracking paradigms exist, of which the most widely used are eye movements during visual-search or picture-scanning tasks, antisaccades, visually guided saccades, memory-guided saccades, and smooth-pursuit eye movements. For example, when combined with a dot-probe or visual-search task (see above), a measure of the participant's eye position is taken approximately every 20 milliseconds (ms), allowing the course of attention to be sampled with a high level of accuracy. Metrics available include fixation count on experimenter-defined "areas of interest" (AOI; e.g., a threat picture in a threat-neutral picture pair), gaze time, time to first fixation on an AOI, and fixation order.

With regard to internalizing disorders, a few studies have begun to unpack components of attentional processing in children and adolescents. In an initial study, Jazbec, McClure, Hardin, Pine, and Ernst (2005) used a monetary reward antisaccade task to investigate cognitive control and error processing to reward and punishment contingency contexts in healthy individuals and in anxious and depressed adolescents. Fulcher, Mathews, and Hammerl (2008) used eye tracking to investigate attentional processing after undertaking an evaluative learning task as a function of differences in child and parental anxiety. They observed that children, regardless of anxiety scores, fixated on frowning faces before smiling faces. Children scoring highly on panic and separation anxiety fixated more on neutral ideographs (Japanese symbols) that had previously predicted a frowning face during the evaluative learning phase than did children scoring low on panic and separation anxiety. Gamble and Rapee (2009) found no evidence for attentional bias to emotionally valenced stimuli in anxious and nonanxious children ages 7–17 years when face pairs were presented for 3,000 ms. At shorter stimulus durations of 500 ms, they observed evidence for a bias in initial orienting. Anxious children directed their first fixation away from happy faces, while anxious adolescents directed their first fixation away from negative faces. In-Albon, Kossowsky, and Schneider (2010) also found evidence for a vigilance–avoidance pattern of attentional bias in children with separation anxiety disorder (SAD) relative to controls. Eye-tracking methodologies have also been used to investigate attentional processes in very young children. Peltola, Leppanen, Vogel-Farley, Hietanen, and Nelson (2009) observed that 7-month-old infants were slower to disengage attention from fearful faces than from happy and neutral faces.

Eye-tracking methodologies have also been employed in conjunction with cognitive tasks to investigate attentional processes in externalizing disorders. For example, Dadds, El Masry, Wimalaweera, and Guastella (2008) used eye tracking to investigate whether psychopathic and CU traits in a sample of male adolescents were associated with reduced attention to the eye region of face stimuli differing in emotional valence. Boys scoring highly on psychopathic traits had poorer recognition of fear faces, and fixated less often and for a shorter duration on the eye region of emotional faces, regardless of valence. Dadds et al. (2008) argue that this deficit in attention to the eyes of faces accounts for the observation that children with high CU traits have deficits in recognizing fear in others. Aggressive children are thought to be hypersensitive to cues of threat and hostility in others' behavior. Horsley, Orobio de Castro, and Van der Schoot (2010) compared the eye movements of a sample of 10- to 13-year-old children with high levels of aggressive behavior to a sample with low levels of aggressive behavior while they viewed cartoon pictures of ambiguous provocation events varying along the dimensions of degree of hostile behavior and emotional response depicted. Eye-tracking indices revealed that aggressive children did not fixate longer on hostile cues or attend less to depictions of nonhostile behavior than children scoring low on aggressive behavior. In fact, aggressive children fixated for longer on nonhostile cues compared to their nonaggressive peers, but in turn attributed more hostile intent to these nonhostile depictions.

Eye movement studies have also been used to investigate the hypothesis that children with ADHD demonstrate problems with response inhibition (Rommelse, Van der Stigchel, & Sergeant, 2008). One of the most robust findings in the ADHD literature is that compared to controls, children with ADHD display increased variability in response latencies in antisaccades (Munoz, Armstrong, Hampton, & Moore, 2003), visually guided saccades (Mostofsky, Lasker, Cutting, Denckla, & Zee, 2001; Mostofsky, Lasker, Singer, Denckla, & Zee, 2001), and memory-guided saccades (Rommelse et al., 2008). More intrusive saccades, defined as inappropriate eye movements, have also been investigated in ADHD with studies using a variety of tasks, including go/no-go tasks (Castellanos et al., 2000), ocular fixation tasks (Gould, Bastain, Israel, Hommer, & Castellanos, 2001), visual-search tasks (Van Der Stigchel et al., 2007), and prolonged fixation tasks (Munoz et al., 2003). For example, Gould et al. (2001) compared the ability of a sample of 53 children with ADHD to 44 healthy controls on a fixation task, in which children had to maintain their fixation on a moving dot for a period of 21 seconds. They observed that the children with ADHD made a significantly greater number of intrusive saccades that interrupted fixation than did control participants.

Methods for Measuring Inhibitory Processes

Inhibitory processes have typically been investigated in the laboratory by using variants of the Stroop and go/no-go tasks. The Stroop task requires participants to ignore the meaning of words or pictures while naming the color in which they are printed or highlighted. The logic is that response times to words/pictures will be slower if the meaning of the word/picture interferes with color naming. In a variant of this task, called the emotional Stroop task, the words or pictures reflect emotional content (such as words that have a threatening meaning or pictures depicting threatening stimuli). The emotional Stroop task has been used widely to study internalizing disorders (for a review, see Bar-Haim et al., 2007), and the conventional Stroop has been used to study externalizing disorders such as ADHD (for a review, see van Mourik, Oosterlaan, & Sergeant, 2005).

The Stroop task is believed to engage various brain regions, including the frontal cortex, which has been implicated in ADHD. Therefore, children with ADHD would be expected to show stronger effects on the Stroop task (indicating poorer control over the interference effect caused by the task) than controls. For internalizing disorders such as anxiety, individuals are expected to respond more slowly when color-naming anxiety-related words. This interference would reflect these individuals' inability to utilize top-down processing to inhibit attention to negative or threat meanings in order to complete the task efficiently (Eysenck, Derakshan, Santos, & Calvo, 2007).

The expected Stroop effects have been shown relative to controls in children with ADHD and in children with both ADHD and oppositional defiant disorder (ODD) (e.g., Perna et al., 1994). However, across studies the evidence is equivocal (Hudziak et al., 1996). A meta-analysis of Stroop interference effects in ADHD found that the effect size for greater Stroop interference in people with ADHD compared to controls was small ($d = 0.35$). More importantly, there was considerable between study variability, with only 5 of the 17 studies showing effect sizes meaningfully different from 0 (see Table 4 in van Mourik et al., 2005).

In children and adolescents with internalizing problems, the emotional Stroop task has looked both at clinical samples, such as youth with PTSD and GAD (e.g., Moradi, Taghavi, Neshat-Doost, Yule, & Dalgleish, 1999; Taghavi, Dalgleish, Moradi, Neshat-Doost, & Yule, 2003), and at normally developing children classified as being high or low in trait anxiety (e.g., Eschenbeck, Kohlmann, Heim-Dreger, Koller, & Leser, 2004; Hadwin, Donnelly, Richards, French, & Patel, 2009; Martin, Horder, & Jones, 1992; Richards, French, Nash, Hadwin, & Donnelly, 2007). Studies typically find longer (though some studies have found shorter) latencies to color naming of threat stimuli for children with specific anxieties, generalized anxiety, and state anxiety, and in both analogue and clinical samples (see Nightingale, Field, & Kindt, 2010, for a review).

A meta-analysis (Bar-Haim et al., 2007) reported a medium effect ($d = 0.50$) of threat-related bias in anxious children, based on 11 studies. Nevertheless, several studies using this paradigm have been unable to demonstrate the basic emotional Stroop effect in anxious nonclinical and clinical samples of children and adolescents (Dalgleish et al., 2003; Eschenbeck et al., 2004; Kindt, Bögels, & Morren, 2003; Kindt & Brosschot, 1999) or have found faster, not slower, color naming to threat stimuli (Morren, Kindt, van den Hout, & van Kasteren, 2003). This variation in results could in part be explained by developmental processes: Kindt suggests in her inhibition hypothesis that a processing bias for threat is a normal part of development that decreases in nonanxious children as they grow older, but increases with age in anxious children. This hypothesis is partly supported by studies that show a general processing bias for threat in all children, at least at a younger age (e.g., Kindt, Brosschot, & Everaerd, 1997).

A second task that measures inhibition is the go/no-go task. In this task, participants are asked to respond to a particular stimulus on some trials (go trials) and avoid responding to any other stimulus on other trials (no-go trials). This task measures both inhibition (using the proportion of presses that they accidentally make on no-go trials) and attentional control (using response times on go trials when no-go trials are relatively sparse).

The go/no-go task has been used to study attentional processes in externalizing disorders. A typical finding would be that children with ADHD (with and without disruptive behavior problems) show less inhibitory control than typically developing children (Diaferia et al., 1993). As selective examples, the go/no-go task has been used to show that differences in inhibition between children with ADHD and controls decrease with age (Diaferia et al., 1993); that inhibition correlates with behavioral problems in preschool children (Mehta et al., 2004); and that the reduced inhibition found in children with ADHD varies as a function of IQ—the lower the IQ, the worse the inhibition (Battaglia et al., 1995). The task has also been used to assess the impact of treatments on behavioral problems in children: Event-related potentials measured during a go/no-go task revealed a reduction in ventral prefrontal activation from pre- to posttreatment in those for whom treatment improved behavior. Treatment improvers showed activation in line with controls after treatment, whereas nonimprovers continued to show higher activation (Brambilla et al., 1992).

In the context of anxiety, the stimuli will be threat-related. For example, girls ages 8–12 years diagnosed with clinical anxiety (compared with typically developing controls) were slower to respond to neutral-face go trials in the context of angry-face (vs. happy-face) no-go trials. There was no corresponding significant effect of anxiety in boys (Waters & Valvoi, 2009). There have been very few studies using the go/no-go task in anxious children, but interesting studies are underway in various laboratories.

Methods for Measuring Automatic Associations

A third family of reaction-time-based tasks that have been used to measure cognition are those measuring automatic associations (see Huijding, Wiers, & Field, 2010, for a review). The most widely investigated measures of automatic associations use the affective priming paradigm, or APP (Fazio, Sanbonmatsu, Powell, & Kardes, 1986); the implicit association test, or

IAT (Greenwald, McGhee, & Schwartz, 1998); and the explicit affective Simon task, or EAST (De Houwer, 2003).

The use of the terms "implicit" and "explicit" in the context of these tasks is often confusing, because different authors use them differently and confound what is being measured with how it is being measured. De Houwer (2006) suggests that these tasks are best described as "indirect" measures, and that the cognitions themselves are referred to as "automatic" rather than "implicit" (to avoid the implication that people are not consciously aware of the cognitions; none of the tasks measure conscious awareness of the cognitions). In keeping with this terminology, we suggest that all three tasks can be used to measure automatically activated cognitions related to psychopathology (whether this is anxiety, depression, aggression, etc.). The main benefit of the tasks is that they are indirect, inasmuch as they rely on reaction times rather than self-report, and so are unlikely to be easily biased by demand awareness; the primary disadvantage is their reliance on reaction time data, which can be noisy due to the presence of errors, outliers, and increased reaction time variability, especially in child samples (Huijding et al., 2010).

The APP, IAT, and EAST are based on similar principles, in that they rely on comparing reaction times to stimuli that are congruent or incongruent. For example, in the APP, two stimuli are presented in quick succession. No response is required to the first stimulus, which is the prime, but an emotional response (usually positive or negative) is required to the second stimulus, which is the target and appears shortly after the prime. If the valence of the prime is congruent with the valence of the target (e.g., the prime is the word "pleasant" and the target is the word "smile"), response times to the target will be faster than when the valence of the prime–target pair is incongruent (i.e., "pleasant–pain"). The valence of the prime can be inferred by comparing response latencies to positive and negative targets that followed the prime.

The APP has been used in child and adolescent samples to measure attitudes to novel cartoon characters following a negative conditioning procedure (Field, 2006a), and to measure negative automatic responses to social situations and animals following verbal threat information (Lawson, Banerjee, & Field, 2007) and observational learning (Askew & Field, 2007). Furthermore, Spence, Lipp, Liberman, and March (2006) used pleasant pictures (e.g., puppies) and threat pictures (e.g., a man with a gun) as primes, and pleasant words (e.g., "friend") and unpleasant words (e.g., "nightmare") as targets, to evaluate emotional priming effects. Surprisingly, younger children (7–10 years of age) showed a reverse priming effect (i.e., faster responses to positive than to negative targets following a negative prime). Spence et al. also did not find the predicted effect of stronger priming effects to threat pictures in anxious children.

The IAT has a more complex procedure: Participants sort stimuli into four different categories, using two response keys. In a typical IAT, two of the categories represent target concepts (e.g., flowers vs. insects), and the remaining categories represent extremes of an emotion or attribute (e.g., "positive" vs. "negative"). The task has five stages:

- *Stage 1: Attribute familiarization.* Participants classify words/pictures along the attribute dimension (e.g., "nice" or "nasty") by pressing a left or right response key.
- *Stage 2: Target concept familiarization.* Words/pictures representing the target concept (e.g., flowers and insects) are classified by pressing a left or right response key.
- *Stage 3: Congruent trials.* Participants classify words/pictures of both the target concept and the attribute concepts. For example, the left response key could be a conjunction of the "nice" attribute and the "positive" target concept (e.g., flowers), whereas the right response key could be a conjunction of the "nasty" attribute and the "negative" target concept (e.g., insects).
- *Stage 4: Reversal.* This is the same as Stage 2, except that the response keys (and categories) for classification swap sides.
- *Stage 5: Incongruent trials.* Participants classify words/pictures of both the target concept and the attribute concepts. For example, the left response key is a conjunction of the "nice" attribute and the "negative" target concept (e.g., insects), whereas the right response key is a conjunction of the "nasty" attribute and the "positive" target concept (e.g., flowers).

The order of the congruent and incongruent trials is reversed for half of the participants. If the participant views the target concepts in the predicted way, then response times to compatible trials should be faster than to incompatible trials.

The IAT has been used to measure children's negative emotional responses to animals about which they have heard threatening information (Field & Lawson, 2003; Field, Lawson, & Banerjee, 2008). Similarly, Teachman and Allen (2007) used the IAT to assess fear of negative evaluation. The IAT assessed the extent to which adolescents associated the category "me" (relative to "not me") with the attributes "liked" versus "rejected." Finally, Sportel, de Hullu, de Jong, Nauta, and Minderaa (described in Huijding et al., 2010) used the IAT to test whether automatic and self-reported evaluations of the self were related to social anxiety in adolescents. Although self-reported self-esteem was significantly related to a self-report measure of social anxiety, IAT responses were not.

In relation to externalizing disorders, an IAT measure has recently been shown to have some predictive validity for aggressive behavior toward peers in children ages 9–11 years (Grumm, Hein, & Fingerle, 2011). In the IAT task, the concepts of "self" (e.g., first name, own month of birth) and "other" (e.g., "other" first name, "other" birth month) were used as target categories. The attribute categories were defined as "aggressive" (e.g., "hit," "argue") and "peaceful" (e.g., "help," "play"). A competitive reaction time task was used as a measure of aggression. In this task, participants were led to believe they were playing a game against an opponent, in which the child who responded faster by pushing a button when a smiley face was presented on the screen would get the chance to withdraw points (between 0 and 100 points) from the opponent. Each child began the game with 1,000 points and played 20 trials, winning 10 and losing 10 rounds. After each loss, a medium-level provocation was introduced by withdrawing 40–60 points. Children were told that they as well as their opponents would receive sweets if they still had at least 450 points left at the end of the game. The results showed that performance on the IAT was a significant predictor of aggressive behavior, with this effect having incremental validity in addition to a measure of explicit aggression (the Aggression subscale of the Youth Rating Scale). Children who showed a stronger association on the IAT between the "self" category and "aggressive" attributes demonstrated greater aggression during the computerized task by withdrawing a larger number of points from their opponents.

The EAST works by training participants in such a way that some extrinsic feature (e.g., a key on a keyboard, or the orientation of a picture) acquires a positive or negative valence, and then having participants use this extrinsically valenced feature when classifying new stimuli. For example, in the original study (De Houwer, 2003), participants sorted positive and negative white words on the basis of their valence, using two response keys. These trials trained the participants so that one response key became extrinsically positive and the other negative. Subsequently, participants sorted blue and green words on the basis of their color, using the same response keys as before. In the critical phase, participants sorted both white and colored words, but they were asked to sort white words on the basis of their valence and the colored words on the basis of their color. As a consequence of the response keys' having acquired extrinsic valence, during the test phase participants had to respond to the colored words by pressing either the (extrinsically) positive or negative key, depending on the print color. Presenting each word equally often in each color made it possible to determine whether participants found it easier to give a positive or a negative response to a certain stimulus, and therefore to infer the participants' affective reaction to it.

The only study of child and adolescent anxiety that has used the EAST is an as yet unpublished doctoral dissertation (Vervoort, 2010). Vervoort used a pictorial version of the EAST in an unselected sample of children (6–12 years old), adolescents (13–18 years old), and adults (older than 18 years). The stimulus materials were general anxiety-relevant and control pictures, and in two experiments no significant reaction time effects were observed (although there was an effect when error rates were examined). To our knowledge, the EAST has not been used to measure constructs directly related to externalizing problems.

All three tasks outlined here are based on the idea of comparing response latencies to a stimulus under different conditions that are manipulated with respect to affect: In the APP, words are primed with stimuli of opposite affective value; in the IAT, participants concurrently categorize affectively opposing stimuli; and in the EAST, participants respond with keys that have an extrinsic affective value. However, the tasks have their pros and cons. For example, the IAT, in its original form, provides a measure of emotional/affective response to one category relative to another. To overcome this limitation, the so-called "single-category" (Karpinski & Steinman, 2006) and "single-attribute" (Penke, Eichstaedt, & Asendorpf, 2006). IATs have been developed. These variants are structurally very similar to the IAT, but use a single target concept or a single attribute category, rather than opposing affective categories. Also, the IAT is affected by attributes *other* than just stimulus valence; for example, some have argued that it is affected by the similarity of the target and attribute concepts, perceptual features, and category salience (De Houwer, Geldof, & De Bruycker, 2005; Rothermund & Wentura, 2004). Also, the IAT effect can be influenced by individual differences in task-switching ability (Mierke & Klauer, 2003), and by the category labels (De Houwer, 2001) and individual stimulus exemplars that are used (Bluemke & Friese, 2006). All three of these tasks may be difficult for younger children because of their cognitive complexity. Of the three, the APP is probably the least complex, because it does not involve categorizing multiple stimuli into multiple categories.

Methods for Measuring Reasoning Processes

"Reasoning" refers to cognitive processes implicated in deducing conclusions, generating judgments, and forming and testing hypotheses in a logical and coherent manner (Muris, 2010). Effective reasoning aids individuals in understanding and responding appropriately to aspects of their internal and external environments. Perhaps the most widely assessed facet of reasoning, especially with regard to internalizing disorders, has been "interpretation bias." This term refers to anxious individuals' tendency to interpret ambiguity in a threatening way relative to nonanxious controls. Various assessment methods have been employed to measure interpretation bias in children. The most commonly used is the ambiguous-vignettes paradigm (see Barrett, Rapee, Dadds, & Ryan, 1996; Bögels & Zigterman, 2000; Creswell & O'Connor, 2006). This task employs short descriptions of everyday situations that a child is likely to encounter (e.g., "On the way to school you feel funny in the tummy") and asks children to give an open-ended response to the question "What do you think is happening?" with responses coded as threatening or nonthreatening by independent raters, and then to choose the response they find most applicable from a choice of threat-related and non-threat-related interpretations (e.g., "You ate some bad food and are going to be really sick at school," or "You did not have enough breakfast and you need to eat something"). In an early study using an ambiguous-vignettes paradigm, Barrett et al. (1996) administered a series of such vignettes to children ages 7–14 years with either an anxiety diagnosis, an ODD diagnosis, or no diagnosis. Both the anxious children and the children with ODD interpreted the situations as more frequently threatening than control children, but the anxious children more often selected avoidant outcomes for the situations, while the children with ODD more frequently chose aggressive outcomes. In two similar studies, youth with anxiety disorders (SAD, GAD, and specific phobia in both studies) interpreted ambiguous stories significantly more negatively than controls and youth (ages 9–18 years) with externalizing disorders (Bögels & Zigterman, 2000), or than children (ages 7–12 years) at risk of anxiety by virtue of having parents with an anxiety diagnosis (Waters, Craske, Bergman, & Treanor, 2008)

"Homophones," words that sound the same but have multiple meanings (e.g., "die–dye"), and "homographs," words that have the same spelling but different meanings (e.g., "beat" [drum beat] vs. "beat" [to beat up]), have also been used to measure interpretation of ambiguity (Hadwin, Frost, French, & Richards, 1997; Taghavi, Moradi, Neshat-Doost, Yule, & Dalgleish, 2000; Waters, Wharton, Zimmer-Gembeck, & Craske, 2008). For the study of anxiety- and depression-related phenotypes, homophones and homographs are used that have a threat and a neutral meaning. Several experimental measures exist for use with homographs/homophones: Children can be asked upon hearing a homograph or homophone to choose between two pictures, one representing the threat meaning and the other representing the neutral meaning, or the children may be asked to use the word in a sentence or to make a drawing of the event to which each word refers. In adolescent samples, participants may be asked to spell the word they hear (for homophones). Hadwin, Frost, French, and Richards (1997) demonstrated that as anxiety increased, the likelihood that a child would select a picture that reflected the threat meaning of a series of homophones also increased. Anxious children and adolescents also produced significantly more sentences using the threat interpretation of a homophone than did control children (Taghavi et al., 2000). Further research has shown that threat interpretation bias measured via homophone tasks decreases in clinically anxious children (ages 8–12) after cognitive-behavioral treatment (CBT) (Waters, Wharton, et al., 2008).

Blended-word paradigms have also been used to assess interpretation bias toward negative stimuli (Dearing & Gotlib, 2009; Lawson, MacLeod, & Hammond, 2002). In these tasks, participants listen to auditory presentations of ambiguous stimuli. The blended-word stimuli are created by acoustically blending together threat-neutral word pairs that differ by only one phoneme (e.g., "cry–dry"). Participants are asked to select from two presented choices the word they thought they heard. In a recent study, Dearing and Gotlib (2009) investigated whether daughters of depressed mothers—a sample at increased risk for experiencing depression—would demonstrate a tendency to interpret ambiguous information in a negative way. Daughters of never-depressed and depressed mothers completed a negative mood induction prior to completing a blended ambiguous-words task. At-risk daughters more often selected the negative word from an ambiguous blended word constructed from a depressotypic and a neutral word (e.g., "sad–sand") than control participants. In contrast, at-risk participants were significantly less likely to select the positive interpretation of positive–neutral blended words (e.g., "joy–boy"), while at-risk and control participants did not differ in their interpretation of social threat-neutral blended words.

Emotional expression tasks have also recently emerged as a means of assessing interpretation bias, particularly related to social anxiety. In these tasks, children are required to interpret the meaning of faces with varying levels of different emotional expressions. These tasks employ a computer technique referred to as "morphing," in which composite stimuli of differing degrees of emotional intensity are created (e.g., 90% angry, 10% neutral). These can be presented as static images or dynamic films in which facial expressions gradually change from neutral to an emotional expression. Such methods provide an opportunity to assess online interpretations by means of reaction times to categorize differing emotions and also accuracy in responses (Battaglia et al., 2010; Broeren, Muris, Bouwmeester, Field, & Voerman, 2011; Creswell et al., 2008; Lau et al., 2009).

Related to interpretation bias is a cognitive distortion referred to as the "reduced evidence for danger" (RED) bias, in which anxious children require only minimal information to decide that a situation is dangerous. This bias may stem from the tendency for even very minor threat cues to trigger hyperarousal in anxious children. This is thought to be a consequence of highly anxious children being acutely vigilant for threat signals in their environment and being more likely to conclude rapidly that these minor cues signal impending danger, without searching for further information that would show that this is not the case (Daleiden & Vasey, 1997). The RED bias is also assessed by using vignette tasks, in which participants are told that they will hear some short stories, some of which will have a scary ending and some will have a happy ending. Each vignette is presented one sentence at a time, with children rating after each sentence whether they think the story will be scary or not. Anxious children may be expected to conclude that the story is going to be scary even with very little information. Muris, Merckelbach, and Damsma (2000) found this to be the case. They exposed 8- to 13-year-old children who were high and low on social anxiety to vignettes of social situations presented to them sentence by sentence. Children with higher levels of social anxiety needed to hear fewer sentences before concluding that a story was going to have a scary ending, thereby demonstrating a lower threshold for threat perception compared to children with lower levels of social anxiety. This bias has been replicated in several other studies and has been found to persist over time (Muris, Kindt, et al., 2000; Muris, Luermans, Merckelbach, & Mayer, 2000; Muris, Rapee, Meesters, Schouten, & Geers, 2003). Higher levels of aggression have also been associated with a RED bias for stories describing ambiguous social situations (Muris, Merckelbach, & Walczak, 2002).

Similar vignette paradigms are also employed to assess emotional reasoning bias in children. "Emotional reasoning" refers to a heuristic by which individuals use physical internal sensations to evaluate the dangerousness of an external situation (see Muris, Mayer, Vermeulen, & Hiemstra, 2007; Muris, Merckelbach, & van Spauwen, 2003; Schneider, Unnewehr, Florin, & Margraf, 2002). In this way, anxiety is strongly related to the notion that "If I feel anxious, then there must be danger," regardless of whether an objective threat is present or not. In emotional reasoning paradigms, children are asked to rate how scary a vignette will be, with the vignettes differing along the dimensions of objective safety and danger information and the presence and absence of physical anxiety symptoms. For each vignette, participants are presented with four scripts: (1) a situation with objective danger information and anxiety response information; (2) a situation with objective danger information but no anxiety response; (3) a situation with objective safety information and an anxiety response; and (4) a situation with objective safety information and no anxiety response.

Several studies have investigated how children with internalizing disorders reason about anxiety-related information. Children were presented with scenarios describing anxiety-related (e.g., giving a talk, getting a report card from a teacher) or everyday (e.g., playing with a ball, drawing, watching TV) situations. The scenarios were manipulated to contain either danger or safety information—for example, "believing a party to be 'fancy dress,' you turn up dressed as a clown, but arrive to discover everyone else is dressed normally [danger]," or "... they too are in costume [safety]." In addition, some vignettes contained anxiety response information (e.g., "You begin to sweat," or "You begin to tremble"). Children ages 7–13 years rated how dangerous they found the vignette. Nonclinical children's danger ratings were affected by whether the vignette contained anxiety information; danger ratings were higher when anxiety response information was given, even for safe stories (Morren, Muris, & Kindt, 2004; Muris, Merckelbach, et al., 2003; Muris, Vermeer, & Horselenberg, 2008). The tendency to use anxiety response information as a heuristic for evaluating the dangerousness of the safe stories was increased by trait anxiety and anxiety sensitivity (Muris, Merckelbach, et al., 2003). Age, cognitive development, and anxiety sensitivity were also positively related to 4- to 13-year-old children's ability to perceive physical symptoms as a signal of anxiety (Muris, Mayer, Freher, Duncan, & van den Hout, 2010).

METHODOLOGICAL CONSIDERATIONS AND PSYCHOMETRIC PROPERTIES

With regard to practical matters, cognitive-based laboratory measures are noninvasive, are relatively easy and quick to administer, and usually require only limited specialist equipment to design and run. Purpose-designed software (e.g., EPrime, Presentation, etc.) is available to assist in the design, running, data collection, and analysis of experimental cognitive tasks. This software also makes it possible to create and run cognitive tasks that can be synchronized with other methodologies (e.g., eye tracking electroencephalography, startle response, and functional magnetic resonance imaging), meaning that there is great flexibility in the design of experiments that can be created. The ability to combine cognitive tasks with other methodologies can also provide a much richer understanding of psychopathology, and we believe that a multimethod approach should continue to be a growing focus of future research. Advances in portable technology (e.g., laptops, hand-held devices, touchscreens) also mean that cognitive measures can be administered in a wide variety of settings—from the laboratory to school, home, and clinic settings. Even eye-tracking methods for assessing selective attention are not limited to use within the lab or to on-screen visual displays. Head-mounted stand-alone systems also allow studies of real-world stimuli, which may be particularly useful for clinical applications.

The use of experimental measures such as the dot-probe task and IAT to measure self-related constructs offers several advantages. First, these tasks provide direct access to facets of individuals' cognitive processing that they are not able to verbalize. These types of tasks have also been demonstrated to have incremental validity over and above explicit self-report measures. Some behaviors and cognitions are also considered socially unacceptable—for example, aggressive or callous thoughts, or extreme anxiety behaviors. As such, self-report explicit measures may be subject to social desirability bias, which may reduce the predictive validity of explicit measures. The use of automatic association measures may therefore help to improve the prediction of internalizing and particularly externalizing behavior. For example, the IAT has been used successfully to assess and predict aggressive behavior (Grumm et al., 2011).

In developing cognitive measures for use with child samples, a number of important methodological factors should be taken into consideration. As with any other type of methodology, the number of experimental trials must be sufficient to ensure adequate reliability and to maximize opportunity to detect an effect, but care must also be taken that children do not become fatigued, as this is likely to have a detrimental effect on performance. For reasoning-based tasks that rely heavily on the use of linguistic stimuli, it is important to ensure that stimuli are appropriate, given the age and anticipated vocabulary of the participant group. This is especially important for homophone and homograph tasks, where participants need to be aware of both meanings of each word and where the opposing meanings should be of approximately equal frequency in the lexicon. One must also be aware of the extent to which task performance may be influenced by demand effects. This is particularly pertinent for reasoning tasks, as they often rely on self-report measures, although there are exceptions (e.g., face morph tasks, which are more experimental in nature).

Another important factor to consider in selecting suitable cognitive tasks that can be used across development, although it is by no means unique to the use of cognitive experimental techniques, is the interplay between task performance and development. This consideration is made all the more difficult by the lack of age norms for tasks measuring facets of cognitive processing. As the maturation of cognitive and neural processes is known to affect performance on cognitive tasks (see Diamond, Kirkham, & Amso, 2002, for an example), researchers should be extremely cautious in interpreting data collected across a wide age range. This is especially the case for tasks that rely on reaction times, as these may be especially problematic in child samples. It is a well-replicated finding that reaction times in general vary as a function of age: Younger children typically have slower reaction times and greater variance. Also, some of the tasks outlined earlier are quite complex and perhaps require cognitive skills and attention spans that younger children do not possess. These problems could help explain many unpublished studies that have failed to find the expected patterns of reaction times on the types of tasks described in this chapter. For example, Askew (2007) reports six studies in which changes in self-reported fear were not mirrored by effects on the APP. Moreover, Huijding, Bos, and Muris (described in Huijding et al., 2010) found no meaningful relations between the IAT and self-report measures of self-esteem. With regard to reasoning tasks, it is established that reasoning abilities increase with age as a result of cognitive development during childhood (e.g., Berk, 2004). We might therefore expect that a minimum level of cognitive maturation may be required before reasoning biases consistently emerge in children (Alfano, Beidel, & Turner, 2002; Field & Lester, 2010). It also means that age-related effects should be considered when one is investigating the manifestation of these biases across a sample with a broad age range.

There has been only very limited focus to date on examining the psychometric properties of cognitive measures. For example, we are not aware of any studies examining the test–retest reliability of interpretation bias tasks with children. Studies investigating the psychometric properties of attentional bias tasks have predominantly been conducted in adult samples so far. Poor test–retest reliability of bias scores has been obtained for the Stroop and dot-probe tasks (Kindt, Bierman, & Brosschot, 1996; Schmukle, 2005; Siegrist, 1997). For example, Schmukle (2005) reported test–retest reliabilities of just .14 over a 1-week interval for a pictorial dot-probe task. The more positive news is that over five experiments, Huijding et al. (2010) reported Spearman–Brown corrected split-half reliabilities of, on average, .63 at the first assessment and around .44 at 1-week and

1-month follow-ups. These values suggest that the internal consistency of the IAT in children is lower than in adult samples, but higher than reliabilities for other latency-based measures. For the EAST, internal consistency for different target pictures (interitem stability) has been show to range from .43 to .54, and the intraclass correlation (interindividual stability) has been shown to be high (.88), suggesting that children's responses are consistent throughout the task (Vervoort, 2010). Also, several of the studies already mentioned showed longitudinal effects on the APP and IAT of up to 6 months, suggesting at least adequate test–retest reliability (Askew & Field, 2007; Field et al., 2008).

Recent work has shown that eye-tracking measures have good internal consistency and test–retest reliability in children and adults (Karatekin, 2007; Klein & Fischer, 2005; O'Driscoll et al., 2005). For example, Klein and Fischer (2005) assessed internal consistency and reliability of pro- and antisaccades across the lifespan. After age was controlled for, reliabilities were high for pro- and antisaccade reaction times (.81–.90 for split-half reliability) and antisaccade errors (.83 for split-half). In 6- to 18-year-olds, test–retest reliability was moderate for pro- and antisaccade reaction times (.65–.66), but relatively low for antisaccade errors (.43). Test–retest reliability over a 3- to 6-week period in a sample of children with ADHD was .79 for antisaccade errors and .62 for predictive saccades (O'Driscoll et al., 2005).

In terms of convergent validity, the correlation between the IAT effect and self-reported fear beliefs in Field's studies was –.035, and that between the IAT and a behavioral avoidance task was –.013. With respect to other measures in this chapter, a handful of studies have looked at the convergent validity of cognitive measures of anxiety and typically reported low correlations. For example, two studies found close to zero correlations ($r = .003$, Dalgleish et al., 2003; $r = -.04$, Heim-Dreger, Kohlmann, Eschenbeck, & Burkhardt, 2006) between interference effects as indexed by the emotional Stroop task and the dot-probe task. This lack of convergence implies that at least one of the measures is unreliable or invalid. In addition, Watts and Weems (2006) found that even word and picture formats of the dot-probe task correlated poorly ($r = -.13$). Moreover, both formats of this task also correlated poorly with memory bias (r's = .14 [word] and .06 [picture]) and measures of cognitive errors (r's = -.04 [word] and .21 [picture]); measures of cognitive errors and memory bias correlated poorly, too ($r = .06$). Although this seems to imply that cognitive measures lack validity, these low correlations are not surprising, given that different measures of anxiety are frequently asynchronous (Lang, 1968; for a review, see Zinbarg, 1998).

In the context of measuring externalizing problems, the go/no-go task correlated fairly well with observational measures of repeating behaviors and difficulty in task switching ($r = -.35$), but not measures of vocalizing frustration ($r = -.21$) or inattentiveness to instructions ($r = -.15$) (Rothenberger et al., 2000). There is also some evidence for modest correlations between inhibition measured with the go/no-go task and with a Stroop-like test: Mehta et al. (2004) reported that correlations between the measures at various time points ranged from .24 to .34. In a study of nonclinical children that used an extensive battery of tests, a factor analysis conducted on scores from the various measures resulted in a factor containing the go/no-go task and a continuous-processing task, in which vigilance to and inhibition in response to certain stimuli must be maintained over a prolonged period of time (Johnstone, Watt, & Dimoska, 2010). This suggests that the go/no-go task has some convergent validity with related tasks. However, the Stroop loaded most strongly on a different factor that included measures of verbal (digit span) and nonverbal working memory (hand movements) and verbal fluency. The highly verbal nature of the Stroop task perhaps makes it unremarkable that it has been shown to share the most variance with other verbal tasks (rather than inhibition tasks); however, a picture version of the Stroop task was employed, which would suggest that even the fact that verbal rather than behavioral responses were recorded means that the task was correlated more strongly with concurrent verbal than with inhibitory measures.

IMPLICATIONS FOR TREATMENT PLANNING AND OUTCOME EVALUATION

In this section, we consider whether the cognitive measures previously described can be used to inform clinical practice by guiding treatment planning and outcome evaluation. In doing so, we apply the framework outlined by Vasey and Lonigan (2000), who propose that a given measure or methodology can have direct or indirect clinical utility. They define "direct utility" as the extent to which the application of a given measure yields benefits in the case of a specific child. Direct clinical utility can be further subdivided to include (1) "diagnostic utility," improving the ability to diagnose a given disorder; (2) "treatment utility," enhancing the ability to match individuals to an optimal treatment; (3) "prevention utility," identifying children by virtue of their increased risk for a condition, who can then be directed to an appropriate prevention program; and (4) "treatment-monitoring utility," improving the measurement of treatment effects and outcomes. These subdivisions are outlined in greater detail in Table 10.1. "Indirect utility" refers to benefits such as advances in understanding the nature, assessment, and treatment of a given clinical problem when the measure is applied in a research setting. Indirect utility can be broken down into (1) "conceptual utility," advancing understanding of the processes and mechanisms underpinning a given form of psychopathology; and (2) "validational utility," improving or confirming the validity of other measures. Table 10.1 provides a more detailed overview of these subdivisions as well. In addition, when determining the potential for the clinical application of assessment methods, we must consider the "incremental utility" of a

TABLE 10.1. Definitions of Direct and Indirect Clinical Utility

Type of utility	Definition
	Direct utility
Diagnostic utility	A measure has diagnostic utility if it helps with accurately identifying and classifying children with a specific disorder or with quantifying an integral characteristic of a diagnostic category (e.g., degree of avoidance of a specific phobic stimulus). However, a measure that leads to more accurate diagnosis only has direct clinical utility if it has a positive impact on treatment selection and outcome. A second component of diagnostic utility is a measure's ability to quantify or validate the degree of impairment associated with a given problem and the need for treatment of that problem.
Treatment utility	A measure or methodology has treatment utility if it has a positive influence on treatment outcome. A measure is likely to have greater direct utility via its effects on treatment utility if it can be shown to provide relevant, reliable and valid information. Assessment measures may contribute to treatment utility by providing information that enhances the selection, design, or implementation of effective treatments ˎ
Treatment-monitoring utility	A measure has treatment-monitoring utility if it is sensitive to treatment response—for example, by measuring change in symptoms or functioning. Such measures are perceived to have greater sensitivity compared to measures that simply consider treatment response in terms of changes in diagnostic status. When measures provide information about moderating, mediating, and causal processes throughout treatment, these can be used to develop empirically informed clinical decision rules to guide treatment cessation, continuation, or modification (Kazdin & Kendall, 1998).
Prevention utility	A measure has prevention utility if it effectively elucidates the causal processes underpinning the development of a given disorder or measures risk factors for a disorder. By assessing causal processes involved in the development of a disorder, a measure may demonstrate prevention utility, inasmuch as it may inform the development of effective interventions that target these causal processes to prevent the emergence of the disorder. By characterizing risk factors for a disorder, a measure may have prevention utility if it can identify children who would benefit most from preventive interventions.
	Indirect utility
Conceptual utility	A measure has conceptual utility if it produces information that, though not providing direct treatment utility, can lead to improved understanding of a disorder and to later improvements in the conceptualization, measurement, treatment, and prevention of a given disorder. An example of an assessment measure with conceptual utility is one that provides information improving the definition of subtypes of a disorder—subtypes that are later found to have important

(continued)

TABLE 10.1. (*continued*)

Type of utility	Definition
	implications for the development and selection of appropriate treatment methods. Assessment methods may also demonstrate conceptual utility by measuring processes that improve construct validity.
Validational utility	A measure has validational utility if the information it yields can be used to validate other measures used in clinical settings—for example, self-report questionnaires or diagnostic interviews. A further example is the use of assessment methods to evaluate the discriminant validity of diagnostic constructs, which is particularly useful when disorders have high rates of observed covariation and comorbidity (Lonigan, Hooe, Kistner, & David, 1999).

Note. Adapted from Vasey and Lonigan (2000). Copyright 2000 by Taylor & Francis Group. Adapted by permission.

measure. This refers to the degree to which a measure can provide useful information in addition to that obtained using standard measures. Regardless of the direct or indirect clinical utility of a given measure, perhaps the most important consideration is the "feasibility" of use in a typical clinical setting.

In this section, we comment on the possible clinical utility of the laboratory-based cognitive methodologies reviewed in this chapter, using the subdivisions of clinical utility proposed by Vasey and Lonigan (2000) as our terms of reference. We use selected examples from the two case studies presented in Chapter 4 to illustrate the possible applications for treatment planning and assessment of outcomes.

Diagnostic Utility

Current diagnostic systems rely predominantly on patients' self-reports of symptoms and their course over time. Cognitive measures are very rarely used in treatment in any diagnostic capacity. However, there is considerable interest in identifying additional diagnostic markers and markers of treatment response, given the potential unreliability of self-report measures, the considerable overlap in diagnostic categories at a symptom level, and the difficulties in defining symptoms for some disorders. Additional diagnostic markers could be obtained by information processing—for example, selective attention to emotional stimuli or interpretive bias toward threat. To date, the closest that cognitive measures have come to having diagnostic utility is in the ability of many of the measures reviewed here to discriminate, for example, between children with high and low levels of trait anxiety or CU traits; between phobic and nonphobic participants; and, in some instances, between groups diagnosed with *Diagnostic and Statistical*

Manual of Mental Disorders (DSM) criteria and normal controls, and between groups with different DSM disorders (e.g., children with anxiety disorders vs. those with major depression or ODD; Vasey & Lonigan, 2000). There is, at best, only limited evidence that these cognitive measures are useful for discriminating at a more nuanced level among different anxiety disorders, for instance. However, a small number of studies have shown evidence of content specificity; for example, adolescents high in social anxiety have demonstrated attentional bias to social-threat-related but not physical-threat-related stimuli (Helzer et al., 2009).

In Sofia's case study, cognitive measures such as the Stroop, dot-probe task, and measures of reasoning and interpretation bias could be used to see whether her anxiety was specific to school or generalized to other situations. These measures might also be useful markers of the degree to which her anxiety affected her attention to threat and interpretation of ambiguity. In other words, they could be used to determine the specific aspects of Sofia's cognition that were affected by anxiety. Likewise, administering similar measures with a range of stimuli to Billy might allow for a differential diagnosis based on his patterns of responses to different classes of stimuli during different tasks. In addition, some anxious children may underreport their level of anxiety and overestimate their ability to cope in anxiety-provoking situations. Cognitive measures, for example, could be helpful for both Billy and Sofia in providing more objective measures of their avoidance behavior or the extent to which they interpreted situations as threatening. These measures could be used to complement and validate self-report and interview-based measures of impairment.

It is also possible that as diagnosis moves toward a transprocess framework (Harvey, Watkins, Mansell, & Shafran, 2004), the laboratory-based measures we have discussed will be used more often in clinics to identify specific cognitive processes that need attention. It has been shown that certain cognitive processes are common to different disorders (Field & Cartwright-Hatton, 2008). In the future, therefore, clinicians may become less concerned with diagnosis than with identifying specific components of cognition and behavior that should be targeted in treatment. The cognitive tasks described in this chapter could prove to be useful ways of identifying the components that need to be targeted.

However, there are problems with applying the tasks in this chapter to the issue of diagnosis. As we have mentioned, there is a considerable issue of signal-to-noise ratio in reaction time techniques, and potential demand effects in self-report reasoning tasks. In addition, there is a lack of standardized assessments with reliable and valid clinical cutoffs, normative data, or information on sensitivity, specificity, and predictive power. It is also unclear for many of the measures outlined in this chapter what the precise degree of relation is between high scores on a measure and level of impairment in functioning. Furthermore, although these methods yield group-level differences, in the absence of clinical norms it is hard to see how reaction time techniques could be used at an individual level to highlight "problem" areas of cognition, to determine level of impairment, or to determine the presence or absence of diagnostic criteria.

Treatment and Treatment-Monitoring Utility

The treatment utility and treatment-monitoring utility of the methods described in this chapter follow directly from the diagnostic utility: If these methods can be honed to isolate specific "problematic" cognitive processes in an individual, then these problematic areas can be targeted in treatment. This enables clinicians to see beyond a diagnostic label and to isolate and treat the specific cognitions and behaviors that cause distress. In the case of Sofia, this might involve showing that she had particular problems disengaging attention from school-related material, or interpreted school-related ambiguity in a threatening way. Her clinician could then usefully implement techniques such as thought or behavioral experiments within a traditional cognitive-behavioral treatment (CBT) framework. Alternatively, drawing on experimental psychopathology research, her clinician could make use of novel computerized "cognitive bias modification" (CBM) techniques, which aim to train individuals to attend to benign stimuli or to interpret ambiguity in a benign way (Mathews & MacLeod, 2002). Such techniques have been shown, at the group level, to be useful ways to reduce internalizing problems in adult populations (Amir, Bomyea, & Beard, 2010; Cowart & Ollendick, 2010; Klumpp & Amir, 2010; Mathews, Ridgeway, Cook, & Yiend, 2007). Recent work has demonstrated that these methods may also have treatment utility in selected child and adolescent samples with high anxiety or clinical anxiety (Eldar et al., 2012; Rozenman, Weersing, & Amir, 2011; Vassilopoulos, Banerjee, & Prantzalou, 2009).

Change in cognitive biases across CBT, and also the magnitude of pretreatment bias (attentional avoidance of severe threat), predict treatment effects in general, suggesting that monitoring these biases throughout treatment might provide useful indications of how successful treatment will be (Legerstee et al., 2009). There is also evidence that reasoning biases toward threat can be reduced by CBT (Bögels & Siqueland, 2006; Waters, Craske, et al., 2008), and that attentional biases to threat are also reduced after successful treatment (Tobon, Ouimet, & Dozois, 2011). Residual biases at posttreatment are also associated with higher anxiety symptomatology (Waters, Wharton, et al., 2008). Therefore, monitoring Sofia's panic-related interpretations throughout the course of treatment or Billy's attitudes to aggression-provoking stimuli might be a useful marker of the extent to which treatment was succeeding. Furthermore, assessing Sofia's patterns of attentional bias toward threat prior to undertaking treatment might be a good indicator of whether CBT was likely to be effective or whether an enhanced treatment package might be needed from the outset. Measures of automatic associations might also prove particularly useful as a way of accessing Sofia's automatic (and possibly implicit) attitudes toward school, or Billy's attitudes toward his family.

Prevention Utility

Rather than rehash the arguments we have already made for diagnostic and treatment utility, we will say only that if laboratory measures could be refined to such an extent that they could identify "problematic" cognitive responses at the individual level, then it is not a huge leap of faith to entertain the possibility that these same measures could be used to identify at-risk children. In the cases of Sofia and Billy, we would simply suggest that if some of these laboratory measures were rolled out as part of a screening program in schools, then perhaps their problems could have been identified earlier and nipped in the bud. It is relatively easy to imagine some of the reaction time tasks that we have discussed being implemented on a mass scale; schools typically have computer rooms, and there would be little cost associated with implementing these tasks on a large scale. However, it would be fair to say that researchers will need to improve the reliability of these tasks and construct individual-level norms before they can be used to identify at-risk children.

Indirect Utility

In terms of validational utility, we have seen throughout this chapter that reaction time measures have frequently been compared against behavioral and self-report measures to cross-validate them. These studies have typically found low cross-validity. This apparent lack of validity may reflect the frequent asynchrony among behavioral, self-report, and physiological measures of internalizing problems (Zinbarg, 1998). This asynchrony raises an important conceptual issue: Should we expect validational utility for cognitive measures with measures tapping different response systems? The other issue is that data from reaction time measures are typically noisy. Until the signal-to-noise ratio is improved, we can expect the correlations between measures across different response systems to be range-restricted.

On a more positive note, there is little doubt that all of the measures have conceptual validity. All of them have been used to elucidate causal and maintaining processes in internalizing and externalizing disorders. We have also provided evidence that they have been employed to identify mechanisms by which treatment might be acting, and are the foundations on which new treatments are developed. One obvious example of this development is the proliferation of CBM tasks to reduce attention to threat and threat interpretations of ambiguity (Amir et al., 2010; Cowart & Ollendick, 2010; Klumpp & Amir, 2010; Mathews et al., 2007). Such interventions are currently being tested around the world and would have never existed without the elegant laboratory tasks that unearthed these cognitive responses in the first place (MacLeod, Campbell, Rutherford, & Wilson, 2004; Mathews & MacLeod, 2002; Wilson, MacLeod, Mathews, & Rutherford, 2006).

SUMMARY

This chapter has taken a selective look at some cognitive tasks that are used in the laboratory to unearth causes and potential treatments of psychological problems in children and adolescents. When planning the chapter, by necessity we have been highly selective and have chosen to review those measures that we believe have the greatest potential for application to both experimental and clinical phenomena in pediatric populations. However, there are many other tasks that, space permitting, we might also have discussed: attentional measures such as the Attentional Network Task, the Children Sustained Attention Task, Conners Continuous Performance Test—II, the Exogenous Cueing Task, the Controlled Oral Word Association Test, and the Trail Making Test; reasoning tasks such as covariation bias tasks, catastrophizing interview tasks, and checking tasks; and methodologies such as habituation, mood induction, bogus pipeline/false feedback, deception, and associative learning/conditioning/causal learning paradigms. This list highlights the range of tasks at laboratory researchers' disposal, as well as the endless creativity of these researchers in devising new and ingenious ways to tap aspects of psychopathology. All of the tasks we discuss have some clinical utility, whether this is diagnostic, treatment, treatment-monitoring, prevention, or conceptual utility. Not all tasks have evidence of utility in all of these domains, but we believe that they will be refined and are the foundations of theory and treatments for child and adolescent mental health for decades ahead—particularly if they are used as part of multimethod assessments in conjunction with the kinds of behavioral and neurophysiological laboratory methods outlined elsewhere in this volume.

REFERENCES

Adalio, C., White, S., & Blair, J. (2011). Youth with conduct disorder and callous-unemotional traits respond differentially in a Posner dot-probe task based on emotional valence and animacy. *Archives of Clinical Neuropsychology*, 26(6), 476–477.

Alfano, C. A., Beidel, D. C., & Turner, S. M. (2002). Cognition in childhood anxiety: Conceptual, methodological, and developmental issues. *Clinical Psychology Review*, 22, 1209–1238.

Amir, N., Bomyea, J., & Beard, C. (2010). The effect of single-session interpretation modification on attention bias in socially anxious individuals. *Journal of Anxiety Disorders*, 24(2), 178–182.

Askew, C. (2007). *Vicarious learning and the development of fear in childhood.* Unpublished doctoral dissertation, University of Sussex, Falmer, East Sussex, UK.

Askew, C., & Field, A. P. (2007). Vicarious learning and the development of fears in childhood. *Behaviour Research and Therapy, 45*(11), 2616–2627.

Bar-Haim, Y., Lamy, D., Pergamin, L., Bakermans-Kranenburg, M. J., & van IJzendoorn, M. H. (2007). Threat-related attentional bias in anxious and nonanxious individuals: A meta-analytic study. *Psychological Bulletin, 133*(1), 1–24.

Barrett, P. M., Rapee, R. M., Dadds, M. M., & Ryan, S. M. (1996). Family enhancement of cognitive style in anxious and aggressive children. *Journal of Abnormal Child Psychology, 24*(2), 187–203.

Battaglia, M., Bertella, S., Politi, E., Bernardeschi, L., Perna, G., Gabriele, A., & Bellodi, L. (1995). Age at onset of panic disorder: Influence of familial liability to the disease and of childhood separation anxiety disorder. *American Journal of Psychiatry, 152*(9), 1362–1364.

Battaglia, M., Zanoni, A., Ogliari, A., Crevani, F., Falzone, L., Bertoletti, E., & Di Serio, C. (2010). Identification of gradually changing emotional expressions in schoolchildren: The influence of the type of stimuli and of specific symptoms of anxiety. *Cognition and Emotion, 24*(6), 1070–1079.

Berk, L. (2004). *Child development.* Boston: Allyn & Bacon.

Blanchette, I. (2006). Snakes, spiders, guns, and syringes: How specific are evolutionary constraints on the detection of threatening stimuli? *Quarterly Journal of Experimental Psychology, 59*, 1484–1504.

Bluemke, M., & Friese, M. (2006). Do features of stimuli influence IAT effects? *Journal of Experimental Social Psychology, 42*(2), 163–176.

Bögels, S. M., & Siqueland, L. (2006). Family cognitive behavioral therapy for children and adolescents with clinical anxiety disorders. *Journal of the American Academy of Child and Adolescent Psychiatry, 45*(2), 134–141.

Bögels, S. M., & Zigterman, D. (2000). Dysfunctional cognitions in children with social phobia, separation anxiety disorder, and generalized anxiety disorder. *Journal of Abnormal Child Psychology, 28*(2), 205–211.

Brambilla, F., Bellodi, L., Perna, G., Battaglia, M., Sciuto, G., Diaferia, G., & Sacerdote, P. (1992). Psychoimmunoendocrine aspects of panic disorder. *Neuropsychobiology, 26*(1–2), 12–22.

Broeren, S., Muris, P., Bouwmeester, S., Field, A. P., & Voerman, J. S. (2011). Processing biases for emotional faces in 4- to 12-year-old non-clinical children: An exploratory study of developmental patterns and relationships with social anxiety and behavioral inhibition. *Journal of Experimental Psychopathology, 2*(4), 454–474.

Brosch, T., & Sharma, D. (2005). The role of fear-relevant stimuli in visual search: A comparison of phylogenetic and ontogenetic stimuli. *Emotion, 5*, 360–364.

Caseras, X., Garner, M., Bradley, B. P., & Mogg, K. (2007). Biases in visual orienting to negative and positive scenes in dysphoria: An eye movement study. *Journal of Abnormal Psychology, 116*(3), 491–497.

Castellanos, F. X., Marvasti, F. F., Ducharme, J. L., Walter, J. M., Israel, M. E., Krain, A. M. Y., & Hommer, D. W. (2000). Executive function oculomotor tasks in girls with ADHD. *Journal of the American Academy of Child and Adolescent Psychiatry, 39*(5), 644–650.

Cowart, M. J. W., & Ollendick, T. H. (2010). Attentional biases in children:

Implications for treatment. In J. A. Hadwin & A. P. Field (Eds.), *Information processing biases and anxiety: A developmental perspective* (pp. 297–319). Chichester, UK: Wiley-Blackwell.

Creswell, C., & O'Connor, T. G. (2006). "Anxious cognitions" in children: An exploration of associations and mediators. *British Journal of Developmental Psychology, 24,* 761–766.

Creswell, C., Woolgar, M., Cooper, P., Giannakakis, A., Schofield, E., Young, A. W., & Murray, L. (2008). Processing of faces and emotional expressions in infants at risk of social phobia. *Cognition and Emotion, 22*(3), 437–458.

Dadds, M. R., El Masry, Y., Wimalaweera, S., & Guastella, A. J. (2008). Reduced eye gaze explains fear blindness in childhood psychopathic traits. *Journal of the American Academy of Child and Adolescent Psychiatry, 47*(4), 455–463.

Daleiden, E. L., & Vasey, M. W. (1997). An information-processing perspective on childhood anxiety. *Clinical Psychology Review, 17*(4), 407–429.

Dalgleish, T., Moradi, A., Taghavi, M., Neshat-Doost, H. T., & Yule, W. (2001). An experimental investigation of hypervigilance for threat in children and adolescents with post-traumatic stress disorder. *Psychological Medicine, 31,* 541–547.

Dalgleish, T., Taghavi, R., Neshat-Doost, H., Moradi, A. R., Canterbury, R., & Yule, W. (2003). Patterns of processing bias for emotional information across clinical disorders: A comparison of attention, memory, and prospective cognition in children and adolescents with depression, generalized anxiety, and posttraumatic stress disorder. *Journal of Clinical Child and Adolescent Psychology, 32*(1), 10–21.

Dearing, K., & Gotlib, I. (2009). Interpretation of ambiguous information in girls at risk for depression. *Journal of Abnormal Child Psychology, 37*(1), 79–91.

De Houwer, J. (2001). A structural and process analysis of the implicit association test. *Journal of Experimental Social Psychology, 37*(6), 443–451.

De Houwer, J. (2003). The extrinsic affective Simon task. *Experimental Psychology, 50*(2), 77–85.

De Houwer, J. (2006). What are implicit measures and why are we using them? In R. W. Wiers & A. W. Stacy (Eds.), *Handbook of implicit cognition and addiction* (pp. 11–28). Thousand Oaks, CA: Sage.

De Houwer, J., Geldof, T., & De Bruycker, E. (2005). The implicit association test as a general measure of similarity. *Canadian Journal of Experimental Psychology/Revue Canadienne de Psychologie Experimentale, 59*(4), 228–239.

Diaferia, G., Sciuto, G., Perna, G., Bernardeschi, L., Battaglia, M., Rusmini, S., & Bellodi, L. (1993). DSM-III-R personality-disorders in panic disorder. *Journal of Anxiety Disorders, 7*(2), 153–161.

Diamond, A., Kirkham, N., & Amso, D. (2002). Conditions under which young children can hold two rules in mind and inhibit a prepotent response. *Developmental Psychology, 38*(3), 352–362.

Donnelly, N., Hadwin, J. A., Menneer, T., & Richards, H. (2010). The use of visual search paradigms to understand attentional biases in childhood anxiety. In J. A. Hadwin & A. P. Field (Eds.), *Information processing biases and anxiety: A developmental perspective* (pp. 109–127). Chichester, UK: Wiley-Blackwell.

Eldar, S., Apter, A., Lotan, D., Perez-Edgar, K., Naim, R., Fox, N. A., & Bar-Haim, Y. (2012). Attention bias modification treatment for pediatric anxiety disorders: A randomized controlled trial. *American Journal of Psychiatry, 169,* 213–220.

Eschenbeck, H., Kohlmann, C. W., Heim-Dreger, U., Koller, D., & Leser, M. (2004). Processing bias and anxiety in primary school children: A modified emotional Stroop colour-naming task using pictorial facial expressions. *Psychology Science, 46*(4), 451–465.

Eysenck, M. W., Derakshan, N., Santos, R., & Calvo, M. G. (2007). Anxiety and cognitive performance: Attentional control theory. *Emotion, 7*(2), 336–353.

Fazio, R. H., Sanbonmatsu, D. M., Powell, M. C., & Kardes, F. R. (1986). On the automatic activation of attitudes. *Journal of Personality and Social Psychology, 50*(2), 229–238.

Field, A. P. (2006a). I don't like it because it eats sprouts: Conditioning preferences in children. *Behaviour Research and Therapy, 44*(3), 439–455.

Field, A. P. (2006b). Watch out for the beast: Fear information and attentional bias in children. *Journal of Clinical Child and Adolescent Psychology, 35*(3), 431–439.

Field, A. P., & Cartwright-Hatton, S. (2008). Shared and unique cognitive factors in social anxiety. *International Journal of Cognitive Therapy, 1*(3), 206–222.

Field, A. P., Hadwin, J. A., & Lester, K. J. (2011). Information processing biases in child and adolescent anxiety: Evidence and origins. In W. K. Silverman & A. P. Field (Eds.), *Anxiety disorders in children and adolescents: Research, assessment and intervention* (2nd ed., pp. 103–128). Cambridge, UK: Cambridge University Press.

Field, A. P., & Lawson, J. (2003). Fear information and the development of fears during childhood: Effects on implicit fear responses and behavioural avoidance. *Behaviour Research and Therapy, 41*(11), 1277–1293.

Field, A. P., Lawson, J., & Banerjee, R. (2008). The verbal threat information pathway to fear in children: The longitudinal effects on fear cognitions and the immediate effects on avoidance behavior. *Journal of Abnormal Psychology, 117*(1), 214–224.

Field, A. P., & Lester, K. J. (2010). Is there room for "development" in developmental models of information processing biases to threat in children and adolescents? *Clinical Child and Family Psychology Review, 13*(4), 315–332.

Fox, E., Griggs, L., & Mouchlianitis, E. (2007). The detection of fear-relevant stimuli: Are guns noticed as quickly as snakes? *Emotion, 7,* 691–696.

Fulcher, E. P., Mathews, A., & Hammerl, M. (2008). Rapid acquisition of emotional information and attentional bias in anxious children. *Journal of Behavior Therapy and Experimental Psychiatry, 39*(3), 321–339.

Gamble, A. L., & Rapee, R. M. (2009). The time-course of attentional bias in anxious children and adolescents. *Journal of Anxiety Disorders, 23*(7), 841–847.

Gould, T. D., Bastain, T. M., Israel, M. E., Hommer, D. W., & Castellanos, F. X. (2001). Altered performance on an ocular fixation task in attention-deficit/hyperactivity disorder. *Biological Psychiatry, 50*(8), 633–635.

Greenwald, A. G., McGhee, D. E., & Schwartz, J. L. K. (1998). Measuring individual differences in implicit cognition: The implicit association test. *Journal of Personality and Social Psychology, 74*(6), 1464–1480.

Grumm, M., Hein, S., & Fingerle, M. (2011). Predicting aggressive behavior in children with the help of measures of implicit and explicit aggression. *International Journal of Behavioral Development, 35*(4), 352–357.

Hadwin, J. A., Donnelly, N., French, C. C., Richards, A., Watts, A., & Daley, D. (2003). The influence of children's self-report trait anxiety and depression on visual search for emotional faces. *Journal of Child Psychology and Psychiatry, 44*(3), 432–444.

Hadwin, J. A., Donnelly, N., Richards, A., French, C. C., & Patel, U. (2009). Childhood anxiety and attention to emotion faces in a modified Stroop task. *British Journal of Developmental Psychology, 27,* 487–494.

Hadwin, J. A., Frost, S., French, C. C., & Richards, A. (1997). Cognitive processing and trait anxiety in typically developing children: Evidence for an interpretation bias. *Journal of Abnormal Psychology, 106*(3), 486–490.

Harvey, A. G., Watkins, E., Mansell, W., & Shafran, R. (2004). *Cognitive behavioural processes across psychological disorders. A transdiagnostic approach to research and treatment.* Oxford, UK: Oxford University Press.

Heim-Dreger, U., Kohlmann, C. W., Eschenbeck, H., & Burkhardt, U. (2006). Attentional biases for threatening faces in children: Vigilant and avoidant processes. *Emotion, 6*(2), 320–325.

Helzer, E. G., Connor-Smith, J. K., & Reed, M. A. (2009). Traits, states, and attentional gates: Temperament and threat relevance as predictors of attentional bias to social threat. *Anxiety, Stress, and Coping, 22*(1), 57–76.

Horsley, T. A., Orobio de Castro, B., & Van der Schoot, M. (2010). In the eye of the beholder: Eye-tracking assessment of social information processing in aggressive behavior. *Journal of Abnormal Child Psychology, 38*(5), 587–599.

Hudziak, J. J., Boffeli, T. J., Kriesman, J. J., Battaglia, M. M., Stanger, C., & Guze, S. B. (1996). Clinical study of the relation of borderline personality disorder to Briquet's syndrome (hysteria), somatization disorder, antisocial personality disorder, and substance abuse disorders. *American Journal of Psychiatry, 153*(12), 1598–1606.

Huijding, J., Wiers, R. W., & Field, A. P. (2010). The assessment of fear-related automatic associations in children. In J. A. Hadwin & A. P. Field (Eds.), *Information processing biases and anxiety: A developmental perspective* (pp. 151–182). Chichester, UK: Wiley-Blackwell.

Hunt, C., Keogh, E., & French, C. C. (2007). Anxiety sensitivity, conscious awareness and selective attentional biases in children. *Behaviour Research and Therapy, 45*(3), 497–509.

In-Albon, T., Kossowsky, J., & Schneider, S. (2010). Vigilance and avoidance of threat in the eye movements of children with separation anxiety disorder. *Journal of Abnormal Child Psychology, 38*(2), 225–235.

In-Albon, T., & Schneider, S. (2010). Using eye tracking methodology in children with anxiety disorders. In J. A. Hadwin & A. P. Field (Eds.), *Information processing biases and anxiety: A developmental perspective* (pp. 129–150). Chichester, UK: Wiley-Blackwell.

Jazbec, S., McClure, E., Hardin, M., Pine, D. S., & Ernst, M. (2005). Cognitive control under contingencies in anxious and depressed adolescents: An antisaccade task. *Biological Psychiatry, 58*(8), 632–639.

Johnstone, S. J., Watt, A. J., & Dimoska, A. (2010). Varying required effort during interference control in children with AD/HD: Task performance and ERPs. *International Journal of Psychophysiology, 76*(3), 174–185.

Karatekin, C. (2007). Eye tracking studies of normative and atypical development. *Developmental Review, 27*(3), 283–348.

Karpinski, A., & Steinman, R. B. (2006). The single category implicit association test as a measure of implicit social cognition. *Journal of Personality and Social Psychology, 91*(1), 16–32.

Kazdin, A. E., & Kendall, P. C. (1998). Current progress and future plans for developing effective treatments: Comments and perspectives. *Journal of Clinical Child Psychology, 27*, 217–226.

Kimonis, E. R., Frick, P. J., Fazekas, H., & Loney, B. R. (2006). Psychopathy, aggression, and the processing of emotional stimuli in non-referred girls and boys. *Behavioral Sciences and the Law, 24*(1), 21–37.

Kimonis, E. R., Frick, P. J., Munoz, L., & Aucoin, K. (2007). Can a laboratory measure of emotional processing enhance the statistical prediction of aggression and delinquency in detained adolescents with callous-unemotional traits? *Journal of Abnormal Child Psychology, 35*(5), 773–785.

Kindt, M., Bierman, D., & Brosschot, J. F. (1996). Stroop versus Stroop: Comparison of a card format and a single-trial format of the standard color–word Stroop task and emotional Stroop task. *Personality and Individual Differences, 21*, 653–661.

Kindt, M., Bögels, S., & Morren, M. (2003). Processing bias in children with separation anxiety disorder, social phobia and generalised anxiety disorder. *Behaviour Change, 20*(3), 143–150.

Kindt, M., & Brosschot, J. F. (1999). Cognitive bias in spider-phobic children: Comparison of a pictorial and a linguistic spider Stroop. *Journal of Psychopathology and Behavioral Assessment, 21*, 207–220.

Kindt, M., Brosschot, J. F., & Everaerd, W. (1997). Cognitive processing bias of children in a real life stress situation and a neutral situation. *Journal of Experimental Child Psychology, 64*(1), 79–97.

Klein, C., & Fischer, B. (2005). Instrumental and test–retest reliability of saccadic measures. *Biological Psychology, 68*(3), 201–213.

Klumpp, H., & Amir, N. (2010). Preliminary study of attention training to threat and neutral faces on anxious reactivity to a social stressor in social anxiety. *Cognitive Therapy and Research, 34*(3), 263–271.

Kuntsi, J., Oosterlaan, J., & Stevenson, J. (2001). Psychological mechanisms in hyperactivity: I. Response inhibition deficit, working memory impairment, delay aversion, or something else? *Journal of Child Psychology and Psychiatry, 42*, 199–210.

Lang, P. J. (1968). Fear reduction and fear behavior: Problems in treating a construct. In J. M. Schlien (Ed.), *Research in psychotherapy* (Vol. 3, pp. 90–103). Washington, DC: American Psychological Association.

Lau, J. Y. F., Burt, M., Leibenluft, E., Pine, D. S., Rijsdijk, F., Shiffrin, N., & Eley, T. C. (2009). Individual differences in children's facial expression recognition ability: The role of nature and nurture. *Developmental Neuropsychology, 34*(1), 37–51.

Lawson, C., MacLeod, C., & Hammond, G. (2002). Interpretation revealed in the blink of an eye: Depressive bias in the resolution of ambiguity. *Journal of Abnormal Psychology, 111*(2), 321–328.

Lawson, J., Banerjee, R., & Field, A. P. (2007). The effects of verbal information on children's fear beliefs about social situations. *Behaviour Research and Therapy, 45*(1), 21–37.

Legerstee, J. S., Tulen, J. H. M., Kallen, V. L., Dieleman, G. C., Treffers, P. D. A., Verhulst, F. C., & Utens, E. (2009). Threat-related selective attention predicts treatment success in childhood anxiety disorders. *Journal of the American Academy of Child and Adolescent Psychiatry, 48*(2), 196–205.

LoBue, V. (2010). What's so scary about needles and knives?: Examining the role of experience in threat detection. *Cognition and Emotion, 24*(1), 180–187.

LoBue, V., & DeLoache, J. S. (2008). Detecting the snake in the grass: Attention to fear-relevant stimuli by adults and young children. *Psychological Science, 19*(3), 284–289.

Lonigan, C. J., Hooe, E. S., Kistner, J. A., & David, C. F. (1999). Positive and negative affectivity in children: Confirmatory factor analysis of a two-factor model and its relation to symptoms of anxiety and depression. *Journal of Consulting and Clinical Psychology, 67*, 374–386.

MacLeod, C., Campbell, L., Rutherford, E., & Wilson, E. (2004). The causal status of anxiety-linked attentional and interpretive bias. In J. Yiend (Ed.), *Cognition, emotion and psychopathology: Theoretical, empirical and clinical directions* (pp. 172–189). Cambridge, UK: Cambridge University Press.

Martin, M., Horder, P., & Jones, G. V. (1992). Integral bias in naming of phobia-related words. *Cognition and Emotion, 6*, 479–486.

Mathews, A., & MacLeod, C. (2002). Induced processing biases have causal effects on anxiety. *Cognition and Emotion, 16*(3), 331–354.

Mathews, A., Ridgeway, V., Cook, E., & Yiend, J. (2007). Inducing a benign interpretational bias reduces trait anxiety. *Journal of Behavior Therapy and Experimental Psychiatry, 38*(2), 225–236.

Mehta, M. A., Goodyer, I. M., & Sahakian, B. J. (2004). Methylphenidate improves working memory and set-shifting in AD/HD: Relationships to baseline memory capacity. *Journal of Child Psychology and Psychiatry, 45*(2), 293–305.

Mierke, J., & Klauer, K. C. (2003). Method-specific variance in the implicit association test. *Journal of Personality and Social Psychology, 85*(6), 1180–1192.

Moradi, A. R., Taghavi, M. R., Neshat-Doost, H. T., Yule, W., & Dalgleish, T. (1999). Performance of children and adolescents with PTSD on the Stroop colour-naming task. *Psychological Medicine, 29*, 415–419.

Morren, M., Kindt, M., van den Hout, M., & van Kasteren, H. (2003). Anxiety and the processing of threat in children: Further examination of the cognitive inhibition hypothesis. *Behaviour Change, 20*(3), 131–142.

Morren, M., Muris, P., & Kindt, M. (2004). Emotional reasoning and parent-based reasoning in normal children. *Child Psychiatry and Human Development, 35*(1), 3–20.

Mostofsky, S. H., Lasker, A. G., Cutting, L. E., Denckla, M. B., & Zee, D. S. (2001). Oculomotor abnormalities in attention deficit hyperactivity disorder. *Neurology, 57*(3), 423–430.

Mostofsky, S. H., Lasker, A. G., Singer, H. S., Denckla, M. B., & Zee, D. S. (2001). Oculomotor abnormalities in boys with Tourette syndrome with and without ADHD. *Journal of the American Academy of Child and Adolescent Psychiatry, 40*(12), 1464–1472.

Mullane, J. C., & Klein, R. M. (2007). Literature review: Visual search by children with and without ADHD. *Journal of Attention Disorders, 12*, 44–53.

Munoz, D. P., Armstrong, I. T., Hampton, K. A., & Moore, K. D. (2003). Altered control of visual fixation and saccadic eye movements in attention-deficit hyperactivity disorder. *Journal of Neurophysiology, 90*(1), 503–514.

Muris, P. (2010). Anxiety-related reasoning biases in children and adolescents. In

J. A. Hadwin & A. P. Field (Eds.), *Information processing biases and anxiety: A developmental perspective* (pp. 21–46). Chichester, UK: Wiley-Blackwell.

Muris, P., Kindt, M., Bögels, S., Merckelbach, H., Gadet, B., & Moulaert, V. (2000). Anxiety and threat perception abnormalities in normal children. *Journal of Psychopathology and Behavioral Assessment, 22*(2), 183–199.

Muris, P., Luermans, J., Merckelbach, H., & Mayer, B. (2000). "Danger is lurking everywhere": The relation between anxiety and threat perception abnormalities in normal children. *Journal of Behavior Therapy and Experimental Psychiatry, 31*(2), 123–136.

Muris, P., Mayer, B., Freher, N. K., Duncan, S., & van den Hout, A. (2010). Children's internal attributions of anxiety-related physical symptoms: Age-related patterns and the role of cognitive development and anxiety sensitivity. *Child Psychiatry and Human Development, 41*(5), 535–548.

Muris, P., Mayer, B., Vermeulen, L., & Hiemstra, H. (2007). Theory-of-mind, cognitive development, and children's interpretation of anxiety-related physical symptoms. *Behaviour Research and Therapy, 45*(9), 2121–2132.

Muris, P., Merkelbach, H., & Damsma, E. (2000). Threat perception bias in nonreferred, socially anxious children. *Journal of Clinical Child Psychology, 29*(3), 348–359.

Muris, P., Merckelbach, H., & van Spauwen, I. (2003). The emotional reasoning heuristic in children. *Behaviour Research and Therapy, 41*(3), 261–272.

Muris, P., Merckelbach, H., & Walczak, S. (2002). Aggression and threat perception abnormalities in children with learning and behavior problems. *Child Psychiatry and Human Development, 33*(2), 147–163.

Muris, P., Rapee, R., Meesters, C., Schouten, E., & Geers, M. (2003). Threat perception abnormalities in children: The role of anxiety disorders symptoms, chronic anxiety, and state anxiety. *Journal of Anxiety Disorders, 17*(3), 271–287.

Muris, P., Vermeer, E., & Horselenberg, R. (2008). Cognitive development and the interpretation of anxiety-related physical symptoms in 4- to 12-year-old nonclinical children. *Journal of Behavior Therapy and Experimental Psychiatry, 39*, 73–86.

Nightingale, Z. C., Field, A. P., & Kindt, M. (2010). The emotional Stroop task in anxious children. In J. A. Hadwin & A. P. Field (Eds.), *Information processing biases and anxiety: A developmental perspective* (pp. 47–75). Chichester, UK: Wiley-Blackwell.

O'Driscoll, G. A., Depatie, L., Holahan, A.-L. V., Savion-Lemieux, T., Barr, R. G., Jolicoeur, C., & Douglas, V. I. (2005). Executive functions and methylphenidate response in subtypes of attention-deficit/hyperactivity disorder. *Biological Psychiatry, 57*(11), 1452–1460.

Öhman, A., Flykt, A., & Esteves, F. (2001). Emotion drives attention: Detecting the snake in the grass. *Journal of Experimental Psychology: General, 130*(3), 466–478.

Peltola, M. J., Leppanen, J. M., Vogel-Farley, V. K., Hietanen, J. K., & Nelson, C. A. (2009). Fearful faces but not fearful eyes alone delay attention disengagement in 7-month-old infants. *Emotion, 9*(4), 560–565.

Penke, L., Eichstaedt, J., & Asendorpf, J. B. (2006). Single-attribute implicit association tests (SA-IAT) for the assessment of unipolar constructs: The case of sociosexuality. *Experimental Psychology, 53*(4), 283–291.

Perez-Olivas, G., Stevenson, J., & Hadwin, J. A. (2008). Do anxiety-related attentional biases mediate the link between maternal over involvement and separation anxiety in children? *Cognition and Emotion, 22*(3), 509–521.

Perna, G., Marconi, C., Battaglia, M., Bertani, A., Panzacchi, A., & Bellodi, L. (1994). Subclinical impairment of lung airways in patients with panic disorder. *Biological Psychiatry, 36*(9), 601–605.

Pine, D. S., Mogg, K., Bradley, B. P., Montgomery, L., Monk, C. S., McClure, E., & Kaufman, J. (2005). Attention bias to threat in maltreated children: Implications for vulnerability to stress-related psychopathology. *American Journal of Psychiatry, 162*(2), 291–296.

Purkis, H. M., Lester, K. J., & Field, A. P. (2011). But what about the Empress of Racnoss?: The allocation of attention to spiders and Doctor Who in a visual search task is predicted by fear and expertise. *Emotion, 11*(6), 1484–1488.

Richards, A., French, C. C., Nash, G., Hadwin, J. A., & Donnelly, N. (2007). A comparison of selective attention and facial processing biases in typically developing children who are high and low in self-reported trait anxiety. *Development and Psychopathology, 19*(2), 481–495.

Rommelse, N. N. J., Van der Stigchel, S., & Sergeant, J. A. (2008). A review on eye movement studies in childhood and adolescent psychiatry. *Brain and Cognition, 68*(3), 391–414.

Rothenberger, A., Banaschewski, T., Heinrich, H., Moll, G. H., Schmidt, M. H., & van't Klooster, B. (2000). Comorbidity in ADHD-children: Effects of coexisting conduct disorder or tic disorder on event-related brain potentials in an auditory selective-attention task. *European Archives of Psychiatry and Clinical Neuroscience, 250*(2), 101–110.

Rothermund, K., & Wentura, D. (2004). Underlying processes in the implicit association test: Dissociating salience from associations. *Journal of Experimental Psychology: General, 133*(2), 139–165.

Roy, A. K., Vasa, R. A., Bruck, M., Mogg, K., Bradley, B. P., Sweeney, M., & Cams, T. (2008). Attention bias toward threat in pediatric anxiety disorders. *Journal of the American Academy of Child and Adolescent Psychiatry, 47*(10), 1189–1196.

Rozenman, M., Weersing, V. R., & Amir, N. (2011). A case series of attention modification in clinically anxious youths. *Behaviour Research and Therapy, 49*(5), 324–330.

Schmukle, S. C. (2005). Unreliability of the dot probe task. *European Journal of Personality, 19*, 595–605.

Schneider, S., Unnewehr, S., Florin, I., & Margraf, J. (2002). Priming panic interpretations in children of patients with panic disorder. *Journal of Anxiety Disorders, 16*(6), 605–624.

Siegrist, M. (1997). Test–retest reliability of different versions of the Stroop test. *The Journal of Psychology, 131*, 299–306.

Sonuga-Barke, E. J. S. (2002). Psychological heterogeneity in AD/HD: A dual pathway model of behaviour and cognition. *Behavioural Brain Research, 130*(1–2), 29–36.

Sonuga-Barke, E. J. S., De Houwer, J., De Ruiter, K., Ajzenstzen, M., & Holland, S. (2004). AD/HD and the capture of attention by briefly exposed delay-related cues: Evidence from a conditioning paradigm. *Journal of Child Psychology and Psychiatry, 45*(2), 274–283.

Sonuga-Barke, E. J. S., Taylor, E., Sembi, S., & Smith, J. (1992). Hyperactivity and delay aversion: I. The effect of delay on choice. *Journal of Child Psychology and Psychiatry, 33*(2), 387–398.

Spence, S. H., Lipp, O. V., Liberman, L., & March, S. (2006). Examination of emotional priming among children and young adolescents: Developmental issues and its association with anxiety. *Australian Journal of Psychology, 58*(2), 101–110.

Taghavi, M. R., Dalgleish, T., Moradi, A. R., Neshat-Doost, H. T., & Yule, W. (2003). Selective processing of negative emotional information in children and adolescents with generalized anxiety disorder. *British Journal of Clinical Psychology, 42*, 221–230.

Taghavi, M. R., Moradi, A. R., Neshat-Doost, H. T., Yule, W., & Dalgleish, T. (2000). Interpretation of ambiguous emotional information in clinically anxious children and adolescents. *Cognition and Emotion, 14*(6), 809–822.

Taghavi, M. R., Neshat-Doost, H. T., Moradi, A. R., Yule, W., & Dalgleish, T. (1999). Biases in visual attention in children and adolescents with clinical anxiety and mixed anxiety-depression. *Journal of Abnormal Child Psychology, 27*(3), 215–223.

Teachman, B. A., & Allen, J. P. (2007). Development of social anxiety: Social interaction predictors of implicit and explicit fear of negative evaluation. *Journal of Abnormal Child Psychology, 35*(1), 63–78.

Tipples, J., Young, A. W., Quinlan, P., Broks, P., & Ellis, A. W. (2002). Searching for threat. *Quarterly Journal of Experimental Psychology: Section A, 55*(3), 1007–1026.

Tobon, J. I., Ouimet, A. J., & Dozois, D. J. A. (2011). Attentional bias in anxiety disorders following cognitive behavioral treatment. *Journal of Cognitive Psychotherapy, 25*(2), 114–129.

Van Der Stigchel, S., Rommelse, N. N. J., Deijen, J. B., Geldof, C. J. A., Witlox, J., Oosterlaan, J., Theeuwes, J. (2007). Oculomotor capture in ADHD. *Cognitive Neuropsychology, 24*(5), 535–549.

van Mourik, R., Oosterlaan, J., & Sergeant, J. A. (2005). The Stroop revisited: A meta-analysis of interference control in AD/HD. *Journal of Child Psychology and Psychiatry, 46*(2), 150–165.

Vasey, M. W., Daleiden, E. L., Williams, L. L., & Brown, L. M. (1995). Biased attention in childhood anxiety disorders: A preliminary-study. *Journal of Abnormal Child Psychology, 23*(2), 267–279.

Vasey, M. W., El Hag, N., & Daleiden, E. L. (1996). Anxiety and the processing of emotionally threatening stimuli: Distinctive patterns of selective attention among high- and low-test-anxious children. *Child Development, 67*(3), 1173–1185.

Vasey, M. W., & Lonigan, C. J. (2000). Considering the clinical utility of performance-based measures of childhood anxiety. *Journal of Clinical Child Psychology, 29*(4), 493–508.

Vassilopoulos, S. P., Banerjee, R., & Prantzalou, C. (2009). Experimental modification of interpretation bias in socially anxious children: Changes in interpretation, anticipated interpersonal anxiety, and social anxiety symptoms. *Behaviour Research and Therapy, 47*, 1085–1089.

Vervoort, L. (2010). *The behavioural inhibition system in childhood and adolescent anxiety: An analysis from the information processing perspective.* Unpublished doctoral dissertation, University of Amsterdam, Amsterdam.

Waters, A. M., Craske, M. G., Bergman, R. L., & Treanor, M. (2008). Threat interpretation bias as a vulnerability factor in childhood anxiety disorders. *Behaviour Research and Therapy, 46*(1), 39–47.

Waters, A. M., Henry, J., Mogg, K., Bradley, B. P., & Pine, D. S. (2010). Attentional bias towards angry faces in childhood anxiety disorders. *Journal of Behavior Therapy and Experimental Psychiatry, 41*(2), 158–164.

Waters, A. M., & Lipp, O. V. (2008). Visual search for emotional faces in children. *Cognition and Emotion, 22*(7), 1306–1326.

Waters, A. M., Lipp, O. V., & Spence, S. H. (2004). Attentional bias toward fear-related stimuli: An investigation with nonselected children and adults and children with anxiety disorders. *Journal of Experimental Child Psychology, 89*(4), 320–337.

Waters, A. M., Lipp, O., & Spence, S. H. (2008). Visual search for animal fear-relevant stimuli in children. *Australian Journal of Psychology, 60*(2), 112–125.

Waters, A. M., Mogg, K., Bradley, B. P., & Pine, D. S. (2008). Attentional bias for emotional faces in children with generalized anxiety disorder. *Journal of the American Academy of Child and Adolescent Psychiatry, 47*(4), 435–442.

Waters, A. M., & Valvoi, J. S. (2009). Attentional bias for emotional faces in paediatric anxiety disorders: An investigation using the emotional go/no go task. *Journal of Behavior Therapy and Experimental Psychiatry, 40*, 306–316.

Waters, A. M., Wharton, T. A., Zimmer-Gembeck, M. J., & Craske, M. G. (2008). Threat-based cognitive biases in anxious children: Comparison with non-anxious children before and after cognitive behavioural treatment. *Behaviour Research and Therapy, 46*(3), 358–374.

Watts, S. E., & Weems, C. F. (2006). Associations among selective attention, memory bias, cognitive errors and symptoms of anxiety in youth. *Journal of Abnormal Child Psychology, 34*(6), 841–852.

Wilson, E. J., MacLeod, C., Mathews, A., & Rutherford, E. M. (2006). The causal role of interpretive bias in anxiety reactivity. *Journal of Abnormal Psychology, 115*(1), 103–111.

Zinbarg, R. E. (1998). Concordance and synchrony in measures of anxiety and panic reconsidered: A hierarchical model of anxiety and panic. *Behavior Therapy, 29*(2), 301–323.

11

Peer Assessment Strategies

Annette M. La Greca, Betty Lai, Sherilynn Chan, and Whitney Herge

Peers play a critical role in the social and emotional development of children and adolescents. During elementary school and even the preschool years, children spend most of their day interacting with peers. In the context of peer relations, children learn to share with others, respond to emotions, and develop social skills (Hodges, Boivin, Vitaro, & Bukowski, 1999; La Greca & Prinstein, 1999; Ladd, 2005). The importance of peers continues to increase through adolescence, as close friends become comparable to and in some ways even surpass parents as adolescents' key source of social support (Furman, 1989; Furman & Buhrmester, 2009). Many of the social skills developed in the context of peer relations set the stage for adult interpersonal relations and adjustment (La Greca & Prinstein, 1999; Parker, Rubin, Erath, Wojslawowicz, & Buskirk, 2006) and for intimacy in later romantic relations (Kuttler & La Greca, 2004; La Greca, Davila, & Siegel, 2009). In fact, there is a substantial literature on the developmentally important and unique aspects of social-psychological functioning that develop in the context of youth's peer relations (see Hartup, 1996; Ladd, 2005; Parker et al., 2006).

At the same time, peer relationships can represent a significant stressor and may contribute to negative psychological outcomes for youth (Ladd, 2005; La Greca & Landoll, 2011; Parker et al., 2006). For example, peer victimization is associated with youth's internalized distress, such as feelings of depression, loneliness, and social anxiety (La Greca & Harrison, 2005; Prinstein, Boergers, & Vernberg, 2001; Siegel, La Greca, & Harrison, 2009; Visconti & Troop-Gordon, 2010; Wang, Iannotti, Luk, & Nansel, 2010). Youth with psychiatric disorders, such as conduct disorder or attention-deficit/hyperactivity disorder (ADHD) (Landau & Moore,

1991), often experience interpersonal difficulties and problems with peer rejection. Moreover, the relationship between peer problems and psychological difficulties appears to be bidirectional: Peer relationship problems can contribute to as well as result from psychological difficulties (Bukowski & Adams, 2005; La Greca & Landoll, 2011; Siegel et al., 2009; Vernberg, Abwender, Ewell, & Beery, 1992; Parker et al., 2006). Given that ample evidence supports the important role of peer relationships in the lives of children and adolescents and the significance of peer relations in developmental psychopathology, it is surprising that peer relationships are often overlooked in clinical treatment settings.

In a clinical context, there are important reasons to evaluate youth's peer relations. Peer relationship difficulties occur at high rates among clinically referred youth and contribute to or maintain behavioral or emotional problems. In fact, deficient or problematic peer relations are a prominent feature of the major psychiatric disorders commonly diagnosed in youth, including conduct problems, ADHD, anxiety disorders, depression, eating disorders, and pervasive developmental disorders (American Psychiatric Association, 2000; Davila, La Greca, Starr, & Landoll, 2010; Kingery, Erdley, Marshall, Whitaker, & Reuter, 2010; La Greca et al., 2009; Parker et al., 2006). Understanding youth's interpersonal functioning will help clinicians develop suitable treatment plans that may include peer-related interventions.

Furthermore, youth may be seen in clinical settings for problems associated with major life stressors and transitions (e.g., parental divorce, serious illness or death in the family, a catastrophic disaster, military deployment of a family member). Such events have the potential to disrupt youth's peer relations, and children may need special assistance in developing new relationships and/or maintaining existing friendship ties. Moreover, building on existing positive peer relations may be an important aspect of treatment, as support from peers (and especially from close friends) represents a significant source of emotional support that buffers the adverse impact of stress (e.g., Adams, Santo, & Bukowski, 2011; Bukowski & Adams, 2005; Heinrich & Shahar, 2008; La Greca, Silverman, Lai, & Jaccard, 2010; Lustig, Wolchik, & Braver, 1992). Friendships and peer relationships may represent an area of strength that clinicians can build on in developing effective treatments for youth.

With these concerns in mind, the present chapter may serve as a beginning primer on the assessment of youth's peer relationships, with the focus on children and adolescents ages 7–18 years (see La Greca & Prinstein, 1999, for a discussion of infants and young children).

Because there are several diverse aspects of peer relations and multiple methods for assessing peer relations, which vary according to youth's age and the purpose of assessment (La Greca & Lemanek, 1996), this chapter is organized somewhat differently from others in this book. In the first main section, we define and review several key aspects of youth's peer relations and discuss why they are important to consider in a clinical context. In the second section, we describe representative measures of the key aspects of peer relationships and their psychometric properties. The third section offers recommendations for assessing youth's peer relationships and presents the two case studies described by McLeod, Jensen-Doss, and Ollendick in Chapter 4 to illustrate how a peer assessment might be conducted in clinical practice. The final section addresses conclusions and further considerations.

KEY ASPECTS OF YOUTH'S PEER RELATIONS: THEORY AND RESEARCH UNDERLYING THE ASSESSMENT

Over the past several decades, researchers have identified several salient aspects of youth's peer relations that make significant contributions to social-psychological adjustment. These aspects of peer relations focus on acceptance, friendship, and victimization (for detailed reviews, see Bukowski & Adams, 2005; Furman, McDunn, & Young, 2009; Kingery et al., 2010; La Greca & Landoll, 2011; La Greca & Prinstein, 1999).

Peer Acceptance/Social Status

"Peer acceptance" refers to the degree to which children or adolescents are accepted by their peer group (La Greca & Landoll, 2011; La Greca & Prinstein, 1999; Nesdale et al., 2007), although both the definition and scope of the "peer group" change with development. During the elementary school years, children spend most of the day in self-contained classrooms with a specific group of classmates—their peer group. However, during middle school and high school, youth's peer networks expand considerably, and the larger peer group may include peers from different classes and different schools (Bowker & Spencer, 2010; La Greca & Prinstein, 1999).

Regardless of the size of the peer group, peer acceptance matters. Peer acceptance provides children and adolescents with a sense of belonging and inclusion (La Greca & Prinstein, 1999; Ladd, 2006). Youth who are not well accepted by their peers, and especially those who are *actively rejected* by peers, have been identified as a vulnerable population. In fact, the separate dimensions of "acceptance" and "rejection" have been used to characterize youth's social status in the larger peer group (Coie, Dodge, & Kupersmidt, 1990; La Greca & Prinstein, 1999).

Specifically, peer nominations of acceptance (or "liking") and rejection (or "disliking") have been used to identify youth's social status. These nominations are combined to identify "popular" youth (those high on liking and low on disliking) and "rejected" youth (those low on liking and high on disliking) (Coie et al., 1990).

During childhood and adolescence, evidence indicates that popular youth often demonstrate good interpersonal skills (e.g., they are helpful and considerate, friendly, cooperative) and personal competencies (e.g., they possess good athletic or academic skills) (Coie et al., 1990; Estell et al., 2008; see Newcomb, Bukowski, & Pattee, 1993, for a review). In contrast, youth who are actively rejected by peers often display maladaptive social behaviors, such as arguing, talking out of turn, and not following rules (Nesdale et al., 2007); high rates of internalizing difficulties, such as depression, social anxiety, and loneliness (Asher & Wheeler, 1985; Hecht, Inderbitzen, & Bukowski, 1998; Inderbitzen, Walters, & Bukowski, 1997; La Greca & Lopez, 1998; La Greca & Stone, 1993); or academic problems and externalizing difficulties, including aggression and disruptive behavior (Hartup, 1996; Ladd, 2006; Stone & La Greca, 1990). In fact, prospective studies indicate that peer-rejected children are at substantial risk for later emotional problems and psychiatric disorders as adults (Kupersmidt & Coie, 1990; Parker & Asher, 1987).

During adolescence, being accepted by the peer group and fitting in with peers become high priorities for most youth (Furman et al., 2009). However, as adolescents' peer networks expand, it is often difficult to gauge their social status via peer nominations. An alternate way to consider adolescents' standing in the larger peer network is to evaluate their "peer crowd affiliation." Affiliating with a peer crowd is a way that adolescents gain peer acceptance and social status (La Greca & Prinstein, 1999). Peer crowds are larger than friendship groups, and peer crowd members are not necessarily friends with one another (Brown, 1990).

Typical peer crowds include "Jocks," "Populars," "Brains," "Burnouts," "Alternatives," and "Loners," although alternative names exist for these groups (Brown, 1990; La Greca, Prinstein, & Fetter, 2001). Some adolescents identify with more than one crowd, and many do not identify with any crowd, or consider themselves to be "normal" or "average" (La Greca et al., 2001; Mackey & La Greca, 2007). Peer crowds' importance appears to peak in midadolescence and then declines as close friends and romantic relationships become more prominent (Brown, 1990).

From an emotional standpoint, peer crowd affiliation provides adolescents with a sense of acceptance, belonging, and identity; peer crowds also provide opportunities for social activities, friendships, and even romantic relationships (Brown, 1990; La Greca & Harrison, 2005; La Greca & Prinstein, 1999). Peer crowds also reflect adolescents' social status in the larger peer group. Typically, the Popular and Jock crowds have the highest social status, with Brains in the middle range, and Alternatives and Burnouts among the least liked (e.g., La Greca et al., 2001).

Peer crowds also have implications for adolescents' social-emotional functioning and health risk behaviors. Adolescents affiliating with high-status peer crowds (e.g., Jocks, Populars) report lower levels of internalized distress (e.g., social anxiety, depressive symptoms) than other youth, whereas adolescents affiliating with low-status crowds (e.g., Burnouts, Alternatives) report significantly more depressive symptoms than other teens (La Greca & Harrison, 2005). For health risk behaviors such as smoking, substance use, unhealthy eating, and risky sex, the low-status crowds report the highest levels of problem behaviors across the board, and Brains the lowest levels of these behaviors (e.g., La Greca et al., 2001; Mackey & La Greca, 2007).

From a clinical perspective, it is extremely important to understand youth's social status and peer acceptance. Such information will provide a clinician with an immediate picture of a youth's day-to-day social context, and can indicate whether peer relations represent an area of strength or an area that needs to be considered in the treatment process. Peer status can also be a marker for the kinds of social opportunities available to the child/adolescent. For example, rejected youth, or adolescents affiliating with the lower-status peer crowds, find it difficult to "break into" more accepted social circles and may only have opportunities to socialize with peers who are also rejected or excluded and who are likely to have negative or undesirable behaviors (Kupersmidt & Coie, 1990; La Greca et al., 2001; La Greca & Prinstein, 1999).

Close Friendships

Although peer group acceptance is important, the ability to form and maintain satisfying and supportive dyadic friendships also represents a critical social adaptation task (Parker & Asher, 1993). Many aspects of children's social lives revolve around "close friendships," defined as dyadic or small-group interactions with their same-age friends (Parker & Asher, 1993).

Both children and adolescents place high value on these close friendships, which provide youth with support, caring, companionship, and intimacy, and also enhance their self-esteem (La Greca & Prinstein, 1999). Close friendships can also buffer the negative impact of peer victimization experiences and of negative family environments (Bukowski & Adams, 2005). Children's close friendships occur almost exclusively between same-sex peers until adolescence, when other-sex close friendships become common and set the stage for romantic relationships (Kuttler, La Greca, & Prinstein, 1999). At all ages, girls are more likely to have a "best friend" and to have more close friends than boys (Parker & Asher, 1993).

From a clinical perspective, three aspects of friendships may be of interest: friendship participation, friendship quality, and the characteristics of youth's close friends. "Friendship participation" is defined as having at least one mutual (i.e., reciprocated) friendship with another peer (Parker & Asher, 1993). Most children and adolescents have at least one mutual friend in school (Bowker & Spencer, 2010; La Greca et al., 2001; Parker & Asher, 1993), and youth with close friends evidence better social-emotional adjustment than those without such ties (Rubin, Bukowski, & Parker, 2006). For example, youth who are friendless report more loneliness and depressive symptoms than do those with friends (Bowker & Spencer, 2010; Brendgen, Lamarche, Wanner, & Vitaro, 2010; Parker & Asher, 1993).

"Friendship quality" is also important, but is often overlooked in clinical settings. Friendships vary on a number of dimensions, including the amount and type of companionship, validation, and support they provide; the degree to which conflict or other negative interactions are present; and their degree of reciprocity (Kuttler et al., 1999; Kuttler & La Greca, 2004; Parker & Asher, 1993; see La Greca & Prinstein, 1999). Increasing levels of intimacy (i.e., sharing private thoughts and feelings, knowing intimate details about one another) are especially evident in adolescents' close friendships (Vernberg, 1990; Vernberg et al., 1992).

Across development, youth with higher-quality friendships (more positive and fewer negative interactions) have fewer behavioral and emotional problems and display greater social competence (La Greca & Prinstein, 1999). Specifically, high-quality friendships are associated with less social anxiety, depression, and loneliness, and with greater self-esteem (e.g., La Greca & Harrison, 2005; La Greca & Lopez, 1998; Vernberg, 1990; Vernberg et al., 1992).

In contrast, friendship problems are typical of youth with behavioral and emotional problems. For example, youth who are aggressive (Brendgen, Vitaro, Turgeon, & Poulin, 2002) have lower-quality friendships than nonaggressive youth do. Youth with ADHD often have multiple peer relation deficits, including difficulties in making and keeping close friends, and being more likely to be rejected (Hoza et al., 2005; Mrug et al., 2009).

Finally, understanding the characteristics of youth's friends can be informative with respect to peer influences. Folk wisdom acknowledges the influence of friends: "You can judge people by the company they keep." In fact, the characteristics of a child's friends are more important for emotional development than whether or not the child has friends (Hartup, 1996).

"Homophily" is a theoretical perspective that provides a useful framework for understanding why the characteristics of children's and adolescents' friends are important. Homophily is the tendency for a person to associate with others who are similar (Kandel, 1978a, 1978b), and it consists of two processes: "selection" (i.e., peers with similar interests and characteristics cluster together and seek one another out) and "socialization" (i.e., peers reward and reinforce similar attitudes and behaviors among group members or friends).

Consistent with the selection process, children choose friends who have similar characteristics, such as age, sex, race, and preference for certain activities (La Greca & Prinstein, 1999). By adolescence, friendship choices are based on subtle factors, such as personality, attitudes, and self-esteem (Aboud & Mendelson, 1998). Friends also *socialize* each other by supporting and reinforcing each other's behaviors and feelings (Deater-Deckard, 2001). For example, Prinstein (2007) found that adolescents whose close friends reported high levels of internalizing symptoms showed increases in their own internalizing symptoms over time. Peer socialization processes also come into play with regard to aggressive or externalizing behaviors (e.g., Bukowski, Brendgen, & Vitaro, 2007; Gifford-Smith, Dodge, Dishion, & McCord, 2005) and health risk behaviors, such as smoking cigarettes (e.g., Kiesner, Poulin, & Dishion, 2010; La Greca et al., 2001). Thus knowing what a youth's friends are like can help a clinician understand the daily socialization influences that play a role in youths' emotions or behaviors.

Considering the developmental and clinical significance of friends, a comprehensive assessment should include an evaluation of whether or not a child/adolescent has friends, the qualities apparent in any close friendships, and what their friends are like. Most clinicians will encounter youth with substantial social dysfunction in their practice, even if it is not articulated as part of the referral problem. For this reason, most clinicians will want to screen for possible social dysfunction early in the assessment process. When friendship problems are evident, a more detailed assessment of social functioning should be pursued (as discussed later). In the event that friendships represent an area of strength for a child or adolescent, the clinician may try to bolster these peer relationships, to help the youth cope with other ongoing life stressors.

Peer Victimization

Peer victimization is a third important aspect of peer influence. The literature on peer victimization initially developed out of efforts to understand peer aggression and its impact (Crick & Bigbee, 1998; Crick & Nelson, 2002). As this area of research evolved, three types of peer aggression/victimization experiences have been identified: (1) "overt" or "physical" (e.g., being hit, pushed, or threatened); (2) "relational" (e.g., being excluded, isolated, or left out by friends); and (3) "reputational" (e.g., being embarrassed or having one's reputation damaged) (Crick & Bigbee, 1998; De Los Reyes & Prinstein, 2004; Prinstein et al., 2001). "Peer victimization" refers to being a recipient of peers' aggressive behaviors.

At this point, the reader may wonder how peer victimization differs from being bullied. "Bullying" is defined as aggressive behavior that is chronic, is systematic, and includes a noted power differential between the aggressor and the victim (Cook, Williams, Guerra, Kim, & Sadek, 2010; Olweus, 1993); bullying also typically focuses on overt aggression (e.g., stalking, physical harm, threats), although teasing and social exclusion can also be part of the picture. In contrast, "peer aggression" and its consequence, "peer victimization," are broader terms that include bullying and forms of overt aggression, but also include the relational and reputational forms of aggression/victimization, which are more subtle and difficult to observe. In addition, peer victimization need not be chronic or imply a power differential, as in the case of bullying. Nevertheless, peer victimization is far more common than bullying, and it has a marked, distressing impact on the victims (Reijntjes, Kamphuis, et al., 2010).

Peer victimization experiences are common among children and adolescents, and even among preschoolers (e.g., Bonnet, Goossens & Schuengel, 2011; Crick, Casas, & Ku, 1999). A 2005–2006 survey indicated that victimization was either a daily or weekly problem for 24% of children in the public schools (Dinkes, Cataldi, & Lin-Kelly, 2007). In fact, peer victimization is a common experience for adolescents, with 20–30% of teens reporting peer victimization on a regular basis (La Greca & Harrison, 2005; Storch, Brassard, & Masia-Warner, 2003; Wang et al., 2010).

Adolescents may also be the targets of "cyber-victimization," which is victimization that occurs through new technologies, such as social networking sites, instant messaging, or text messages (Landoll & La Greca, 2009; Slonje & Smith, 2008; Wang et al., 2010). Studies of adolescents (ages 12–17 years) reveal that 93% go online, 75% own a mobile phone, and over 54% text daily (Lenhart, 2010). Thus it is not surprising that 32% of online teens report experiencing victimization via the Internet, such as by having private material (text, images) forwarded or posted without permission, or having someone spread rumors about them (Lenhart, 2008). Many forms of cyber-victimization may be extensions of reputational victimization, as the intent is often to embarrass others or damage their reputation (Landoll, La Greca, & Lai, 2012).

Among school-age children, girls report more relational and less overt victimization than boys (Crick & Bigbee, 1998). Similarly, adolescent boys report more overt victimization (and overt aggression) than adolescent girls (De Los Reyes & Prinstein, 2004; La Greca & Harrison, 2005; Siegel et al., 2009). However, among adolescents, gender differences are less clear for the other types of peer victimization (Coyne, Archer, & Eslea, 2006; De Los Reyes & Prinstein, 2004; La Greca & Harrison, 2005; Prinstein et al., 2001; Siegel et al., 2009).

In terms of psychological impact, evidence strongly indicates that peer victimization has an adverse impact on youth and contributes to both internalizing and externalizing problems. Among children, peer victimization predicts behavioral adjustment difficulties and internalizing problems (Crick & Bigbee, 1998; Crick & Nelson, 2002; Crick, Ostrov, & Werner, 2006), especially anxiety and depression (Hawker & Boulton, 2000). For example, a recent prospective study (Rudolph, Troop-Gordon, Hessel, & Schmidt, 2011) revealed that peer victimization that occurred in the second grade, and increased over time, predicted children's depressive symptoms and aggressive behavior in the fifth grade; moreover, girls who were victimized were especially likely to engage in relational aggression. Other evidence indicates that youth who are victimized may retaliate and become "bully-victims" (e.g., Nansel et al., 2001).

Research with adolescents similarly demonstrates that peer victimization experiences contribute to internalizing symptoms, especially the interpersonal forms of peer victimization (i.e., relational and reputational victimization). Specifically, relational victimization contributes to adolescent social anxiety and depressive affect, even when other types of peer victimization are controlled for (La Greca & Harrison, 2005; Siegel et al., 2009; Vernberg et al., 1992). Other studies link reputational victimization and cyber-victimization to depressive affect among adolescents (e.g., La Greca,

Chan, Landoll, & Siegel, 2012; Landoll & La Greca, 2012; Wang, Iannotti, & Nansel, 2009). Moreover, prospective studies indicate that interpersonal forms of peer victimization lead to significant *increases* in adolescents' symptoms of social anxiety and depression over time (Reijntjes, Kamphuis, et al., 2010; Siegel et al., 2009; Storch, Masia-Warner, Crisp, & Klein, 2005; Vernberg et al., 1992), and that adolescents with internalizing problems also are more likely to be the targets of such peer victimization experiences (e.g., Reijntjes et al., 2010; Siegel et al., 2009). Interpersonal forms of peer victimization may be particularly damaging for adolescents because the aggressors may be close friends, and when victimization occurs in the context of friendships, it can interfere with the quality of the friendships and reduce social support (La Greca & Harrison, 2005; Vernberg et al., 1992). (For further discussion, see Davila et al., 2010; La Greca et al., 2009; La Greca & Landoll, 2011.)

From a clinical standpoint, assessing youth's peer victimization experiences would be extremely useful, especially whenever social anxiety, depression, or aggressive behavior is part of the clinical picture. As the literature review above indicates, interpersonal problems with peers that manifest as peer victimization experiences could well contribute to or maintain anxious or depressive affect, and lead to further interpersonal difficulties as well as aggressive (retaliatory) behaviors. Peer victimization experiences may be evident for youth with externalizing problems and aggressive behavior (see Cook et al., 2010). In such cases, the children or adolescents may be *peer aggressors* as well as *victims* of peers' aggression; in fact, youth who are both aggressors and victims often display high levels of both internalizing and externalizing problems and have more maladjustment overall than nonvictimized youth (Cook et al., 2010).

In sum, a comprehensive clinical assessment should include at least a brief evaluation of whether or not a youth is experiencing victimization, and if so, what type (i.e., overt, relational, reputational). Obtaining direct input from the youth is critical. Although overt victimization (e.g., pushing, shoving) may be obvious to others, youth rarely disclose relational and reputational peer victimization, other than to close friends (La Greca, Herge, & Bailey, 2012; Vernberg, Ewell, Beery, Freeman, & Abwender, 1995). Assessing peer aggression is also important for youth with externalizing problems, as such aggression is likely to interfere with their interpersonal relationships and could be a result of prior or ongoing peer victimization.

ASSESSING YOUTH'S PEER RELATIONSHIPS

Peer relationships are important to consider in a clinical context, but can be challenging to evaluate. Reports from parents, teachers, peers, and youth themselves have been used to evaluate various aspects of above youth's peer relations (La Greca & Prinstein, 1999). However, the "best informant" and the "best measure" will vary, depending on a youth's age or developmental level and on the purpose of the assessment (i.e., screening, comprehensive assessment, evaluating treatment outcome) (La Greca & Lemanek, 1996). As a general rule of thumb, it is always advisable to get input directly from the child or adolescent and, if possible, also from an adult.

Developing an Assessment Strategy

Self-ratings are widely used to assess youth's perceptions of social acceptance, the number and qualities of close friendships, and peer victimization. For children, peer nominations are useful for evaluating acceptance–rejection and for identifying mutual close friendships. Ratings by teachers are also useful for evaluating children's acceptance–rejection, whereas parents may be useful informants for children's peer status and social skills. However, the overall utility of teacher and parent reports declines during adolescence (La Greca & Lemanek, 1996).

For adolescents, self-reports are the most common assessment method. Peer nominations are impractical, as adolescents have large peer networks that extend across multiple classes and grades; thus school-based peer nominations for social acceptance or mutual friendships may be difficult to obtain. Teachers also are poor informants for adolescents' peer relations, as they may have little contact with adolescents in social contexts. Although used infrequently, parents have served as informants for aspects of adolescents' peer relations, such as peer rejection, the number of close friends, and social skills (Bagwell, Molina, Pelham, & Hoza, 2001; Gresham & Elliot, 1990). Unless it is extreme, parents may not be aware of adolescents' victimization experiences, as youth rarely disclose these events to parents, except when the victimization is overt or when there is a supportive parent–child relationship (La Greca, Herge, & Bailey, 2012; Vernberg et al., 1992).

Below we provide a representative sample of measures that have been used to evaluate youth's peer relations and that could be used in clinical settings (see Tables 11.1 and 11.2). We focus on measures that are widely used and have good psychometric properties, as a comprehensive review of all available peer measures is beyond the scope of this chapter.

Measures of Peer Acceptance–Rejection

Peer Reports

In research contexts, peer nomination procedures (e.g., Coie et al., 1990; La Greca & Stone, 1993; Newcomb et al., 1993) are commonly used to evaluate children's peer acceptance or rejection. Typically, children's classmates are asked to nominate three peers they like most and three they like least; based on the average number of nominations children in the class

TABLE 11.1. Summary of Representative Measures of Peer Assessment Measures

Peer domain	Measure (alphabetically listed)
Acceptance–rejection	• Child Behavior Checklist for Ages 6–18 (CBCL/6–18), Teacher Report Form (TRF), and Youth Self-Report (YSR), individual items; CBCL/6–18 and YSR, Social Competence subscale • Peer Crowd Questionnaire (PCQ) • Peer nominations (for children and adolescents) • Self-Perception Profile for Adolescents (SPPA), Social Acceptance, Romantic Appeal subscales • Self-Perception Profile for Children (SPPC), Social Acceptance subscale • Teacher nominations
Close friendships	• CBCL/6–18 and YSR, Social Competence subscale • Friendship Qualities Measure (FQM) • Friendship Qualities Scale (FQS) • Friendship Quality Questionnaire (FQQ) • Networks of Relationships Inventory—Revised (NRI-R) • Peer nominations of best friends • Self Perception Profile for Adolescents, Close Friends subscale
Peer victimization and aggression	• CBCL/6–18, YSR, and TRF, individual items • Cyber Victimization Scale for Adolescents • FQM • Revised Peer Experiences Questionnaire (R-PEQ) • Social Experiences Questionnaire (SEQ, Self, Peer, and Teacher Report)
Social support	• Child and Adolescent Social Support Scale (CASSS) • Social Support Scale for Children and Adolescents (SSSCA) • Survey of Children's Social Support (SCSS)
Other peer constructs	• Children's Depression Inventory • Loneliness Scale and the Revised UCLA Loneliness Scale • Social Anxiety Scale for Adolescents; Social Anxiety Scale for Children—Revised • Social Skills Rating System

receive, these "like most" and "like least" nominations are converted into standard scores, to determine the degree to which a child is liked (accepted) or disliked (rejected).

Peer nominations also have been used to assess adolescents' peer acceptance–rejection (e.g., Hecht et al., 1998; Inderbitzen et al., 1997; Prinstein & Aikins, 2004), but nominations are more complicated to use as adolescents' peer networks expand. As an illustration, Prinstein and Aikins (2004) used peer nominations in the context of a longitudinal study of 158 adolescents, ages 15–17 years. Adolescents were given a roster of all students in the same grade and asked to nominate an unlimited number of peers whom they "liked to spend time with the most" and "liked to spend time with the least." For each adolescent, a standardized score was computed for their "liked most" and "liked least" nominations, based on

TABLE 11.2. Summary of Measures of Peer Relationships (Listed Alphabetically)

Measure name	Domain	Age/grade for which scale was developed	Informant (number of items)
Child and Adolescent Social Support Scale (CASSS; Demaray & Malecki, 2002; Malecki, Demeray, & Elliot, 2000)	Social support	3rd–12th grades	Self (40)
Achenbach System of Empirically Based Assessment (ASEBA; Achenbach, 2009)	Acceptance–rejection	6–18 years	Self (2), teacher (2), parent (2)
• Child Behavior Checklist for Ages 6–18 (CBCL/6–18) • Teacher Report Form (TRF) • Youth Self-Report (YSR)	Close friendships (CBCL/6–18 and YSR only)		Self (7), parent (7)
Children's Depression Inventory (Kovacs, 1992)	Depression	7–17 years	Self (28), teacher (12), parent (17)
Cyber Victimization Scale for Adolescents (Landoll & La Greca, 2012)	Peer victimization	13–19 years	Self (16)
Friendship Qualities Measure (FQM; Grotpeter & Crick, 1996)	Peer victimization Close friendships	3rd–6th grades	Self (43)
Friendship Qualities Scale (FQS; Bukowski, Hoza, & Boivin, 1994)	Close friendships	5th–7th grades	Self (30)
Friendship Quality Questionnaire (FQQ; Parker & Asher, 1993)	Close friendships	3rd–5th grades	Self (40)
Loneliness Scale (Asher et al., 1984; Asher & Wheeler, 1985)	Loneliness	Elementary school	Self (24)
Networks of Relationships Inventory—Revised (NRI-R; Furman, 1998)	Close friendships	5th–6th grades	Self (30)
Peer Crowd Questionnaire (PCQ; La Greca et al., 2001)	Acceptance–rejection	15–19 years	Self (5)
Peer nominations (e.g., Coie et al., 1990; Prinstein & Aikins, 2004)	Acceptance–rejection Close friendships	Elementary–high school	Peer (2)
Peer nominations of best friends (Crick & Nelson, 2002)	Close friendships	3rd–6th grades	Peer (1)
Revised Peer Experiences Questionnaire (R-PEQ; De Los Reyes & Prinstein, 2004)	Peer victimization	15–17 years	Self (18)

(continued)

TABLE 11.2. (*continued*)

Measure name	Domain	Age/grade for which scale was developed	Informant (number of items)
Revised UCLA Loneliness Scale (Mahon, Yarcheski, & Yarcheski, 1995)	Loneliness	12–21 years	Self (20)
Self-Perception Profile for Adolescents (SPPA; Harter, 1988)	Acceptance–rejection Close friendships	8th–11th grades	Self (6)
Self-Perception Profile for Children (SPPC; Harter, 1985a)	Acceptance–rejection	3rd–8th grades	Self (6)
Social Anxiety Scale for Adolescents (La Greca & Lopez, 1998)	Social anxiety	10th–12th grades	Self (22)
Social Anxiety Scale for Children—Revised (La Greca & Lopez, 1998)	Social anxiety	4th–6th grades	Self (22)
Social Experiences Questionnaire (SEQ; Crick & Bigbee, 1998; Crick & Grotpeter, 1996)	Peer victimization	3rd–6th grades 4th–5th grades 4th grade	Self (15), peer (14), teacher (15)
Social Skills Rating System (Gresham & Elliot, 1990)	Social skills	3–18 years	Self, teacher, parent[a]
Social Support Scale for Children and Adolescents (SSSCA; Harter, 1985b)	Social support	3rd–12th grades	Self (24)
Survey of Children's Social Support (SCSS; Dubow & Ullman, 1989)	Social support	3rd–5th grades	Self (72)
Teacher nominations (Anthonysamy & Zimmer-Gembeck, 2007)	Acceptance–rejection	4–8 years	Teacher (4)

[a]Number of items varies, depending on scales employed.

the average number of nominations the adolescent received. The difference between "like most" and "like least" standardized scores was also used to create a measure of "social preference," with higher scores indicating greater acceptance and lower scores reflecting greater peer rejection.

Peer nominations are considered the "gold standard" for assessing youth's acceptance and rejection (Newcomb et al., 1993; La Greca & Prinstein, 1999); they have strong psychometric properties, including concurrent and predictive validity with youth's mental health problems (Coie et al., 1990; Hoza, 2007; Parker & Asher, 1987). However, because of the time demands involved (and challenges in obtaining parental consent for participants), nomination procedures may not be practical to use in many clinical situations.

Self-Reports

Youth's self-reports may be the place to start for assessing peer acceptance. Several well-validated measures have items that would allow a clinician to assess a child's or adolescent's peer acceptance from the youth's perspective. The measures described below assess youth's perceptions of social acceptance and also adolescents' reports of their peer crowd affiliation, which can reflect their status in the larger peer group (as discussed earlier).

Susan Harter (1985a, 1988) developed two widely used measures for assessing youth's perceptions of social acceptance, as well as other aspects of their competence and self-worth. The Self-Perception Profile for Children (SPPC; Harter, 1985a) contains 36 items and can be used with children in third–eighth grades. It contains six subscales: Social Acceptance, Scholastic Competence, Athletic Competence, Physical Appearance, Behavioral Conduct, and Global Self-Worth. The six-item Social Acceptance subscale assesses children's perceptions of their peer acceptance; internal consistency (alpha) has been adequate, ranging from .75 to .80 across samples (Harter, 1985a). The response format is complicated; for each item, children first decide which of two statements better describes them (e.g., "Some kids are popular with others their age" but "Other kids are not very popular") and then decide whether their chosen statement is "sort of true" or "really true" for them. Each item receives a score of between 1 (negative statement, "really true") and 4 (positive statement, "really true"), with summary scores created for each subscale. A parallel teacher rating scale also exists (Harter, 1985a).

The Self-Perception Profile for Adolescents (SPPA; Harter, 1988) is a similar measure designed for adolescents 13 years of age and older. It contains 45 items and nine subscales; six are the same as for the SPPC, with three additional subscales: Job Competence, Romantic Appeal, and Close Friends. The six-item Social Acceptance subscale assesses adolescents' perceptions of their peer acceptance, and the response format and scoring are identical to those for the SPPC. The Romantic Appeal and Close Friends subscales may also be of interest for assessing adolescents' perceptions of other close peer relationships (e.g., see La Greca & Lopez, 1998). The internal consistencies of the SPPA subscales have been adequate, ranging from .74 to .93 (Harter, 1988). A parallel teacher rating scale also exists (Harter, 1988).

The SPPC and SPPA are quick and practical methods for obtaining youth's perceptions of their social acceptance. With adolescents, it also may be useful to evaluate whether or not they affiliate with any particular peer crowd and, if so, which one. The Peer Crowd Questionnaire (PCQ; La Greca et al., 2001; La Greca & Harrison, 2005; La Greca & Mackey, 2007) was developed for that purpose. Adolescents are asked whether any of the following crowds are present in their school (and the terms used to identify the crowds, if these differ from the terms given): Jocks (those who are athletic, are on a school team), Brains (those who do well in school, enjoy academics), Burnouts (those who skip school, get into trouble), Populars (those who are very social, involved in many activities, concerned about their image), Nonconformists or Alternatives (those who rebel against the norm in clothing or ideas, who do not conform to social ideals), and None or Average (no affiliation, "just average"). They also are asked whether any other crowds are present in their school. Then adolescents indicate which crowd they most identify with, how that crowd is viewed (to index acceptance–rejection), and their best friends' crowd affiliations. The PCQ was developed on a sample of 250 high school students, 15–19 years of age (La Greca et al., 2001). Peer crowd affiliation has been linked with adolescents' mental health and health risk behaviors, as discussed earlier. Assessing youth's peer crowd affiliations can also provide the clinician with an idea of what the youth's friends are like, as most adolescents' close friends affiliate with similar peer crowds (La Greca et al., 2001).

Finally, for youth ages 11–18 years, items from the Youth Self-Report (YSR; Achenbach, 2009) may also prove useful for obtaining a brief assessment of youth's peer functioning. The YSR is the youth report instrument in the Achenbach System of Empirically Based Assessment (ASEBA; Achenbach, 2009), described in detail by Achenbach in Chapter 6 of this volume, and contains a Social Competence subscale (part of the Competence Scales that precede the behavior problems portion of the ASEBA) that can be used to index youth's peer relations. In addition, several items from the Social Problems subscale of the YSR reflect peer rejection and peer victimization; these items are also contained on the teacher and parent report versions of the ASEBA, as described below. The YSR, including the Social Competence subscale, has strong psychometric properties and age-based norms. If the YSR is administered as part of clinical assessment protocol, it could serve as an initial screening for youth's peer relation problems.

Teacher Reports

Teacher nominations have been used to assess younger children's acceptance–rejection in conjunction with or as an alternative to peer nominations. Anthonysamy and Zimmer-Gembeck (2007) provide an illustration of this approach; they obtained teacher nominations for 400 children (ages 4–8 years) that involved 24 teachers from 22 schools. Teachers nominated three children in the class whom others "most liked to play with" (acceptance) and three whom others "least liked to play with" (rejection). Teachers also rated how well other children liked to play with each child on a 5-point scale (1 = "very little," 5 = "very much"). Acceptance and rejection nominations and likeability ratings were standardized within each classroom, to index each child's peer status. The teacher ratings of peer likeability were significantly correlated with both peer and teacher nominations of acceptance and rejection (absolute value of $r = .15–.59$); teacher and child reports also were significantly related (absolute value of r's = .20–.47). These findings suggest that teachers using this approach may provide reasonable estimates of children's acceptance, rejection, and likeability, especially for younger elementary school children.

Aside from classroom-based teacher nominations and ratings, the Teacher Report Form (TRF; Achenbach, 2009) from the ASEBA can be used to obtain input on children's peer acceptance. The TRF can be used with youth ages 6–18 years and has strong psychometric support (see Achenbach, Chapter 6). As with each of the ASEBA measures, specific items from the Social Problems subscale can be used to assess peer rejection ("Is not liked by other kids") and potential peer victimization ("Gets teased a lot"). (Note that the TRF does not have a Social Competence subscale prior to the behavior problem ratings.) Other teacher measures containing items or subscales that tap youth's peer relations include the Child Behavior Scale (see Ladd, Herald-Brown, & Andrews, 2009) and the Pupil Evaluation Inventory (see La Greca, 1981; Pekarik, Prinz, Liebert, Weintraub, & Neale, 1976).

Parent Report

Parents often report on their children's acceptance and friendships as part of a broader assessment of youth's behavioral and emotional problems. Widely used measures of youth's behavioral functioning—such as the Child Behavior Checklist for Ages 6–18 Years (CBCL/6–18; Achenbach, 2009; Achenbach & Rescorla, 2001), which is the parent report form from the ASEBA—contain items that can serve as proxies for assessing peer rejection, friendships, and peer victimization, and can be used for screening purposes.

Specifically, as with both the TRF and YSR, the CBCL/6–18 contains an item that reflects peer rejection (i.e., "Is not liked by other kids") and one that reflects potential peer victimization (i.e., "Gets teased a lot"). These items have been used to index peer relations in studies of youth with ADHD (e.g., Bagwell et al., 2001; Cardoos & Hinshaw, 2011). Although these items are part of the Social Problems subscale on the CBCL/6–18 (and also on the TRF and YSR), we do not recommend using the Social Problems subscale to index youth's peer relationship problems. This is because many of the items in this subscale either do not reflect peer relations (e.g., "clumsy," "speech problems," and "accident prone") or do not reflect the key aspects of peer relationships (e.g., "jealous," "dependent," "prefers younger children").

The CBCL/6–18 (like the YSR, as noted above) also contains a Social Competence subscale that provides an overall assessment of a child's competence in peer relationships, such as whether or not the child has friends and "gets along with other kids." The Social Competence subscale of the CBCL/6–18 has strong psychometric properties and moderate to high cross-informant agreement (see Achenbach, Chapter 6). The CBCL/6–18 items and the Social Competence subscale can be administered as part of a standard screening of youth's interpersonal functioning.

Measures of Close Friendships

Aside from acceptance–rejection, understanding youths' friendships is also important. Clinically, it is useful to know whether a child/adolescent has friends, what the qualities of the friendships are like, and what the friends are like.

As noted above, the YSR and CBCL/6–18 contain a Social Competence subscale that provides a general index of youth's friendships. Structured diagnostic interviews also may contain items that assess youth's friendships. For example, five items from the Anxiety Disorders Interview Schedule for Children (Parent Interview; Silverman & Nelles, 1988) were used in one study to evaluate anxious children's friendships (Festa & Ginsburg, 2011). These items included "Does your child have a best friend?" and "Does your child have more friends than most kids, fewer, or the same?" Asking youth (and their parents) directly who their friends are and what they are like would also be a good starting point for evaluating youth's close friendships. In fact, most measures of youth's friendship qualities begin by asking the youth to list their closest friends.

When youth are having social difficulties, a detailed assessment of their friendships may be indicated. Below we describe several measures with good psychometric properties that assess positive and negative qualities in youth's friendships—from the youth's perspective. Measures assessing youth's perceptions of social support from close friends also could be used to gauge the positive qualities of youth's friendships. None of the measures assess what the friends *are like*; thus it may be useful simply to ask a youth and parent (or teacher) about this. (Note that the PCQ [La Greca et al., 2001] also provides an idea of what adolescents' friends may be like, since youth's close friends often affiliate with similar crowds.)

Self-Reports of Friendship Qualities

Several measures assess children's close friendships. The Friendship Quality Questionnaire (FQQ; Parker & Asher, 1993) contains 40 items that evaluate the qualities of a child's best friendship across six domains: Validation and Caring; Conflict and Betrayal; Companionship and Recreation; Help and Guidance; Intimate Exchange; and Conflict Resolution. Sample items include "[Friend's name] makes me feel good about my ideas" and "[Friend's name] tells me I am good at things." Children indicate how true each item is for their friendship (0 = "not at all true," 4 = "really true"). The FQQ was developed with 484 children in the third–fifth grades. A principal-components analysis supported the six-factor structure; internal consistencies of the factors are adequate (alphas = .73–.90). Children who were low on peer acceptance reported significantly less help and guidance, less validation and caring, and more difficulty resolving conflict in their friendships than did high-accepted and average-accepted peers, and less intimate disclosure than high-accepted peers (Parker & Asher, 1993). These findings indicate that youth who are low in peer acceptance also have difficulties in their close friendships. Brendgen et al. (2002) also used this measure with fourth through sixth graders, shortening the scale to 27 items across five domains: Companionship and Recreation; Help and Guidance; Validation and Caring; Intimate Exchange; Conflict Resolution; and Conflict. These authors created summary scales for positive (alpha = .93) and negative (alpha = .77) friendship qualities.

Similar to the FQQ, the 30-item Friendship Qualities Scale (FQS; Bukowski, Hoza, & Boivin, 1994) was developed to assess the quality of older children's and young adolescents' best friendships. The FQS contains five factors: Companionship, Conflict, Help/Aid, Closeness, and Security. Sample items include "If I have a problem at school or at home, I can talk to my friend about it." Youth answer each item in relation to their best friend; items are scored 1 ("not true about the relationship") to 5 ("really true about the relationship"). The internal consistencies for the factors have been adequate (alphas = .71–.86). Reciprocal friends report greater companionship, help, security, and closeness, and less conflict than nonreciprocal friends; youth with stable friendships (6 months or longer) report greater companionship, help, security, and closeness than youth with nonstable friendships (Bukowski et al., 1994).

As another option, Grotpeter and Crick (1996) developed the 43-item Friendship Qualities Measure (FQM), which combines subscales from both the FQQ (Parker & Asher, 1993) and the FQS (Bukowski et al., 1994). It also contains new items that evaluate relational and overt aggression and victimization within youth's friendships. As in its predecessors, items are rated in reference to the youth's best friendship (1 = "not at all true," 5 = "almost always true"). The FQM was developed for youth in the third–sixth grades and contains 14 subscales: Validation and Caring; Conflict I (Friend Mad); Conflict II (Subject Mad); companionship and Recreation; Help and Guidance; Intimate Exchange I (Subject Intimacy); Intimate Exchange II (Friend Intimacy); Ease of Conflict Resolution; Relational Aggression within the Friendship; Overt Aggression within the Friendship; Relational Aggression towards Others; Overt Aggression towards Others; Exclusivity I (Subject Desire); and Exclusivity II (Friend Demand). Sample items include "[Friend's name] makes me feel good about my ideas." Items have strong factor loadings, ranging from .78 to .91, although the internal consistencies of the subscales range from .61 to .87.

For adolescents, a widely used measure for assessing close relationships, including best friendships and (if applicable) romantic relationships, is the 42-item Network of Relationships Inventory—Revised (NRI-R;

Furman, 1998; Furman & Buhrmester, 1985, 1992; Furman et al., 2009). The NRI-R measures nine positive relationship qualities (Companionship, Affection, Disclosure, Nurturance, Instrumental Aid, Approval, Support, Reliable Alliance, and Satisfaction) and five negative interactions (Conflict, Criticism, Exclusion, Dominance, and Pressure). Three items assess each quality; all items are rated on a 5-point scale (1 = "little or none" and 5 = "the most"). Items include "How much do you and this person get upset with or mad at each other?" Substantial support exists for the reliability and validity of this scale (Furman & Buhrmester, 1992; Kuttler & La Greca, 2004; La Greca & Harrison, 2005). The NRI-R subscales can be useful for pinpointing specific areas that are strengths or weaknesses in youth's close friendships.

There is also good psychometric support for the NRI-R summary scores, based on average scores across the positive and the negative items (La Greca & Harrison, 2005; La Greca & Mackey, 2007). Others have used shortened forms of the NRI-R. For example, based on factor analysis, Kuttler and La Greca (2004) used four positive scales (Companionship, Affection, Disclosure/Support, Reliable Alliance/Satisfaction) and two negative scales (Conflict, Pressure) to assess adolescents' friendships and romantic relationships, and demonstrated good validity and internal consistency with this approach. Finally, an alternative version of the NRI (the NRI—Behavioral Systems Version) was recently developed to assess how relationships fulfill three behavioral systems functions: Attachment, Caregiving, and Affiliation (Furman & Buhrmester, 2009).

Self-Reports of Social Support

Several measures of youth's social support contain subscales that reflect support from peers. These measures are especially useful when support from "classmates" (which may reflect peer acceptance) is differentiated from support from "close friends" (which may reflect positive qualities of close friendships).

The Social Support Scale for Children and Adolescents (SSSCA; Harter, 1985b), a widely used measure, was developed to assess perceived support from significant others in youth's lives, and has been used with youth in third through twelfth grades. The SSSCA contains 24 items that assess support from four sources (6 items each): parents, classmates, teachers, and close friends. Sample items include "Some kids have classmates who like them the way they are" but "Other kids have classmates who wish they were different." Items are scored in the same manner as for the Self-Perception Profiles, with scores ranging from 1 ("low support") to 4 ("high support"). Psychometric properties for the SSSCA are strong. Subscale internal reliabilities range from .72 to .86, and factor loadings following oblique rotation (.30–.80) have been adequate; the SSSCA subscales also correlate as expected with scores on the Self-Perception Profiles (Harter, 1985b).

Another measure, the Child and Adolescent Social Support Scale (CASSS; Demaray & Malecki, 2002), was also developed for youth in third–twelfth grades. It contains 40 items that assess support from parents, teachers, classmates, and close friends. Sample items include "My classmates treat me nicely," and items are rated on frequency (1 = "never," 6 = "always") and importance (1 = "not important," 3 = "very important"). Factor analysis supported the four subscales, with item loadings ranging from .55 to .86; across subscales, internal consistencies ranged from .87 to .94, and test–retest stability across 8 weeks ranged from .60 to .76 (Malecki & Demaray, 2002). The CASSS correlates with other measures of support, such as the SSSCA ($r = .70$).

Finally, the Survey of Children's Social Support (SCSS) provides a comprehensive picture of children's social support networks (Dubow & Ullman, 1989). This 72-item measure has three subscales: the frequency of supportive behaviors available from a child's support network (SAB) (38 items); the child's subjective appraisals of family, teacher, and peer support (APP) (31 items); and the size of the child's support network (NET) (3 items). In particular, the APP subscale has been used to evaluate youth's perceptions of support from key sources (e.g., La Greca et al., 2010). Items are rated on a 5-point scale (0 = "never," 4 = "always") and include "Do you think your friends care about you?" and "Are you well liked by your classmates?" For the NET items, youth list significant others who provide them with emotional, tangible, and informational support. Dubow and Ullman (1989) report good psychometric support for the measure among third through fifth graders. Internal consistencies ranged from .88 (APP) to .94 (SAB); test–retest reliability (3–4 weeks) for the NET was moderate (.52–.54); and construct validity was demonstrated via correlations with other measures of social support (SSSCA) and with children's self-perceptions on SPPCA (Harter, 1985a).

Peer Nominations

Although peer nominations are rarely used in clinical situations to assess mutual friendships, they are commonly used in research with children and early adolescents (e.g., Bowker & Spencer, 2010; Brendgen et al., 2002); thus we describe the method here. An advantage of peer nominations is that they reveal whether youth's friendships are reciprocated. In clinical situations, one could ask a youth, parents, and teacher (for a child) who the youth's closest friends are, to see whether there is consistent reporting across sources.

Crick and Nelson (2002) assessed the presence of children's mutual friendships by using a standardized peer nomination procedure (see also Grotpeter & Crick, 1996). Children were given class rosters and asked to indicate their top three friends (listed as first, second, and third best friends). Children were identified as having a mutual best friend if any of the children they listed as best friends also nominated them as best friends. If a target child was not also listed as a best friend by any of his or her choices, the child was noted as not having a mutual best friend. Bowker and Spencer (2010) used a similar procedure with early adolescents, asking youth to name their three very best same-sex friends in the same grade and school; they found that 68% of the youth had at least one mutual same-grade friend, and that girls were more likely to have such mutual friends than boys. Mutual friendships appear to buffer the negative impact of adverse peer and family experiences (Bukowski & Adams, 2005; Crick & Nelson, 2002).

Measures of Peer Victimization

Victimization experiences mainly have been assessed from youth's perspective. In fact, as noted earlier, youth often do not disclose victimization experiences to others, especially adults. Thus, unless peer victimization is extreme, adults may not be the best informants.

Self-Reports

For children and early adolescents, the Friendship Qualities Measure (FQM; Grotpeter & Crick, 1996) has been widely used to assess overt and relational peer victimization. The FQM assesses youths' friendships, but also contains subscales that assess peer victimization within the friendship. One subscale is Friendship Relational Aggression (four items; Cronbach's alpha = .73; a sample item is "Ignores me when s/he is mad at me"). The other is Friendship Overt Aggression (three items; Cronbach's alpha = .79; a sample item is "Hits and pushes me"). (The FQM also assesses relational and overt *aggression* toward others.) The FQM was developed with third–fifth graders from diverse backgrounds, and also has been used with early adolescents (Paquette & Underwood, 1999; Storch, Zelman, Sweeney, Danner, & Dove, 2002).

Another measure for children and adolescents is the Social Experiences Questionnaire—Self-Report (SEQ-S; Crick & Grotpeter, 1996; Crick & Bigbee, 1998). This 15-item measure contains three subscales: Relational Victimization (e.g., "How often does another kid say they won't like you unless you do what they want you to do?"), Overt Victimization (e.g., "How often do you get hit by another kid at school?"), and Receipt of Prosocial Acts (e.g., "How often does another kid give you help when you need it?"). Responses range from 1 ("never") to 5 ("all the time"). Factor analysis supports the three-factor model of the SEQ-S, with item loadings ranging from .69 to .88 (Crick & Grotpeter, 1996). Note that the SEQ-S evaluates peer victimization experiences more generally than does the FQQ, which focuses on victimization by *friends*. The SEQ-S was initially developed for third through sixth graders, and subscales range in internal consistency from .77 to .80. In addition, recent studies reveal that the three subscales of the SEQ-S also have good psychometric properties with adolescents ages 13–17 years (Storch, Crisp, Roberti, Bagner, & Masia-Warner, 2005; Storch & Masia-Warner, 2004). Peer and teacher report forms of the SEQ also have been developed and are described below.

With adolescents, a widely used measure is the Revised Peer Experiences Questionnaire (R-PEQ; De Los Reyes & Prinstein, 2004; Prinstein et al., 2001). It contains 18 items and has subscales for Overt, Relational, and Reputational Victimization (three items each) as well as for prosocial acts. Items include "A peer hit, kicked, or pushed me in a mean way" (Overt), "Some peers left me out of an activity that I really wanted to be included in" (Relational), and "A teen gossiped about me so others would not like me" (Reputational). Adolescents rate the frequency of each event over the past two months (1 = "never" to 5 = "a few times a week"). Overt, Relational, and Reputational Aggression can also be measured with parallel items (i.e., rating how often the adolescent *did these things* to other peers). The R-PEQ has satisfactory reliability and validity (De Los Reyes & Prinstein, 2004; Siegel et al., 2009). Internal consistencies range from .59 to .87 for the Victimization subscales and from .68 to .83 for the Aggression subscales. The initial PEQ contained subscales for Overt and Relational Peer Victimization and demonstrated satisfactory test–retest stability (r's = .48–.52) over 6 months (Prinstein et al., 2001).

At present, there is no well-developed measure of youth's cyber-victimization. However, development is ongoing for the 16-item Cyber Victimization Scale for Adolescents (Landoll & La Greca, 2012; for youth ages 13–19 years), which assesses peer victimization that occurs through technology, such as cell phones and the Internet. Initial psychometric data are promising; cyber-victimization appears to be distinct from other types of peer victimization, and contributes uniquely to the prediction of youth's depressive symptoms (Landoll & La Greca, 2012).

Peer Reports

Studies of children's peer victimization have often used peer nomination procedures (e.g., Cardoos & Hinshaw, 2011; Crick & Bigbee, 1998). Specifically, the Social Experiences Questionnaire—Peer Report (SEQ-P; Crick & Bigbee, 1998) was developed with fourth and fifth graders to assess peers' perceptions of children's positive and negative peer experiences. The SEQ-P is similar to peer nominations of acceptance–rejection: Children are given a class roster and asked to nominate up to three classmates who fit each descriptor; children's scores are then summed and standardized within classrooms. The SEQ-P has subscales for victims of relational aggression (five items; alpha = .86; "Gets ignored by other kids when someone is mad at them"); victims of overt aggression (five items; alpha = .93; "Gets beat up"); and recipients of caring acts (four items; alpha = .77; "Other kids help them when they need it"). Principal-components factor analysis supported the three-factor model, with loadings ranging from .60 to .87. Peer reports of overt and relational victimization correlate moderately with self-reported victimization on the SEQ-S (r's = .31–.39) (Crick & Bigbee, 1998).

Teacher Reports

A teacher version of the SEQ, the Social Experiences Questionnaire—Teacher Report (SEQ-T; Cullerton-Sen & Crick, 2005), was developed with fourth graders. The SEQ-T contains two subscales: Physical Victimization (three items; alpha = .93; "This child gets hit or kicked by peers") and Relational Victimization (three items; alpha = .82; "This child gets ignored by other children when a peer is mad at them"). Teachers rate each item on a 5-point scale (1 = "never" to 5 = "almost always"). Teacher and peer reports correlated modestly for Relational Victimization (r = .34) and Physical Victimization (r = .21). Teacher reports and self-reports were also modestly correlated (r = .29 for Relational and r = .22 for Physical Victimization). However, even after controls for self- and peer-reported victimization, teacher reports of Physical Victimization predicted children's externalizing behaviors, and their reports of Relational Victimization predicted both internalizing and externalizing behaviors. Thus findings suggest that teacher input contributes unique information to the assessment of children's victimization.

Parent Report

To our knowledge, no specific measures have been developed to obtain parents' reports of their children's peer victimization. As noted earlier, items from the CBCL/6–18 may provide a general estimate of victimization. Some investigators have used brief questions to assess parents' (and teachers') perceptions of children's peer victimization. For example, in a study of youth in the first–tenth grades, Lohre, Lydersen, Paulsen, Maehle, and Vatten (2011) asked parents (and teachers) two questions: "During recess, do others tease or bother your daughter (son)/this child?" and "Does your daughter (son)/this child experience being left out from being together with peers?" Items were scored from 1 ("never") to 5 ("about every day"). Parent–child agreement was low to moderate, and child reports of victimization were more strongly associated with their emotional and somatic symptoms than parent or teacher reports were. These data suggest caution in using adult informants for youth's peer victimization experiences.

Other Peer-Related Areas to Consider Assessing

When youth encounter peer relations problems as assessed with the measures described above, it may also be useful to assess their (1) level of distress, particularly as reflected in symptoms of social anxiety, depression, and/or loneliness; (2) social skills; and (3) levels of peer aggression. These areas may aid the clinician in identifying potential mechanisms contributing to peer relationship problems and selecting relevant targets for intervention. For example, an adolescent who is experiencing considerable peer victimization, especially from friends (i.e., relational victimization), may be very socially anxious and/or depressed. If this is the case, the intervention will need to address the teen's affect as well as the victimization, so that the adolescent does not avoid social situations or withdraw from peers completely, further compromising her or his social functioning. As another example, poor social skills could contribute to a child's difficulty in making and keeping close friends; in this case, coaching in social skills might be incorporated into the treatment plan to improve the child's friendships and support system. Assessing a child's level of peer aggression can also be helpful in determining a suitable treatment plan.

Although it is beyond the scope of this chapter to review these additional areas of assessment in detail, we note a few well-developed measures that may be useful in clinical settings. To assess internal distress, available measures for social anxiety, depression, and loneliness include (1) the Social Anxiety Scale for Children—Revised (La Greca & Stone, 1993; for ages 7–13 years) and the Social Anxiety Scale for Adolescents (La Greca & Lopez, 1998; for ages 13–19 years); (2) the Children's Depression Inventory (Kovacs, 1992; for ages 7–17 years); (3) the Loneliness Scale (Asher, Hymel, & Renshaw, 1984; Asher & Wheeler, 1985; for elementary school youth); and (4) the Revised UCLA Loneliness Scale (Mahon, Yarcheski, & Yarcheski, 1995; for ages 12–21 years). To assess social skills, the child, parent, and teacher versions of the Social Skills Rating System (Gresham & Elliot, 1990) assess these social skills in five areas: Cooperation, Empathy, Assertion, Self-Control, and Responsibility. Finally, to assess peer aggression, many of the previously described measures of peer victimization also assess how often children or adolescents are the perpetrators of aggressive acts; for example, the R-PEQ asks youth not only how often these experiences have occurred to them, but how often they have done them to others.

IMPLICATIONS FOR TREATMENT PLANNING AND OUTCOME EVALUATION

Now that we have reviewed key peer relationship constructs and measures, how can clinicians use this information to sharpen their assessment and treatment of youth? We recommend brief screening for peer relationship problems for all youth seen in clinical settings. If problems are identified in any area (acceptance, friendships, peer victimization), a more detailed assessment should reveal strengths and weaknesses that could be addressed and incorporated into treatment planning. Finally, peer measures may be useful for tracking treatment outcome, depending on the specific treatment plan. Below we elaborate and offer specific recommendations.

Screening

At the beginning of treatment, it would be useful to administer a brief screening battery of peer relationship measures. For children, this might include their reports of (1) acceptance–rejection, such as the six-item Social Acceptance subscale of the SPPC; (2) close friendships, such as the Close Friends subscale of the SSSCA; (3) peer victimization, such as the 10 items from the SEQ-S that assess overt and relational victimization; and (4) internal distress, such as the 18-item Social Anxiety Scale for Children— Revised. For adolescents, screening might include the adolescent versions of these measures, plus youth's report of their peer crowd affiliation on the PCQ. Also, for adolescents, the nine items from the R-PEQ assessing Overt, Relational, and Reputational Victimization might be used instead of the SEQ-S.

In addition to youth reports, parents and/or teachers could complete items from the CBCL/6–18 or TRF, respectively, that index peer rejection or victimization (e.g., "Is not liked by other kids," "Gets teased a lot"). In addition, the Social Competence subscale of the CBCL/6–18 could provide general information on youth's friendships (e.g., number of close friends). As noted earlier, structured diagnostic interviews (e.g., the Anxiety Disorders Interview Schedule for DSM-IV: Child and Parent Versions; see Marin, Rey, & Silverman, Chapter 5, this volume) also may contain some items that provide an idea of youth's friendships. Finally, as a screen for peer victimization, parents or teachers might be asked whether (and how often) other peers (1) tease or bother the child; (2) leave the child out or excluded the child from activities; and (3) embarrass the child or try to damage his or her reputation.

Assessment for Treatment Planning

If the screening reveals a problem area, a detailed assessment of all three key areas of peer functioning (i.e., acceptance–rejection, friendships, victimization) would be indicated. This is because the three areas are interrelated, so a child or adolescent may have multiple peer relationship issues to address in treatment. However, it is also the case that some youth may have an area of strength (e.g., one close, high-quality friendship) in the context of other problems (e.g., peer victimization), and this area of strength could be useful in developing a treatment plan.

The measures described in this chapter (and in Tables 11.1 and 11.2) should provide ideas of appropriate measures for follow-up. In general, a comprehensive assessment might include both youth and adult reports (including teacher reports, at least for preadolescents). It might also include measures that provide details on the number and quality of the youth's friendships (e.g., the FQQ or the NRI-R) and on peer victimization *and* aggression (e.g., subscales from a version of the SEQ or the R-PEQ). Moreover, it may be useful to evaluate a youth's level of distress or discomfort with peers, using a measure of social anxiety, depressive symptoms, and/or loneliness (if not completed at screening). It also will be useful to evaluate factors contributing to the identified peer relationship problems (e.g., poor social skills, peer aggression). Finally, understanding the youth's sources of social support, whether it be from classmates, friends, parents, or teachers, could help identify areas of strength that could be built upon in treatment.

Evaluation of Treatment Outcome

The detailed peer assessment should provide information that is useful for treatment planning. For example, if a child has few or no close friends, is socially anxious, and has poor social skills, the child may be a good candidate for Social Effectiveness Therapy for Children, a cognitive-behavioral intervention that focuses on socially anxious children 8–12 years of age (Beidel, Turner, & Morris, 2000; Beidel et al., 2007). Or, an adolescent who shows signs of being victimized by peers, feels depressed, and has poor-quality friendships might be an appropriate candidate for Interpersonal Psychotherapy for Adolescents (Mufson, Dorta, Moreau, & Weissman, 2004). As another illustration, a child who has behavior problems due to a contentious parental divorce (or other family stressor), but who has good peer relations and a few close friendships, might benefit from a treatment plan that includes efforts to build upon and maintain her or his friendship ties. In tracking treatment outcome for youth, it would be useful to include measures not only of the presenting problem(s) (e.g., social anxiety, depression, behavior problems), but also of the peer area(s) addressed in the intervention (e.g., building social skills, improving friendship qualities, enhancing social support).

APPLICATION TO THE CASE OF BILLY

Billy was a 10-year-old boy with oppositional, negativistic, and noncompliant behaviors at home and school. Problematic peer relationships appeared to be a key aspect of Billy's behaviors at presentation. Billy had difficulty getting along with peers and might be experiencing peer rejection at school; he reported that "it seems like everyone is picking on" him. It was unclear whether Billy had good-quality close friendships, as "even his friends . . . just want to get [him] in trouble." Furthermore, Billy had experienced overt peer victimization, in the form of physical and verbal bullying from older students. Billy might also have social skill deficits, as he reported not understanding why classmates did not like or get along with him. Billy's history revealed that he had a speech delay and was very shy around strangers as a young child.

Billy's referral information provided clear signs that he was experiencing problems in all three areas of peer functioning: acceptance–rejection, close friendships, and victimization. Thus screening measures of Billy's peer functioning would not be sufficient. Instead, a clinician would need a detailed assessment of Billy's peer relations and related constructs right from the start.

With respect to peer acceptance–rejection, it was unclear whether Billy was being actively rejected. It would help to obtain Billy's perspective on his social acceptance (e.g., with the SPPC), as well as input from his teacher and mother (e.g., with specific items from the TRF and the CBCL/6–18, respectively, that assess peer rejection). Several pieces of clinically relevant information might emerge from these measures. If Billy's teacher or mother reported that he was rejected, then countering the peer rejection would need to be a key focus of treatment, as it could be chronic and as ample evidence points to strong associations between peer rejection and aggression/maladjustment in youth (e.g., Parker & Asher, 1987). Billy's perspective would also be important. The SPPC would provide information about Billy's areas of competence, which might be developed and used to increase Billy's positive peer interactions and his sense of acceptance and belonging in school. For example, if Billy reported athletic competence, he might join an after-school sports team to help him highlight his strengths, interact with peers in a positive context, and look forward to school. Therapy also might address Billy's emotions and responses to peer rejection, to ensure that he would not retaliate in ways that could make the problem worse.

With respect to close friendships, Billy did not feel supported by his friends, and he rarely sought out friends for companionship. Thus the quality of Billy's close friendships was questionable and would need to be evaluated with a measure such as the FQM. If Billy reported no areas of strengths in his friendships, treatment might need to focus, in part, on helping him build close friendships. It would also will be important to know about the characteristics of Billy's friends, as he might have friends who displayed aggressive or undesirable behaviors. Part of the plan to improve Billy's friendships might include identifying suitable peers for friendship development. Tracking Billy's close friendships would be particularly important throughout treatment.

With respect to peer victimization, Billy had experienced overt victimization in school. Thus it would be important to assess his peer victimization experiences and peer aggression, using a measure like the FQM. Two scenarios should be seen as important "red flags." First, if Billy reported high levels of victimization in all areas (e.g., overt, relational), this would be important to monitor and address in treatment. Children who are polyvictimized often have chronic, stable trajectories of victimization (Wang et al., 2010). Second, if Billy reported both aggression and victimization, his peer experiences would need to be addressed in therapy. As noted earlier, youth who are both victims and aggressors often display high levels of both internalizing and externalizing problems (Cook et al., 2010); thus if Billy reported aggression as well as victimization, treatment might focus on reducing his aggressive behavior (Ybrant & Armelius, 2010) and also improving his peer relations. If Billy primarily reported peer victimization, treatment might focus on strategies to help him avoid internalizing negative experiences with peers (Lopez & DuBois, 2005), in addition to improving peer relations and close friendships.

Finally, more information would be needed about Billy's social skills, given some evidence that his social skills might be deficient and also because Billy might be rejected by his peers (rejection is associated with maladaptive social behaviors; Nesdale et al., 2007). Billy's social skills could be assessed with the Social Skills Rating System, and skill deficits could be addressed in treatment.

With regard to tracking treatment progress, the clinician could select measures targeting the peer areas addressed in intervention; thus the progress and outcome measures would depend on the initial detailed assessment (e.g., they would track social skills, friendship qualities, and/or peer victimization–aggression, depending on the treatment focus). This strategy would allow for repeated measurement of the same constructs, which could be graphically represented to discuss therapy progress and outcome with Billy and his mother.

APPLICATION TO THE CASE OF SOFIA

Sofia was a 15-year-old girl with internalizing difficulties, for whom treatment was being sought to address her anxiety about attending school. Sofia had been having school attendance issues for the previous 8 months. She first stopped attending school because of panic attacks, and after treatment for panic symptoms, she returned to school. However, she had recently learned that she would have to repeat a grade due to academic problems. When told this, Sofia stopped attending school altogether, reporting embarrassment about retention and concern that peers would know about her academic difficulties. Sofia had withdrawn from her friends, although she remained close with one friend.

School refusal problems are often linked to youth's social functioning and this might be the case with Sofia, whose internal distress and social avoidance increased while her peer functioning and school attendance decreased. Thus improving Sofia's peer relations would probably be an important therapy goal, to help her return to school. Being held back a grade would also represent a potentially large disruption in Sofia's existing peer relationships. Sofia might need help maintaining her peer relationships or developing new ones. Thus, based on the information provided, a detailed analysis of Sofia's peer relationships was needed; screening would not be sufficient.

Sofia was concerned about peer acceptance, and especially whether she would "fit in" after being held back a year in school. Thus understanding her current social status might provide a useful starting point for assessment. Sofia might complete the SPPA and the PCQ. The SPPA would provide information about social acceptance and areas of competence. Sofia was already reporting low academic competence, so it would be important to identify other areas of competence, which might be used to strengthen her feelings of belonging in school. The PCQ would provide information about Sofia's current peer crowd affiliation(s). Given her nonattendance at school, Sofia might feel isolated and not a part of any peer crowd. Moreover, reports suggested that Sofia used to be affiliated with the Popular crowd at school, and she now might feel left out or excluded by Popular peers (also a sign of relational victimization, which should also be examined closely). A better understanding of Sofia's peer crowd affiliation(s) would provide valuable information about her current social context and the social opportunities accessible to her. For example, if Sofia reported that she used to be affiliated with the Popular crowd, but that Popular youth now ignored her, this would represent a large shift in her peer network and would need consideration during treatment. If, however, Sofia continued to feel affiliated with the Popular crowd, this could represent a potential area of strength for Sofia.

With respect to her close friendships, Sofia had one close friend, but it was unclear whether Sofia felt supported by her friends or by others in her life. One of the social support measures, such as the CASSS, would help identify Sofia's support from classmates, friends, teachers, and parents. A measure of friendship quality, such as the NRI-R, would also be useful to identify the strengths and weaknesses in her close friendship(s). Identifying and enhancing a close, supportive friendship in the school setting might facilitate Sofia's school attendance. Moreover, Sofia's friends could help support her through the next year's school transition. Thus therapeutic interventions for Sofia could involve developing or building on the strength of her supportive relationships.

It would be especially important to understand whether Sofia was experiencing peer victimization. A measure such as the R-PEQ would be useful and would reveal the specific types of peer victimization Sofia might be experiencing. Peer victimization, especially interpersonal victimization (e.g., social exclusion, embarrassment by others), might be contributing to Sofia's social avoidance and internalizing difficulties (Siegel et al., 2009). If so, treatment might address ways for Sofia to handle these experiences, using cognitive-behavioral strategies such as identifying emotions, appraising threats, and developing strategies for coping with threats (e.g., Ehrenreich, Goldstein, Wright, & Barlow, 2009).

Finally, Sofia worried about how peers perceived her. Thus administering the Social Anxiety Scale for Adolescents would provide normative and clinically useful information for treatment. If Sofia reported high levels of social anxiety, the clinician might focus on improving Sofia's interpersonal functioning and reducing her anxiety in social situations (Masia-Warner, Fisher, Shrout, Klein, & Rathor, 2007). If Sofia reported fear of negative evaluation from peers (an aspect of social anxiety), treatment could focus on cognitive restructuring of the fears and her appraisal of threats. If, on the other hand, Sofia reported distress related to new situations or unfamiliar peers, treatment could focus on exposure to these types of situations; it also would be important to prepare Sofia for a new peer group with her upcoming grade retention in school.

For Sofia, measures used to evaluate treatment progress would depend on the areas targeted in therapy. Most likely, because Sofia and her mother were seeking treatment for Sofia's school refusal, it would be important to track her perception of social acceptance and social support from peers, as well as her friendships and levels of social anxiety over time. Conducting peer assessments might also provide a starting point for discussing Sofia's peer relationships in therapy. For example, a clinician could review Sofia's results with her and ask her to identify her own peer functioning goals. Some of the measures administered at the start of therapy could be used to track treatment outcomes over time. Clinically, it would be important to see that Sofia's perceptions of her acceptance and social support increased over time (Rigby, 2000).

CONCLUSIONS

In closing, we note a few additional points that may be relevant for understanding youth's peer relations. First, adolescents' romantic relationships are another aspect of peer functioning that may be important to consider. By age 16 years, most youth report having had at least one romantic relationship, and such relationships are often associated with strong emotions but also can be key sources of support (for details, see Davila et al., 2009; Furman et al., 2009; La Greca, Davila, Landoll, & Siegel, 2011; La Greca et al., 2009; Starr, Davila, La Greca, & Landoll, 2011)

Second, we have not discussed atypical youth, such as sexual minority youth or those with obvious cognitive limitations; yet these youth are often rejected, neglected, and even victimized by peers (e.g., Williams, Connolly, Pepler, & Craig, 2005). For such youth, monitoring their peer relations and building their sources of support from friends (and adults) may be critical for their adaptive functioning.

Third, technology is rapidly changing how we communicate and socialize, and this is especially true for youth. Text messaging is now the predominant form of daily friendship communication for youth 12–17 years of age, whereas talking face to face has declined dramatically (Lenhart, 2010). Texting and cell phone use are also major areas of teen–parent conflict

(Lenhart, 2010). Clinicians need to keep abreast of youth's technology use in their peer relations and to understand the potential consequences (e.g., youth who are heavy technology users may be less skilled at developing in-person social skills or negotiating conflict).

In summary, this chapter has provided an overview of youth's peer relationships, strategies for assessing important peer constructs, and suggestions for how to integrate youth's peer relationships into a comprehensive assessment of their emotional and psychological functioning and treatment planning. We hope that the information will encourage and empower clinicians to routinely take into account youth's peer relationships in clinical contexts.

REFERENCES

Aboud, F. E., & Mendelson, M. J. (1998). Determinants of friendship selection and quality: Developmental perspectives. In W. M. Bukowski, A. F. Newcomb, & W. W. Hartup (Eds.), *The company they keep: Friendships in childhood and adolescence* (pp. 87–112). New York: Cambridge University Press.

Achenbach, T. M. (2009). *The Achenbach System of Empirically Based Assessment (ASEBA): Development, findings, theory, and applications.* Burlington: University of Vermont, Research Center for Children, Youth, and Families.

Achenbach, T. M., & Rescorla, L. (2001). *Manual for the ASEBA School-Age Forms & Profiles.* Burlington: University of Vermont, Research Center for Children, Youth, and Families.

Adams, R. E., Santo, J. B., & Bukowski, W. M. (2011). The presence of a best friend buffers the effects of negative experiences. *Developmental Psychology, 47*, 1786–1791.

American Psychiatric Association. (2000). *Diagnostic and statistical manual of mental disorders* (4th ed., text rev.) Washington, DC: Author.

Anthonysamy, A., & Zimmer-Gembeck, M. J. (2007). Peer status and behaviors of maltreated children and their classmates in the early years of school. *Child Abuse and Neglect, 31*, 971–991.

Asher, S., Hymel, S., & Renshaw, P. D. (1984). Loneliness in children. *Child Development, 55*, 1456–1464.

Asher, S. R., & Wheeler, V. A. (1985). Children's loneliness: A comparison of rejected and neglected peer status. *Journal of Consulting and Clinical Psychology, 53*, 500–505.

Bagwell, C. L., Molina, B. S., Pelham, W. E., & Hoza, B. (2001). Attention-deficit hyperactivity disorder and problems in peer relations: Predictions from childhood to adolescence. *Journal of the American Academy of Child and Adolescent Psychiatry, 40*(11), 1285–1292.

Beidel, D. C., Turner, S. M., & Morris, T. L. (2000). Behavioral treatment of childhood social phobia. *Journal of Consulting and Clinical Psychology, 68*, 1072–1080.

Beidel, D. C., Turner, S. M., Sallee, F. R., Ammerman, R. T., Crosby, L. A., & Pathak, S. (2007). SET-C versus fluoxetine in the treatment of childhood social phobia. *Journal of the American Academy of Child and Adolescent Psychiatry, 46*, 1622–1632.

Bonnet, M., Goossens, F., & Schuengel, C. (2011). Parental strategies and trajectories of peer victimization. *Journal of School Psychology, 49*, 385–398.

Bowker, J. C., & Spencer, S. V. (2010). Friendship and adjustment: A focus on mixed-grade friendships. *Journal of Youth and Adolescence, 39*, 1318–1329.

Brendgen, M., Lamarche V., Wanner, B., & Vitaro, F. (2010). Links between friendship relations and early adolescents' trajectories of depressed mood. *Developmental Psychology, 46*, 491–501.

Brendgen, M., Vitarao, F., Turgeon, L., & Poulin, F. (2002). Assessing aggressive and depressed children's social relations with classmates and friends: A matter of perspective. *Journal of Abnormal Child Psychology, 30*(6), 609–624.

Brown, B. B. (1990). Peer groups and peer cultures. In S. S. Feldman & G. R. Elliot (Eds.), *At the threshold: The developing adolescent* (pp. 171–196). Cambridge, MA: Harvard University Press.

Bukowski, W. M., & Adams, R. (2005). Peer relationships and psychopathology: Markers, moderators, mediators, mechanisms, and meanings. *Journal of Clinical Child and Adolescent Psychology, 34*(1), 3–10.

Bukowski, W. M., Brendgen, M., & Vitaro. F. (2007). Peers and socialization. In J. E. Grusec & P. D. Hastings (Eds.), *Handbook of socialization: Theory and research* (pp. 355–381). New York: Guilford Press.

Bukowski, W. M., Hoza, B., & Boivin, M. (1994). Measuring friendship quality during pre- and early adolescence: The development and psychometric properties of the Friendship Qualities Scale. *Journal of Social and Personal Relationships, 11*(3), 471–484.

Cardoos, S. L., & Hinshaw, S. P. (2011). Friendship as protection from peer victimization for girls with and without ADHD. *Journal of Abnormal Child Psychology, 39*(7), 1035–1045.

Coie, J. D., Dodge, K. A., & Kupersmidt, J. B. (1990). Peer group behavior and social status. In S. R. Asher & J. D. Coie (Eds.), *Peer rejection in childhood* (pp. 17–59). New York: Cambridge University Press.

Cook, C. R., Williams, K. R., Guerra, N. G., Kim, T. E., & Sadek, S. (2010). Predictors of bullying and victimization in childhood and adolescence: A meta-analytic investigation. *School Psychology Quarterly, 25*(2), 65–83.

Coyne, S. M., Archer, J., & Eslea, M. (2006). "We're not friends anymore! Unless . . .": The frequency and harmfulness of indirect, relational and social aggression. *Aggressive Behavior, 32*, 294–307.

Crick, N. R., & Bigbee, M. A. (1998). Relational and overt forms of peer victimization: A multi-informant approach. *Journal of Consulting and Clinical Psychology, 66*, 337–347.

Crick, N., Casas, J., & Ku, H. (1999). Relational and physical forms of peer victimization in preschool. *Developmental Psychology, 35*(2), 376–385.

Crick, N. R., & Grotpeter, J. K. (1996). Children's treatment by peers: Victims of relational and overt aggression. *Development and Psychopathology, 8*, 367–380.

Crick, N. R., & Nelson, D. A. (2002). Relational and physical victimization within friendships: Nobody told me there'd be friends like these. *Journal of Abnormal Child Psychology, 30*, 599–607.

Crick, N. R., Ostrov, J. M., & Werner, N. E. (2006). A longitudinal study of relational aggression, physical aggression, and children's social-psychological adjustment. *Journal of Abnormal Child Psychology, 34*, 131–142.

Cullerton-Sen, C., & Crick, N. R. (2005). Understanding the effects of physical and relational victimization: The utility of multiple perspectives in predicting social-emotional adjustment. *School Psychology Review, 34*, 147–160.

Davila, J., La Greca, A. M., Starr, L. R., & Landoll, R. (2010). Anxiety disorders in adolescence. In J. G. Beck (Ed.), *Interpersonal processes in the anxiety disorders: Implications for understanding psychopathology and treatment* (pp. 97–124). Washington, DC: American Psychological Association.

Davila, J., Steinberg, S. J., Ramsay, M., Stroud, C. B., Starr, L., & Yoneda, A. (2009). Assessing romantic competence in adolescence: The Romantic Competence Interview. *Journal of Adolescence, 32*, 55–75.

De Los Reyes, A., & Prinstein, M. J. (2004). Applying depression–distortion hypotheses to the assessment of peer victimization in adolescents. *Journal of Clinical Child and Adolescent Psychology, 33*, 325–335.

Deater-Deckard, K. (2001). Annotation: Recent research examining the role of peer relationships in the development of psychopathology. *Journal of Child Psychology and Psychiatry, 42*, 565–579.

Demaray, M. K., & Malecki, C. (2002). The relationship between perceived social support and maladjustment for students at risk. *Psychology in the Schools, 39*(3), 305–316.

Dinkes, R., Cataldi, E. F., & Lin-Kelly, W. (2007). *Indicators of school crime and safety: 2007* (NCES Publication No. 2008-021/NCJ 219553). Washington, DC: National Center for Education Statistics, Institute of Education Sciences, U.S. Department of Education; and Bureau of Justice Statistics, Office of Justice Programs, U.S. Department of Justice.

Dubow, E. F., & Ullman, D. G. (1989). Assessing social support in elementary school children: The Survey of Children's Social Support. *Journal of Clinical Child Psychology, 18*, 52–64.

Ehrenreich, J. T., Goldstein, C. R., Wright, L. R., & Barlow, D. H. (2009). Development of a unified protocol for the treatment of emotional disorders in youth. *Child and Family Behavior Therapy, 31*(1), 20–37.

Estell, D. B., Jones, M. H., Pearl, R., Van Acker, R., Farmer, T. W., & Rodkin, P. C. (2008). Peer groups, popularity, and social preference: Trajectories of social functioning among students with and without learning disasbilities. *Journal of Learning Disabilities, 41*, 5–14.

Festa, C., & Ginsburg, G. (2011). Parental and peer predictors of social anxiety in youth. *Child Psychiatry and Human Development, 42*, 291–306.

Furman, W. (1989). The development of children's social networks. In D. Belle (Ed.), *Children's social networks and social supports* (pp. 151–172). New York: Wiley.

Furman, W. (1998). The measurement of friendship perceptions: Conceptual and methodological issues. In W. M. Bukowski, A. F. Newcomb, & W. W. Hartup (Eds.), *The company they keep: Friendships in childhood and adolescence* (pp. 41–65). New York: Cambridge University.

Furman, W., & Buhrmester, D. (1985). Children's perceptions of the personal relationships in their social networks. *Developmental Psychology, 21*(6), 1016–1024.

Furman, W., & Buhrmester, D. (1992). Age and sex differences in perceptions of networks of personal relationships. *Child Development, 63*, 103–115.

Furman, W., & Buhrmester, D. (2009). Methods and measures: The Network of Relationships Inventory: Behavioral Systems Version. *International Journal of Behavioral Development, 33*(5), 470–478.

Furman, W., McDunn, C., & Young, B. (2009). The role of peer and romantic relationships in adolescent affective development. In N. Allen & L. Sheeber (Eds.), *Adolescent emotional development and the emergence of depressive disorders* (pp. 318–336). New York: Cambridge University Press.

Gifford-Smith, M., Dodge, K., Dishion, T., & McCord, J. (2005). Peer influence in children and adolescents: Crossing the bridge from developmental to intervention science. *Journal of Abnormal Child Psychology, 33*(3), 255–265.

Gresham, F. M., & Elliot, S. N. (1990). *Social Skills Rating System manual.* Circle Pines, MN: American Guidance Service.

Grotpeter, J. K., & Crick, N. R. (1996). Relational aggression, overt aggression, and friendship. *Child Development, 67*, 2328–2338.

Harter, S. (1985a). *Manual for the Self-Perception Profile for Children.* Denver, CO: University of Denver.

Harter, S. (1985b). *Manual for the Social Support Scale for Children.* Denver, CO: University of Denver.

Harter, S. (1988). *Manual for the Self-Perception Profile for Adolescents.* Denver, CO: University of Denver.

Hartup, W. W. (1996). The company they keep: Friendships and their developmental significance. *Child Development, 67*, 1–13.

Hawker, D. S. J., & Boulton, M. J. (2000). Twenty years' research on peer victimization and psychosocial maladjustment: A meta-analytic review of cross-sectional studies. *Journal of Child Psychology and Psychiatry, 41*, 441–455.

Hecht, D. B., Inderbitzen, H. M., & Bukowski, A. L. (1998). The relationship between peer status and depressive symptoms in children and adolescence. *Journal of Abnormal Child Psychology, 26*, 153–160.

Heinrich, C. C., & Shahar, G. (2008). Social support buffers the effects of terrorism on adolescent depression: Findings from Sderot, Israel. *Journal of the American Academy of Child and Adolescent Psychiatry, 47*, 1073–1076.

Hinshaw, S. P., & Lee, S. S. (2003). Conduct and oppositional defiant disorders. In E. J. Mash & R. A. Barkley (Eds.), *Child psychopathology* (pp. 144–198). New York: Guilford Press.

Hodges, E., Boivin, M., Vitaro, F., & Bukowski, W. (1999). The power of friendship: Protection against an escalating cycle of peer victimization. *Developmental Psychology, 35*(1), 94–101.

Hoza, B. (2007). Peer functioning in children with ADHD. *Journal of Pediatric Psychology, 32*(6), 655–663.

Hoza, B. B., Mrug, S., Gerdes, A. C., Hinshaw, S. P., Bukowski, W. M., Gold, J. A., & Arnold, L. E. (2005). What aspects of peer relationships are impaired in children with attention-deficit/hyperactivity disorder? *Journal of Consulting and Clinical Psychology, 73*, 411–423.

Inderbitzen, H. M., Walters, K. S., & Bukowski, A. L. (1997). The role of social anxiety in adolescent peer relations: Differences among sociometric status groups and rejected subgroups. *Journal of Clinical Child Psychology, 26*, 338–348.

Kandel, D. B. (1978a). Homophily, selection, and socialization in adolescent friendships. *American Journal of Sociology, 84*, 427–436.

Kandel, D. B. (1978b). Similarity in real-life adolescent friendship pairs. *Journal of Personality and Social Psychology, 36*, 306–312.

Kiesner, J., Poulin, F., & Dishion, T. (2010). Adolescent substance use with friends: Moderating and medicating effects of parental monitoring and peer activity contexts. *Merrill Palmer Quarterly, 56*(4), 529–556.

Kingery, J., Erdley, C., Marshall, K., Whitaker, K., & Reuter, T. (2010). Peer experiences of anxious and socially withdrawn youth: An integrative review of the developmental and clinical literature. *Clinical Child and Family Psychology Review, 13*(1), 91–128.

Kovacs, M. (1992). *Manual of the Children's Depression Inventory.* Toronto: Multi-Health Systems.

Kupersmidt, J. B., & Coie, J. D. (1990). Preadolescent peer status, aggression, and school adjustment as predictors of externalizing problems in adolescence. *Child Development, 61*, 1350–1362.

Kuttler, A. F., & La Greca, A. M. (2004). Adolescents' romantic relationships: Do they help or hinder close friendships? *Journal of Adolescence, 27*, 395–414.

Kuttler, A. F., La Greca, A. M., & Prinstein, M. J. (1999). Friendship qualities and social-emotional functioning of adolescents with close, cross-sex friendships. *Journal of Research on Adolescence, 9*(3), 339–366.

Ladd, G. W. (2005). *Children's peer relations and social competence: A century of progress.* New Haven, CT: Yale University Press.

Ladd, G. W. (2006). Peer rejection, aggressive or withdrawn behavior, and psychological maladjustment from ages 5 to 12: An examination of four predictive models. *Child Development, 77*(4), 822–846.

Ladd, G. W., Herald-Brown, S. L., & Andrews, R. K. (2009). The Child Behavior Scale (CBS) revisited: A longitudinal evaluation of CBS subscales with children, preadolescents, and adolescents. *Psychological Assessment, 21*(3), 325–339.

La Greca, A. M. (1981). Peer acceptance: The correspondence between children's sociometric scores and teachers' ratings of peer interactions. *Journal of Abnormal Child Psychology, 9*, 167–178.

La Greca, A. M., Chan, S., Landoll, R. R., & Siegel, R. (2012, April). *Interpersonal peer victimization: Unique contributions to adolescents' symptoms of social anxiety and depression.* Poster presented at the meeting of the International Society for Affective Disorders, London.

La Greca, A. M., Davila, J., Landoll, R., & Siegel, R. (2011). Social anxiety and romantic relationships. In C. Alfano & D. Beidel (Eds.), *Social anxiety in adolescents and young adults: Translating developmental science into practice* (pp. 93–106). Washington, DC: American Psychological Association.

La Greca, A. M., Davila, J., & Siegel, R. (2009). Peer relations, friendships, and romantic relationships: Implications for the development and maintenance of depression in adolescents. In N. Allen & L. Sheeber (Eds.), *Adolescent emotional development and the emergence of depressive disorders* (pp. 299–317). New York: Cambridge University Press.

La Greca, A. M., & Harrison, H. M. (2005). Adolescent peer relations, friendships, and romantic relationships: Do they predict social anxiety and depression? *Journal of Clinical Child and Adolescent Psychology, 34*(1), 49–61.

La Greca, A. M., Herge, W., & Bailey, L. (2012, March). *Disclosure of peer victimization experiences: Who do adolescents tell?* Poster presented at the Society for Research on Adolescence Conference, Vancouver, British Columbia, Canada.

La Greca, A. M., & Lai, B. S. (in press). The role of peer relationships in youth psychopathology: A transdiagnostic approach. In B. Chu & J. Ehrenreich-May (Eds.), *Transdiagnostic mechanisms and treatment of youth psychopathology.* New York: Guilford Press.

La Greca, A. M., & Landoll, R. R. (2011). Peer influences. In W. K. Silverman & A. Field (Eds.), *Anxiety disorders in children and adolescents: Research, assessment and intervention* (2nd ed., pp. 323–346). Cambridge, UK: Cambridge University Press.

La Greca, A. M., & Lemanek, K. L. (1996). Assessment as a process in pediatric psychology. *Journal of Pediatric Psychology, 21,* 137–151.

La Greca, A. M., & Lopez, N. (1998). Social anxiety among adolescents: Linkages with peer relations and friendships. *Journal of Abnormal Child Psychology, 26,* 83–94.

La Greca, A. M., & Mackey, E. (2007). Adolescents' anxiety in dating situations: The potential role of friends and romantic partners. *Journal of Clinical Child and Adolescent Psychology, 36,* 522–533.

La Greca, A. M., & Prinstein, M. J. (1999). The peer group. In W. K. Silverman & T. H. Ollendick (Eds.), *Developmental issues in the clinical treatment of children and adolescents* (pp. 171–198). Needham Heights, MA: Allyn & Bacon.

La Greca, A. M., Prinstein, M. J., & Fetter, M. D. (2001). Adolescent peer crowd affiliation: Linkages with health-risk behaviors and close friendships. *Journal of Pediatric Psychology, 26*(3), 131–143.

La Greca, A. M., Silverman, W. K., Lai, B. S., & Jaccard, J. (2010). Hurricane-related exposure experiences and stressors, other life events, and social support: Concurrent and prospective impact on children's persistent posttraumatic stress symptoms. *Journal of Consulting and Clinical Psychology, 78,* 794–805.

La Greca, A. M., & Stone, W. L. (1993). The Social Anxiety Scale for Children—Revised: Factor structure and concurrent validity. *Journal of Clinical Child Psychology, 22,* 17–27.

Landau, S., & Moore, L. A. (1991). Social skills deficits in children with attention deficit hyperactive disorder. *School Psychology Review, 20,* 235–251.

Landoll, R. R., & La Greca, A. M. (2009, November). Peer victimization in a new generation: Understanding victimization via social networking sites. In A. M. La Greca & J. Davila (Chairs), *Interpersonal processes contributing to adolescent's internalizing symptoms: Implications for research and intervention.* Symposium conducted at the meeting of the Association for Behavioral and Cognitive Therapies, New York.

Landoll R. R., La Greca, A. M., & Lai, B. S. (in press). Aversive peer experiences on social networking sites: Development of the Social Networking Peer Experiences Questionnaire (SN-PEQ). *Journal of Research on Adolescence.*

Lenhart, A. (2008, June 30). *Teens, online stranger contact and cyberbullying: What the research is telling us.* Pew Internet and American Life Project. Retrieved from *www.slideshare.net/PewInternet/teens-online-stranger-contact-cyberbullying*

Lenhart, A. (2010, April 20). *Teens, cell phones and texting: Text messaging becomes centerpiece communication*. Pew Internet and American Life Project. Retrieved from *http://pewresearch.org/pubs/1572/teens-cell-phones-text-messages*

Lohre, A., Lydersen, S., Paulsen, B., Maehle, M., & Vatten, L. (2011). Peer victimization as reported by children, teachers, and parents in relation to children's health symptoms. *Biomed Central Public Health, 11*, 278.

Lopez, C., & DuBois, D. L. (2005). Peer victimization and rejection: Investigation of an integrative model of effects on emotional, behavioral, and academic adjustment in early adolescence. *Journal of Clinical Child and Adolescent Psychology, 34*(1), 25–36.

Lustig, J. L., Wolchik, S. A., & Braver, S. L. (1992). Social support in chumships and adjustment of children of divorce. *American Journal of Community Psychology, 20*, 393–399.

Mackey, E. R., & La Greca, A. M. (2007). Adolescents' eating, exercise, and weight control behaviors: Does peer crowd affiliation play a role? *Journal of Pediatric Psychology, 32*, 13–23.

Mahon, N., Yarcheski, T., & Yarcheski, A. (1995). Validation of the Revised UCLA Loneliness Scale for adolescents. *Research in Nursing and Health, 18*, 263–270.

Malecki, C. K., & Demaray, M. K. (2002). Measuring perceived social support: Development of the Child and Adolescent Social Support Scale (CASSS). *Psychology in the Schools, 3*, 305–316.

Malecki, C. K., Demaray, M. K., & Elliot, S. N. (2000). *The Child and Adolescent Social Support Scale*. DeKalb: Northern Illinois University.

Masia-Warner, C., Fisher, P. H., Shrout, P. E., Klein, R. G., & Rathor, S. (2007). Treating adolescents with social anxiety disorder in school: An attention control trial. *Journal of Child Psychology and Psychiatry, 48*, 676–686.

Mrug, S., Hoza, B., Gerdes, A. C., Hinshaw, S., Arnold, L. E., Hechtman, L., & Pelham, W. E. (2009). Discriminating between children with ADHD and classmates using peer variables. *Journal of Attention Disorders, 12*, 372–380.

Mufson, L., Dorta, K. P., Moreau, D., & Weissman, M. M. (2004). *Interpersonal psychotherapy for depressed adolescents*. (2nd ed.). New York: Guilford Press.

Nansel, T., Overpeck, M., Pilla, R., Ruan, J., Simons-Morton, B., & Scheidt, P. (2001). Bullying behaviors among U.S. youth: Prevalence and association with psychosocial adjustment. *Journal of the American Medical Association, 285*(16), 2094–2100.

Nesdale, D. D., Maass, A., Kiesner, J., Durkin, K., Griffiths, J., & Ekberg, A. (2007). Effects of peer group rejection, group membership, and group norms, on children's outgroup prejudice. *International Journal of Behavioral Development, 31*(5), 526–535.

Newcomb, A. F., Bukowski, W. M., & Pattee, L. (1993). Children's peer relations: A meta-analytic review of popular, rejected, neglected, controversial, and average sociometric status. *Psychological Bulletin, 113*, 99–128.

Olweus, D. (1993). *Bullying at school: What we know and what we can do*. Cambridge, MA: Blackwell.

Paquette, J., & Underwood, M. (1999). Gender differences in young adolescents' experiences of peer victimization: Social and physical aggression. *Merrill–Palmer Quarterly, 45*, 242–266.

Parker, J., & Asher, S. (1987). Peer relations and later personal adjustment: Are low-accepted children at risk? *Psychological Bulletin, 102*(3), 357–389.

Parker, J., & Asher, S. (1993). Friendship and friendship quality in middle childhood: Links with peer group acceptance and feelings of loneliness and social dissatisfaction. *Developmental Psychology, 29*(4), 611–621.

Parker, J., Rubin, K., Erath, S., Wojslawowicz, J., & Buskirk, A. (2006). Peer relationships, child development, and adjustment: A developmental psychopathology perspective. In D. Cicchetti & D. Cohen (Eds.), *Developmental psychopathology: Vol. 1. Theory and method* (2nd ed., pp. 419–493). Hoboken, NJ: Wiley.

Pekarik, E. G., Prinz, R. J., Liebert, D. E., Weintraub, S., & Neale, J. M. (1976). The Pupil Evaluation Inventory: A sociometric technique for assessing children's social behavior. *Journal of Abnormal Child Psychology, 4*(1), 83–97.

Prinstein, M. J., & Aikins, J. W. (2004). Cognitive moderators of the longitudinal association between peer rejection and adolescent depressive symptoms. *Journal of Abnormal Child Psychology, 32,* 147–158.

Prinstein, M. J., Boergers, J., & Vernberg, E. M. (2001). Overt and relational aggression in adolescents: Social-psychological adjustment of aggressors and victims. *Journal of Clinical Child and Adolescent Psychology, 30*(4), 479–491.

Reijntjes, A., Kamphuis, J. H., Prinzie, P., & Telch, M. J. (2010). Peer victimization and internalizing problems in children: A meta-analysis of longitudinal studies. *Child Abuse and Neglect, 34,* 897–976.

Reijntjes, A., Thomaes, S., Bushman, B., Boelen, P., de Castro, B., & Telch, M. (2010). The Outcast-lash-out-effect in youth: Alienation increases aggression following peer rejection. *Association for Psychological Science, 21*(10), 1394–1398.

Rigby, K. (2000). Effects of peer victimization in schools and perceived social support on adolescent well being. *Journal of Adolescence, 23*(1), 57–68.

Rubin, K., Bukowski, W., & Parker, J. (2006). Peer interactions, relationships, and groups. In W. Damon & R. Lerner (Series Ed.) & N. Eisenberg (Vol. Ed.), *Handbook of child psychology: Vol. 3. Social, emotional, and personality development* (6th ed., pp. 571–645). Hoboken, NJ: Wiley.

Rudolph, K., Troop-Gordon, W., Hessel, E., & Schmidt, J. (2011). A latent growth curve analysis of early and increasing peer victimization as predictors of mental health across elementary school. *Journal of Clinical Child and Adolescent Psychology, 40*(1), 111–122.

Siegel, R. S., La Greca, A. M., & Harrison, H. M. (2009). Peer victimization and social anxiety in adolescents: Prospective and reciprocal relationships. *Journal of Youth and Adolescence, 38*(8), 1096–1109.

Silverman, W., & Nelles, W. (1988). The Anxiety Disorders Schedule for Children. *Journal of the American Academy of Child and Adolescent Psychiatry, 27*(6), 772–778.

Slonje, R., & Smith, P. K. (2008). Cyberbullying: Another main type of bullying? *Scandinavian Journal of Psychology, 49,* 147–154.

Starr, L. R., Davila, J., La Greca, A., & Landoll, R. (2011). Social anxiety and depression: The teenage and early adult years. In C. Alfano & D. Beidel (Eds.), *Social anxiety in adolescents and young adults: Translating developmental science into practice* (pp. 75–92). Washington, DC: American Psychological Association.

Stone, W., & La Greca, A. M. (1990). The social status of children with learning disabilities: A reexamination. *Journal of Learning Disabilities, 23*(1), 32–37.

Storch, E. A., Brassard, M. R., & Masia-Warner, C. L. (2003). The relationship of peer victimization to social anxiety and loneliness in adolescence. *Child Study Journal, 33*, 1–18.

Storch, E., Crisp, H., Roberti, J., Bagner, D., & Masia-Warner, C. (2004). Psychometric evaluation of the Social Experience Questionnaire in adolescents: Descriptive data, reliability, and factorial validity. *Child Psychiatry and Human Development, 36*(2), 167–176.

Storch, E., & Masia-Warner, C. (2004). The relationship of peer victimization to social anxiety and loneliness in adolescent females. *Journal of Adolescence, 27*(3), 361–362.

Storch, E., Masia-Warner, C., Crisp, H., & Klein, R.G. (2005). Peer victimization and social anxiety in adolescence: A prospective study. *Aggressive Behavior, 31*, 437–452.

Storch, E., Zelman, E., Sweeney, M., Danner, G., & Dove, S. (2002). Overt and relational victimization and psychosocial adjustment in minority preadolescents. *Child Study Journal, 32*, 73–80.

Vernberg, E. M. (1990). Psychological adjustment and experiences with peers during early adolescence: Reciprocal, incidental, or unidirectional relationships? *Journal of Abnormal Child Psychology, 18*, 187–198.

Vernberg, E. M., Abwender, D. A., Ewell, K. K., & Beery, S. H. (1992). Social anxiety and peer relationships in early adolescence: A prospective analysis. *Journal of Clinical Child Psychology, 21*(2), 189–196.

Vernberg, E. M., Ewell, K. K., Beery, S. H., Freeman, C. M., & Abwender, D. A. (1995). Aversive exchanges with peers and adjustment during early adolescence: Is disclosure helpful? *Child Psychiatry and Human Development, 26*(1), 43–59.

Visconti, K. J., & Troop-Gordon, W. (2010). Prospective relations between children's responses to peer victimization and their socioemotional adjustment. *Journal of Applied Developmental Psychology, 31*(4), 261–272.

Wang, J. J., Iannotti, R. J., Luk, J. W., & Nansel, T. R. (2010). Co-occurrence of victimization from five subtypes of bullying: Physical, verbal, social exclusion, spreading rumors, and cyber. *Journal of Pediatric Psychology, 35*(10), 1103–1112.

Wang, J. J., Iannotti, R. J., & Nansel, T. R. (2009). School bullying among U.S. adolescents: Physical, verbal, relational, and cyber. *Journal of Adolescent Health, 45*(4), 368–375.

Williams, T., Connolly, J., Pepler, D., & Craig, W. (2005). Peer victimization, social support, and psychosocial adjustment of sexual minority adolescents. *Journal of Youth and Adolescence, 34*, 471–482.

Ybrant, H., & Armelius, K. (2010). Peer aggression and mental health problems: Self-esteem as a mediator. *School Psychology International, 31*, 146–163.

12

Parent and Family Assessment Strategies

David J. Hawes and Mark R. Dadds

The effective treatment of child and adolescent problems relies on a sufficient understanding of the family environments in which those problems occur. This chapter is concerned with the assessment data that inform this understanding, and with core strategies for their collection. The methods of family assessment selected by a therapist carry implications for the breadth and quality of the data available to inform conceptualizations of childhood problems and subsequent treatment planning. At the same time, the process through which family assessment data are collected may either reinforce or reduce a family's motivation to join a therapist in pursuing the treatment goals that arise from this assessment. In this chapter we address the clinical assessment of parenting and family factors within an evidence-based framework, giving special attention to the initial interview, self-report inventories, and observational procedures. We advocate for a process-oriented approach to this assessment, in which multi-informant and multimethod measurement is guided by an awareness of the consultation and family process issues that may affect family members' participation and engagement.

DEFINITIONS

The subject of this chapter necessitates that we first define our use of the terms "family" and "parent." Throughout this chapter, "family" refers to the individuals who are responsible for meeting the developmental needs of a child. We use the term "parent" to refer to an individual in a primary caregiver role, who performs executive functions for a family. Our use of these terms recognizes the multiplicity of contemporary forms of family structure, and the impact of recent social trends (and reproductive technologies) on the ways in which families are formed and structured. As such, the individuals represented by such terms potentially include not only biological parents and siblings (i.e., nuclear family members), but those who assume family membership through legal processes of divorce, remarriage, custody change, foster care, and adoption, as well as through informal arrangements (e.g., extended family members, live-in partners).

FUNCTIONS OF FAMILY ASSESSMENT

The assessment of parenting and family factors serves a number of critical functions across various stages of clinical practice with children and adolescents. First—and somewhat paradoxically—information about the impact of child symptoms on family functioning (e.g., disruptions to family routine, distress to family members) can provide important indications of clinical significance, and is therefore a key consideration in the diagnosis of childhood disorders. Second, family assessment is essential to formulation-driven clinical practice, informing functional hypotheses about the controlling variables (e.g., patterns of social rewards and punishment) commonly targeted in evidence-based interventions. Third, a range of family factors represent potential barriers to treatment, and so data on those factors are often needed to guide the effective implementation of planned interventions with families. Such factors include a family's resources for change (e.g., relationship quality, self-regulatory skills), as well as parents' readiness for change and motivation for treatment (Geffken, Keeley, Kellison, Storch, & Rodrique, 2006). Fourth, judgments about a child's prognostic status—potentially within the context of high-risk scenarios involving neglect or maltreatment—require reliable data on parents' capacities to meet the child's current and future developmental needs, and the appropriateness of the demands being made by the child's environment. Finally, the ongoing assessment of parent and family factors plays a key role in the evaluation of treatment progress and outcomes. Such data may allow a therapist faced with poor adherence to treatment to understand and address barriers to change (e.g., parents' self-defeating cognitions, interference from other family members), and may inform important revisions to problem formulation across therapy.

EVIDENCE-BASED ASSESSMENT OF PARENTING AND THE FAMILY

An evidence-based framework for the assessment of clinic-referred children and their families concerns not only the use of methods with established psychometric properties, but the use of empirically supported theory to guide the focus and scope of this assessment (see Hunsley & Mash, 2007). As no formal diagnostic criteria exist with which to define and operationalize family disturbance, there is a need to look to the broader literature in order to "diagnose" it. Evidence-based models of childhood disorders represent means to map out the domains of the family that are of most clinical importance to children and adolescents with various diagnostic and developmental features. These models specify the optimal starting points from which to plan the assessment of parenting and family variables, and they guide the interpretation of the resulting data in relation to data on a child's behavior and development.

The role of parenting in the emergence and maintenance of externalizing problems (primarily the disruptive behavior disorders) has been investigated extensively in recent decades (see Hawes & Dadds, 2005a). Across early to middle childhood, these problems have been associated most directly with high levels of harsh and inconsistent discipline, and low levels of parental warmth and involvement. The parent–child dynamics through which these parenting practices operate include the modeling of aggression, as well as escalating cycles of coercion based on escape/avoidance mechanisms. These cycles function as "reinforcement traps" that reward both parents' and children's use of aversive control tactics (e.g., whining, nagging, shouting, hitting), and that extinguish positive family interactions. The participation of siblings in this coercion also contributes to family-based risk for conduct problems. With these ongoing exchanges, children become increasingly skilled in the use of coercion and in turn more difficult to discipline, as the quality of parenting and family relationships is progressively eroded. Outside the family, peers play an increasing role in the amplification and transformation of externalizing problems across development, through interactions characterized by rejection, coercion, and the selective reinforcement of deviant talk in friendships with antisocial peers. Importantly, parenting processes remain vital to externalizing trajectories across adolescence; however, the precise parent–child dynamics of proximal importance in this period shift from those related to setting limits on behavior in the home, to those related to the regulation of children's peer activities in external settings. As such, the parenting practices of most clinical importance to adolescent conduct problems are considered to be monitoring and supervision (Dishion & Patterson, 2006).

The critical/rejecting parenting associated with coercive cycles in the families of children with conduct problems has also been associated with risk for internalizing problems—in particular, child and adolescent depression (Rapee, 1997; McLeod, Weisz, & Wood, 2007). Alternatively, risk for anxiety disorders has been associated most strongly with overprotective/overcontrolling parenting, wherein parents excessively restrict children's engagement with situations or behaviors based on anticipation of potential threat (Rapee, Schniering, & Hudson, 2009). This may extend to psychological control expressed through intrusive or passive–aggressive parenting behaviors that inhibit autonomy granting. Such parents may withdraw affection or induce guilt as means of discipline, creating a family environment in which acceptance is contingent on a child's behavior (Barber, 1996). Meta-analytic research has not found the association between such parenting practices and child anxiety to be moderated by age, suggesting that they may confer risk across development (McLeod, Wood, & Weisz, 2007). These parenting behaviors are thought to confer risk through a number of mechanisms, potentially functioning to (1) model anxious responding to innocuous events, (2) enhance children's threat interpretations, (3) prevent the habituation of anxious arousal by limiting children's exposure to fear-provoking events, and (4) interfere with the adaptive development of children's emotion regulation skills (Ollendick, Costa, & Benoit, 2010).

The parenting factors that shape child psychopathology often interact and transact with child factors in pathways of risk and protection. There is growing evidence that child characteristics play an important role in moderating the causal effects of parenting on a range of child outcomes. For example, a number of studies suggest that it is only among children characterized by high levels of behavioral inhibition that parenting risk factors for child anxiety produce such outcomes (Degnan, Almas, & Fox, 2010). More complex interactions have been described in emerging research based on the subtyping of childhood conduct problems (e.g., Hawes, Brennan, & Dadds, 2009). Findings suggest that for a subgroup of antisocial children characterized by high levels of callous–unemotional (CU) traits (i.e., lack of guilt and empathy), the patterns of harsh/inconsistent parenting generally associated with childhood conduct problems do not explain such outcomes (see Frick & Viding, 2009). Conversely, the conduct problems of this subgroup appear to be primarily accounted for by low levels of parental warmth (Pasalich, Dadds, Hawes, & Brennan, 2011).

Child characteristics have also been implicated in bidirectional parent–child dynamics in pathways to various childhood disorders. We (Hawes, Dadds, Frost, & Hasking, 2011), for example, found that childhood CU traits uniquely predicted longitudinal deterioration in parental involvement, which in turn uniquely accounted for increased levels of CU traits over time. Likewise, twin data suggest that genetically based child anxiety evokes overcontrolling parenting practices (Eley, Napolitano, Lau, & Gregory, 2010), which in turn account for longitudinal growth in child anxiety above and beyond that predicted by child factors (Edwards, Rapee, & Kennedy, 2010). Similar bidirectional parent–child dynamics have been implicated in childhood pathways to depression (e.g., Dietz et al., 2008).

PRELIMINARY PROCESS ISSUES

Given the influence that parents exert on child outcomes across development—including their role in regulating the involvement of children and adolescents in social contexts outside the home—the most effective

interventions for problems in either home or peer settings generally emphasize family-based targets (Dishion & Stormshak, 2007). Importantly, we
assume that accurate data on family dynamics are essential, but not sufficient, prerequisites for a therapist to act on those dynamics effectively. We
assume that the process of therapeutic change is also driven by the process
of consultation, the most important part of which is the initial assessment
of the family. When a therapist is dealing with a distressed, multiprob-
lem family, the effective management of this process is particularly crucial
(Scott & Dadds, 2009).

Our approach to managing this process (see Dadds & Hawes, 2006)
draws on a structural model of the family system. According to Minuchin
(1974), a healthy family is characterized by overlapping but independent
parent, child, and extended family subsystems, which are organized hierarchically. Most importantly, parents act as an executive subsystem, wherein
they maintain a positive relationship independent of the parenting role and
can function cooperatively to solve family problems. Although there are
few data to show that problematic structural dynamics are direct causal
variables for child psychopathology, evidence suggests that these dynamics
may confer broad risk for childhood problems. In the families of children
with conduct problems, for example, it has been found that the boundaries
between parent and child subsystems often become unclear; the parents'
relationship becomes conflicted; and extended family members get drawn
into failed attempts to manage the children's behavior (Green, Loeber, &
Lahey, 1992; Shaw, Criss, Schonberg, & Beck, 2004). We assume that the
first critical aim of the therapy process is to join with the parental subsystem of the family to form a therapeutic team, and that a therapist is best
placed to influence the broader family system through this parent-centered
partnership.

In our work, we have found that the process difficulties encountered
by therapists in the assessment of parenting and family issues often stem
from a failure to structure initial contacts that are compatible with this aim
(Dadds & Hawes, 2006). The effective management of the consultation process begins with the first telephone contact, at which point it is important
to clarify who is involved in the parenting of the child, and to take the necessary steps to ensure that the relevant members of the parenting subsystem
attend the initial assessment session whenever possible. Many therapists
trained in family systems approaches believe that the first session should
involve all family members, so that the system as a whole can be observed.
This opportunity for observation can come at a significant cost, however. A
therapist's attempts to explore issues beyond those directly associated with
the child are in many cases rejected by parents whose experiences and perceptions of the problem have not first been sufficiently validated. This relies
on parents' being free to express and explore their experiences in the family, no matter how distressing or controversial. Complaints about the effect
of the child's behavior on the parents' lives and marriage, catastrophic fears
about the child's future, and hostile feelings toward the child are common

themes. Parents may withhold such disclosures in the presence of the target child and siblings, while the therapist may be forced to restrict the scope of the interview similarly when such expressions intensify. We therefore recommend scheduling the initial assessment interview with parents alone, in order to allow for the full expression and exploration of the issues and their impact on the family, and for the planning of future contacts as an adult team. There can be important benefits to including an older child or adolescent in the initial assessment session; however, this is generally most advantageous within a session structure that permits the therapist to build relationships with the adolescent and his or her parents separately (e.g., dividing the session to accommodate one-on-one time with respective subsystems). We recommend not proceeding to more formal assessments of family dynamics until open and trusting relationships have been established with all relevant family members. This generally means conducting family observations no earlier than the second assessment session.

THE INITIAL INTERVIEW

The collection of interview data on parenting and family issues typically occurs in the course of a broader clinical interview that also addresses a range of other topics pertaining more directly to the referred child (e.g., dimensions of the presenting problem, developmental and treatment history, social and academic functioning). The effective collection of family-focused data from parents often relies on effective strategies for managing these respective child and family foci in relation to one another. In our consultation model, these strategies are based around the central aim of building a shared perception of the presenting problem with parents. The process through which these data are collected shifts parents away from definitions of the presenting problem as a child issue, and toward a perspective that allows this problem to be considered alongside other issues in the family and their own lives. This is reflected by the structure of the initial interview, within which an initial focus on the child's presenting problem gradually expands to encompass issues of importance to the broader family system. As such, careful attention is paid to the order in which topics are raised, and the management of transitions between these topics (Sanders & Dadds, 1993; Dadds & Hawes, 2006).

The Presenting Problem in the Context of the Family

The initial discussion of the child's presenting problem—typically the first major topic of the clinical interview—is important not only for characterizing its components and typography, but also for establishing the impact of those problems on family members. It also allows for the preliminary assessment of the contextual dynamics and related functions of a child's current behavior and distress. Functional hypotheses are most likely to be

informed by prioritizing attention to the current moment-to-moment interactions of family members, particularly those specific to the settings in
which the child's problem is apparent.

This line of questioning can be facilitated by asking parents to recount
a recent episode involving the problem. What is important is that the
account of such an example is not restricted to the child's problem behavior, but specifies those actions of the child and other family members that
preceded and followed the manifestation of the problem. To emphasize our
interest in understanding these events as they unfold sequentially, we may
ask a parent, "Walk me through the incident, beginning with what was
happening leading up to it, and what happened afterwards, so I can see the
full story." The increasing use of closed-ended questions provides a means
to proceed through this material efficiently, while eliciting appropriately
detailed behavioral data (e.g., "How long did that continue for? . . . What
did he do next? . . . What did you say then? . . . What happened next? . . .").
Follow-up questions can then explore how typical this example may be,
and how such events may differ at other times.

For example, a mother of an aggressive preschool-age girl in our clinic
recently recounted an incident involving her daughter's aggression toward
a sibling, and described placing the child in time out very appropriately.
Follow-up questions, however, revealed that although this was currently
typical for approximately half of these occurrences, at the remaining times
the parent would typically respond by imitating the child's behavior (e.g.,
pinching her back); these occasions were characterized by child aggression
of greater severity, as well as increased levels of parental frustration. The
preliminary hypotheses informed by this line of questioning may guide the
more explicit exploration of family relationship dynamics and related systemic factors at later stages of the interview.

Historical Aspects of Child and Family Functioning

Historical dimensions of the presenting problem, as well as child developmental history, can have significant implications for treatment planning.
For the purpose of assessment, it is important that these historical child
data can be related to historical events in the family environment, especially
events associated with family-based transitions. Such transitions include
those associated with biological maturity, which often involve changes in
context. These changes may result from the effects of maturation on family
dynamics, such as the parenting demands associated with supporting and
setting limits on a child's emerging independence in the toddler years. Other
important transitions result from changes to the structure and composition
of families through various events, including separation and remarriage,
as well as births and deaths. Such events may require children to adjust to
significant change in their relationships with caregivers, including losses
of various kinds, and the formations of new relationships with stepparents
and siblings (Cowan & Hetherington, 1991).

In the developmental psychopathology literature, transitions are conceptualized as salient environmental stress points (Sameroff, 1981). The reorganization that occurs with the stress of transitions can produce both positive and negative outcomes—growth or maladjustment. Importantly, there appear to be important individual differences related to children's sensitivity to the stress of such transitions. For example, children who exhibit developmental characteristics related to poor self-regulation—specifically, low effortful control—appear to be particularly vulnerable to the effects of divorce (Bakker, Ormel, Verhulst, & Oldehinkel, 2011). When a clinician is assessing patterns of historical change concerning the onset and temporal stability of the presenting problem, it is therefore valuable to inquire into concurrent family-based events that may have precipitated this change. It is important that these questions be direct and nonleading (e.g., "You have said that Abigail's worries seemed to escalate soon after her sixth birthday. Can you tell me what else was happening in her life at that time? . . . Were there any changes to family life around that time? . . ."). A similar line of questioning is appropriate when a child's developmental history indicates disruptions or deviations from a typical trajectory (e.g., regression associated with previously achieved milestones, or problems forming attachments).

Parent and Family Issues

The assessment of the various issues that may be adversely affecting a family system represents a distinct challenge within the parent interview. Included here are issues related to parents' mental health and substance use, social support, feelings and attributions about the parent–child relationship, family history of mental health problems, and distress or violence in the marital relationship. These issues may be sensitive, highly emotional, or frightening—to parents and therapists alike. They can also be the issues that carry the most critical implications for the planning and delivery of family-based interventions with complex cases. We find that problems in the assessment of these issues usually lie at two extremes. At one extreme, problems can arise when a therapist fails to raise these issues for discussion, perhaps due to fear of confronting intimate family details or due to conceptual biases about the role of these variables. At the other extreme, problems can occur when these issues are raised in such a way that causes parents to deny their importance, their existence, or the therapist's right to focus on them.

A number of steps can be taken—both before and during this component of the interview—to maximize the likelihood that parents will be receptive to the assessment of these issues. First and foremost, we advise that inquiries about other problems or stressors in the family be initiated only after parents' presenting concerns about the child have been adequately addressed. Doing so reflects a basic respect for those concerns, while at the same time allowing elementary rapport to be established before more sensitive issues are broached. In our assessment model, the focus on these issues is therefore reserved for the final topic of the interview.

Second, the manner in which this component of the interview is introduced to parents can be an important factor in their willingness to shift the focus of discussion from the referred child to their own lives. Parents are often not expecting to be faced with personal questions of this kind when seeking help for their child, and may react adversely when caught off guard. The smooth transition to this focus can be facilitated by first summarizing the child-focused information gathered up to this point, and providing a plain-language rationale for turning to issues in the broader family system (e.g., "With my questions today, I've been trying to build a complete picture of Nicholas's difficulties and his life in general, which is what will allow me to work out the best way that I can help. As part of this, I was also hoping to also ask some standard questions about yourselves and family life more generally, so I can really understand the big picture of what's important. Is that all right with you?"). We make it a rule to explicitly ask parents' permission to proceed at this point—a gesture that should not be underestimated.

Third, by structuring the order in which these issues are raised, it is possible to confront those more sensitive issues most gradually. Although the specific parent and family issues addressed in such an interview may vary, depending on the nature of the referral and the clinical setting, we recommend always proceeding from the least to the most potentially threatening. The flow of this discussion can also be facilitated by organizing these issues around related domains. We typically begin with parents' physical health (e.g., any recent or current illnesses or medical conditions), which follows naturally into parents' mental health (e.g., stress, mood problems, coping strategies) and in turn social support and quality of life (e.g., availability of social networks, pleasant events outside the parenting role). This is typically followed by questions pertaining to parents' relationships in the family, beginning with the parent–child relationship. This can commence with inquiries into how each parent's time with the child is spent, and this parent's role in relation to various caregiver duties, before moving on to the parents' feelings and attributions about the child and the presenting problem. Broader relationships in the family may then be explored—in particular, the parents' own relationship, and the child's relationships with significant others. It is also important to invite parents to identify any additional issues that may qualify as stressors in the family, such as financial strain, problematic work schedules, or difficulties related to broader social contexts (e.g., interference from relatives, neighborhood safety).

Fourth, when a therapist is exploring these issues in an interview attended by two (or more) parents, it is important that each be allowed to respond to these questions without interruption. Given the nature of these issues, the comments provided by one parent can at times evoke strong responses from the other. Although the discussion of such responses can be important to the aim of forming a shared perception of the problem, it is not generally compatible with eliciting necessary details about these issues. Our strategy for facilitating this questioning is to set up a process whereby the respective sequence of issues is addressed with each parent in turn. This can be introduced with a simple rationale and invitation (e.g., "To help me keep track of the things that may be important for me to know, I would like to ask these next questions first to one of you and then the other. Who would like to go first?"). Any interruptions from the other parent can then be dealt with through reminders that she or he will soon have a chance to comment, and while appealing for patience as firmly as necessary.

Recommendations for Assessing Family Relationships

Unique sensitivities related to the parent–child relationship and the marital relationship warrant distinct interviewing strategies. From a clinical perspective, parents' cognitive attributions about their child and the meaning of the presenting problem represent a critical aspect of the parent–child relationship—one that is associated with risk for both externalizing and internalizing disorders (Dadds, Mullins, McAllister, & Atkinson, 2003; Snyder, Cramer, Afrank, & Patterson, 2005; Chen, Johnston, Sheeber, & Leve, 2009). These attributions may include ideas that a child's behavior/ emotion is intentional and under the child's control, is deliberately designed to upset the parent, is a sign of serious mental problems, is inherited from other (disliked) family members (e.g., an abusive ex-spouse), or is in some way a punishment that the parent deserves. Parental attributions may be directly incompatible with the assumptions of the respective treatment model (e.g., expectations that exposure to anxiety-provoking stimuli will cause the child harm). These attributions may also be associated with intense emotion, including explosive anger in reaction to provocative child behavior, and intense guilt following impulses of rejection and resentment toward the child. The intensity of such emotion can easily "flood" parents' capacity to manage child behavior and emotion effectively, and can overwhelm their attempts to initiate and maintain change (Snyder, Edwards, McGraw, Kilgore, & Holton, 1994).

Although therapy may later target such attributions through various means, the critical process at the initial assessment stage is often to help parents to make these thoughts explicit. This can usually be done via a line of questioning that begins with direct, open-ended inquiries (e.g., "How would you describe your feelings toward Oscar at the moment?"), and progresses to closed-ended questions oriented toward the parents' distress (e.g., "How did you feel the last time he really tried to hurt you?", "In those moments when you are really struggling with Oscar's behavior, how bad does it get? . . . What is the worst thought that you have had at that time?", "What is your greatest fear about Oscar's behavior?", "In your darkest moments, what do you think is happening with Oscar?"). The rationale for actively eliciting parent cognitions in this way does not simply concern the collection of important parenting data; it also includes the therapeutic gains associated with expressing these largely unspoken ideas. We advise against attempts to challenge the irrational cognitions of parents at this point, which may be countertherapeutic. It is usually more appropriate that the fears and concerns presented by parents be simply responded to empathically, normalized, and explored openly. As suggested by Scott and Dadds (2009), the most appropriate way to conclude a discussion of these attributions may be with a simple acknowledgment of their importance (e.g., "OK, so let's keep an eye on how you are going with these thoughts and feelings").

In the initial assessment of the marital relationship, we recommend erring on the side of inquiring about how this relationship has been affected by the child's problem, rather than how marital issues may be contributing to the problem. This can be done by first summarizing the child's problem, and then referring to the considerable stress that dealing with such a problem often places on the rest of the family—particularly the marital relationship—in such a way that it is normalized. Parents can then simply be invited to comment on how this may apply to themselves. When the inquiry is approached with a parent-centered process of this kind, emphasis can often be smoothly shifted from notions that the child's issues are causing marital distress, to a more reciprocal conceptualization as the discussion progresses. When signs of significant relationship discord are evident, a more comprehensive assessment (including risk assessment) may be indicated.

Screening for family violence is an important objective for this component of the interview. An effective strategy for this involves responding to any indications of relationship discord, however minor, with probing questions such as "How bad do those disagreements/fights get? . . . What is the worst it has ever gotten?" This line of questioning can then escalate to match the indicated level of risk, with follow-up queries such as "Has anyone ever gotten hurt? . . . What did that involve?" and "How often does it get that bad?" During this discussion, it is important to integrate parents' reports with other forms of assessment regarding family functioning. It is not unknown for parents to report the absence of such problems during this discussion, but to report noteworthy marital distress on relevant inventories. Any discrepancies should be addressed with careful consideration of the individuals concerned. For example, one parent may have been coerced by the other into not talking about any problems beyond those concerning the child, and confronting parents with this information within a session may in some cases increase the risk of violence afterward. When this is suspected, it is advisable to schedule a visit with the spouse reporting marital distress (or depression, etc.) alone—perhaps in the context of assessing the child—to explore the extent of conflict, violence, and the possible implications of discussing these issues openly.

SELF-REPORT INVENTORIES

Self-report inventories are used widely in the collection of parent and child report data on a range of parenting and family variables. These questionnaires benefit from the advantages commonly associated with analogous measures of child characteristics and psychopathology, such as efficiency; the capacity to assess a broad range of domains and levels of functioning; the comparison of an individual against various normative and clinical reference groups; and the potential to facilitate disclosure about events and experiences that respondents may be reluctant to discuss with an interviewer or with another person present. A review of psychometric studies of eight well-recognized measures of parenting by Morsbach and Prinz (2006) generally supported the convergent validity between parental self-report and other methods of measurement in this area. Moderate levels of concordance between parent and child report data were identified, particularly in the area of discipline, with estimates ranging from .23 to .37. Convergence between parental self-report and observational data was generally higher, ranging from .15 to .63.

It has been argued, however, that these instruments may also be particularly vulnerable to the distortions inherent in self-report measurement, due to the nature of the constructs they represent. According to Morsbach and Prinz (2006), this vulnerability stems from three broad issues. First, such measures often require parents to make estimates of potentially high-frequency behaviors (e.g., yelling, ignoring misbehavior) over lengthy periods of time (e.g., a month or more). Second, these measures often rely on parents' accurate interpretation of potentially ambiguous parenting terms (e.g., "time out"). Third, many items on such measures can be considered highly sensitive in nature, due to issues of social desirability, intrusiveness, or risk of disclosure to third parties. A number of strategies may be useful in minimizing the limitations of self-report measures of parenting and family environment; the most important of these is a multimethod measurement approach, in which self-report data are integrated with data collection through clinical interviews and direct observation. The collection of multi-informant self-report data is also beneficial in this respect. In other clinical areas (e.g., addiction), it has been found that respondents tend to report more accurately when they know or believe that corroborating evidence will be collected (e.g., Del Boca & Noll, 2000). In addition, issues related to the potential sensitivity of self-report questions in this area can often be addressed effectively in the context of the clinical interview.

The self-report inventories of parenting and family variables reviewed below are not intended to represent the many such measures that are presently available. Rather, we have selected a small number of established and highly practical measures upon which to focus. Key details (including reliability statistics) are reported for these measures in Table 12.1.

TABLE 12.1. Self-Report Inventories of Parenting and Family Domains

Variable	Rating scale	Description	Reliability
Parenting practices	Alabama Parenting Questionnaire (APQ; Shelton et al., 1996)	42 items. Assesses parenting practices, from parent and child report. Five subscales: Poor Monitoring/Supervision, Inconsistent Discipline, Corporal Punishment, Parental Involvement, and Positive Parenting.	Internal consistency: Subscales range from .45 to .80. Test–retest reliability: Subscales range from .84 to .90.
Parenting practices	Parenting Scale (PS; Arnold et al., 1993)	30 items. Assesses dysfunctional discipline practices, from parent report. Three subscales: Laxness, Overreactivity, and Verbosity.	Internal consistency: Subscales range from .63 to .84. Test–retest reliability: Subscales range from .79 to .83.
Parenting practices	Family Accommodation Scale—Parent Report (FAS-PR; Peris et al., 2008)	13 items. Assesses parent/family accommodation of a child's OCD-related behavior, from parent report. Four subscales: Modification of Routines, Participation in Rituals, Informant Distress Associated with Accommodating, and the target child's reactions (Consequences).	Internal consistency: Subscales range from .75 to .83. Test–retest reliability: .76.
Parent–child relationship	Issues Checklist (IC; Robin & Foster, 1989)	44 items. Assesses sources of conflict in the parent–adolescent relationship, from parent and child report.	Test–retest reliability: Ranges from .47 to .81 across parent–child informants.
Parent–child relationship	Children's Report of Parent Behavior Inventory (CRPBI-30; Schludermann & Schludermann, 1988)	30 items. Assesses perceptions of parents' behaviors toward child, from child and parent report. Three subscales: Psychological Control, Acceptance, and Firm Control.	Internal consistency: Subscales range from .68 to .73. Test–retest reliability: Subscales range from .79 to .89.
Parent–child relationship	Conflict Behavior Questionnaire (Prinz et al., 1979)	20 items. Assesses parent–adolescent communication (positive and negative) and conflict behavior from child and parent report.	Internal consistency: Total scale ranges from .88 to .95.
Parental distress	Parenting Stress Index—Short Form (PSI-SF; Abidin, 1995)	36 items. Assesses stressors related to parenting, from parent report. Three scales: Parental Distress, Parent–Child Dysfunctional Interaction, and Difficult Child.	Internal consistency: Subscales range from .80 to .87. Test–retest reliability: Subscales range from .68 to .85.

(continued)

TABLE 12.1. *(continued)*

Variable	Rating scale	Description	Reliability
Parental distress	Child Abuse Potential Inventory (CAPI), 2nd ed. (Milner, 1986)	160 items. Assesses parental behavior associated with risk for child abuse. Includes a composite Abuse scale comprising six subscales (Distress, Rigidity, Unhappiness, Problems with Child, Problems with Family, and Problems with Others).	Internal consistency: Abuse scale ranges from .92 to .96. Test–retest reliability: Abuse scale ranges from .75 (1 day) to .91 (3 months).
Marital relationship	Dyadic Adjustment Scale (DAS; Spanier, 1976)	32 items, parent report. Assesses marital satisfaction and discord. Four subscales: Dyadic Consensus, Dyadic Satisfaction, Dyadic Cohesion, and Affectional Expression.	Internal consistency: Subscales range from .73 to .94. Test–retest reliability: Subscales range from .75 to .87.
Marital relationship	Revised Conflict Tactics Scales (CTS2; Straus et al., 1996)	39 item pairs, parent report. Assesses the strategies couples use to resolve conflict, ranging from calm discussion to extreme verbal and physical aggression. Five subscales: Negotiation, Psychological Aggression, Physical Assault, Injury, and Sexual Coercion.	Internal consistency: Subscales range from .79 to .95. Test–retest reliability: Subscales range from .60 to .76.
Marital relationship	O'Leary–Porter Scale (Porter & O'Leary, 1980)	10 items. Assesses marital conflict in the presence of the target child, from parent report.	Internal consistency: .86. Test–retest reliability: .96.
Marital relationship	Parent Problems Checklist (PPC; Dadds & Powell, 1991)	16 items, parent report. Assesses interparental conflict over parenting duties, including disagreement about child discipline, open conflict over child rearing, and undermining each other's relationship with the child.	Internal consistency: .70. Test–retest reliability: .90.

Externalizing Presentations

Self-report inventories are commonly used to assess parenting practices related to child discipline and behavior management in the families of children referred for externalizing problems. The Alabama Parenting Questionnaire (APQ; Shelton, Frick, & Wootton, 1996) is a 42-item measure that assesses the positive and negative parenting practices most directly related to child and adolescent conduct problems. These parenting practices are represented by five subscales: Poor Monitoring/Supervision, Inconsistent Discipline, Corporal Punishment, Parental Involvement, and Positive Parenting (i.e., responding to desirable child behavior with positive reinforcement). The measure was originally developed for use with parents of children ages 6–17 years, but an empirically supported preschool revision of the measure is now also available (Clerkin, Marks, Policaro, & Halperin, 2007). Support for a 9-item short form of the APQ has also been demonstrated (Elgar, Waschbusch, Dadds, & Sigvaldason, 2007). We (Hawes & Dadds, 2006) found that APQ scores converged with observations of parents' use of praise, and harsh/aversive parenting, in families of boys with clinic-referred conduct problems. APQ scores were also found to reflect change in parenting practices across treatment, and to covary with clinical child outcomes following parenting intervention.

The Parenting Scale (PS; Arnold, O'Leary, Wolff, & Acker, 1993) is a 30-item parent report measure of dysfunctional parenting practices related to disciplining of children ages 2–16 years. The measure consists of a Laxness scale, which assesses how often parents are aware of their children's misbehavior but do not provide discipline; an Overreactivity scale, which assesses parents' emotional reactivity when disciplining; and a Verbosity scale, which assesses how often parents discipline by using detailed explanations or verbal persuasion. Scores on the PS have been found to be related to observations of ineffective discipline (Arnold et al., 1993) and are sensitive to treatment effects (e.g., Whittingham, Sofronoff, Sheffield, & Sanders, 2009).

Another focus of self-report measurement in this area concerns sources of stress or conflict in the parent–child/adolescent relationship. The Issues Checklist (IC; Prinz, Foster, Kent, & O'Leary, 1979; Robin & Foster, 1989) measures the intensity and sources of conflict between parents and adolescents (ages 12–16 years), from parent and child report. It comprises a 44-item list of issues on which adolescents and parents often disagree, with respondents indicating the frequency and intensity of anger with which each topic was discussed in the past month. Issues include those related to chores, curfews, friends, homework, and drugs. Parents and adolescents typically complete identical forms of the measure, with a referred adolescent potentially completing one in relation to each parent. The IC produces three scores for each family member: (1) the quantity of issues discussed; (2) the mean anger intensity level of the endorsed issues; and (3) the weighted average of the frequency and anger intensity level of the endorsed issues (i.e., an estimate of the intensity of anger per discussion). Responses on the IC are commonly used to identify appropriate stimuli for observations of family problem-solving communication. Discrepancies between parent and adolescent responses may also be used to explore differential perceptions of issues within the family system.

Internalizing Presentations

In guidelines for the evidence-based assessment of childhood anxiety, Silverman and Ollendick (2005) recommended five measures of the variables maintaining child and adolescent anxiety, only two of which were measures of family variables: the Children's Report of Parent Behavior Inventory (CRPBI-30; Schludermann & Schludermann, 1988); and the Conflict

Behavior Questionnaire (Prinz et al., 1979). The CRPBI-30 assesses children's perceptions of their mothers' accepting and controlling behaviors toward them. The 30-item questionnaire consists of three subscales: Psychological Control (e.g., "Says, if I really care for her, I would not do things that cause her to worry"), Firm Control (e.g., "Insists that I must do exactly as I am told"), and Acceptance (e.g., "Cheers me up when I am sad"). The Conflict Behavior Questionnaire assesses parent–adolescent communication and conflict behavior during the preceding 2 weeks. It uses 20 (yes–no) items to characterize dissatisfaction with the other family member's behavior and evaluate interactions between the two members.

In addition to these established measures, some promising self-report measures of anxiety-specific aspects of parenting have emerged in recent years. One prominent example is the Family Accommodation Scale—Parent Report (FAS-PR; Peris et al., 2008). This 13-item parent report measure was designed to assess family members' accommodation of a child's behaviors related to obsessive–compulsive disorder (OCD) over the previous month, and is derived from a therapist-rated measure of the degree to which relatives of adults with OCD have accommodated the individual's OCD rituals (Calvocoressi et al., 1995). The FAS-PR measures both the behavioral involvement of family members in the child's OCD (e.g., modification of daily routines, participation in rituals) and the level of family distress and disruption associated with this involvement, via four subscales: Modification of Routines, Participation in Rituals, Informant Distress Associated with Accommodating, and the target child's reaction (Consequences) to family attempts to refrain from accommodation. High scores on the FAS-PR have been found to be predicted by both child symptoms (compulsion severity, oppositional behavior, frequency of washing behavior) and parent anxiety (Flessner et al., 2011).

Parental Stress and Risk

Self-report measures are also used in the assessment of parents' distress and negativity toward their child, including that associated with risk for child maltreatment. The Parenting Stress Index (PSI; Abidin, 1986) assess stressors related to parenting in the family context of children up to the age of 12 years. The Parenting Stress Index—Short Form (PSI-SF; Abidin, 1995) has 36 items and correlates highly with the original 151-item PSI. In addition to producing a total score representing parents' overall experience of parenting stress, the PSI-SF comprises three scales: Parental Distress (the distress a parent feels due to personal factors, such as a lack of social support or parental depression); Parent–Child Dysfunctional Interaction (parent perceptions of interactions with the child as being positive or negative); and Difficult Child (behavioral characteristics of the child that make him or her easy or difficult to manage, due to either temperament and/or noncompliant, defiant, or demanding behavior).

The Child Abuse Potential Inventory (CAPI, second edition) (Milner,

1986) is a 160-item parent report instrument designed to measure parental behavior associated with risk for physical abuse of children. The CAPI produces a composite Abuse scale comprising six primary subscales: a Distress scale (assessing parental anger, frustration, impulse control, anxiety, and depression); a Rigidity scale (assessing the flexibility and appropriateness of parents' expectations of children's behavior); an Unhappiness scale (assessing a parent's personal fulfillment as an individual, as a parent, as a spouse, and as a friend); a Problems with Children and Self scale (assessing parents' perceptions of their child's behavior and their perceptions of their own self-concept as parents); a Problems with Family scale (assessing levels of conflict in the extended family); and a Problems with Others scale (assessing conflict with persons outside the family or community agencies). The composite Abuse scale has been shown to discriminate between proven perpetrators of abuse and control participants (Milner & Wimberley, 1980), and to be sensitive to the effects of interventions for high-risk parents (Wolfe, Edwards, Manion, & Koverola, 1988). Ondersma, Chaffin, Mullins, and LeBreton (2005) developed a brief 24-item version of the CAPI that correlates highly with the original.

The Marital Relationship

Many different self-report inventories have been developed to assess aspects of the marital relationship, including risk of violence. Although such measures are generally not routine in the clinical assessment of a child's family, they provide an efficient means to quantify issues in this domain when indicated. The Dyadic Adjustment Scale (DAS; Spanier, 1976) is a 32-item parent report measure of marital satisfaction and discord comprising four subscales: Dyadic Consensus (spouses' agreement regarding various marital issues); Dyadic Satisfaction (overall evaluation of the marital relationship and level of commitment to the relationship); Dyadic Cohesion (extent to which partners involve themselves in joint activities); and Affectional Expression (degree of affection and sexual involvement in the relationship). Various short forms of the DAS have been developed over time; among the most evaluated and established of these is the seven-item DAS-7 (Sharpley & Cross, 1982; Hunsley, Best, Lefebvre, & Vito, 2001).

The Conflict Tactics Scales (CTS; Straus, 1979) measure the strategies couples use to resolve conflict, ranging from calm discussion to extreme verbal and physical aggression. These scales have been used widely in studies of marital violence, and have undergone extensive measurement research and revision over time (see Straus, Hamby, & Warren, 2003). The CTS2 consists of 39 item pairs (each item is asked once for the respondent and once for the partner), and comprises five subscales: Negotiation, Psychological Aggression, Physical Assault, Injury, and Sexual Coercion. The response categories gauge the frequency with which acts were used during conflict with a partner in the past year.

Other measures address aspects of marital discord that involve a target child. The O'Leary–Porter Scale (Porter & O'Leary, 1980) is a 10-item parent report scale developed to assess the frequency with which overt parental conflict occurs in the presence of the child. High levels of internal consistency (.86) and 2-week test–retest reliability (.96) have been reported for the scale. The Parent Problem Checklist (PPC; Dadds & Powell, 1991) is a 16-item parent report measure of interparental conflict over parenting duties. Six items assess the extent to which parents disagree over rules and discipline for child misbehavior; six items measure the amount of open conflict over child-rearing issues; and four items focus on the extent to which parents undermine each other's relationship with their children. The total number of items rated as problematic in the previous 4 weeks provides an overall Problem scale, while parents' ratings of the intensity of these problems contributes to an Extent scale. The PPC has been used widely in parenting intervention research with families of children with conduct problems; this research has demonstrated that parenting conflict of this kind influences children's outcomes independently of either general marital conflict or marital satisfaction (Morawska & Thompson, 2009).

OBSERVATIONAL PROCEDURES

Direct observation has long been a cornerstone of behavior therapy practice and research, allowing for the systematic analysis of the functional relationships between problematic child behavior and the family environment in which it occurs (e.g., Patterson, 1974). Indeed, much of what we now know about risk and protective processes within the relationship contexts of couples, parents and children, and siblings has its origins in data coded from direct observation. Current conceptualizations of these relationship processes suggest an integral role for direct observation in the multimethod assessment of the family. Notably, it is now widely recognized that the behaviors of functional importance to many psychological disorders occur in highly overlearned patterns (Dishion & Stormshak, 2007; Gottman, 1998). That is, as a result of frequent repetition, they are often performed somewhat automatically and outside of conscious awareness. This means, for example, that the overreactive parenting behavior that characterizes families of children with conduct problems may often be enacted with the same automaticity of other overlearned behaviors, such as driving a car. Importantly, the perspective afforded by the observational coding of these family dynamics is neither limited by family members' explicit awareness of their behavior, nor contaminated by the other biases inherent in self-report.

A primary consideration associated with the observational assessment of the family is "accessibility"—the notion that some events are more amenable to direct observation than others. In fields where dysfunction is associated with highly overt or "public" behavioral events (e.g., parent–child interactions associated with conduct problems, marital conflict), observational coding systems have proliferated. In contrast, systems for observing clinical populations characterized by more covert or "private" behavioral events—such as the families of children and adolescents with anxiety disorders—are far less well established (Silverman & Ollendick, 2005). With regard to the observational setting, there is considerable evidence that the observation of family members in home-based (naturalistic) assessment—traditionally favored by clinical psychologists—is not confounded by the presence of an observer. Although clinic-based (analogue) observations offer a range of advantages (e.g., convenience, control over the conditions under which behavior is observed), measurement research suggests that not all such procedures are representative of typical interactions in the home (see Gardner, 2000).

Planning Observations of the Family

Sanders and Dadds (1993) outlined five key steps in planning and implementing an observational assessment of a clinic-referred family. The first step in this process is the generation of hypotheses about the nature of the family's problem, formulated in terms of directly observable and testable patterns of behavior. These hypotheses—informed where possible by evidence-based models of child psychopathology—guide the subsequent selection of observational strategies.

The second step is to select the target behaviors to be coded. These generally include the features of the child's problems that have prompted the referral, as well as other behaviors of the child, parents or siblings that are hypothesized to be involved in maintaining the problem. Targets can be expressed as discrete behaviors or as interactional sequences, and should be operationalized in terms that are most conducive to direct observation. This is often facilitated by existing observational coding systems, three examples of which are described shortly. The development of such manualized systems is typically data-driven, resulting in behavior codes that are both reliable and economical. These systems vary considerably in terms of the specificity or precision with which codes are operationalized. Molecular (or microsocial) coding systems are the most intensive, specifying discrete, fine-grained behavioral units (e.g., eye contact, criticize, whine); such coding is particularly suited to describing behavior as it unfolds over time. An example of a system based on such coding is the Dyadic Parent–Child Interaction Coding System (DPICS), third edition (Eyberg, Nelson, Duke, & Boggs, 2005). At the other end of the spectrum are molar (or global/ macro-level) coding systems, based on more inclusive behavioral categories. As global or molar systems are often better able than microsocial coding to take the broader context of behavior into account, such ratings have the potential to capture some constructs more appropriately than molecular codes. Examples of such coding can be seen in the Family Problem Solving Code (FAMPROS; Forbes, Vuchinich, & Kneedler, 2001) and the Rapid Marital Interaction Coding System (RMICS; Heyman, 2004).

The third step is the selection of the procedures used to schedule and structure the observation. This includes any task to be given to family members, the means of instructing the family to engage in this task, and the activities of the therapist throughout the process. Structure that deliberately directs a parent to interact with a child is often necessary when the goal is to sample the immediate antecedents and consequences of child behavior. Where the therapist is more interested in the natural topography of parent–child interaction, a less structured approach can be useful in providing data on the extent to which the parent structures activities for the child, provides routine, and gives attention. The most effective procedures for observing patterns of dysfunctional behavior are usually those that best approximate the natural occurrence of these patterns, while providing sufficient procedural structure to prevent conflict or aggression from escalating to a level that may be unusually distressing for participants.

Table 12.2 summarizes the two most widely used observational procedures for eliciting problem behaviors and the family interactions in which they are embedded. The first is a three-part parent–child play task designed to vary the degree of control required by the parent. This approach is suited to young children up to the age of 89 years or so, and is often used in conjunction with a range of coding systems, including the DPICS, the Family Observation Schedule (Sanders, Dadds, & Bor, 1989), and the Family Process Code (Dishion, Gardner, Patterson, Reid, & Thibodeaux, 1983). As children approach middle childhood and adolescence, they become far more conscious of being observed and are less likely to engage in open conflict with parents and siblings. The procedures that are most likely to elicit clinically informative interactions in the families of referred adolescents and older children are those that direct family members to discuss stress-provoking issues, generally in the context of a family problem-solving discussion. Established originally as a method for observing distressed couples, problem-solving discussions can facilitate the sampling of a range of important communication and relationship dynamics within the family. The major points for observation are the extent to which family members actively listen to each other's point of view, take time to agree on a problem definition, and generate solutions and action strategies—or, conversely, interrupt each other, criticize, talk tangentially, and prevent problem solving through vagueness, concreteness, and the expression of hopelessness and despair. Systems for the coding of such discussions include the FAMPROS and the RMICS, as described below.

The fourth step is the selection of a data collection method. The behavior of family members may be recorded and interpreted descriptively (i.e., qualitatively); however, quantitative data are often better suited to clinical purposes such as the evaluation of behavior change. The collection of such data requires that the behavior in question be quantified using appropriate units of measurement, and that a compatible strategy be used to record it. A number of parameters or dimensions of family members' behavior may be useful to index for clinical purposes. The most common of these are frequency, intensity, and temporal properties (e.g., duration). Strategies

TABLE 12.2. Procedures for the Observational Assessment of the Family

Task and age group	Component	Procedural details
Structured play task Parents and young children (ages 2–8 years)	Free play/child-led play	Show the family to a room equipped with age-appropriate toys and table/chairs. Ask the parents to engage the child in free play (e.g., "Let Jimmy choose any activity he wishes. You just play along as you usually would"). (5 minutes)
	Structured task/ parent-led play	Ask the parents and the child to try to complete a goal-directed activity (e.g., puzzle) that is age-appropriate for the child. (5 minutes)
	Cleanup	Ask the parents to supervise the child in cleaning up the toys and materials used in the previous play (e.g., "Please have Jimmy put all the toys away by himself"). (5 minutes)
Family problem-solving discussion Older children (ages 8+ years) and adult couples	Select problem	Ask the parents and child to complete the IC. Alternatively, for the purpose of couple observation, ask each member to nominate three or so topics of recent disagreement.
	Establish setting	Seat the family in a comfortable room with video or two-way mirror facilities, with chairs facing each other in an equidistant circular formation.
	Provide instructions	Ask the family to discuss and attempt to find solutions to the nominated problems. Spend 5–10 minutes on the child's problem and 5–10 minutes on the parents' problems. Ask the family to begin discussing the problem as soon as you (the therapist) leave the room and to continue until you return.
	Debrief	Discuss the attempts to find solutions with the family, and deal with any distress that has arisen. Inform the family that the results of the assessment will be used for treatment planning and that they will be fully informed of the results. Thank the family.

commonly used to record these units include event records (in which every occurrence is recorded), and interval-based methods, including partial-interval, whole-interval, and momentary time sampling (for recommendations regarding these approaches, and recent innovations related to family observation, see Hawes, Dadds, & Pasalich, in press).

The fifth and final step in the use of clinical observation with families is the evaluation of initial hypotheses regarding the role of the family context in the presenting problem. This may be facilitated by using written summaries (e.g., tables, figures), which may in turn facilitate the subsequent communication of results to family members. The five steps outlined here may be repeated with a family at numerous points, in an ongoing process of hypothesis testing.

Observational Coding Systems

Dyadic Parent–Child Interaction Coding System, Third Edition

The third edition of the DPICS (Eyberg et al., 2005) was designed to assess parent–child relationship quality, as expressed through overt verbal and physical behaviors during dyadic interactions. The child behaviors coded by the DPICS are intended to reflect social reciprocity and cooperation in dyadic interaction. The parent codes concern behaviors that express reciprocity, nurturance, and parental control. These codes were developed for use with families of children ages 3–6 years, and are typically applied to parent–child dyads observed in a three-part (child-led play, parent-led play, cleanup) procedure similar to that described in Table 12.2. The DPICS and other closely related coding systems have been used extensively in the evaluation of parenting interventions (e.g., Hawes & Dadds, 2005b, 2006; Thomas & Zimmer-Gembeck, 2007).

The parent and child codes in the DPICS are organized into categories of Verbalization, Vocalization, Physical Behavior, and Response. Parent behavior is captured predominantly in verbalization codes, the broadest of which is Negative Talk; this is defined as any verbal expression of disapproval of the child or the child's attributes, activities, products, or choices. Other parent Verbalization codes (and their respective variants) include Command (Direct, Indirect), Praise (Labeled, Unlabeled), Information Question, Descriptive/Reflective Question, Reflective Statement, Behavioral Description, and Neutral Talk. The remaining parent codes appear in the Physical Behavior categories of Positive Touch and Negative Touch. The codes applied to child behavior are fewer in number, comprising the Verbalization categories of Negative Talk, Command, Question, and Prosocial Talk; the Vocalization categories of Yell, Whine; and the Physical Behavior categories of Negative Touch, Positive Touch. Also coded for children (and potentially parents, where desired) are a range of behaviors classed as Response Categories, which capture sequences of behavior.

These child behaviors are coded in part on the basis of the parent behaviors that precede them, as seen in child responses to parent questions (Answer, No Answer, No Opportunity for Answer) and to parent commands (Comply, Noncomply, No Opportunity for Compliance).

To facilitate the application of these codes, the DPICS specifies an established "priority order" for determining which code applies in instances where a behavior contains elements of more than one category within a class of behavior (e.g., when a parent's praise is phrased as a question). Also included are a set of "decision rules" for the coding of ambiguous behaviors that potentially qualify for more than one code within a category (e.g., when it is uncertain whether a parent's comment is praise or a question). These codes are typically recorded by using a continuous frequency count (event record) of all behaviors observed during each 5-minute component of the observation; however, interval sampling may also be used, especially in live observations. The authors suggest that, depending on the specific purpose of a parent–child assessment, it may be appropriate to use only a subset of the DPICS codes, or to add more target behaviors.

Successive revisions to the DPICS have been conducted to improve the reliability of its codes, and considerable support for this reliability has been reported in research to date (Eyberg et al., 2005). The reliable use of a comprehensive microsocial coding system such as the DPICS typically requires an intensive and ongoing training process. DPICS coder training is most often conducted in the context of broader therapist training in parent–child interaction therapy, as part of approximately 40 hours of basic training across 3–6 months (McNeil & Hembree-Kigin, 2009).

Family Problem Solving Code

The FAMPROS (Forbes et al., 2001) was designed to assess problem-solving characteristics and relationship dynamics in the families of children ages 8 years and older. In addition to drawing on research and theory in family problem solving, this coding system integrates principles from learning theory and family systems theory. The FAMPROS consists of six coding domains—Positive Behavior, Negative Behavior, Participation, Relationships, Coalitions, and Problem Solving—each of which comprises several codes (25 in total). Positive Behavior codes for how much positive behavior (e.g., affection, warmth, agreement, support) each family member directs toward each other family member. Negative Behavior refers to displays of criticism, anger, disagreement, rejection, or the like. The Participation code is used to rate how active each person is in the discussion. The Relationship code is used to rate the amount of interpersonal closeness displayed for each dyad in the sessions (in terms of bidirectional interaction). The Coalitions code captures the extent to which two family members "gang up" on a third family member. Finally, four specific Problem Solving codes are used to characterize the family's efforts: Definition of the Problem, Extent of Resolution, Quality of Proposed Solutions, and Problem Solving Process (i.e., the extent to which family members are able to effectively engage in perspective taking, compromise, and build on each other's suggestions).

The basis for assigning these codes is typically a family problem-solving discussion such as that outlined in Table 12.2. In contrast to a molecular coding system such as the DPICS, the FAMPROS is based on global codes. A coder will view a 10- to 20-minute discussion, either live or recorded, taking into account all variations in speech and expression (e.g., intonation, tone of voice, facial gestures, body gestures, etc.) as well as frequency of behaviors. The dimensions of the respective codes are then rated on a scale from 1 to 7. According to its authors, the FAMPROS typically requires approximately 40 hours of coder training to be used reliably, after which coders can often reliably code a 10-minute observation in 10–15 minutes after one viewing. The FAMPROS has been used in research with a diverse range of families, in which high levels of reliability have been reported (see Forbes et al., 2001).

The Rapid Marital Interaction Coding System

The RMICS (Heyman, 2004) is used in the observational assessment of a couple's relationship quality, and may therefore be used to supplement other measures of the parental relationship in clinic-referred families. The 11-code RMICS was adapted from the 40-code Marital Interaction Coding System–IV (MICS-IV; Heyman, Weiss, & Eddy, 1995), based on a factor analysis of 1,088 couples coded with the MICS over a 5-year period. In doing so, the authors aimed to develop a parsimonious coding system that could be implemented with high reliability, and with greater ease than the full MICS-IV.

The RMICS is typically used to code a couple's behavior during a problem-solving discussion, similar in structure to those already addressed. Specific problems for discussion may be selected by using partners' responses on the DAS to identify topics that each have listed as generating frequent disagreements of late. The basic coding unit in the RMICS is the speaker turn. The RMICS includes five negative codes (Psychological Abuse, Distress-Maintaining Attribution, Hostility, Dysphoric Affect, Withdrawal), four positive codes (Acceptance, Relationship-Enhancing Attribution, Self-Disclosure, Humor), and one neutral code (Constructive Problem Discussion–Solution). These codes are ordered hierarchically in order of decreasing importance to marital conflict, and if a member of the couple emits more than one code during a speaker turn, she or he receives the code highest on the hierarchy. Speaker turns that last more than 30 seconds are interval-coded in 30-second segments (i.e., coded as if a new speaker turn occurs every 30 seconds). The RMICS has been shown to demonstrate strong psychometric properties, and to predict attrition and improvement in interventions for partner aggression. Coders who undertake a weekly training schedule comprising 2 hours of supervised coding and 4 hours of homework can typically use the RMICS reliably after approximately 3 months (Heyman, 2004).

APPLICATION TO THE CASE OF SOFIA

The family assessment principles outlined in this chapter draw attention to the process of the intake assessment already conducted for the case of Sofia (see McLeod, Jensen-Doss, & Ollendick, Chapter 4, this volume). This intake session was attended by Sofia and her mother, Adriana, who reported that Sofia's father (Sergio) was unavailable to attend due to his work schedule. The consultation guidelines we have presented point to various risks associated with this commonplace scenario, which can often be avoided. Most importantly, there was a risk that Sergio would be more reluctant to attend future sessions once he was aware (or simply assumed) that his wife and daughter had already discussed their perspectives on his behavior (including his disagreements with Adriana over the management of the problem, and his arguments with Sofia). This would potentially limit not only the ongoing assessment of these issues, but the potential for the therapist to join with the executive parental subsystem of the family. Given the apparent discord in this subsystem, the process of jointly engaging and assessing Sofia's parents not only might be critical to subsequent therapy, but might only be possible if dealt with at the earliest stage of consultation. For example, Sergio might well have attended the first session if the importance of this had been addressed more explicitly in the initial telephone contact, and relevant logistical issues had been discussed with Adriana or Sergio directly.

In addition, it might have been advantageous to structure this session to include one-on-one interview time with Sofia and each of her parents. This might have facilitated the parent-centered exploration and validation of Adriana's and Sergio's perceptions of the problem, including aspects that might be countertherapeutic to explore in their daughter's presence. These might have included parental attributions about the problem (e.g., Sergio's interpretation of his daughter's avoidance as laziness) and discord in the parents' own relationship (e.g., feelings of blame; disagreement over the definition and management of the problem). Likewise, one-on-one interview time with Sofia might have facilitated the assessment of her perception of the problem in relation to broader family issues and relationships. A key focus for further assessment would be the impact of various issues on the family system, which (in addition to the parental attributions and marital discord already noted) would potentially include maternal anxiety and mood problems, as well as stress related to the language barrier. In line with the interviewing principles we have outlined, issues of this kind would be first explored with Sofia's parents only after their presenting concerns about her had been fully addressed. This component of the interview would commence with a clear rationale, and would be structured in such a way that inquiries about potentially important parent and family issues would be made with each parent in turn, moving from those least to most confronting.

Clinically useful data on Sofia's relationships with her parents might be acquired through interviews, self-report inventories, and structured observation. Theoretically relevant self-report measures, such as the CRPBI and the Conflict Behavior Questionnaire, might be given to Sofia at the end of the interview. The collection of relevant observational data might be achieved by scheduling a family problem-solving discussion for the following session. This could be used to provide descriptive qualitative data on the family's interactions, or video-recorded and coded quantitatively with the FAMPROS. Initial interview data might also indicate some benefit to using self-report and observational methods to further assess the conflict in Adriana and Sergio's own relationship. Sofia's parents might each be asked to complete the DAS, thereby providing data on the quality of their relationship, as well as issues that might form the basis for an observation of their communication in a problem-solving discussion. Should quantitative data be sought on the couple's interactions, this structured discussion might be video-recorded and coded with the RMICS.

APPLICATION TO THE CASE OF BILLY

From a structural perspective, Billy's mother (Mary) alone seemed to function as the executive parental subsystem, and to be relatively unsupported within the broader system of the family. There were also some indications of interference from the extended family subsystem (e.g., accusations that her parenting had contributed to the behavior problems of her children), and she appeared to hold negative attributions about herself as a parent that were consistent with this (e.g., "I have failed my children"). The high levels of distress she was exhibiting might also be associated with attributions she held about the meaning of Billy's behavior for his future (e.g., "Billy is just like Mike, and will therefore also end up in juvenile detention"), and with some potential mood disturbance. Not only are issues of this kind surprisingly common among the families of children referred for conduct problems, but they are also often associated with poor engagement and subsequent treatment dropout. As discussed in this chapter, engagement is most likely to succeed when parents are free to express and explore their concerns, attributions, and emotions openly in the context of an empathic and validating parent-centered interview. In order to conduct such an interview, we would ask Billy's mother to attend the initial assessment session without him (as we usually would all parents of children his age).

Prior to exploring the impact of various issues on the family system—such as Mary's general health and functioning (including her mood and social support), family relationship issues, and financial strain—the interview would be used to assess the impact of the problem on the family, and the family contexts in which Billy's problem behaviors were apparent. Mary would be asked to detail examples of recent incidents that could provide preliminary data on the various parent and sibling behaviors that commonly featured as antecedents and consequences. At the conclusion of this interview, Mary might be asked to complete some self-report inventories (e.g., the APQ) concerning parenting practices that are theoretically associated with conduct problems; this measure might also be given to Billy, who was old enough to complete the youth report form. Depending on the symptoms of mood disturbance reported by Mary during the interview, she might also be given a self-report inventory to assess this more formally (e.g., the Beck Depression Inventory–II; Beck, Steer, & Brown, 1996); similarly, if indications of harsh/abusive parenting were apparent, she might also be asked to complete the CAPI.

An observation session involving Billy and his mother would also probably be scheduled for the following week. If Billy were younger, this might involve a structured play procedure; however, given his age, a family problem-solving discussion would be likely to provide more informative observational data. At the beginning of the session, Billy and his mother would be asked to complete the IC, which the therapist would review to identify appropriate issues for discussion. Billy and his mother would be observed first aiming to resolve his nominated problem, and then hers. This discussion might be used to derive descriptive data on the observed parent–child interactions, or video-recorded and coded quantitatively with the FAMPROS.

SUMMARY AND RECOMMENDATIONS

Clinical assessment of parenting and the family is often complicated by the nature of these domains. By the time many children and adolescents are referred to clinical services, their parents have suffered a long history of failed attempts to manage the presenting problem. In addition to the distress associated with this, many of the family factors implicated in parenting problems (e.g., parental psychopathology, negative parental attributions and feelings toward the child, marital conflict, lack of social support) are distressing in their own right. Such factors are also often associated with poor engagement in child and adolescent mental health services. For these reasons, the most valuable strategies in the assessment of parenting and family domains are those that support the dual aim of eliciting valid and reliable data while building a strong therapeutic relationship with parents. Chief are strategies for structuring and managing the process of family consultation in relation to the participation of family (subsystem) members, and the attention devoted to child versus family issues in relation to one another.

Our key recommendations are to (1) ensure that parents have sufficient space to express and explore perceptions of the presenting problem in the absence of children; (2) apply interview structures that facilitate the integration of a parent's worldview with one in which child issues are considered alongside the other issues affecting the family system; (3) use self-report inventories where appropriate to supplement the perspectives of parents and children obtained via interview; (4) use structured observational procedures to elicit clinically relevant family interactions, and in turn to measure family process variables that may not otherwise be accessible; and (5) draw on empirically supported theories of child development and psychopathology to map out the parenting and family domains of priority to the assessment of children and adolescents with specific diagnostic and developmental features.

REFERENCES

Abidin, R. R. (1986). *Parenting Stress Index* (2nd ed.). Charlottesville, VA: Pediatric Psychology Press.

Abidin, R. R. (1995). *Parenting Stress Index: Test manual* (3rd ed.). Odessa, FL: Psychological Assessment Resources.

Arnold, D. S., O'Leary, S. G., Wolff, L. S., & Acker, M. M. (1993). The Parenting Scale: A measure of dysfunctional parenting in discipline situations. *Psychological Assessment, 5*, 137–144.

Bakker, M. P., Ormel, J., Verhulst, F. C., & Oldehinkel, A. J. (2011). Adolescent family adversity and mental health problems: The role of adaptive self-regulation capacities. The TRAILS study. *Journal of Abnormal Child Psychology, 39*(3), 341–350.

Barber, B. K. (1996). Parental psychological control: Revisiting a neglected construct. *Child Development, 67*, 3296–3331.

Beck, A. T., Steer, R. A., & Brown, G. K. (1996). *Manual for the Beck Depression Inventory–II*. San Antonio, TX: Psychological Corporation.

Calvocoressi, L., Lewis, B., Harris, M., Trufan, S. J., Goodman, W. K., McDougle, C. J., & Price, L. H. (1995). Family accommodation in obsessive–compulsive disorder. *American Journal of Psychiatry, 152*, 441–443.

Chen, M., Johnston, C., Sheeber, L., & Leve, C. (2009). Parent and adolescent depressive symptoms: The role of parental attributions. *Journal of Abnormal Child Psychology, 37*, 119–130.

Clerkin, S. M., Marks, D. J., Policaro, K. L., & Halperin, J. M. (2007). Psychometric properties of the Alabama Parenting Questionnaire—Preschool Revision. *Journal of Clinical Child and Adolescent Psychology, 36*, 19–28.

Cowan, P. A., & Hetherington, E. M. (1991). *Family transitions*. Hillsdale, NJ: Erlbaum.

Dadds, M. R., & Hawes, D. J. (2006). *Integrated family intervention for child conduct problems*. Brisbane, Queensland, Australia: Australian Academic Press.

Dadds, M. R., Mullins, M., McAllister, R. A., & Atkinson, E. (2003). Attributions, affect, and behavior in abuse-risk mothers: A laboratory study. *Child Abuse and Neglect, 27*, 5–45.

Dadds, M. R., & Powell, M. B. (1991). The relationship of interparental conflict and global marital adjustment to aggression, anxiety, and immaturity in aggressive and nonclinic children. *Journal of Abnormal Child Psychology,* 19, 553–567.

Degnan, K. A., Almas, A. N., & Fox, N. A. (2010), Temperament and the environment in the etiology of childhood anxiety. *Journal of Child Psychology and Psychiatry,* 51, 497–517.

Del Boca, F. K., & Noll, J. A. (2000). Collecting valid data from community sources. Truth or consequences: The validity of self-report data in health services research on addictions. *Addiction,* 95, 347–360.

Dietz, L. J., Birmaher, B., Williamson, D. E., Silk, J. S., Dahl, R. E., Axelson, D. A., & Ryan, N. D. (2008). Mother–child interactions in depressed children and children at high risk and low risk for future depression. *Journal of the American Academy of Child and Adolescent Psychiatry,* 47(5), 574–582.

Dishion, T. J., Gardner, K., Patterson, G. R., Reid, J. B., & Thibodeaux, S. (1983). *The Family Process Code: A multidimensional system for observing family interaction.* Unpublished coding manual. (Available at *www.oslc.org/ resources/codemanuals/familyprocesscode.pdf*).

Dishion, T. J., & Patterson, G. R. (2006). The development and ecology of antisocial behavior. In D. Cicchetti & D. J. Cohen (Eds.), *Developmental psychopathology: Vol. 3. Risk, disorder, and adaptation* (2nd ed., pp. 503–541). Hoboken, NJ: Wiley.

Dishion, T. J., & Stormshak, E. (2007). *Intervening in children's lives: An ecological, family-centered approach to mental health care.* Washington, DC: American Psychological Association.

Edwards, S. L., Rapee, R. M., & Kennedy, S. (2010). Prediction of anxiety symptoms in preschool-aged children: Examination of maternal and paternal perspectives. *Journal of Child Psychology and Psychiatry,* 51(3), 313–321.

Eley, T. C., Napolitano, M., Lau, J. Y., & Gregory, A. M. (2010). Does childhood anxiety evoke maternal control?: A genetically informed study. *Journal of Child Psychology and Psychiatry,* 51, 772–779.

Elgar, F. J., Waschbusch, D. A., Dadds, M. R., & Sigvaldason, N. (2007). Development and validation of a short form of the Alabama Parenting Questionnaire. *Journal of Child and Family Studies,* 16, 243–259.

Eyberg, S., Nelson, M., Duke, M., & Boggs, S. (2005). *Manual for the Dyadic Parent–Child Interaction Coding System* (3rd ed.). Retrieved May 10, 2010, from *www.pcit.org*

Flessner, C. A., Freeman, J. B., Sapyta, J., Garcia, A., Franklin, M. E., March, J., & Foa, E. (2011). Predictors of parental accommodation in pediatric obsessive–compulsive disorder: Findings from the Pediatric Obsessive Compulsive Disorder Treatment Study (POTS) trial. *Journal of the American Academy of Child and Adolescent Psychiatry,* 50(7), 716–725.

Forbes, C., Vuchinich, S., & Kneedler, B. (2001). Assessing families with the Family Problem Solving Code. In P. K. Kerig & K. M. Lindahl (Eds.), *Family observational coding systems* (pp. 59–75). Mahwah, NJ: Lawrence Erlbaum.

Frick, P. J., & Viding, E. (2009). Antisocial behavior from a developmental psychopathology perspective. *Development and Psychopathology,* 21, 1111–1131.

Gardner, F. (2000). Methodological issues in the direct observation of parent–child interaction: Do observational findings reflect the natural behavior of participants? *Clinical Child and Family Psychology Review,* 3, 185–198.

Geffken, G. R., Keeley, M., Kellison, I., Storch, E. A., & Rodrigue, J. R. (2006). Parental adherence to child psychologists' recommendations from psychological testing. *Professional Psychology: Research and Practice, 37,* 499–505.

Gottman, J. M. (1998). Psychology and the study of marital processes. *Annual Review of Psychology, 49,* 169–197.

Green, S. M., Loeber, R., & Lahey, B. B. (1992). Child psychopathology and deviant family hierarchies. *Journal of Child and Family Studies, 1,* 341–349.

Hawes, D. J., Brennan, J., & Dadds, M. R. (2009). Cortisol, callous–unemotional traits, and antisocial behaviorbehavior. *Current Opinion in Psychiatry, 22,* 357–362.

Hawes, D. J., & Dadds, M. R. (2005a). Oppositional and conduct problems. In J. Hudson & R. Rapee (Eds.), *Current thinking on psychopathology and the family* (pp. 73–91). New York: Elsevier.

Hawes, D. J., & Dadds, M. R. (2005b). The treatment of conduct problems in children with callous–unemotional traits. *Journal of Consulting and Clinical Psychology, 73*(4), 737–741.

Hawes, D. J., & Dadds, M. R. (2006). Assessing parenting practices through parent-report and direct observation during parent-training. *Journal of Child and Family Studies, 15*(5), 555–568.

Hawes, D. J., Dadds, M. R, Frost, A. D. J., & Hasking, P. A. (2011). Do childhood callous–unemotional traits drive change in parenting practices? *Journal of Clinical Child and Adolescent Psychology, 40*(4), 1–12.

Hawes, D. J., Dadds, M. R., & Pasalich, D. (in press). Observational coding strategies. In J. Comer & P. Kendall (Eds.), *The Oxford handbook of research strategies for clinical psychology.* New York: Oxford University Press.

Heyman, R. E. (2004). Rapid Marital Interaction Coding System (RMICS). In P. K. Kerig & D. H. Baucom (Eds.), *Couple observational coding systems* (pp. 67–93). Mahwah, NJ: Erlbaum.

Heyman, R. E., Weiss, R. L., & Eddy, J. M. (1995). Marital Interaction Coding System: Revision and empirical evaluation. *Behavioral Research and Therapy, 33,* 737–746.

Hunsley, J., Best, M., Lefebvre, M., & Vito, D.(2001). The seven-item short form of the Dyadic Adjustment Scale: Further evidence for construct validity. *American Journal of Family Therapy, 29,* 325–335.

Hunsley, J., & Mash, E. J. (2007). Evidence-based assessment. *Annual Review of Clinical Psychology, 3,* 29–51.

McLeod, B. D., Weisz, J. R., & Wood, J. J. (2007). Examining the association between parenting and childhood depression: A meta-analysis. *Clinical Psychology Review, 27*(8), 986–1003.

McLeod, B. D., Wood, J. J., & Weisz, J. R. (2007). Examining the association between parenting and childhood anxiety: A meta-analysis. *Clinical Psychology Review, 27,* 155–172.

McNeil, C. B., & Hembree-Kigin, T. L. (2010). *Parent–child interaction therapy* (2nd ed.). New York: Springer.

Milner, J. S. (1986). *The Child Abuse Potential Inventory: Manual* (2nd ed.). Webster, NC: Psyctec.

Milner, J. S., & Wimberley, R. C. (1980). Prediction and explanation of child abuse. *Journal of Clinical Psychology, 36,* 875–884.

Minuchin, S. (1974). *Families and family therapy.* Cambridge, MA: Harvard University Press.

Morawska, A., & Thompson, E. (2009). The Parent Problem Checklist: Examining the effects of parenting conflict on children. *Australian and New Zealand Journal of Psychiatry, 43*(3), 260–269.

Morsbach, S., & Prinz, R. (2006). Understanding and improving the validity of self-report of parenting. *Clinical Child and Family Psychology Review, 9*(1), 1–21.

Ollendick, T. H., Costa, N. M., & Benoit, K. E. (2010). Interpersonal processes and the anxiety disorders of childhood. In G. Beck (Ed.), *Interpersonal processes in the anxiety disorders: Implications for understanding psychopathology and treatment* (pp. 71–95). Washington, DC: American Psychological Association.

Ondersma, S. J., Chaffin, M., Mullins, S. M., & LeBreton, J. M. (2005). The Brief Child Abuse Potential Inventory: Development and validation. *Journal of Clinical Child and Adolescent Psychology, 34,* 301–311.

Pasalich, D. S., Dadds, M. R., Hawes, D. J., & Brennan, J. (2011). Do callous–unemotional traits moderate the relative importance of parental coercion versus warmth in child conduct problems?: An observational study. *Journal of Child Psychology and Psychiatry, 52*(12), 1308–1315.

Patterson, G. F. (1974). A basis for identifying stimuli which control behaviors in natural settings. *Child Developmental, 45,* 900–911.

Peris, T. S., Bergman, R. L., Langley, A., Chang, S., McCracken, J. T., & Piacentini, J. (2008). Correlates of accommodation of pediatric obsessive–compulsive disorder: Parent, child, and family characteristics. *Journal of the American Academy of Child and Adolescent Psychiatry, 47*(10), 1173–1181.

Porter, B., & O'Leary, K. D. (1980). Marital discord and childhood behavior problems. *Journal of Abnormal Child Psychology, 8,* 287–295.

Prinz, R. J., Foster, S. L., Kent, R. N., & O'Leary, K. D. (1979). Multivariate assessment of conflict in distressed and nondistressed mother–adolescent dyads. *Journal of Applied Behavior Analysis, 12,* 691–700.

Rapee, R. M. (1997). Potential role of childrearing practices in the development of anxiety and depression. *Clinical Psychology Review, 17,* 47–67.

Rapee, R. M., Schniering, C. A., & Hudson, J. L. (2009). Anxiety disorders during childhood and adolescence: Origins and treatment. *Annual Review of Clinical Psychology, 5,* 335–365.

Robin, A. L., & Foster, S. L. (1989). *Negotiating parent–adolescent conflict: A behavioral–family systems approach.* New York: Guilford Press.

Sameroff, A. J. (1981). Development and the dialectic: The need for a systems approach. In W. A. Collins (Ed.), *Minnesota Symposium on Child Psychology* (Vol. 15, pp. 83–103). Hillsdale, NJ: Erlbaum.

Sanders, M. R., & Dadds, M. R. (1993). *Behavioral family intervention.* Needham Heights, MA: Allyn & Bacon.

Sanders, M. R., Dadds, M. R., & Bor, W. (1989). Contextual analysis of child oppositional and maternal aversive behaviors in families of conduct disordered and non-problem children. *Journal of Clinical Child Psychology, 18,* 72–83.

Schludermann, E. H., & Schludermann, S. M. (1988). *Children's Report of Parent Behavior Inventory (CRPBI-108, CRPBI-30) for older children and adolescents* (Technical report). Winnipeg, Manitoba, Canada: University of Manitoba, Department of Psychology.

Scott, S., & Dadds, M. R. (2009). When parent training doesn't work: Theory-driven strategies. *Journal of Child Psychology and Psychiatry, 50,* 1441–1450.

Sharpley, C. F., & Cross, D. G. (1982). A psychometric evaluation of the Spanier Dyadic Adjustment Scale. *Journal of Marriage and the Family, 44,* 739–741.

Shaw, D. S., Criss, M., Schonberg, M., & Beck, J. (2004). Hierarchies and pathways leading to school-age conduct problems. *Development and Psychopathology, 16,* 483–500.

Shelton, K. K., Frick, P. J., & Wootton, J. (1996). The assessment of parenting practices in families of elementary school-aged children. *Journal of Clinical Child Psychology, 25,* 317–327.

Silverman, W. K., & Ollendick, T. H. (2005). Evidence-based assessment of anxiety and its disorders in children and adolescents. *Journal of Clinical Child and Adolescent Psychology, 34,* 380–411.

Snyder, J., Cramer, A., Afrank, J., & Patterson, G. R. (2005). The contributions of ineffective discipline and parental hostile attributions of child misbehavior to the development of conduct problems at home and school. *Developmental Psychology, 41,* 30–41.

Snyder, J., Edwards, P., McGraw, K., Kilgore, K., & Holton, A. (1994). Escalation and reinforcement in mother–child conflict: Social processes associated with the development of physical aggression. *Development and Psychopathology, 6,* 305–321.

Spanier, G. B. (1976). Measuring dyadic adjustment: New scales for assessing the quality of marriage and similar dyads. *Journal of Marriage and the Family, 38,* 15–28.

Straus, M. A. (1979). Measuring intrafamily conflict and violence: The Conflict Tactics (CT) Scales. *Journal of Marriage and the Family, 41,* 75–88.

Straus, M. A., Hamby, S. L., & Warren, W. L. (2003). *The Conflict Tactics Scales handbook.* Los Angeles: Western Psychological Services.

Thomas, R., & Zimmer-Gembeck, M. J. (2007). Behavioral outcomes of parent–child interaction therapy and Triple P—Positive Parenting Program: A review and meta-analysis. *Journal of Abnormal Child Psychology, 35,* 475–495.

Whittingham, K., Sofronoff, K., Sheffield, J., & Sanders, M. R. (2009). Stepping Stones Triple P: A randomized controlled trial with parents of a child with an autism spectrum disorder. *Journal of Abnormal Child Psychology, 37,* 469–480.

Wolfe, D. A., Edwards, B., Manion, I., & Koverola, C. (1988). Early intervention for parents at risk of child abuse and neglect: A preliminary investigation. *Journal of Consulting and Clinical Psychology, 56*(1), 40–47.

13

Toward Evidence-Based Clinical Assessment of Ethnic Minority Youth

Armando A. Pina, Nancy A. Gonzales, Lindsay E. Holly,
Argero A. Zerr, and Henry Wynne

This chapter focuses on the clinical assessment of ethnic minority and culturally diverse youth (hereafter referred to as "ethnic minority youth"). Given the field's increased emphasis on utilizing evidence-based assessments, we believe that a chapter on this segment of the child and adolescent population is timely for at least two primary reasons. First, comprehensive information about theoretical, methodological, and practical issues in the assessment of ethnic minority youth is scant, and as such this chapter helps fill a significant gap in the literature. Second, current population estimates show that these youth (both immigrant and U.S.-born) constitute a significant proportion of the nation's existing and growing population. For instance, estimates suggest that there are about 18 million Hispanic/Latino, 12 million African American, 3 million Asian American, and 1 million Native American youth in the United States (U.S. Census Bureau, 2010, 2011). Moreover, Census Bureau projections indicate that the number of ethnic minority youth in the United States will increase significantly over time (e.g., an increase of almost 7 million for Hispanic/Latino, 1 million for African Americans, and 2 million for Asian Americans is expected by 2020).

Emphasis on utilizing evidence-based assessments and the prominent growth of ethnic minority youth in the United States has prompted urgency for determining and establishing *whether* and *how* currently available clinical assessment tools developed for one cultural group can be used with other cultural groups. This is an important issue because data derived from a cultural group may be artifactual if the measures used in the assessment, including diagnostic interviews and rating scales, yield nonequivalent information. More specifically, according to Okazaki and Sue (1995), nonequivalent cross-ethnic information can arise from variations in respondents' values, attitudes, language, and worldviews. As such, we have sought in this chapter to review evidence for the validity/reliability of clinical assessment tools for ethnic minority youth.

Whereas the focus of the chapter is on broadly defined groups of minority youth, it is important to note that variations exist within broad ethnic groups. As such, these groups should not be viewed as homogeneous or "pan-ethnic" (Knight, Roosa, & Umaña-Taylor, 2009), although very few studies report data about ethnic/cultural subgroups (e.g., youth from the Navajo Nation, Filipino youth, etc.). Our broad emphasis is on Hispanic/Latino, African American, Asian American, and Native American youth because these cultural groups are better represented in the extant literature. It is also important to note that although we primarily highlight clinical measures in this chapter, the conceptual issues presented are relevant to other areas (e.g., the assessment of emotion regulation; see Sulik et al., 2010).

In our review of the literature for this chapter, we found a modest body of culturally grounded, sophisticated research. A growing number of methodological and empirical pieces are focusing on two key issues very relevant to the clinical assessment of ethnic minority youth: "measurement equivalence" and "method bias." In an effort to keep within the space constraints of this chapter, but most importantly to advance the knowledge base, we have focused largely on these two issues; in addition, we have sought to fill gaps in the literature relevant to the assessment of ethnic minority youth. Moreover, we found a few studies that reported on the reliability and validity of diagnoses and symptoms ascertained via interviews, along with several studies that reported on the reliability and validity of rating scales for a single minority group. Because this body of research is critical to the process of establishing evidence-based clinical assessments for minority youth, we have also reviewed it briefly herein. Thus we begin with a brief conceptual overview of measurement equivalence and method bias. Then we review quantitative findings for clinical diagnostic measures and rating scales. We conclude with an overview of critical issues in the clinical assessment of ethnic minority youth—issues that must be considered because quantitative demonstration of validity and cross-ethnic equivalence is necessary but not sufficient for culturally sensitive clinical assessment.

MEASUREMENT EQUIVALENCE AND METHOD BIAS

Hui and Triandis (1985) discuss measurement equivalence by focusing on "item equivalence" and "construct validity equivalence" (Knight & Hill, 1998; Knight, Tein, Prost, & Gonzales, 2002; Millsap, 1997; Widaman &

Reise, 1997). Item equivalence (or "factorial invariance") can be evaluated from least restrictive to most restrictive—that is, "configural," "metric," "threshold," and "item uniqueness invariance." "Functional equivalence" and "scalar equivalence" (two main types of construct validity equivalence) can be evaluated by testing the relation of the construct in question to other constructs (Knight et al., 2002; Millsap & Kwok, 2004).

"Configural invariance" refers to whether the same factors of a measure exist across groups (Ghorpade, Hattrup, & Lackritz, 1999; Millsap & Tein, 2004; Vandenberg & Lance, 2000). For example, finding support for the configural invariance of the Revised Children's Manifest Anxiety Scale (RCMAS; Reynolds & Richmond, 1978) (a child-completed measure that assesses negative affect/manifest anxiety) would mean that the three factors found in past research with European American youth (i.e., Physiological Anxiety, Worry/Oversensitivity, and Social Concerns/Concentration) would similarly be found in ethnic minority youth, thereby indicating that both groups share the same concept of negative affect/manifest anxiety. Conversely, lack of support for configural invariance would mean that some scale items do not load on the same factor for minority and European American youth. The RCMAS, for instance, includes a Physiological Anxiety factor scale. If physiological anxiety is noted by Asian American youth as "poor concentration," and not as having "sweaty hands" or "bad dreams" (as represented for European American youth), this would indicate that a different set of items would be needed for Asian American youth. Clearly, evidence supporting configural invariance is important, although not sufficient to support the use of a measure across groups. In fact, other levels relevant to item equivalence and construct validity equivalence are likely to yield more clinically and culturally meaningful information. For instance, metric invariance may be more informative than configural invariance, because it can yield information about important nuances in the presentation of clinical problems that might need to be considered in deriving a diagnosis and designing a treatment plan for a minority child. Below, we explore these issues and possibilities in greater depth.

"Metric invariance" refers to the meaning of scale items across groups (Labouvie & Ruetsch, 1995; Raykov, 2004), and it focuses on item-level factor loadings. Non-invariance in factor loadings could reflect differences in the presentation of a clinical problem or differences in semantic/linguistic interpretation of an item. A semantic/linguistic example can be demonstrated with the RCMAS item "I feel nervous when things don't go the right way." If Puerto Rican youth interpret the word "nervous" as meaning the same as *nervios* (e.g., as in *ataques de nervios,* a culture-bound syndrome),[1] which is distinct from "nervous" (Baer et al., 2003; Guarnaccia,

---

[1]*Ataques de nervios* are intense episodes of emotional distress typically expressed through trembling, crying, and screaming. Episodes often result from disruptions in familial bonds, such as a parent–child conflict or bereavement (see López, Rivera, Ramirez, Guarnaccia, Canino, & Bird, 2009).

Lewis-Fernández, & Marano, 2003; Salgado de Snyder, Diaz-Perez, & Ojeda, 2000), then the loading of this item on the Worry/Oversensitivity factor would be different across these groups, indicating that the RCMAS would lack metric invariance. Clinically, the distinction between "nervous" and *nervios* is important, because for some Hispanic/Latino youth these terms denote anxiety and depression, respectively.

When it comes to the next two invariance levels, "threshold invariance" refers to the severity of the construct needed before a respondent endorses a given categorical item on a scale (Widaman & Reise, 1997), whereas "item uniqueness invariance" refers to the error or unexplained variance in the endorsement of an item (Byrne, Shavelson, & Muthén, 1989). Continuing with the RCMAS, let us suppose that threshold invariance is not supported for the item "I have trouble making up my mind"; this would mean that greater indecisiveness is needed in youth from one group than in youth from another to provide positive endorsement. When it comes to item uniqueness invariance, the focus is on whether the errors in measurement associated with any specific item are the same or different across ethnic groups. As such, variations (or differential measurement error) could differentially attenuate the observed relations between the construct as measured by the focal scale and other related measures across groups. Hence any cross-group differences (or similarities) found could be due to measurement artifact.

Construct validity equivalence—consisting of "functional equivalence" and "scalar equivalence"—is quite important as well. These latter two terms mean that the construct being assessed has similar precursors, consequences, and/or correlates across groups (Knight & Hill, 1998; Knight et al., 2002). More specifically, functional and scalar equivalence refer to the equivalence of the slopes and intercepts, respectively, of the construct validity relations. Thus, to evaluate these two types of equivalence, theoretically relevant predictors need to be utilized in the analyses (Knight, Little, Losoya, & Mulvey, 2004; Pina, Little, Knight, & Silverman, 2009). For the RCMAS, construct validity equivalence could be evaluated by examining cross-group relations to measures of the same construct (i.e., negative affect/manifest anxiety) or related constructs (e.g., depression). If supported, functional and scalar equivalence would indicate that RCMAS anxiety is related to other constructs (e.g., depression) equivalently across groups. Functional equivalence would indicate cross-group similarity in the slopes of the construct validity relations, whereas scalar equivalence would indicate cross-group similarity in the intercepts of these relations. Support for functional and scalar equivalence would indicate that the RCMAS has potential utility for advancing theory—for example, about the relation between negative affect/anxiety and depression in the particular ethnic group being studied. If construct validity equivalence is not supported, this could indicate that the RCMAS has potential limitations, and other clinical measures might need to be used/developed for this ethnic group.

In addition to measurement equivalence, a brief note on method bias is warranted as we work to move closer to securing clinical tools for the assessment of ethnic minority youth. Van de Vijver and colleagues (e.g., Van de Vijver & Poortinga, 1997; Van de Vijver & Tanzer 2004; Van de Vijver & Leung, 2011) point to the problem of method bias, or the degree to which assessment methods (e.g., interviews, questionnaires) yield (non)equivalent information. For instance, data show variability in ethnic differences based on assessment method. In interviews, for example, Asian Americans score significantly lower on social anxiety than European Americans, but they score significantly higher on social anxiety than European Americans on questionnaires; on peer reports and behavioral indices of social anxiety, no significant differences between the two groups typically emerge (Hwu, Yeh, & Chang, 1989; Okazaki, 1997, 2000, 2002; Okazaki, Liu, Longworth, & Minn, 2002; Somers, Goldner, Waraich, & Hsu, 2006; Sue, Ino, & Sue, 1983; Lee et al., 1987; Wittchen & Fehm, 2001). In other words, the assessment method may partially account for cross-cultural differences in the construct being measured. As explained by Matsumoto and Kupperbusch (2001), method differences with Asians may be due to cultural values that discourage display of emotions, especially to outsiders. Since Asian cultures typically value emotional discretion, the use of interviews, peer reports, and behavioral observations may underestimate emotional distress, whereas self-rating scales may yield better information. Given this knowledge, should interviews (and the like) be barred in the clinical assessment of Asian American youth? We do not have a concrete answer to this question. However, we suggest that the role cultural values may play in the clinical assessment of ethnic minority youth needs to be carefully considered, and in this case it seems prudent to give preference to self-rating scales (alone or in combination with other methods) for assessing internalizing symptoms with this population.

PROMISING TOOLS FOR THE ASSESSMENT OF CLINICAL ISSUES IN ETHNIC MINORITY YOUTH

In regard to diagnostic tools for the clinical assessment of ethnic minority youth, we should note that although the knowledge base is growing, little is known about most assessment procedures. For instance, we identified the most widely used and cited child diagnostic interview schedules; however, studies reporting on the validity and reliability of these tools in ethnic minority youth are scant (see Table 13.1). We found several studies reporting on the reliability (and validity; Bravo, Woodbury-Farina, Canino, & Rubio-Stipec, 1993) of *Diagnostic and Statistical Manual of Mental Disorders* (DSM) diagnoses among certain segments of ethnic minority youth, with the Diagnostic Interview Schedule for Children (DISC; Costello, Edelbrock, Dulcan, Kalas, & Klaric, 1984; DISC for DSM-III-R: Fisher et al., 1993; Shaffer et al., 1996; DISC for DSM-IV: Shaffer, Fisher, Lucas,

TABLE 13.1. Diagnostic Interview Schedules Evaluated with Ethnic Minority Youth

Interview	Study	Sample	Reliability	Validity
Preschool Age Psychiatric Assessment (PAPA): DSM-IV	Egger et al. (2006) (English; ~11-day retest); parent estimates provided.	Community sample of 307 youth (ages 2–5 years); 46% girls; 55% African American, 35% European American, 2% Hispanic/Latino, 1% Asian American, 7% other; lay interviewers used.	Kappas were excellent for attention-deficit/hyperactivity disorder and elimination disorders; good for depression, separation anxiety disorder, posttraumatic stress disorder, conduct disorder, and serious emotional disturbance. Remaining kappas were largely fair and a few poor. No significant differences (kappas or ICCs) between African Americans and non-African Americans were found.	Not evaluated.
Diagnostic Interview Schedule for Children (DISC): DSM-IV.	Bravo et al. (2001) (Spanish; ~12-day retest); child and parent estimates provided.	Clinical sample of 146 youth (ages 4–17 years); 33% girls; 100% Puerto Rican; lay interviewers used.	Kappas were excellent for parent-reported separation anxiety disorder (with impairment) and depression in younger children, and for older-youth-reported substance use; kappas were good for parent-reported oppositional defiant disorder in younger children, and for older-youth-reported alcohol abuse. Remaining kappas were largely fair and some poor.	Not evaluated.
DISC: DSM-III-R	Bravo, Woodbury-Fariña, Canino, & Rubio-Stipec (1993); Ribera et al. (1996); Rubio-Stipec et al. (1994) (Spanish; ~2-week retest); child, parent, combined child–parent (c/p) estimates provided.	Community sample of 248 youth, and clinical sample of 74 youth (ages 9–17 years); 58% girls; 100% Puerto Rican; psychiatrist and lay interviewers used.	For combined c/p, community: Kappas were excellent for disruptive disorders, poor for anxiety and depression. For combined c/p, clinical: Kappas were good for depression and disruptive disorders, fair for anxiety. Parent reports about younger children were generally more reliable.	For combined c/p using "best diagnostic estimate" criterion, community: Psychiatrist kappas were good for depression and disruptive disorders, fair for anxiety; lay kappas were fair for disruptive disorders, poor for anxiety and depression. For combined *(continued)*

353

TABLE 13.1. (*continued*)

Interview	Study	Sample	Reliability	Validity
				c/p as above, clinical: Psychiatrist kappas were good for depression and disruptive disorders, fair for anxiety; lay kappas were fair for depression and disruptive disorders, poor for anxiety.
				Clinicians' reports were most concordant with child-reported depression and with parent-reported disruptive disorders.
DISC: DSM-III-R	Roberts, Solovitz, Chen, & Casat (1996) (mostly English; 7- to 14-day retest); adolescent estimates provided.	Clinical sample of 101 youth (ages 12–17 years); ~60% girls; Mexican American, African American, European American; lay interviewers used.	Kappas for separation anxiety disorder, dysthymia, oppositional defiant disorder, conduct disorder, and attention-deficit/ hyperactivity disorder were good. Remaining kappas were largely fair and a few poor. Kappas were slightly better for African Americans (compared to the other two groups) on anxiety, disruptive, and substance use disorders, although the differences were nonsignificant. Kappas were slightly better for Mexican Americans (compared to the other two groups) on affective disorders.	Not evaluated.

Note. Criteria provided by Landis and Koch (1977) were used to evaluate kappa coefficients. The criteria are as follows: kappa > 0.74 indicates excellent reliability; kappa between .59 and .74 indicates good reliability; kappa between .40 and .58 indicates fair reliability; and kappa < 0.40 indicates poor reliability. These criteria are generally consistent with those reported by Shrout (1998). ICC, intraclass correlation coefficient.

Dulcan, & Schwab-Stone, 2000) receiving by far the most research attention. Canino and colleagues (e.g., Bravo et al., 1993; Bravo et al., 2001; Ribera et al., 1996; Rubio-Stipec et al., 1994) translated the DISC (for DSM-III-R and DSM-IV) into Spanish and reported on its (Spanish) reliability and validity in community and clinic samples from Puerto Rico, with lay interviewers versus psychiatrists, and across various time points (e.g., 2 weeks) (see Table 13.1). Roberts, Solovita, Chen, and Casat (1996) evaluated the reliability of diagnoses using the DISC with Mexican American and African American adolescents.

Overall, DISC data suggest that diagnoses of separation anxiety disorder, disruptive disorders, substance use disorders, and mood disorders can be reliably derived among Hispanic/Latino and African American youth (DSM-III-R and DSM-IV). Among preschoolers, the Preschool Age Psychiatric Assessment (PAPA; Egger & Angold, 2004; Egger, Ascher, & Angold, 1999) was found to yield reliable diagnoses for elimination disorder, conduct disorder, attention-deficit/hyperactivity disorder, depression, separation anxiety disorder, posttraumatic stress disorder, and serious emotional disturbance among African Americans. Data also suggest that reliability estimates across sources (child, parent) are typically similar across certain minority and European American populations (see Table 13.1; McClellan & Werry, 2000). Reliability is better when diagnoses are derived by experts (e.g., psychiatrists) than when derived by lay diagnosticians. When diagnoses are based on parent reports, reliability is better for younger children, but self-report data from older children yield better reliability about substance use. However, the reliability of children's diagnoses has not been evaluated in certain U.S. ethnic minority groups (i.e., Asian Americans, Native Americans). In addition, the reliability of minority children's diagnoses has not been systematically evaluated with many other diagnostic interviews, including the Schedule for Affective Disorders and Schizophrenia for School-Age Children (K-SADS; Chambers et al., 1985), the Dominic-R: A Pictorial Interview (Valla, Bergeron, Bidaut-Russell, St.-Georges, & Gaudet, 1997), and the Anxiety Disorders Interview Schedule for DSM-IV: Child and Parent Versions (ADIS-IV: C/P; Silverman & Albano, 1996). The ADIS-IV: C/P reliability study did include 32 Hispanic/Latino participants (Silverman, Saavedra, & Pina, 2001) and Pina and Silverman (2004) found reliability for the Spanish version of the ADIS-IV: C/P to range from .64 to .92 (no additional details were reported). As such, caution is recommended when deriving diagnoses or symptom scores for minority youth, and certainly in using the K-SADS or the Dominic-R for this purpose.

In regard to rating scales, data are scant when it comes to cross-ethnic measurement equivalence and basic reliability (interitem) and validity (concurrent). Tables 13.2 and 13.3 summarize findings from our comprehensive search of the literature, in which we identified studies reporting basic reliability/validity estimates and a few measurement equivalence studies reporting on widely used clinical measures. Most studies reporting basic reliability/validity focused on broad measures of child behavior problems (e.g., the Achenbach System of Empirically Based Assessment [ASEBA]), with several others reporting on measures for specific clinical problems (e.g., the Children's Depression Inventory [CDI]). Across measures, studies typically reported on samples of African American youth, followed by Hispanic/Latino youth. Notably, some studies reported basic reliability/validity in the acceptable range for specific clinical measures, whereas others reporting on the same measures showed lack of cross-ethnic invariance (i.e., failed some measurement equivalence tests). For example, the Center for Epidemiologic Studies Depression Scale (CES-D) has been found to yield adequate alpha reliability estimates for Hispanic/Latino youth (see Table 13.2), but Crockett, Randall, Shen, Russell, and Driscoll (2005) obtained no support for the configural or metric invariance of the CES-D with this same group.

Between-study variability can occur for several reasons, including possible variations in within-group cultural heterogeneity and the fact that alpha reliability estimates are based on "basic" interitem correlations, whereas invariance tests are more robust (based on item-level factor loadings, errors, and slopes). Nonetheless, the measurement equivalence studies reviewed in Table 13.3 indicate a number of promising clinical measures for minority youth.

Briefly, we found this literature to be characterized by studies that relied on adequate sample sizes (with some exceptions; e.g., Varela & Biggs, 2006) and scales designed to measure mood problems/negative affect. A small number of studies also evaluated the cross-ethnic measurement equivalence of disruptive behavior problem scales (e.g., the IOWA Conners Teacher Rating Scale). Most studies reported on samples of Hispanic/Latino and European American youth (e.g., Crockett et al., 2005; Knight, Virdin, Ocampo, & Roosa, 1994; Pina, Little, et al., 2009), followed by studies reporting on African American and European American youth (e.g., Reid, Casat, Norton, Anastopoulos, & Temple, 2001; Tyson, Teasley, & Ryan, 2011). Remarkably, only one study reported on a sample of Native American youth (Beiser, Dion, & Gotowiec, 2000)—a population that is largely underrepresented in the research literature as a whole. Lastly, Gross et al. (2007) and Prenoveau et al. (2009) reported measurement equivalence data of somewhat limited utility, because minority youth were aggregated pan-ethnically for the analyses. Unfortunately, findings from these types of studies cannot be generalized to any particular ethnic minority group.

It also is important to note that across most studies, configural invariance was supported (i.e., the same factors of a measure were found to exist across groups—the "weakest" index of measurement equivalence), with some notable exceptions. For instance, the configural invariance of the Child Behavior Checklist for Ages 6–18 (CBCL/6–18; Internalizing and Externalizing scales) across European American and African American

TABLE 13.2. Selected Rating Scales for Assessing Clinical Problems in Ethnic Minority Youth

Clinical measures	Hispanic/ Latino	African American	Native American	Asian American	Selected studies
			Comprehensive rating scales		
ASEBA: Child Behavior Checklist for Ages 6–18	V R	V R	R	V R	Dionne, Davis, Sheeber & Madrigal (2009); Lau et al. (2004)
ASEBA: Teacher's Report Form	V R	V R	R	V R	Dionne et al. (2009); Lau et al. (2004)
ASEBA: Youth Self-Report	V R	V R	R	V R	Lau et al. (2004); Silmere & Stiffman (2006)
Behavior Assessment System for Children	R	V			McCloskey, Hess, & D'Amato (2003); Jastrowski Mano, Davies, Klein-Tasman, & Adesso (2009)
Behavior Problem Index	R	R	R		Momper & Jackson (2007); Spencer, Fitch, Grogan-Kaylor, & McBeath (2005)
			Internalizing rating scales		
Center for Epidemiologic Studies Depression Scale	V R	R	V R	R	Brown, Meadows, & Elder (2007); Thrane, Whitbeck, Hoyt, & Shelley (2004); Umaña-Taylor & Updegraff (2007)
Children's Depression Inventory	V R	V R	V R	R	Cole, Martin, Peeke, Henderson, & Harwell (1998); Davanzo et al. (2004); Hamill, Scott, Dearing, & Pepper (2009); Kistner, David-Ferdon, Lopez, & Dunkel (2007); Randall & Bohnert (2009); Rieckmann, Wadsworth, & Deyhle (2004)
Fear Survey Schedule for Children—Revised	V R				Varela, Sanchez-Sosa, Biggs, & Luis (2008)
Multidimensional Anxiety Scale for Children	V R	V R	R		Goodkind, LaNoue, & Milford (2010); McLaughlin, Hilt, & Nolen-Hoeksema (2007)

(*continued*)

TABLE 13.2. (continued)

Clinical measures	Hispanic/ Latino	African American	Native American	Asian American	Selected studies
Revised Child Anxiety and Depression Scale				V R	Chorpita, Yim, Moffitt, Umemoto, & Francis (2000)
Revised Children's Manifest Anxiety Scale	V R	R			Argulewicz & Miller (1984); Pina, Little, et al. (2009)
Reynolds Adolescent Depression Scale	V R	V R	V R		LaFromboise, Medoff, Lee, & Harris (2007); Stein et al. (2010)
Social Phobia and Anxiety Inventory for Children	V R	V R			McLaughlin et al. (2007)
State–Trait Anxiety Inventory for Children	R	R			Ortiz, Silverman, Jaccard, & La Greca (2011); Walton, Johnson, & Algina (1999)
State–Trait Anxiety Inventory for Children		R			Walton et al. (1999)
Externalizing rating scales					
Eyberg Child Behavior Inventory	V R	V R	R		Dionne et al. (2009); Gross et al. (2007)
IOWA Conners Rating Scale		V			Reid, Casat, Norton, Anastopoulos, & Temple (2001)
Sutter–Eyberg Student Behavior Inventory		V R			Floyd, Rayfield, Eyberg, & Riley (2004)
Swanson, Nolan, and Pelham–IV		V R			Bussing et al. (2008)

Note. ASEBA, Achenbach System of Empirically Based Assessment; R, reliability demonstrated; V, validity demonstrated. No published report showing inadequate reliability/validity was found.

youth was not supported in one study (Tyson et al., 2011). If these findings are replicated, it may be the case that (1) these measures have lower accuracy in capturing the underlying construct in the cultural groups of interest; (2) there are cultural and contextual factors influencing the basic nature of the construct; or (3) both. As also shown in Table 13.3, threshold, item uniqueness, functional, and scalar equivalence remain largely unexamined in the literature.

ADDITIONAL ISSUES IN THE CLINICAL ASSESSMENT OF ETHNIC MINORITY YOUTH

As noted earlier, quantitative demonstration of validity and cross-ethnic equivalence is necessary but not sufficient for culturally sensitive clinical assessment. For this reason, we articulate a few further critical issues that must be considered in the clinical assessment of ethnic minority youth.

1. *Clinical measures need to be evaluated in the context of informed theory.* That is, they need to be evaluated in terms of the degree to which constructs being assessed conform to theory about the population being measured (e.g., Knight, Tein, et al., 2002; Knight & Zerr, 2010; Pina, Little, et al., 2009). A main implication of informed theory is that a measure may fail certain measurement equivalence tests and still be useful with minority youth. Knight, Roosa, et al. (2009) explain that whereas an item assessing the frequency of suicidal ideation may be appropriate on a scale measuring depression, there may be less variability in responses to this item in a given ethnic group because of a strong religious prohibition against suicide. As a result, the suicidal item may load on different factors for different ethnic groups, due to differences in response variance. Dropping the item due to lack of factorial invariance, however, is not recommended (not only clinically, but also culturally). Instead, if there is a culturally related phenomenon that explains ethnic differences on the item(s), accepting partial invariance on the basis of informed theory would be more appropriate than dropping the "offending" item to secure full invariance.

A related implication of informed theory is that interpretations of expressed emotion in ethnic minority youth need to be considered in the context of culture. We found a general lack of theory-driven and culturally grounded explanations for variations in severity/endorsement of expressed emotions among ethnic minority youth. In the literature, a typical interpretation of such variations is that certain segments of ethnic minority youth are at increased risk for poor mental health outcomes. On the basis of informed theory, however, assigning culturally grounded meaning to clinical phenomena is sometimes worth considering. For instance, among African American youth, emerging evidence shows that physiological arousal is especially intense among those suffering from anxiety (e.g., Carter,

Study	Sample	Clinical measures	Findings
		Comprehensive rating scales	
Guttmannova, Szanyi, & Cali (2008)	Community sample of 1,099 youth (ages 5–11 years); sex not reported; 47% European American, 32% African American, 21% Hispanic/Latino	Behavior Problem Index (BPI; Internalizing and Externalizing scales; Peterson & Zill, 1986).	Results showed no support for the configural invariance of the two BPI scales across Hispanic/Latino, African American, and European American youth. For the short version of the BPI (17 items identical to some from the CBCL), results showed support for the configural, metric, and threshold invariance of the two scales across the three ethnic groups. Item uniqueness, functional, and scalar equivalence were not examined.
Spencer, Fitch, Grogan-Kaylor, & McBeath (2005)	Community sample of 1,691 youth (M age = 10.45 years, SD = 2.83); 49% girls; 53% European American, 28% African American, 19% Hispanic/Latino.	BPI (Internalizing and Externalizing scales; Antisocial, Anxious/Depressed, Dependent, Headstrong, Hyperactive, and Peer Problems subscales).	Results showed no support for the configural invariance of the two-factor or six-factor model of the BPI across Hispanic/Latino, African American, and European American youth.
Tyson, Teasley, & Ryan (2011)	Community sample of 910 adopted youth (ages 6–18 years); sex not reported; 68% European American, 32% African American.	Child Behavior Checklist for Ages 6–18 (CBCL/6–18; Internalizing and Externalizing scales; Achenbach & Rescorla, 2001).	Results showed no support for the cross-ethnic configural or metric invariance of the two CBCL/6–18 broad-band scales.
		Internalizing rating scales	
Crockett, Randall, Shen, Russell, & Driscoll (2005)	Community sample of 10,691 youth (ages 12–18 years); 51% girls; 80% European American, 12% Mexican American, 4% Cuban American, 4% Puerto Rican living in mainland United States.	Center for Epidemiologic Studies Depression Scale (CES-D; Negative Affect, Positive Affect, Somatic Symptoms, and Interpersonal Aspects subscales; Radloff, 1977).	Results showed support for the configural and (partial) metric invariance of the four CES-D subscales across European American and Mexican American youth. There was no support for the configural or metric invariance of the CES-D between European American and Cuban youth or between European American and Puerto Rican (mainland) youth.

Study	Sample	Measure	Findings
			After establishment of configural and metric invariance for the Add Health Self-Esteem Scale between European American and Mexican American youth and European American and Puerto Rican (mainland) youth, and of configural invariance between European American and Cuban American youth, functional and scalar equivalence were supported for the CES-D total score (after controls for sex, age, parental education, and receipt of public assistance) across European American, Mexican American, Cuban American, and Puerto Rican (mainland) American youth. Threshold and item uniqueness invariance were not examined.
Gonzalez, Weersing, Warnick, Scahill, & Woolston (2012)	Clinic sample of 808 parents of youth (ages 5–18 years); 38% girls; 60% European American, 40% African American. Clinic sample of 374 youth (ages 11–18 years); 46% girls; 60% European American, 40% African American.	Screen for Child Anxiety Related Emotional Disorders, Parent and Child Report (SCARED-P, SCARED-C; General Anxiety, Separation Anxiety, Panic/Somatic, Social Phobia, and School Phobia subscales; Birmaher et al., 1999).	Results showed support for the cross-ethnic configural and (partial) metric invariance of the five SCARED-P and five SCARED-C subscales. Threshold, item uniqueness, functional, and scalar equivalence were not examined.
Knight, Virdin, Ocampo, & Roosa (1994)	Community sample of 968 youth (ages 9–13 years); sex not reported; 72% European American, 28% Hispanic/Latino (mostly Mexican American).	Children's Depression Inventory (CDI; Kovacs, 1985).	Results showed support for the cross-ethnic functional and scalar equivalence of the CDI (total scale) with the Child Hostility Scale (Cook, 1986), the Global Self-Worth scale from the Self-Perception Profile for Children (Harter, 1985), and the General Life Events Schedule for Children (Sandler et al., 1986). Configural, metric, threshold, and item uniqueness invariance were not examined.

(continued)

TABLE 13.3. (continued)

Study	Sample	Clinical measures	Findings
Pina, Little, Knight, & Silverman (2009)	Clinic sample of 677 youth referred for anxiety (ages 6–16 years); 47% girls; 59% Hispanic/Latino, 41% European American	Revised Children's Manifest Anxiety Scale (RCMAS; Physiological Anxiety, Worry/ Oversensitivity, and Social Concerns/Concentration subscales; Reynolds & Richmond, 1978); CDI; Fear Survey Schedule for Children—Revised (FSSC-R; Ollendick, 1983).	After the configural, metric, threshold, and item uniqueness invariance of the RCMAS were established across sex and age, results showed support for the cross-ethnic configural, metric, threshold, and item uniqueness invariance of the three RCMAS subscales. After configural, metric, threshold, and item uniqueness invariance were evaluated for the CDI total and the FSSC-R subscales, functional and scalar equivalence for the RCMAS Total Anxiety scale were supported.
Prenoveau et al. (2009)	Community sample of 542 youth (M age = 16.9 years, $SD = 0.81$; 68% girls; 50% European American, 15% Hispanic/Latino, 12% African American, 4% Asian American, 1% Pacific Islander, 13% mixed race/ethnicity, 5% other.	Dysfunctional Attitude Scale, Form A (DAS-A; Dysfunctional Attitudes about Achievement, Dysfunctional Attitudes about Needing Approval, Reverse-Worded Items subscales; Weissman & Beck, 1978; Weissman, 1979).	After the configural and (partial) metric invariance of the DAS-A were established across sex, results showed support for the cross-ethnic (European American and non-European American) configural and (partial) metric invariance of the three DAS-A subscales and the Total scale. Threshold, item uniqueness, functional, and scalar equivalence were not examined.
Russell, Crockett, Shen, & Lee (2008)	Community sample of 9,262 youth (ages 12–18 years); 51% girls; 92% European American, 5% Filipino American, 3% Chinese American.	CES-D (Negative Affect, Positive Affect, Somatic Symptoms, and Interpersonal Aspects subscales).	Results supported the configural, metric, (partial) threshold, and (partial) item uniqueness invariance of the four CES-D subscales between European American and Filipino American youth. Configural invariance was not supported between European American and Chinese American youth for the four CES-D subscales. An alternative three-factor model was found for Chinese American youth, consisting of Negative Affect/Somatic, Positive Affect, and Interpersonal Aspects. Functional and scalar equivalence were not examined.

Varela & Biggs (2006)	Community sample of 150 youth (ages 10–14 years); 47% girls; 35% Mexican, 34% European American, 31% Mexican American.	RCMAS (Physiological Anxiety, Worry/Oversensitivity, Social Concerns/Concentration, and Lie subscales).	Results showed support for the configural, metric, and (partial) item uniqueness invariance of the four RCMAS subscales across Mexican, Mexican American, and European American youth. Functional equivalence also was supported among the four RCMAS subscales across the three groups. Threshold and scalar equivalence were not examined.
Varela, Sanchez-Sosa, Biggs, & Luis (2008)	Community sample of 217 youth (ages 7–16 years); 46% girls; 46% Mexican, 33% Hispanic/Latino, 21% European American.	RCMAS (Physiological Anxiety, Worry/Oversensitivity, Social Concerns/Concentration, and Lie subscales); FSSC-R (Failure and Criticism, Unknown, Injury and Small Animals, Danger and Death, and Medical Phenomena subscales); Multidimensional Anxiety Scale for Children (MASC; Physical Symptoms, Harm Avoidance, Social Anxiety, and Separation Anxiety subscales; March, Parker, Sullivan, Stallings, & Conners, 1997).	Results showed support for the configural invariance of the child- and mother-completed versions of the four RCMAS subscales across Mexican, other Hispanic/Latino, and European American youth. Configural invariance was supported for the child- and mother-completed versions of the five FSSC-R subscales and the four MASC subscales across the three groups. Functional equivalence of the child-completed FSSC-R (total score and five subscales) was supported with the child-completed MASC (total and four subscales) and RCMAS (total and four subscales). Functional equivalence of the mother-completed FSSC-R was not examined. Threshold, item uniqueness, and scalar equivalence were not examined.

Externalizing rating scales

Beiser, Dion, & Gotowiec (2000)	Community sample of 2,044 youth (second and fourth graders; for second graders, M age = 8.5 years, $SD = 0.65$; for fourth graders, M age = 10.6 years, $SD = 0.50$; 52% girls; 76% Native American, 23% European American, 1% Hispanic/Latino, Asian American, or African American.	Child's Assessment by a Parent—Attention-Deficit/Hyperactivity Disorder (CAP-ADHD; Attention-Deficit and Hyperactivity/Impulsivity subscales); Teacher Interview Form—ADHD (TIF-ADHD; Attention-Deficit and Hyperactivity/Impulsivity subscales); Student's Observation of Self—ADHD (SOS-ADHD; Combined ADHD subscale).	Results showed support for the cross-ethnic (Native American and non-Native American) metric invariance of the two CAP-ADHD subscales, the two TIF-ADHD subscales, and the SOS-ADHD scale. Configural, threshold, item uniqueness, functional, and scalar equivalence were not examined.

(continued)

TABLE 13.3. (*continued*)

Study	Sample	Clinical measures	Findings
Gross et al. (2007)	Community sample of 682 youth (ages 2–4 years); 52% girls; 47% Hispanic/Latino, 29% African American, 24% European American	Eyberg Child Behavior Inventory, Intensity subscale (ECBI-I; Eyberg & Ross, 1978; Eyberg & Pincus, 1999).	Results supported the configural invariance of the ECBI-I subscale for European American and non-European American youth (African American and Hispanic/Latino). Threshold, item uniqueness, functional, and scalar equivalence were not examined.
Reid, Casat, Norton, Anastopoulos, & Temple (2001)	Community sample of 3,998 youth (ages 5–11 years); sex not reported; 53% African American, 47% European American	IOWA Conners Teacher Rating Scale (Inattention/Overactivity and Aggression subscales; Loney & Milich, 1982; Pelham, Milich, Murphy, & Murphy, 1989).	Results showed support for the cross-ethnic configural invariance of the two IOWA Conners subscales. Metric, threshold, item uniqueness, functional, and scalar equivalence were not examined.

Miller, Sbrocco, Suchday, & Lewis, 1999; Kingery, Ginsburg, & Alfano, 2007; Lambert, Cooley, Campbell, Benoit, & Stansbury, 2004; Nishina, Juvonen, & Witkow, 2005). Higher levels of physiological arousal among anxious African American youth could be viewed as an acceptable way to express suffering while avoiding the stigma associated with mental illness in the culture (Kingery et al., 2007; Nishina et al., 2005), or even avoiding institutionalization (especially given African Americans' discrimination and segregation history). As such, to assign culturally grounded meaning to anxiety-related physiological symptom levels in African American youth, historical trends and culture may prove more useful than the overpathologizing of these youth.

2. *Measurement equivalence studies need to move beyond cross-ethnic comparisons.* Using ethnicity as the main focal variable in measurement equivalence studies probably offers limited information about a measure's performance. For example, since within-ethnic-group variations exist, it should not be expected that a measure would perform equivalently when administered to U.S.-born Mexican American youth versus recent-immigrant Mexican youth. Immigration status, generational status, ethnic identity, racial/ethnic socialization, and acculturation may prove to be meaningful indicators of a measure's performance among youth within certain broad ethnic groups, especially if the construct targeted by the measure can be influenced by the contextual indicator. As such, explanatory variables may need to be considered as focal variables in equivalence studies.

3. *Cultural norms need to be carefully considered in the clinical assessment of ethnic minority youth.* As illustrated in the discussion of method bias, cultural norms and values can influence outcomes measured by various methods (e.g., self-report, observations). Whereas most method bias research has focused on youth of Asian origin, additional data suggest that this type of bias may also be relevant in the assessment of other minority youth. Native American youth, for example, may appear nonassertive, nonspontaneous, and quiet; make limited eye contact; and appear reluctant to disclose their problems—all of which may be linked to the fact that many Native cultures emphasize perfection and actively reinforce these behaviors (Manson, Bechtold, Novins, & Beals, 1997). Hispanic/Latino children also may present as less expressive, may look down, and may speak softly. Again, these behaviors probably reflect the fact that Latino families typically strive to raise children who are *bien educados* (well mannered) and *respetuosos* (respectful). Both of these concepts translate into being calm, quiet, and agreeable, especially in social situations with adults and authority figures; naturally, English-language ability may also influence these youth's expressiveness (Canino & Guarnaccia, 1997). Therefore, Native American and Latino youth may perform differently during behavior observation tasks and interviews compared to questionnaires. For these reasons, systematic research examining method bias in these groups is needed.

4. *For some clinical issues among ethnic minority youth, new measures need to be developed.* When it comes to negative affect, there is evidence that cross-ethnic variations in expressed emotion may arise when cultures selectively emphasize and elaborate experiential aspects of emotional distress. Outcomes from these cultural processes include distress syndromes that vary from Western taxonomy, as well as differences in the way distress is labeled or emphasized. For example, Guarnaccia and colleagues (Guarnacchia, Martinez, Ramirez, & Canino, 2005; López et al., 2009) surveyed Puerto Rican youth's experiences with *ataques de nervios*. In adults, *ataques* are characterized by screaming uncontrollably, crying spells, trembling, and becoming verbally and/or physically aggressive (Guarnaccia, Rivera, Franco, & Neighbors, 1996). *Ataques* typically occur after a stressful family life event (e.g., death, separation; Guarnaccia et al., 1996). *Ataques* in adults also may include dissociative experiences, seizure-like episodes followed by fainting, and suicidal gestures (Guarnaccia, Canino, Rubio-Stipec, & Bravo, 1993; Lewis-Fernandez, Garrido-Castillo, et al., 2002). One feature that differentiates an *ataque* from a panic disorder episode is its temporal association with the stressful event and the absence of acute fear symptoms (Lewis-Fernandez, Guarnaccia, et al., 2002). In children, research on *ataques* is scant, but data show that *ataques* tend to occur among those who meet DSM criteria for a psychiatric disorder, especially depression rather than anxiety. The only two research studies on *ataques* in children published to date have relied on a single item: "Have you ever had an *ataque de nervios*?" (Guarnaccia et al., 2005; Lopez et al., 2009). Clearly, this is one example where a comprehensive and culturally grounded measure of expressed emotion for youth needs to be developed.

APPLICATION TO THE CASE OF SOFIA

Our review and evaluation of the research literature suggest that practitioners can use selected measures in the assessment of ethnic minority youth, but should do so cautiously. Some measures are especially promising (e.g., the CES-D), but should not be applied across ethnic groups equivalently (see Table 13.3). And, just as in the assessment of nonminority youth, clinicians should rely on the use of multiple measures and informants in assessing minority youth.

For example, in the case of Sofia (the Guatemalan-origin girl experiencing affective difficulties and school refusal behavior as described by McLeod, Jensen-Doss, & Ollendick, Chapter 4, this volume), the CBCL/6–18 could be completed by her parent(s), and Sofia might complete the Reynolds Adolescent Depression Scale, the CDI, and/or the RCMAS. Given evidence from "basic" psychometric and measurement equivalence studies, the CDI and the RCMAS probably would offer good clinical information.

In addition, a thorough clinical assessment of Sofia's case should include a cultural component (i.e., a focus on cultural values, practices, affiliation, and identity) to help guide case conceptualization and treatment plans (see Pina, Villalta, & Zerr, 2009), with particular attention to within-ethnic-group variation or cultural heterogeneity (Knight, Roosa, et al., 2009). One way to gather basic information on cultural factors that could influence minority youth's responses is to use open-ended follow-up questions about emotions, behaviors, and cognitions endorsed at the item level on a given measure. For example, suppose Sofia were to endorse the CDI item "I do not like being with people many times." With follow-up questions, the clinician could learn how, if at all, this feeling was related to a family-referent cultural script (e.g., children should be taught to be good at all times because they represent the family; Knight et al., 2010). That is, Sofia might feel she had disappointed her family by not going to school—especially her father, who, like many Hispanics/Latinos, probably migrated to the United States to offer his children the opportunity to attend college. Moreover, if the family referent cultural script was related to Sofia's distress, then the clinician could probably determine how interpersonal therapy for depression (see Bernal & Rosselló, 2008) might help Sofia and her family. In short, the practitioners might find several mainstream measures useful in Sofia's case, albeit culturally guided probing would be an essential part of the evaluation.

CONCLUDING COMMENTS

A growing number of assessment tools appear to be promising for use with ethnic minority youth, although research remains scant when it comes to the evaluation of such tools with robust methodological strategies. At the very least, studies that include significant proportions of minority youth must report reliability estimates for measures completed by the specific ethnic group(s) being studied. In addition, cross-ethnic comparison studies should report measurement invariance results for the scales used, to assist the process of primary hypothesis testing. In studies focusing on a single ethnic group (e.g., Mexican Americans), it will be important for future research to explore whether within-group variability along theory-relevant cultural variables (e.g., cultural orientation, ethnic/racial socialization) attenuates a measure's ability to assess a focal construct in the study. For example, findings from a study aimed at testing the relations between control, stress reactivity, and anxiety may be biased if the measure used to assess control yields nonequivalent information for less acculturated versus highly acculturated Mexican adolescents. As we move forward with all these endeavors, we can improve our knowledge about mental health issues relevant to minority youth in the United States, and subsequently can help to improve the lives of these youth and their families.

ACKNOWLEDGMENTS

This chapter was supported in part by Grant Nos. K01MH086687 and L60MD001839 from the National Institute of Mental Health and the National Center on Minority Health and Health Disparities, awarded to Armando A. Pina. The content is solely our own responsibility and does not represent the official views of the funding agencies.

REFERENCES

Achenbach, T. M., & Rescorla, L. A. (2001). *Manual for the ASEBA School-Age Forms and Profiles*. Burlington: University of Vermont, Research Center for Children, Youth, and Families.

Argulewicz, E. N., & Miller, D. C. (1984). Self-report measures of anxiety: A cross-cultural investigation of bias. *Hispanic Journal of Behavioral Sciences, 6*, 397–406.

Baer, R. D., Weller, S. C., de Alba Garcia, J. G., Glazer, M., Trotter, R., Pachter, L., & Klein, R. E. (2003). A cross-cultural approach to the study of the folk illness *nervios*. *Culture, Medicine, and Psychiatry, 27*, 315–337.

Beiser, M., Dion, R., & Gotowiec, A. (2000). The structure of attention-deficit and hyperactivity symptoms among Native and non-Native elementary school children. *Journal of Abnormal Child Psychology, 28*, 425–437.

Bernal, G., & Rosselló, J. (2008). Depression in Latino children and adolescents: Prevalence, prevention, and treatment. In S. A. Aguilar-Gaxiola & T. P. Gullotta (Eds.), *Depression in Latinos: Assessment, treatment, and prevention* (pp. 263–275). New York: Springer.

Birmaher, B., Brent, D. A., Chiappetta, L., Bridge, J., Monga, S., & Baugher, M. (1999). Psychometric properties of the Screen for Child Anxiety Related Emotional Disorders (SCARED): A replication study. *Journal of the American Academy of Child and Adolescent Psychiatry, 38*, 1230–1236.

Bravo, M., Ribera, J., Rubio-Stipec, M., Canino, G., Shrout, P., Ramirez, R., & Martinez Taboas, A. (2001). Test–retest reliability of the Spanish version of the Diagnostic Interview Schedule for Children (DISC-IV). *Journal of Abnormal Child Psychology, 29*, 433–444.

Bravo, M., Woodbury-Farina, M., Canino, G. J., & Rubio-Stipec, M. (1993). The Spanish translation and cultural adaptation of the Diagnostic Interview Schedule for Children (DISC) in Puerto Rico. *Culture, Medicine, and Psychiatry, 17*, 329–344.

Brown, J. S., Meadows, S. O., & Elder, G. H. (2007). Race–ethnic inequality and psychological distress: Depressive symptoms from adolescence to young adulthood. *Developmental Psychology, 43*, 1295–1311.

Bussing, R., Fernandez, M., Harwood, M., Hou, W., Garvan, C. W., Eyberg, S. M., & Swanson, J. M. (2008). Parent and teacher SNAP-IV ratings of attention deficit hyperactivity disorder symptoms: Psychometric properties and normative ratings for a school district sample. *Assessment, 15*, 317–328.

Byrne, B. M., Shavelson, R. J., & Muthén, B. (1989). Testing for the equivalence of factor covariance and mean structures: The issue of partial measurement invariance. *Psychological Bulletin, 105*, 456–466.

Canino, G., & Guarnaccia, P. (1997). Methodological challenges in the assessment of Hispanic children and adolescents. *Applied Developmental Science, 1,* 124–134.

Carter, M. M., Miller, O., Sbrocco, T., Suchday, S., & Lewis, E. L. (1999). Factor structure of the Anxiety Sensitivity Index among African American college students. *Psychological Assessment, 11,* 525–533.

Chambers, W. J., Puig-Antich, J., Hirsch, M., Paez, P., Ambrosini, P. J., Tabrizi, M., & Davies, M. (1985). The assessment of affective disorders in children and adolescents by semistructured interview: Test–retest reliability of the K-SADS-P. *Archives of General Psychiatry, 42,* 696–702.

Chorpita, B. F., Yim, L., Moffitt, C., Umemoto, L. A., & Francis, S. E. (2000). Assessment of symptoms of DSM-IV anxiety and depression in children: A Revised Child Anxiety and Depression Scale. *Behaviour Research and Therapy, 38,* 835–855.

Cole, D. A., Martin, J. M., Peeke, L., Henderson, A., & Harwell, J. (1998). Validation of depression and anxiety measures in white and black youths: Multi-trait–multimethod analyses. *Psychological Assessment, 10,* 261–276.

Cook, A. (1986). *The Youth Self Report Hostility scale.* Unpublished manuscript, Program for Prevention Research, Arizona State University, Tempe.

Costello, A. J., Edelbrock, C. S., Dulcan, M. D., Kalas, R., & Klaric, S. H. (1984). *Report of the NIMH Diagnostic Interview Schedule for Children (DISC).* Washington, DC: National Institute of Mental Health.

Crockett, L. J., Randall, B. A., Shen, Y., Russell, S. T., & Driscoll, A. K. (2005). Measurement equivalence of the Center for Epidemiological Studies Depression Scale for Latino and Anglo adolescents: A national study. *Journal of Consulting and Clinical Psychology, 73,* 47–58.

Davanzo, P., Kerwin, L., Nikore, V., Esparza, C., Forness, S., & Murrelle, L. (2004). Spanish translation and reliability testing of the Children's Depression Inventory. *Child Psychiatry and Human Development, 35,* 75–92.

Dionne, R., Davis, B., Sheeber, L., & Madrigal, L. (2009). Initial evaluation of a cultural approach to implementation of evidence-based parenting interventions in American Indian communities. *Journal of Community Psychology, 37,* 911–921.

Egger, H. L., & Angold, A. (2004). The Preschool Age Psychiatric Assessment (PAPA): A structured parent interview for diagnosing psychiatric disorders in preschool children. In R. DelCarmen-Wiggins & A. Carter (Eds.), *Handbook of infant, toddler, and preschool mental health assessment* (pp. 223–243). New York: Oxford University Press.

Egger, H. L., Ascher, B. H., & Angold, A. (1999). *The Preschool Age Psychiatric Assessment: Version 1.1. Unpublished Interview Schedule.* Durham, NC: Center for Developmental Epidemiology, Department of Psychiatry and Behavioral Sciences, Duke University Medical Center.

Egger, H. L., Erkanli, A., Keeler, G., Potts, E., Walter, B. K., & Angold, A. (2006). Test–retest reliability of the Preschool Age Psychiatric Assessment (PAPA). *Journal of the American Academy of Child and Adolescent Psychiatry, 45,* 538–549.

Eyberg, S., & Pincus, D. (1999). *Eyberg Child Behavior Inventory and Sutter–Eyberg Student Behavior Inventory—Revised: Professional manual.* Odessa, FL: Psychological Assessment Resources.

Eyberg, S., & Ross, W. A. (1978). Assessment of child behavior problems: The validation of a new inventory. *Journal of Clinical Child Psychology, 7,* 113–116.

Eysenck, S. B. G., Eysenck, H. J., & Barrett, P. (1985). A revised version of the Psychoticism scale. *Personality and Individual Differences, 6,* 21–29.

Fisher, P., Shaffer, D., Piacentini, J., Lapkin, J., Kafantaris, V., Leonard, H., & Herzog, D. B. (1993). Sensitivity of the Diagnostic Interview Schedule for Children, 2nd edition (DISC 2.1) for specific diagnoses of children and adolescents. *Journal of the American Academy of Child and Adolescent Psychiatry, 32,* 666–673.

Floyd, E. M., Rayfield, A., Eyberg, S. M., & Riley, J. L. (2004). Psychometric properties of the Sutter–Eyberg Student Behavior Inventory with rural middle school and high school children. *Assessment, 11,* 64–72.

Ghorpade, J., Hattrup, K., & Lackritz, J. R. (1999). The use of personality measures in cross-cultural research: A test of three personality scales across two countries. *Journal of Applied Psychology, 84,* 670–679.

Gonzalez, A., Weersing, V. R., Warnick, E., Scahill, L., & Woolston, J. (2012). Cross-ethnic measurement equivalence of the SCARED in an outpatient sample of African American and non-Hispanic white youths and parents. *Journal of Clinical Child and Adolescent Psychology, 41*(3), 361–369.

Goodkind, J. R., LaNoue, M. D., & Milford, J. (2010). Adaptation and implementation of cognitive behavioral intervention for trauma in schools with American Indian youth. *Journal of Clinical Child and Adolescent Psychology, 39,* 858–872.

Gross, D., Fogg, L., Young, M., Ridge, A., Cowell, J., Sivan, A., & Richardson, R. (2007). Reliability and validity of the Eyberg Child Behavior Inventory with African-American and Latino parents of young children. *Research in Nursing and Health, 30,* 213–233.

Guarnaccia, P. J., Canino, G., Rubio-Stipec, M., & Bravo, M. (1993). The prevalence of *ataques de nervios* in the Puerto Rico Disaster Study: The role of culture in psychiatric epidemiology. *Journal of Nervous and Mental Disease, 181,* 159–167.

Guarnaccia, P. J., Lewis-Fernandez, R., & Marano, M. R. (2003). Toward a Puerto Rican popular nosology: *Nervios* and *ataque nervios. Culture, Medicine, and Psychiatry, 27,* 339–366.

Guarnaccia, P. J., Martinez, I., Ramirez, R., & Canino, G. (2005). Are *ataques de nervios* in Puerto Rican children associated with psychiatric disorder? *Journal of American Academy for Child and Adolescent Psychiatry, 44,* 1184–1192.

Guarnaccia, P. J., Rivera, M., Franco, F., & Neighbors, C. (1996). The experiences of *ataques de nervios*: Towards an anthropology of emotion in Puerto Rico. *Culture, Medicine, and Psychiatry, 20,* 343–367.

Guttmannova, K., Szanyi, J. M., & Cali, P. W. (2008). Internalizing and externalizing behavior problem scores: Cross-ethnic and longitudinal measurement invariance of the Behavior Problem Index. *Educational and Psychological Measurement, 68,* 676–694.

Hamill, S. K., Scott, W. D., Dearing, E., & Pepper, C. M. (2009). Affective style and depressive symptoms in youth of a North American Plains tribe: The moderating roles of cultural identity, grade level, and behavioral inhibition. *Personality and Individual Differences, 47,* 110–115.

Harter, S. (1985). *Manual for the Self-Perception Profile for Children.* Denver, CO: University of Denver.

Hui, H. C., & Triandis, H. C. (1985). The instability of response sets. *Public Opinion Quarterly, 49,* 253–260.

Hwu, H. G., Yeh, E. K., & Chang, L. Y. (1989). Prevalence of psychiatric disorders in Taiwan defined by the Chinese Diagnostic Interview Schedule. *Acta Psychiatrica Scandinavica, 79*, 136–147.

Jastrowski Mano, K. E., Davies, W. H., Klein-Tasman, B. P., & Adesso, V. J. (2009). Measurement equivalence of the Child Behavior Checklist among parents of African American adolescents. *Journal of Child and Family Studies, 18*, 606–620.

Kingery, J. N., Ginsburg, G. S., & Alfano, C. A. (2007). Somatic symptoms and anxiety among African American adolescents. *Journal of Black Psychology, 33*, 363–378.

Kistner, J. A., David-Ferdon, C., Lopez, C. M., & Dunkel, S. B. (2007). Ethnic and sex differences in children's depressive symptoms. *Journal of Clinical Child and Adolescent Psychology, 36*, 171–181.

Knight, G. P., Gonzales, N. A., Saenz, D. S., Bonds, D. D., Germán, M., Deardorff, J., & Updegraff, K. A. (2010). The Mexican American Cultural Values Scale for Adolescents and Adults. *The Journal of Early Adolescence, 30*(3), 444–481.

Knight, G. P., & Hill, N. E. (1998). Measurement equivalence in research involving minority adolescents. In V. C. McLoyd & L. Steinberg (Eds.), *Studying minority adolescents: Conceptual, methodological, and theoretical issues* (pp. 183–210). Mahwah, NJ: Erlbaum.

Knight, G. P., Little, M., Losoya, S., & Mulvey, E. P. (2004). The self-report of offending among serious juvenile offenders. *Youth Violence and Juvenile Justice, 2*, 273–295.

Knight, G. P., Roosa, M. W., & Umaña-Taylor, A. J. (2009). *Studying ethnic minority and economically disadvantaged populations: Methodological challenges and best practices.* Washington, DC: American Psychological Association.

Knight, G. P., Tein, J., Prost, J. H., & Gonzales, N. A. (2002). Measurement equivalence and research on Latino children and families: The importance of culturally informed theory. In J. M. Contreras, K. A. Kerns, & A. M. Neal-Barnett (Eds.), *Latino children and families in the United States: Current research and future directions* (pp. 181–201). Westport, CT: Praeger/Greenwood.

Knight, G. P., Virdin, L. M., Ocampo, K. A., & Roosa, M. (1994). An examination of the cross-ethnic equivalence of measures of negative life events and mental health among Hispanic and Anglo-American children. *American Journal of Community Psychology, 22*, 767–783.

Knight, G. P., & Zerr, A. A. (2010). Informed theory and measurement equivalence in child development research. *Child Development Perspectives, 4*, 25–30.

Kovacs, M. (1985). The Children's Depression Inventory (CDI). *Psychopharmacology Bulletin, 21*, 995–999.

Labouvie, E., & Ruetsch, C. (1995). Testing for equivalence of measurement scales: Simple structure and metric invariance reconsidered. *Multivariate Behavioral Research, 30*, 63–76.

LaFromboise, T. D., Medoff, L., Lee, C. C., & Harris, A. (2007). Psychosocial and cultural correlates of suicidal ideation among American Indian early adolescents on a Northern Plains reservation. *Research in Human Development, 4*, 119–143.

Lambert, S. F., Cooley, M. R., Campbell, K. D. M., Benoit, M. Z., & Stansbury, R. (2004). Assessing anxiety sensitivity in inner-city African American children: Psychometric properties of the Childhood Anxiety Sensitivity Index. *Journal of Clinical Child and Adolescent Psychology, 33*, 248–259.

Landis, J. R., & Koch, G. G. (1977). The measurement of observer agreement for categorical data. *Biometrics, 33,* 159–174.

Lau, A. S., Garland, A. F., Yeh, M., McCabe, K. M., Wood, P. A., & Hough, R. L. (2004). Race/ethnicity and inter-informant agreement in assessing adolescent psychopathology. *Journal of Emotional and Behavioral Disorders, 12,* 145–156.

Lee, C. K., Kwak, Y. S., Rhee, H., Kim, Y. S., Han, J. H., Choi, J. O., & Lee, Y. H. (1987). The nationwide epidemiological study of mental disorders in Korea. *Journal of Korean Medical Science, 2,* 19–34.

Lewis-Fernandez, R., Garrido-Castillo, P., Bennasar, M., Parrilla, E. M., Laria, A. J., Ma, G., & Petkova, E. (2002). Dissociation, childhood trauma, and *ataque de nervios* among Puerto Rican psychiatric outpatients. *American Journal of Psychiatry, 159,* 1603–1605.

Lewis-Fernandez, R., Guarnaccia, P., Martinez, I. E., Salman, E., Schmidt, A., & Liebowitz, M. (2002). Comparative phenomenology of *ataques de nervios,* panic attacks, and panic disorder. *Culture, Medicine, and Psychiatry, 26,* 199–223.

Loney, J., & Milich, R. (1982). Hyperactivity, inattention and aggression in clinical practice. In M. Woolraich & D. K. Routh (Eds.), *Advances in developmental and behavioral pediatrics* (Vol. 3, pp. 113–147). Greenwich, CT: JAI Press.

López, I., Rivera, F., Ramirez, R., Guarnaccia, P. J., Canino, G., & Bird, H. (2009). *Ataques de nervios* and their psychiatric correlates in Puerto Rican children from two different contexts. *Journal of Nervous and Mental Disease, 197,* 923–929.

Manson, S. M., Bechtold, D. W., Novins, D. K., & Beals, J. (1997). Assessing psychopathology in American Indian and Alaska Native children and adolescents. *Applied Developmental Science, 1,* 135–144.

March, J. S., Parker, J. D. A., Sullivan, K., Stallings, P., & Conners, C. K. (1997). The Multidimensional Anxiety Scale for Children (MASC): Factor structure, reliability, and validity. *Journal of the American Academy of Child and Adolescent Psychiatry, 36,* 554–565.

Matsumoto, D., & Kupperbusch, C. (2001). Idiocentric and allocentric differences in emotional expression, experience, and the coherence between expression and experience. *Asian Journal of Social Psychology, 4,* 113–131.

McClellan, J. M., & Werry, J. S. (Eds.). (2000). Research psychiatric diagnostic interviews for children and adolescents [Special section]. *Journal of the American Academy of Child and Adolescent Psychiatry, 39,* 19–99.

McCloskey, D. M., Hess, R. S., & D'Amato, R. C. (2003). Evaluating the utility of the Spanish version of the Behavior Assessment System for Children—Parent Report System. *Journal of Psychoeducational Assessment, 21,* 325–337.

McLaughlin, K. A., Hilt, L. M., & Nolen-Hoeksema, S. (2007). Racial/ethnic differences in internalizing and externalizing symptoms in adolescents. *Journal of Abnormal Child Psychology, 35,* 801–816.

Millsap, R. E. (1997). Invariance in measurement and prediction: Their relationship in the single-factor case. *Psychological Methods, 2,* 248–260.

Millsap, R. E., & Kwok, O. M. (2004). Evaluating the impact of partial measurement invariance on selection in two populations. *Psychological Methods, 9,* 93–115.

Millsap, R. E., & Tein, J. (2004). Assessing factorial invariance in ordered-categorical measures. *Multivariate Behavioral Research, 39,* 479–515.

Momper, S. L., & Jackson, A. P. (2007). Maternal gambling, parenting, and child behavioral functioning in Native American families. *Social Work Research, 31,* 199–209.

Mor, N., Zinbarg, R. E., Craske, M. G., Mineka, S., Uliaszek, A., Rose, R., & Waters, A. M. (2008). Evaluating the invariance of the factor structure of the EPQ-R-N among adolescents. *Journal of Personality Assessment, 90,* 66–75.

Nishina, A., Juvonen, J., & Witkow, M. R. (2005). Sticks and stones may break my bones, but names will make me feel sick: The psychosocial, somatic, and scholastic consequences of peer harassment. *Journal of Clinical Child and Adolescent Psychology, 34,* 37–48.

Okazaki, S. (1997). Sources of ethnic differences between Asian American and White American college students on measures of depression and social anxiety. *Journal of Abnormal Psychology, 106,* 52–60.

Okazaki, S. (2000). Asian American and White American differences on affective distress symptoms: Do symptom reports differ across reporting methods? *Journal of Cross-Cultural Psychology, 31,* 603–625.

Okazaki, S. (2002). Beyond questionnaires: Conceptual and methodological innovations in Asian American psychology. In N. Hall, C. Gordon, & S. Okazaki (Eds.), *Asian American psychology: The science of lives in context* (pp. 13–39). Washington, DC: American Psychological Association.

Okazaki, S., Liu, J. F., Longworth, S. L., & Minn, J. Y. (2002). Asian American–white American differences in expressions of social anxiety: A replication and extension. *Cultural Diversity and Ethnic Minority Psychology, 8,* 234–247.

Okazaki, S., & Sue, S. (1995). Methodological issues in assessment research with ethnic minorities. *Psychological Assessment, 7,* 367–375.

Ollendick, T. H. (1983). Reliability and validity of the revised Fear Survey Schedule for Children (FSSC-R). *Behavior Research and Therapy, 21,* 685–692.

Ortiz, C. D., Silverman, W. K., Jaccard, J., & La Greca, A. M. (2011). Children's state anxiety in reaction to disaster media cues: A preliminary test of a multivariate model. *Psychological Trauma: Theory, Research, Practice, and Policy, 3,* 157–164.

Pelham, W. E., Jr., Milich, R., Murphy, D., & Murphy, H. A. (1989). Normative data on the IOWA Conners Teacher Rating Scale. *Journal of Clinical Child Psychology, 18,* 259-262.

Peterson, J. L., & Zill, N. (1986). Marital disruption, parent–child relationships, and behavior problems in children. *Journal of Marriage and the Family, 48,* 295–307.

Pina, A. A., Little, M., Knight, G. P., & Silverman, W. K. (2009). Cross-ethnic measurement equivalence of the RCMAS in Latino and white youth with anxiety disorders. *Journal of Personality Assessment, 91,* 58–61.

Pina, A. A., & Silverman, W. K. (2004). Clinical phenomenology, somatic symptoms, and distress in Hispanic/Latino and European American youths with anxiety disorders. *Journal of Clinical Child and Adolescent Psychology, 33,* 227–236.

Pina, A. A., Villalta, I. K., & Zerr, A. A. (2009). Exposure-based cognitive behavioral treatment of Anxiety in youth: A culturally-prescriptive framework. *Behavioral Psychology, 17,* 111–135.

Prenoveau, J. M., Zinbarg, R. E., Craske, M. G., Mineka, S., Griffith, J. W., & Rose, R. D. (2009). Evaluating the invariance and validity of the structure of dysfunctional attitudes in an adolescent population. *Assessment, 16,* 258–273.

Radloff, L. S. (1977). The CES-D Scale: A self-report depression scale for research in the general population. *Applied Psychological Measurement, 1,* 385–401.

Randall, E. T., & Bohnert, A. M. (2009). Organized activity involvement, depressive symptoms, and social adjustment in adolescents: Ethnicity and socioeconomic status as moderators. *Journal of Youth and Adolescence, 38,* 1187–1198.

Raykov, T. (2004). Behavioral scale reliability and measurement invariance evaluation using latent variable modeling. *Behavior Therapy, 35,* 299–331.

Reid, R., Casat, C. D., Norton, H. J., Anastopoulos, A. D., & Temple, E. P. (2001). Using behavior rating scales for ADHD across ethnic groups: The IOWA Conners. *Journal of Emotional and Behavioral Disorders, 9,* 210–218.

Reynolds, C., & Richmond, B. (1978). "What I think and feel": A revised measure of children's manifest anxiety. *Journal of Abnormal Child Psychology, 6,* 271–280.

Ribera, J. C., Canino, G., Rubio-Stipec, M., Bravo, M., Bauermeister, J. J., Alegria, M., & Guevara, L. M. (1996). The Diagnostic Interview Schedule for Children (DISC-2.1) in Spanish: Reliability in a Hispanic population. *Journal of Child Psychology and Psychiatry, 37,* 195–204.

Rieckmann, T. R., Wadsworth, M. E., & Deyhle, D. (2004). Cultural identity, explanatory style, and depression in Navajo adolescents. *Cultural Diversity and Ethnic Minority Psychology, 10,* 365–382.

Roberts, R. E., Solovitz, B. L., Chen, Y., & Casat, C. (1996). Retest stability of DSM-III-R diagnoses among adolescents using the Diagnostic Interview Schedule for Children (DISC-2.1C). *Journal of Abnormal Child Psychology, 24,* 349–362.

Rubio-Stipec, M., Canino, G. J., Shrout, P., Dulcan, M., Freeman, D., & Bravo, M. (1994). Psychometric properties of parents and children as informants in child psychiatry epidemiology with the Spanish Diagnostic Interview Schedule for Children (DISC.2). *Journal of Abnormal Child Psychology, 22,* 703–720.

Russell, S. T., Crockett, L. J., Shen, Y., & Lee, S. (2008). Cross-ethnic invariance of self-esteem and depression measures for Chinese, Filipino, and European American adolescents. *Journal of Youth and Adolescence, 37,* 50–61.

Salgado de Snyder, V. N., Diaz-Perez, M. J., & Ojeda, V. D. (2000). The prevalence of *nervios* and associated symptomatology among inhabitants of Mexican rural communities. *Culture, Medicine, and Psychiatry, 24,* 453–470.

Sandler, I. N., Ramirez, R., & Reynolds, K. (1986). *Life events for children of divorce, bereaved, and asthmatic children.* Poster presented at the meeting of the American Psychological Association, Washington, DC.

Shaffer, D., Fisher, P., Dulcan, M.K., Davies, M., Piacentini, P., Schwab-Stone, M. E., & Regier, D. A. (1996). The NIMH Diagnostic Interview Schedule for Children Version 2.3 (DISC-2.3): Description, acceptability, prevalence rates, and performance in the MECA study. *Journal of the American Academy of Child and Adolescent Psychiatry, 35,* 865–877.

Shaffer, D., Fisher, P., Lucas, C. P., Dulcan, M. K., & Schwab-Stone, M. E. (2000). NIMH Diagnostic Interview Schedule for Children Version IV (NIMH

DISC-IV): Description, differences from previous versions, and reliability of some common diagnoses. *Journal of the American Academy of Child and Adolescent Psychiatry, 39*, 28–38.

Shrout, P. E. (1998). Measurement reliability and agreement in psychiatry. *Statistical Methods in Medical Research, 7*, 301–317.

Silmere, H., & Stiffman, A. R. (2006). Factors associated with successful functioning in American Indian youths. *Journal of the National Center for American Indian and Alaska Native Mental Health Research, 13*, 23–47.

Silverman, W. K., & Albano, A. M. (1996). *Anxiety Disorders Interview Schedule for DSM-IV: Child and Parent Versions.* San Antonio, TX: Psychological Corporation.

Silverman, W. K., Saavedra, L. M., & Pina, A. A. (2001). Test–retest reliability of anxiety symptoms and diagnoses with the Anxiety Disorders Interview Schedule for DSM-IV: Child and Parent Versions. *Journal of the American Academy of Child and Adolescent Psychiatry, 40*, 937–944.

Somers, J. M., Goldner, E. M., Waraich, P., & Hsu, L. (2006). Prevalence and incidence studies of anxiety disorders: A systematic review of the literature. *The Canadian Journal of Psychiatry, 51*, 100–113.

Spencer, M. S., Fitch, D., Grogan-Kaylor, A., & McBeath, B. (2005). The equivalence of the Behavior Problem Index across U.S. ethnic groups. *Journal of Cross–Cultural Psychology, 36*, 573–589.

Stein, G. L., Curry, J. F., Hersh, J., Breland-Noble, A., March, J., Silva, S. G., & Jacobs, R. (2010). Ethnic differences among adolescents beginning treatment for depression. *Cultural Diversity and Ethnic Minority Psychology, 16*, 152–158.

Sue, D., Ino, S., & Sue, D. M. (1983). Nonassertiveness of Asian Americans: An inaccurate assumption? *Journal of Counseling Psychology, 30*, 581–588.

Sulik, M. J., Huerta, S., Zerr, A. A., Eisenberg, N., Spinrad, T. L., Valiente, C., & Taylor, H. B. (2010). The factor structure of effortful control and measurement invariance across ethnicity and sex in a high-risk sample. *Journal of Psychopathology and Behavioral Assessment, 32*, 8–22.

Thrane, L. E., Whitbeck, L. B., Hoyt, D. R., & Shelley, M. C. (2004). Comparing three measures of depressive symptoms among American Indian adolescents. *American Indian and Alaska Native Mental Health Research, 11*(3), 20–42.

Tyson, E. H., Teasley, M., & Ryan, S. (2011). Using the Child Behavior Checklist with African American and Caucasian American adopted youth. *Journal of Emotional and Behavioral Disorders, 19*, 17–26.

Umaña-Taylor, A. J., & Updegraff, K. A. (2007). Latino adolescents' mental health: Exploring the interrelations among discrimination, ethnic identity, cultural orientation, self-esteem, and depressive symptoms. *Journal of Adolescence, 30*, 549–567.

U.S. Census Bureau. (2010). *Annual estimates of the American Indian and Alaska Native Alone Resident Population by sex and age for the United States: April 1, 2000 to July 1, 2009.* Retrieved September 8, 2011, from *www.census.gov/popest/national/asrh/NC-EST2009-asrh.html*

U.S. Census Bureau. (2011). *Minority population in the United States: 2010 tables* (Current Population Survey, Annual Social and Economic Supplement). Retrieved September 8, 2011, from *www.census.gov/newsroom/minority_links/minority_links.html*

Valla, J. P., Bergeron, L., Bidaut-Russell, M., St.-Georges, M., & Gaudet, N. (1997). Reliability of the Dominic-R: A young child mental health questionnaire combining visual and auditory stimuli. *Journal of Child Psychology and Psychiatry, 38,* 717–724.

Vandenberg, R. J., & Lance, C. E. (2000). A review and synthesis of the measurement invariance literature: Suggestions, practices, and recommendations of organization research. *Organizational Research Methods, 3,* 4–70.

Van de Vijver, F., & Leung, K. (2011). Equivalence and bias: A review of concepts, models, and data analytic procedures. In D. Matsumoto & F. J. R. Van de Vijver (Eds.), *Cross-cultural research methods in psychology* (pp. 17–45). New York: Cambridge University Press.

Van de Vijver, F., & Poortinga, Y. H. (1997). Towards an integrated analysis of bias in cross-cultural assessment. *European Journal of Psychological Assessment, 13,* 29–37.

Van de Vijver, F., & Tanzer, N. K. (2004). Bias and equivalence in cross-cultural assessment: An overview. *European Review of Applied Psychology, 54,* 119–135.

Varela, R. E., & Biggs, B. K. (2006). Reliability and validity of the Revised Children's Manifest Anxiety Scale (RCMAS) across samples of Mexican, Mexican American, and European American children: A preliminary investigation. *Anxiety, Stress and Coping, 19,* 67–80.

Varela, R. E., Sanchez-Sosa, J., Biggs, B. K., & Luis, T. M. (2008). Anxiety symptoms and fears in Hispanic and European American children: Cross-cultural measurement equivalence. *Journal of Psychopathology and Behavioral Assessment, 30,* 132–145.

Walton, J. W., Johnson, S. B., & Algina, J. (1999). Mother and child perceptions of child anxiety: Effects of race, health status, and stress. *Journal of Pediatric Psychology, 24,* 29–39.

Weissman, A. N. (1979). The Dysfunctional Attitude Scale: A validation study. *Dissertation Abstracts International, 40,* 1389B–1390B.

Weissman, A. N., & Beck, A. T. (1978). *Development and validation of the Dysfunctional Attitude Scale: A preliminary investigation.* Paper presented at the meeting of the Association for the Advancement of Behavior Therapy, Chicago.

Widaman, K. F., & Reise, S. P. (1997). Exploring the measurement invariance of psychological instruments: Applications in the substance use domain. In K. J. Bryant, M. Windle, & S. G. West (Eds.), *The science of prevention: Methodological advances from alcohol and substance abuse research* (pp. 281–324). Washington, DC: American Psychological Association.

Wittchen, H., & Fehm, L. (2001). Epidemiology, patterns of comorbidity, and associated disabilities of social phobia. *Psychiatric Clinics of North America, 24,* 617–641.

14

Assessment of Therapy Processes

Stephen R. Shirk, John Paul M. Reyes, and Patrice S. Crisostomo

Assessment of treatment progress is a fundamental principle of evidence-based practice. Regardless of the strength of evidence for a particular treatment, the assessment of progress over the course of therapy is essential for determining whether a treatment is having its expected effect. Treatments for disorders are translated into treatments for individuals through assessment of individual progress.

Although progress assessment is essential for evidence-based practice, the assessment of therapy processes has not attained similar status. Why, then, is the assessment of therapy process important for evidence-based practice? Just as *research* on therapy process is in the service of improving outcome (Shirk & Karver, 2006), assessment of process in clinical practice serves a similar function. It is our view that the assessment of therapy processes provides a direct path to *personalizing* evidence-based treatments for children and adolescents. Treatment manuals typically provide scripts of varying levels of specificity to guide the delivery of therapy. But therapy is not a monologue. A therapist's actions are met with varying client reactions, and these responses shape the therapist's subsequent behaviors (Patterson & Chamberlain, 1994; Jungbluth & Shirk, 2009). The manual-based script, then, is like the melody in a jazz composition; it is both the starting and ending point for improvisation, or, to paraphrase Kendall and colleagues, the manual provides boundaries for therapist flexibility (Kendall, Chu, Gifford, Hayes, & Nauta, 1998). Because there is substantial variation in clients' responses to interventions outlined in treatment manuals (Chu & Kendall, 2004; Jungbluth & Shirk, 2009), therapists are tasked with personalizing interventions in order to maximize potential benefits (Chu & Kendall, 2009). The assessment of therapy processes can guide this task.

To be useful, assessment of treatment processes and progress requires systematic data collection and feedback to therapists. A growing body of evidence indicates that systematic feedback regarding client progress improves treatment outcomes in routine-care settings (Shimokawa, Lambert, & Smart, 2010), although virtually all of this work has been done with adults. Importantly, feedback about treatment process—specifically, the strength of the therapeutic alliance—is associated with improved outcomes (Lambert & Shimokawa, 2011). Our focus, then, is on measures of process that have the potential to contribute to better outcomes in youth therapy by serving as feedback.

A basic assumption of this chapter is that personalized treatment requires more than the assessment of symptom profiles, diagnostic features, and comorbidities. Although these characteristics are important for treatment *selection*, personalized treatment *delivery* requires the assessment of ongoing processes and the evaluation of factors that affect treatment process. Therefore, we focus on two sets of constructs: nondiagnostic predictors of treatment process (i.e., psychological variables that can affect the successful delivery of evidence-based treatments), and processes emerging during treatment delivery that may signal a need for therapy adaptation. Both participant report and observational approaches to assessing these constructs are considered. We realize that we are casting a rather broad net, and in order to retain reasonable scope, we have selected constructs that have an emerging or sound research base. Thus, in keeping with our view of process research, we focus on constructs that have either a direct or an indirect impact on treatment outcomes.

ASSESSMENT CONSTRUCTS

Pretreatment Constructs

Many different client and family characteristics are associated with child and adolescent treatment outcomes (see Shirk & McMakin, 2007, for a review). At present, there is little consensus about the most important constructs for personalizing treatment, though the development of age-related protocols for specific disorders indicates the importance of developmental level. In this section, we focus on three pretreatment constructs that are related to process and outcome, including attrition, in child and adolescent therapy: treatment expectancies, barriers to treatment, and readiness for change.

Treatment Expectancies

"Treatment expectancies" are anticipatory beliefs about the likelihood of treatment success or the amount of improvement that will be achieved through an intervention (Kazdin, 1979). Expectancies have been shown to predict treatment outcomes across diverse therapies for varied psychological problems (Devilly & Borkovec, 2000; Dew & Bickman, 2005).

Clients who enter therapy with positive expectancies tend to show better treatment responses in both psychosocial and pharmacological treatments (Stewart-Williams, 2004). The conventional explanation for this association highlights the link between positive expectancies and active treatment participation. Individuals who hold positive beliefs about a particular treatment are more likely to adhere to specific treatment demands, either by consistently taking medications or by completing prescribed therapy tasks (Nock, Ferriter, & Holmberg, 2007). Research has demonstrated an association between expectancies and the therapeutic alliance in both psychotherapy (Constantino, Arnow, Blasey, & Agras, 2005) and pharmacotherapy (Krupnick et al., 1996). A number of studies have shown that the alliance partially mediates the association between expectancies and outcomes (Krupnick et al., 1996). For example, among patients receiving pharmacotherapy for bipolar disorder, the alliance partially mediated the link between expectancies and outcomes assessed over a 28-month period following an acute episode (Guadiano & Miller, 2006).

Despite the importance of expectancies for treatment process and outcome, expectancies have been relatively neglected in the child and adolescent literature. Early studies largely focused on children's knowledge about the structure and content of therapy, rather than expectations about potential treatment benefits (see Shirk & Russell, 1998, for a review). Such expectations failed to produce consistent associations with therapy process or outcome, including early attrition (Shirk & Russell, 1998). Fortunately, there has since been renewed interest in the role of treatment expectancies in child and adolescent therapy. For the most part, interest has shifted to *parent (caregiver)* expectancies, primarily in the context of parent management training. For example, in a series of studies, Nock and colleagues (Nock & Kazdin, 2001; Nock et al., 2007) showed that parent expectancies predict treatment adherence, treatment attendance, and premature dropout in parent management training for youngsters with disruptive disorders. In a study of multisystemic therapy (MST), Ellis, Weiss, Han, and Gallop (2010) found that parent expectancies were associated with therapist adherence to treatment principles. Given that parents play a critical role in treatment initiation and continuation, parent expectations represent an important assessment target in youth treatment. Less is known about the role of child or adolescent expectancies (Dew & Bickman, 2005). In one of the few studies to evaluate youth expectancies in the context of a clinical trial, Curry et al. (2006) found that adolescent expectancies predicted treatment outcomes across cognitive-behavioral treatment (CBT), pharmacotherapy, and combined therapy conditions in the Treatment for Adolescents with Depression Study (TADS).

Barriers to Treatment

Premature termination is a significant problem for outpatient youth psychotherapy. An estimated 40–60% of youth clients terminate therapy prematurely (Kazdin, 1996; Wierzbicki & Pekarik, 1993). Not surprisingly, premature terminators have been shown to have fewer clinical gains than clients who remain in therapy (Prinz & Miller, 1994).

Although various demographic factors are associated with premature termination (e.g., parental stress and psychopathology, lower socioeconomic status, and membership in a minority group), perceived barriers to treatment have been shown to mediate the link between these variables and early dropout. Research by Kazdin and colleagues (Kazdin & Mazurick, 1994; Kazdin, Mazurick, & Bass, 1993) on the "barriers-to-treatment" model (Kazdin, Holland, & Crowley, 1997; Kazdin, Holland, Crowley, & Breton, 1997) links premature termination to client and family characteristics through perceptions and judgments. According to this model, families may experience varied obstacles related to active participation in therapy, and these obstacles increase the risk for premature termination. These barriers fall under four general categories: practical obstacles (e.g., difficulties scheduling treatment sessions, lack of transportation to sessions); a parent's or youth's perception that treatment is too demanding (e.g., information or topics discussed in sessions are perceived as confusing or unclear); perceived irrelevance of treatment to the child's functioning; and negative relationship with treatment providers (i.e., poor therapeutic alliance). In brief, the degree to which treatment is perceived as stressful, burdensome, or irrelevant can undermine active participation and continuation.

Research has shown that parent- and therapist-reported perceived barriers to treatment significantly predict early treatment termination (Kazdin et al., 1993). In another study, Kazdin (2000) found that perceived barriers were related to perceived treatment acceptability (e.g., the degree to which consumers viewed the treatment as palatable and necessary) by both youth and parents who were involved in outpatient treatment for antisocial behavior. In this study, treatment acceptability was found to be associated with symptom change over the course of therapy. In addition, perceived barriers to treatment have been linked to clinical outcomes (Kazdin & Wassell, 2000); greater perceived barriers were directly related to fewer treatment gains in a treatment for antisocial behavior. The authors found that in particular, parents' perception of treatment relevance and demands largely accounted for the relationship between perceived barriers and treatment outcome.

In summary, existing research on barriers to treatment points to the importance of assessing families' perceptions of treatment relevance and burden at the outset of therapy. Identifying and addressing specific barriers for each family could improve retention and optimize clinical gains. Hoberman (1992) highlighted the need to understand barriers to treatment as part of culturally sensitive mental health care for ethnic minority youth and their families. For example, Kazdin and colleagues (1993) suggested that addressing parental expectations and making explicit connections between therapeutic practices that address youth problems might strengthen participation and prevent dropout. Nock and Kazdin (2005) have developed initial treatment modules to address parental expectations and perceived barriers as a method of personalizing treatment.

Readiness for Change

Prochaska and DiClemente (1982) developed a transtheoretical model of readiness to change, identifying four distinct stages: "precontemplation," "contemplation," "action," and "maintenance." Briefly, individuals in the precontemplation stage remain unaware of problems or do not want to change. Individuals in the contemplation stage are more aware of some difficulties or distress and are considering whether their problems can be resolved; however, there is no commitment to change. Those in the action stage are taking steps to solve the difficulties, but the desired changes have yet to be achieved. Finally, being in the maintenance stage indicates that change goals have been achieved, and these individuals are either looking to prevent relapse or seeking to consolidate these positive changes. In effect, these stages of change provide a means of classifying client motivation for therapy.

Low motivation is associated with poorer treatment outcomes, including early termination and decreased adherence to treatment, whereas high motivation is associated with better outcomes (e.g., Miller & Rollnick, 2013). Furthermore, research has demonstrated that interventions aimed at increasing motivation leads to better treatment participation and outcomes (e.g., Miller & Rollnick, 2013; Prochaska & Norcross, 2002). Although most research on treatment motivation has focused on adults, there is an emerging literature exploring readiness for change in youth treatment. Motivation may play an even more important role in youth treatment, insofar as caregivers typically initiate referral, often without any interest on the youth's part in pursuing therapy. Thus an action orientation to treatment cannot be assumed with many youth.

Consistent with the adult literature, research with adolescents has shown links between change stage and outcome (e.g., Gusella, Butler, Nichols, & Bird, 2003; Lewis et al., 2009; Littell & Girvin, 2005; Maisto, Chung, Cornelius, & Martin, 2003). For example, Lewis et al. (2009) found in the TADS that higher scores on the Action subscale of a stages-of-change measure (discussed in more detail later) were associated with greater reductions in depressive symptoms. Fitzpatrick and Irannejad (2008) found that higher scores on the Precontemplation subscale of this measure predicted poorer alliance, and that higher scores on the Action subscale predicted more positive alliance. As these examples indicate, readiness for change has been shown to predict both process and outcomes with adolescents.

In-Session Constructs

Over the last 20 years, there has been growing interest in constructs related to engagement and participation in child and adolescent therapy (Shirk,

Jungbluth, & Karver, 2011). This focus makes sense for two reasons: First, as noted above, children rarely refer themselves for treatment and may be less than enthusiastic participants; and second, efficacious treatments uniformly require active client participation. Therefore, constructs of alliance, involvement, and resistance have received increasing attention from youth process researchers (Shirk et al., 2011). On the therapist side, treatment integrity has emerged as a critical construct, both in clinical trials and for the transportation of evidence-based treatments to usual-care settings. Treatment integrity also is integral for assessing the impact of clinical training. Our focus, then, is on constructs related to clients' participation in therapy and therapists' skillful delivery of treatment components.

The Therapeutic Alliance

Bordin (1979) proposed a three-component alliance construct: "bond" (i.e., the affective experience, such as warmth, trust, and acceptance); "agreement on goals" (i.e., collaboratively deciding on the aims of treatment), and "task collaboration" (i.e., working together on treatment-specific activities). This transtheoretical model has informed both adult and youth alliance research. However, three studies support a single-factor model of alliance (DiGiuseppe, Linscott, & Jilton, 1996; Faw, Hogue, Johnson, Diamond, & Liddle, 2005; Fjermestad et al., 2012) among adolescents, and studies of child alliance measures indicate high correlations among subscales (Shirk & Saiz, 1992). Thus youth therapeutic alliance may be a unitary construct—what has been called "collaborative bond" (Kazdin, Marciano, & Whitley, 2005).

Child and adolescent therapeutic relationship variables have demonstrated modest but consistent associations with treatment outcome in the youth literature (e.g., Karver, Handelsman, Fields, & Bickman, 2006; Shirk & Karver, 2003). The youth alliance literature has often suggested that a positive therapeutic bond may facilitate treatment collaboration (e.g., Shirk & Saiz, 1992; Shirk & Russell, 1996; Shirk, Gudmundsen, Kaplinski, & McMakin, 2008). Shirk and Karver (2006) asserted that initial interactions between youth and therapists influence alliance formation, which then influences active treatment involvement, such that a positive therapeutic alliance may promote treatment continuation, active involvement in sessions, and homework completion. Shirk and Saiz (1992) found that therapy bond was associated with treatment collaboration, and therapeutic alliance has been shown to be associated with treatment involvement (Karver et al., 2008), treatment dropout (Garcia & Weisz, 2002; Hawley & Weisz, 2005; Kazdin, Holland, & Crowley, 1997), and treatment completion (Florsheim, Shotorbani, Guest-Warnick, Barratt, & Hwang, 2000; Robbins et al., 2006). Furthermore, Kazdin and Whitley (2006) found that parent–clinician alliance is associated with improvements in parenting practices.

The mechanisms linking alliance and outcome remain largely unexamined. Some investigators have proposed a direct causal relationship between alliance and outcome, suggesting that alliance is an active component of treatment. For example, a client may experience a corrective interpersonal relationship with a therapist thereby resulting in a change in negative interpersonal schema or core representation of self (Shirk & Russell, 1996; Wright, Everett, & Roisman, 1986). Others contend that alliance promotes active participation in the specific tasks of psychotherapy, which results in better outcomes (Kendall et al., 2009; Shirk & Karver, 2006; Shirk & Russell, 1996). Whether the association is direct or indirect, alliance monitoring is critical for gauging changes in therapy process.

Involvement and Resistance

"Client involvement" refers to a client's level of in-session participation and collaboration with therapists in the treatment process (e.g., Braswell, Kendall, Braith, Carey, & Vye, 1985; Karver et al., 2006). Behaviors such as verbal self-disclosure, initiation of therapy topics, demonstration of enthusiasm, or providing feedback to a therapist about therapy tasks are viewed as markers of involvement. The construct of client involvement is particularly important in youth treatments, given the intersection of treatment demands of cognitive and behavioral treatments and notable variation in youth motivation (Curry et al., 2006; Shirk & Saiz, 1992). For example, a primary assumption of youth CBT is that beneficial effects depend on active youth involvement in therapy (Chu & Kendall, 2004).

Overall, results suggest a positive association between youth involvement and treatment outcome. Results from a meta-analysis by Karver et al. (2006) revealed a medium effect size ($r_w = .27$) for the association between youth involvement and outcomes in child and adolescent. Karver et al. (2006) observed that the range of treatments, problem types, and settings as well as the variety of measures of involvement and outcome suggest a rather robust process variable. For example, Braswell et al. (1985) found that client in-session involvement predicted changes in teacher ratings of youth's disruptive classroom behavior among impulsive children. In another study, Chu and Kendall (2004) found associations between child involvement in CBT for anxiety (e.g., the Coping Cat program) and the absence of primary anxiety diagnoses and reductions in anxiety impairment ratings at posttreatment. Karver et al. (2008) found a substantial association between in-session client involvement in specific CBT tasks and change in depressive symptoms ($r = .56$); however, the correlation was only marginally significant, due to a small sample size. In addition, Karver et al. (2006) noted the positive association between youth involvement and other relevant process variables ($r_w = .30$) such as therapeutic alliance (Creed & Kendall, 2005; Tryon & Kane, 1995), as well as measures of therapist behaviors and flexibility (Chu & Kendall, 2009; Siler, Crisostomo, & Jungbluth, 2010).

Other researchers have focused on the "flip side" of involvement: client disengagement or resistance. For example, research by Patterson and Chamberlain (1994) on parent management training showed that parent resistance developed over the course of treatment as a function of specific therapist interventions. Importantly, the trajectory of resistance, as opposed to its mean level, was a better predictor of treatment outcome. Parents who failed to resolve heightened resistance during the middle of therapy often failed to attain beneficial treatment effects. It is not clear whether disengagement or resistance is simply the other pole of engagement or involvement, or a distinct construct. For example, Jungbluth and Shirk (2009) found a large association between independently coded measures of resistance and client involvement. To be sure, resistance appears to involve distinctive behavioral indicators ranging from active defiance and hostility to passive withdrawal. Although both can interfere with completion of treatment tasks, such behaviors differ in the degree to which they reflect disengagement and may predict different treatment trajectories or outcomes.

A number of studies have indicated that early resistance predicts more difficult process and poorer outcomes. For example, among a sample of 69 adolescents referred to inpatient hospital treatment, patients with high ratings of "treatment difficulty" were associated with poorer treatment outcomes (Colson et al., 1990). In a school-based CBT program for adolescent depression, a high level of observed hostile resistance during the first session significantly predicted low client involvement in treatment tasks, treatment completion, and both observed and therapist-reported alliance (Peterson, Jungbluth, Siler, & Shirk, 2010). Either high initial levels or emerging resistance may signal the need for treatment modification and interventions that target treatment

Treatment Integrity

To the degree that change is catalyzed by specific components defined by treatment manuals, effective therapy hinges on delivery of these components in practice in a manner that closely approximates delivery in clinical trials (McHugh, Murray, & Barlow, 2009). "Treatment integrity," then, refers to the degree to which therapists skillfully implement prescribed treatment components and limit their use of proscribed methods. As this definition suggests, treatment integrity consists of three features: "adherence," the degree to which the therapist implements the treatment as intended; "competence," how skillfully the therapist implements the treatment; and "differentiation," the degree to which the therapist refrains from including proscribed interventions as part of treatment (Perepletchikova & Kazdin, 2005; Perepletchikova, Treat, & Kazdin, 2007).

Research linking treatment integrity and treatment outcome in youth therapy is quite limited. Studies of MST have shown predictive associations between therapist adherence to MST principles (as reported by treatment recipients) and treatment outcomes (Huey, Henggeler, Brondino, & Pickrel, 2000; Schoenwald, Carter, Chapman, & Sheidow, 2008). Similarly, in a study of CBT and multidimensional family therapy for adolescent substance abuse, both linear and curvilinear relations between adherence and outcome were reported (Hogue, Henderson, et al., 2008). The curvilinear association is particularly interesting, in that moderate levels of adherence were associated with better outcomes than either high or low adherence. This pattern has been replicated in the treatment of adult cocaine dependence (Barber et al., 2006) and suggests that evidence-based treatments may produce beneficial effects at lower thresholds than anticipated—a finding that could have positive implications for treatment transportation. Alternatively, the curvilinear association might indicate that therapist flexibility is potentially more important than strict adherence, once an adherence threshold has been crossed (McHugh et al., 2009).

The association between therapist competence and treatment outcomes has received even less attention than adherence in the child and adolescent literature. In the adult literature, relations between competence and outcome have been relatively weak and inconsistent (McHugh et al., 2009). In one of the only studies to examine competence–outcome relations in youth treatment, Hogue, Dauber, et al. (2008) did not find a significant association between therapist competence and outcome in CBT or family therapy for adolescent substance abuse. However, it seems premature to conclude that therapist competence is unrelated to treatment outcomes. Lack of consensus about the nature of therapist competence is a likely contributor to weak results. For example, there is disagreement about whether the competence construct should include both technical and relational features of therapy (McLeod, Southam-Gerow, & Weisz, 2009), or both treatment formulation and implementation of specific components (Hogue, Henderson, Dauber, Barajas, Fried, & Liddle, 2008). One emerging view of competence underscores the importance of therapist flexibility in the context of treatment adherence (McHugh et al., 2009). In essence, a therapist's ability to apply treatment procedures and principles in a highly flexible and responsive manner *while maintaining an adequate level of adherence* represents highly skillful therapy. Studies on the relationship between flexibility and outcome have produced mixed results (McHugh et al., 2009). In the youth literature, therapist-reported flexibility in implementing CBT procedures for child anxiety was not related to treatment outcomes (Kendall & Chu, 2000), but therapist flexibility has been shown to predict subsequent child involvement in treatment, which in turn predicts symptom reduction (Chu & Kendall, 2009).

Finally, research on treatment differentiation in youth therapy is virtually nonexistent. Efforts to describe usual-care therapy and to distinguish it from therapies delivered in clinical trials have used observational methods to characterize treatment content (Garland, Hurlburt, & Hawley, 2006). Both therapist report (Weersing, Weisz, & Donenberg, 2002) and observational systems (McLeod & Weisz, 2010) have been developed for characterizing treatment methods and procedures. Given the limited associations between therapist reports and independent observations, it should not be assumed that these methods are equivalent (Hurlburt, Garland, Nguyen, & Brookman-Frazee, 2010).

In summary, despite the importance of treatment integrity for clinical trials and clinical practice, research on this multidimensional construct is only beginning to emerge. Fundamentally, it is hard to imagine a more important process construct. Knowing what therapists are doing and not doing, and how well they are doing what they do, seems to be at the heart of psychotherapy process research. Moreover, treatment integrity seems especially important for implementation of evidence-based treatments in usual-care settings, as well as for supervision of therapists in training.

ASSESSMENT INSTRUMENTS

The evaluation of youth therapy process is an emerging field, and many instruments have been used in only one study (Karver et al., 2006; Shirk & Karver, 2003). Our aim, then, is not to review each and every instrument, but rather to focus on promising measures of each construct, and (where possible) to highlight instruments that have been used in multiple studies.

Measurement of Pretreatment Constructs

Treatment Expectancies

Early studies of expectations typically focused on child and parent beliefs about the structure and content of therapy, rather than expectations about potential effects (Shirk & Russell, 1998). Recent research on adolescent expectancies has utilized single-item indicators. For example, in the TADS, expectancies were measured with one item on a 7-point Likert scale ranging from "very much improved" to "very much worse" (Curry et al., 2006). Although the item appears face-valid, predicts outcome in the expected direction, and has the virtue of simplicity, relatively little is known about its reliability or validity.

Two measures of parent expectancies have been developed, the Parent Expectancies for Therapy Scale (PETS; Kazdin & Holland, 1991) and the Credibility/Expectancies Questionnaire—Parent Version (CEQ-P; Nock, Ferriter, & Holmberg, 2007). The reliability and validity of both measures have been evaluated in clinical samples of children with disruptive behavior problems and their parents/caregivers.

The PETS is a 25-item scale containing items related to a parent's beliefs about the credibility of treatment (e.g., "I believe this treatment sounds reasonable for the problems that I have been experiencing with my child"), potential treatment benefits (e.g., "Once therapy begins, I believe my child's problems will improve"), and the parent's role in therapy (e.g., "I believe I will have to do a lot of work outside the sessions in order for my child to improve"). Items are rated on a 5-point scale. Initial reliability and validity were established with an ethnically diverse sample of 405 parents/ caregivers who were referred for the treatment of their children's opposi- tional, aggressive, or antisocial behavior (Nock & Kazdin, 2001).

A factor analysis produced a three-factor solution consistent with the three hypothesized dimensions. The first factor, Credibility, consisted of 13 items and accounted for approximately 25% of the variance; the second, Child Improvement, included six items and explained nearly 8% of the variance; the third, Parent Involvement, was composed of six items and accounted for roughly 6.5% of the variance. There were moderate posi- tive correlations among the factors. The overall scale showed good internal consistency (alpha = .79), and the three subscales evidenced comparable, though slightly lower, levels of internal consistency. Because overall inter- nal consistency was high, validity was examined with the full scale.

Two studies have examined the validity of the PETS. Correlations with parent, child, and family characteristics showed that socioeconomic disad- vantage, parenting stress, and higher levels of child dysfunction were asso- ciated with lower expectancies, but not so highly related as to be redundant and threaten divergent validity (Nock & Kazdin, 2001). A second study showed that PETS scores predicted number of sessions attended and early termination after the researchers controlled for child, parent, and family characteristics, including barriers to treatment, thus supporting both the predictive and incremental validity of the scale.

In order to provide a brief measure of parent beliefs about treatment credibility and expectancies that could be readily administered in clinical practice, Nock et al. (2007) adapted the original Credibility/Expectancy Questionnaire (Borkovec & Nau, 1972) for parent use. Items were modi- fied to be appropriate for parents with a child in therapy. Three items assess parent beliefs about credibility (e.g., "How much does the therapy offered to you seem to make sense?"), and three items assess expectancies about treatment outcome (e.g., "By the end of treatment, how much improvement in your child's behavior do you think will have occurred?"). Internal and test–retest reliability as well as convergent and predictive validity of the scale were assessed with a sample of 76 parents or caregivers who were referred for treatment for their children's disruptive problems in a specialty clinic.

A factor analysis of the CEQ-P produced a two-factor solution that accounted for 80% of the variance in the scale. Factors corresponded to Credibility and Outcome expectancies. Although the two factors were highly related ($r = .58$), other results indicate that they should be considered separately. Internal consistency and test–retest reliability for the total scale and the subscales were highly comparable. For internal consistency, coef- ficient alpha ranged from .82 to .88; for test–retest reliability correlations, it ranged from .34 to .52.

Convergent validity of the CEQ-P was supported by a significant correlation with parent motivation for treatment. As predicted, parents with more positive beliefs about treatment credibility and potential outcomes reported greater motivation for treatment. Predictive validity was supported by prospective associations between parent attendance in therapy and utilization of parent management skills. Results indicated that the CEQ-P, specifically the Outcome Expectancies subscale, predicted significant variance in treatment utilization after the researchers controlled for child, parent, and family characteristics, as well as treatment motivation. For attendance, outcome expectancies showed a nonsignificant, but medium, linear association with attendance.

In summary, relatively little research has been done on treatment expectancies in child and adolescent therapy. However, preliminary findings are consistent with research with adults that show links between expectancies and treatment attendance and utilization. Thus far, existing measures assess parent expectancies; this seems justified, insofar as parents manage treatment attendance. However, a complementary measure of child and adolescent expectancies is conspicuously missing.

Barriers to Treatment

The Barriers to Treatment Participation Scale (BTPS; Kazdin, Holland, Crowley, & Breton, 1997; Kazdin, Holland, & Crowley, 1997), a 44-item measure rated on a 5-point Likert scale, offers a systematic way to assess perceived barriers to treatment participation. In this measure, the four BTPS subscales reflect barrier types as described earlier, and are summed to create a total barriers score. The BTPS also includes a list of separate events that may also lead to premature drop out, but are not necessarily related to the treatment itself (e.g., parental separation, death of a caregiver or close relative). In the initial validation and relationship to outcome study, the BTPS was administered at the end of treatment via telephone and in-person interviews; however, there appears to be clinical utility in the use of the BTPS Stressors and Obstacles subscale at the start of therapy (Kazdin, 1997).

The psychometric properties of the BTPS have been evaluated with clinical samples of youth with disruptive and antisocial behaviors and their parents (e.g., Kazdin, 1997; Kazdin, Marciano, & Whitley, 2005; Kazdin & Wassell, 2000). The BTPS demonstrated good to excellent psychometric properties (Kazdin, Holland, & Crowley, 1997; Kazdin, Holland, Crowley, & Breton, 1997). The BTPS Total Barriers score demonstrated excellent internal consistency (alpha = .86 and .93 for parent and therapist report, respectively). The authors utilized factor analyses to evaluate the structure of the BTPS, and these analyses supported the use of the BTPS Total Barriers score rather than individual subscale scores in evaluating relationships to clinical outcomes.

For both parent and therapist reports, the BTPS Total Barriers score has shown a consistent pattern of significant positive associations between barriers and treatment dropout, attendance, and the number of cancellations and "no-shows." In addition, the BTPS Total Barriers score has been associated with other therapeutic processes, such as child–therapist and parent–therapist alliance in CBT for children with oppositional, aggressive, and antisocial behavior (e.g., Kazdin et al., 2005). The BTPS showed adequate divergent validity, as it had small or nonsignificant correlations with contextual factors (family, parent, or child characteristics) found in previous research to be correlated with early dropout (Armbruster & Kazdin, 1994; Gould, Shaffer, & Kaplan, 1985). For the variables that were significantly correlated (e.g., parental stress, adverse child-rearing practices, and psychopathology), the small but significant correlations might be attributable to common-rater variance. The BTPS has also evidenced incremental validity, because perceived barriers significantly predicted early treatment termination when contextual characteristics were controlled for (e.g., Armbruster & Kazdin, 1994; Gould et al., 1985).

It is important to note that the original BTPS study (Kazdin et al., 1993) included a relatively diverse socioeconomic and ethnic/racial sample of families. Given previous research indicating that treatment dropout is associated with cultural factors, one limitation of the scale is the lack of culturally specific items related to treatment attendance.

Readiness for Change

Multiple measures have been developed or adapted from the adult literature to assess stages of change in adolescent samples. Many of these measures are problem-specific, such as the Stages of Change Readiness and Treatment Eagerness Scale (Miller & Tonigan, 1996; Maisto et al., 2003) for alcohol abuse, and the Motivational Stages of Change for Adolescents Recovering from an Eating Disorder (Gusella et al., 2003). The most widely studied stages of change measure in the youth and adult literature is the University of Rhode Island Change Assessment (URICA; McConnaughy, Prochaska, & Velicer, 1983), previously known as the Stages of Change Scale. As opposed to the previously mentioned problem-specific measures, the URICA is not anchored to any particular type of difficulty. More recently, Nock and Photos (2006) developed a measure of parent motivation for youth treatment called the Parent Motivation Inventory (PMI). The reliability and validity of both measures have been evaluated in the context of youth treatment.

University of Rhode Island Change Assessment

The URICA is a 32-item scale consisting of four subscales purported to measure the four stages of change: Precontemplation, Contemplation, Action, and Maintenance. Items are rated on a 5-point Likert scale from 1 ("strongly agree") to 5 ("strongly disagree"). The URICA was originally developed with an adult sample by McConnaughy et al. (1983) and demonstrated adequate reliability and validity for adult psychotherapy samples (McConnaughy, DiClemente, Prochaska, & Velicer, 1989; McConnaughy, Prochaska, & Velicer, 1983). Greenstein, Franklin, and McGuffin (1999) adapted the URICA for use with adolescents. The authors amended the directions and nine items to improve relevance and ease of understanding.

Reliability and validity analyses were performed on a sample of 89 adolescents ages 12–16, who were admitted to a private psychiatric facility with varied psychopathology. The internal consistency of the subscales was adequate and similar to that found with adults. Correlations between the subscales were also similar to those found in adult samples and consistent with the transtheoretical model. Cluster analyses revealed that a three-cluster solution best characterized the data. The results placed adolescents into groups termed in this study Precontemplation, Uninvolved, and Participation. A Maintenance group was not identified.

More recently, studies have examined the psychometric properties of the URICA, using different adolescent populations: adolescent offenders (Hemphill & Howell, 2000), Taiwanese adolescents who abused methamphetamine (Yen, Huang, Chang, & Cheng, 2010), and adolescent males incarcerated in a juvenile detention facility (Cohen, Glaser, Calhoun, Bradshaw, & Petrocelli, 2005). The results supported the use of the URICA in these adolescent populations. Cohen et al. (2005) performed preliminary factor analyses for the URICA with an adolescent sample. Results suggested a three-factor solution. The Precontemplation factor accounted for 8.56% of item variance, the Contemplation/Action factor accounted for 19.34%, and the Maintenance component accounted for 14.82%. Altogether, the three-factor solution accounted for 42.72% of the item variance.

An abbreviated version of the URICA (Bellis, 1994) was modified for an adolescent sample by altering the wording of directions and selected items (Lewis et al., 2009). This 18-item measure, referred to as the Stages of Change Questionnaire (SOCQ), includes items from each of the four stages of change. Lewis et al. (2009) examined the psychometric properties of the SOCQ, using a sample of 332 depressed adolescents. The authors reported adequate internal consistency, and an exploratory factor analysis yielded a four-component solution accounting for 56.5% of the variance. These four components mapped directly onto the Precontemplation, Contemplation, Action, and Maintenance stages of change.

In order to examine the convergent and divergent validity of the measure, correlations between subscale scores and previously identified predictors and moderators of treatment response were examined (Lewis et al., 2009). Higher Precontemplation scores were related to lower treatment expectations and age. Contemplation scores were positively associated with higher treatment expectations and age. Higher Action scores showed significant associations with lower depression severity and hopelessness, as well as higher treatment expectations and age. Maintenance scores were positively correlated with age. Regarding predictive validity, the authors reported that Action scores were positively associated with better outcomes (e.g., lower depression severity), and that increases in Action scores during the course of treatment mediated treatment effects, predicting greater improvement.

The results of these studies support the use of the URICA to measure stages of change in youth therapy. Replication of these findings to examine the predictive validity of the URICA and further confirm the predictive validity of the SOCQ in adolescent populations may be useful. In addition, the use of the URICA and SOCQ with varied samples to explore the multicultural sensitivity of these measures would further strengthen their validity.

Parent Motivation Inventory

The PMI is a 25-item self-report measure aiming to capture three aspects of parents' motivation: hope for change in their children's behavior (e.g., "I want my child's behavior to improve"), willingness to change themselves for the purposes of impacting child behavior (e.g., "I am willing to change my current parenting techniques and try new ones"), and confidence in their ability to change (e.g., "I believe that I am capable of learning the skills needed to change my child's behavior").

Nock and Photos (2006) examined the factor structure, internal reliability, and convergent and predictive validity of the PMI, using a sample of 76 caregivers presenting for outpatient psychotherapy for children with oppositional, aggressive, and antisocial behavior. A principal-components analysis showed that a single-factor solution accounting for 56% of the variance in scores best represented the PMI. Both the internal consistency and test–retest reliabilities for the PMI were adequate for the overall measure. The PMI did not demonstrate significant correlations with child, caregiver, or family demographic variables.

Nock and Photos (2006) also found that though level of parent motivation at the first and fifth sessions was not significantly related to parent experiences of barriers to treatment, change in parent motivation between these two sessions significantly predicted barriers to treatment. In addition, parent motivation did not predict treatment attendance, but barriers to treatment did predict treatment attendance, suggesting that a relationship between parent motivation and treatment attendance may be mediated by barriers to treatment. Therefore, the PMI demonstrates substantial potential as a measure of parent motivation. Results indicated adequate reliability and suggest some predictive validity. Further examination of convergent, divergent, and predictive validity will be needed to strengthen support for this measure.

Overall, research indicates that youth and parent readiness for change can be measured by the URICA, SOCQ, or PMI in child and adolescent therapy. Each measure has demonstrated acceptable reliability and validity in youth samples; however, further research is needed for a better understanding of accurately and efficiently measuring youth and parent readiness for change in psychotherapy.

Measurement of In-Session Constructs

The Therapeutic Alliance

A large number of measures have been developed or adapted from the adult literature to measure child, adolescent, and caregiver alliance in youth psychotherapy. These measures include forms for therapists, caregivers, and observers, and youths themselves. Research indicates that each type of reporter is able to rate therapeutic alliance with adequate reliability and validity. Some of the most prominent and promising measures are reviewed here.

Therapeutic Alliance Scale for Children

The 12 items of the Therapeutic Alliance Scale for Children (TASC) were based on Bordin's (1979) transtheoretical model of the therapeutic alliance and adapted by Shirk and Saiz (1992) to be developmentally appropriate for children. TASC items distinguish between bond and work aspects of alliance. Furthermore, the TASC aims to capture both the positive and negative features of the therapeutic bond. For example, the Positive Bond subscale includes items such as "I like spending time with my therapist," and the Negative Bond subscale includes items such as "When I am with my therapist, I want the session to end quickly." The Work scale items aim to assess the level of collaboration on tasks of treatment. Shirk and Saiz (1992) also developed a parallel form of the measure for therapists to complete. This version includes the same items reworded for therapist response (e.g., "The child likes spending time with you, the therapist"). Hawley and Weisz (2005) developed a parallel parent report version with similarly reworded items (e.g., "I like spending time with my child's therapist"). All items are rated on a 4-point scale ranging from 1 ("not at all") to 4 ("very much").

Reliability and validity analyses have been performed for the TASC and support its use with multiple samples of children, their therapists, and their caregivers, representing a wide range of ethnicities, races, and presenting problems (e.g., DeVet, Kim, Charlot-Swilley, & Ireys, 2003; Creed & Kendall, 2005; Hawley & Weisz, 2005; Kronmuller et al., 2003; Shirk & Saiz, 1992). Shirk and Saiz (1992) examined the psychometric properties of the TASC with 62 hospitalized children (ages 7–12 years, with significant internalizing and externalizing problems) and their therapists. They found that subscale alphas ranged from .67 to .74 on the child report version and from .72 to .88 on the therapist report version. As expected, the Bond and Work scales were significantly related within each version of the TASC. However, the Work scale was not related across the child and therapist report versions. Still, the client and therapist reports of alliance did demonstrate a moderate degree of convergence.

Using an ethnically and racially diverse sample of 65 youth and their caregivers, Hawley and Weisz (2005) reported excellent internal consistency on a shortened form of the TASC child report version (alpha = .93) and good internal consistency on the parent report version (alpha = .81). The abbreviated TASC showed adequate 7- to 14-day test–retest reliability on both the child and parent report measures. Parent and youth alliances were correlated ($r = .32$, $N = 65$) in this sample. The TASC also demonstrated predictive validity. Hawley and Weisz (2005) found that parent alliance was related to therapy retention variables, including family involvement, frequency of cancellations and missed appointments, and therapist agreement on treatment termination, but that child alliance did not reveal significant associations with therapy retention variables. The child alliance did, however, demonstrate significant associations with greater decreases in symptom severity, while the parent alliance did not.

Creed and Kendall (2005) reported good internal consistency for the TASC, with alphas ranging from .88 to .92 on the 12-item child report and .94 to .96 on the therapist report version. This more recent version of the TASC involved minor modifications to Work items to make the scale applicable to a wide range of child therapies. Though Creed and Kendall (2005) did not examine the predictive validity of the TASC, they did examine associations between observer-rated therapist alliance-building behaviors and therapeutic alliance. Results indicated that working toward collaboration predicted higher ratings of child- and therapist-reported alliance; that finding common ground and pushing the client to talk predicted lower ratings of child-reported alliance; and that being overly formal predicted lower ratings of therapist-reported alliance. Research by McLeod and Weisz (2005) has supported the convergent validity of the TASC by showing significant associations with observer-rated alliance.

Working Alliance Inventory

The Working Alliance Inventory (WAI; Horvath & Greenberg, 1989) consists of 36 items measuring the quality of the therapeutic relationship. It has three subscales: Bonds, Tasks, and Goals. Though the WAI was designed for use with adults, it has been adapted for use with adolescents in several studies (Dennis, Ives, White, & Muck, 2008; Fitzpatrick & Irannejad, 2003; Florsheim et al., 2000; Glueckauf et al., 2002; Tetzlaff et al., 2005; Linscott, DiGiuseppe, & Jilton, 1993). Adolescent self-report, therapist report, and observer report versions have been developed. Raters respond to each item by using a 7-point Likert-type scale. Shortened 12-item versions of the adolescent and therapist report versions (WAI-S) have also been developed. With the exception of Linscott et al. (1993), these modifications consisted of relatively minor wording alterations. Linscott et al. (1993) further amended the WAI by modifying the content of the items in order to reflect adolescent treatment more closely, and thus created the Adolescent WAI. Despite the more substantial changes made to develop the Adolescent WAI, the measure maintains the original three-subscale structure.

Adolescent and therapist report versions of the WAI, modified versions of the WAI, and the WAI-S have all demonstrated good internal consistency with alphas ranging from .81 to .97 across multiple studies. The three-factor structure of the WAI has been confirmed with adult samples; however, a single-factor solution emerged from analyses of the structure of the Adolescent WAI (Linscott et al., 1993). Analyses of the structure of the WAI-S yielded similar results. This suggests that adolescents may perceive the therapeutic relationship as a general positive or negative construct, but do not further distinguish between different aspects of the therapeutic relationship (Linscott et al., 1993).

Analyses of the WAI's test–retest reliability revealed significant stability for the measure (e.g., Florsheim et al., 2000; Hawley & Garland, 2008). Cross-informant agreement has also been examined in several studies, with variable results. These results appear to vary regardless of the version of the WAI or the specific adolescent sample. For example, within the substance abuse literature, Auerbach, May, Stevens, and Kiesler (2008) found that correlations between client and therapist reports of alliance ranged from .07 to .28; however, Diamond et al. (2006) reported a higher correlation of .50. The youth literature has provided some support for the convergent validity of the WAI. Sapyta, Karver, and Bickman (1999) found that subscale correlations of the Context Specific Therapeutic Alliance Scale with the WAI ranged from .19 to .59, and that the total scale correlated with the WAI at .46. For the WAI-S, correlations have been demonstrated above .50 with the Client Affiliation axis of the Impact Message Inventory—Circumplex (a measure of dyadic interactions in psychotherapy), as well as with the Counselor Affiliation axis. In addition, a .85 correlation was found between the adolescent report WAI-S and scores on the Alliance Observation Coding System.

The divergent validity of the WAI has received limited attention. However, scores on the WAI-S and a treatment satisfaction measure showed only a moderate positive correlation, indicating that alliance and satisfaction are separate constructs. Regarding predictive validity, analyses revealed that scores on the WAI were associated with treatment completion (Florsheim et al., 2000). Furthermore, studies have shown significant relationships with scores on the WAI and multiple outcome indicators: decreased symptoms, lower relapse rates, improved family relationships, increased self-esteem, higher levels of perceived social support, and therapy satisfaction (e.g., Florsheim et al., 2000; Hawley & Garland, 2008).

Therapy Process Observational Coding System—Alliance Scale

The Therapy Process Observational Coding System—Alliance Scale (TPOCS-A; McLeod & Weisz, 2005) is a nine-item observational coding measure consisting of child and parent forms. It is designed to provide the field with a comprehensive observational system capable of objectively describing the child–therapist and parent–therapist alliances. The measure comprises two dimensions: Bond (e.g., "experience therapist as supportive" and "act hostile toward therapist") and Task (e.g., "not comply with tasks" and "work together equally on tasks"). Coders rate items after observing full sessions of therapy. Psychometric properties were examined with a sample of 22 children presenting for outpatient treatment of an anxiety or depressive disorder (McLeod & Weisz, 2005).

The child items of the TPOCS-A demonstrated excellent internal consistency (alpha = .95) and moderate test–retest reliability, with a correlation of .54 between early and late alliance. The parent items of the TPOCS-A also demonstrated good internal consistency (alpha = .89) and high test–retest reliability, with a correlations of .88 between early and late alliance. McLeod and Weisz (2005) reported acceptable interrater reliability for both the child and parent items. The child items showed an average intraclass correlation coefficient (ICC) of .59, and the parent items showed an average ICC of .61. Significant correlations between the Bond and Task subscales were found for both the child and parent items. Despite the similar psychometric properties listed above, the child and parent items did not demonstrate a significant correlation, thus indicating that the child–therapist and parent–therapist alliances may be separate and distinct. Also, Chiu, McLeod, Har, and Wood (2009) reported adequate internal consistency and interrater reliability for the TPOCS-A in another sample of children with anxiety difficulties, and Fjermestad et al. (2012) reported acceptable interrater reliability in a Norwegian sample of youth. Fjermestad et al. (2012) further conducted a factor analysis of the TPOCS-A. Results indicated a single-factor solution accounting for nearly 65% of the total variance, with item loadings ranging from .44 to .87.

McLeod and Weisz (2005) also examined the convergent validity of the TPOCS-A, using the TASC. Though stronger associations were present for the child alliance than for the parent alliance, analyses supported the convergent validity of the TPOCS-A and the TASC for both child and parent alliance. Specifically, the correlations between the TPOCS-A child items and the child report version of the TASC were as follows: .53 for the overall measures, .51 for the bond items, and .66 for the task items. The correlations between the TPOCS-A parent items and the parent report TASC were as follows: .29 for the overall measures, .24 for the bond items, and .45 for the task items. Fjermestad et al. (2012) also found significant correlations between the TPOCS-A and the child and parent versions of the TASC. However, no significant correlations were found between the

TPOCS-A and a client motivation measure or a measure of client belief in treatment, thus providing some evidence of divergent validity (Fjermestad et al., 2012).

Regarding predictive validity, associations between the TPOCS-A child and parent items and a general measure of internalizing symptoms were assessed (McLeod & Weisz, 2005). A positive parent–therapist alliance assessed during treatment was associated with a reduction in total internalizing symptoms following treatment. Associations between the TPOCS-A child and parent forms and anxiety-specific measures were also examined, and both the child and parent forms exhibited significant associations with a reduction in anxiety symptomatology at the end of treatment. Finally, relations between the child and parent forms and measures of depressive symptomatology were examined, and results revealed that the parent–therapist alliance scores, but not the child–therapist alliance scores, were related to reductions in depressive symptoms. Chiu et al. (2009) similarly found that the TPOCS-A measured early in treatment correlated with symptom reduction at midtreatment and treatment satisfaction. Therapeutic alliance improvement over the course of treatment was also associated with symptom reduction.

In summary, multiple measures of alliance have demonstrated adequate reliability and validity. At present, among participant report measures, the TASC seems most appropriate for children and the WAI for adolescents. Among observational measures, the TPOCS-A has been used with multiple samples and has accrued solid reliability and validity support.

Involvement and Resistance

Emerging research indicates that level of client involvement predicts beneficial outcomes in both child-focused and parent-focused forms of youth therapy (Karver et al., 2006). Given the early stage of this research, only a few measures of involvement and resistance have been developed and evaluated for youth therapy. Two of the more widely used and empirically supported measures of involvement are reviewed below. (Readers are advised to refer to Karver et al., 2006, for a more comprehensive list of measures.)

The Child Involvement Rating Scale (CIRS; Chu & Kendall, 2004) is an empirically supported six-item observational rating scale developed to evaluate involvement in therapy activities. Items are rated on a 6-point Likert scale and summed to compute an overall CIRS involvement score. In the original study, involvement was coded from two randomly selected audiotaped sessions (two 10-minute segments per session) from the early and later phases of treatment. Therefore, the involvement score is based on ratings of a child's verbal behavior and participation, which in turn are based on excerpts from in-session action (e.g., therapist's comments on child's behavior).

The psychometric properties of the CIRS are described further by

Chu and Kendall (2004). The CIRS showed moderate internal consistency (alpha = .73), adequate interrater reliability (ICC = .61), and moderate test–retest reliability (ICC = .59). Construct validity of the CIRS was established by evaluating correlations between involvement in early and later phases of treatment with demographic and diagnostic variables. Nonsignificant associations were found between involvement scores and demographic features or pretreatment diagnoses, thereby demonstrating adequate divergent validity. Evidence for convergent validity has not been reported. The original CIRS was developed for use in individual outpatient CBT for anxious children, implemented in university-based clinics. The CIRS was more recently used in a study of group CBT for anxious youth in a community setting, and demonstrated similar psychometric properties to those found in the original study (Tobon et al., 2011).

A second measure of involvement that has been used with youth is the Patient Participation subscale of the Vanderbilt Psychotherapy Process Scales (VPPS; O'Malley, Suh, & Strupp, 1983). This subscale is an eight-item observational rating scale developed to evaluate involvement in the therapeutic interaction. Items are scored on a 5-point scale and summed to compute a composite score. Suh and colleagues (1989) recommended the use of 15-minute segments to code VPPS subscales. The subscale demonstrated excellent internal consistency (alpha = .93) and interrater reliability (ICC = .91). The VPPS was developed for research with adults and has been shown to predict symptom improvement (O'Malley et al., 1983; Lane & Strupp, 1987; Windholz & Silberschatz, 1988). However, it has also been modified to evaluate level of involvement in CBT tasks with depressed adolescents. Both internal consistency and interrater reliability were high with this youth sample (Jungbluth & Shirk, 2009).

Research on the measurement of resistance in youth therapy is scanty. The Child Psychotherapy Process Scales (Estrada & Russell, 1999) and the CIRS (Chu & Kendall, 2004) each include a few global, observationally coded items to evaluate disengagement or low involvement. The psychometric properties of these scales have been evaluated on the basis of total scale scores; thus the reliability and validity of items tapping disengagement are not known. In contrast, the Client Resistance Code (CRC), an observationally coded measure developed by Kavanagh, Gabrielson, and Chamberlain (1982) for the assessment of resistance in parent training, includes multiple behavioral indicators, demonstrates excellent interrater reliability, and sound evidence for validity. Specifically, resistance as measured by the CRC changes in intensity over the course of treatment as predicted by the parent management model, and predicts both early dropout and therapists' ratings of treatment success (Chamberlain, Patterson, Reid, Kavanagh, & Forgatch, 1984). It is not known, however, whether similar patterns of results would be obtained with child and adolescent clients.

In summary, observational methods for assessing involvement and resistance seem most promising at present. Reliable and valid participant-based measures have yet to emerge. Although observational methods are feasible in research trials, the time and cost of such methods make them less feasible in routine practice. The development of participant-based measures of these constructs would be beneficial for assessment in clinical practice.

Treatment Integrity

The assessment of treatment integrity is a critical component of randomized controlled trials, but most studies with children and adolescents have focused exclusively on the measurement of therapist adherence (McLeod et al., 2009). A brief review of the efficacy literature suggests that using adherence checklists and reporting overall adherence rates represent typical practice. However, some variation in measurement strategies exists. In terms of *content*, measures vary in whether they assess adherence to discrete procedures or to general therapeutic principles. In terms of *source*, both observational and participant measures have been developed. We consider two prominent approaches to the assessment of adherence.

Observation of Discrete Procedures

Observational checklists appear to be the most common method for evaluating therapist adherence to specific treatment procedures. Checklists vary in their degree of specificity, with some targeting molar units such as relaxation training, and others focusing on specific intervention elements (e.g., "Therapist presented the rationale for relaxation skills, demonstrated breathing techniques, engaged the client in practice with feedback, and encouraged practice outside the session"). Although most empirically evaluated treatment manuals have a corresponding adherence measure of this type, surprisingly few data have been reported on the reliability or validity of such measures. Their virtue resides in their specificity: An adherence checklist is directly tied to a specific treatment manual. Of course, their primary limitation is also specificity: An adherence checklist devised for one manual cannot be used with another.

Other concerns have been raised as well. Perhaps the most important is the lack of sensitivity of simply assessing completion or noncompletion of specific treatment elements. Such ratings fail to account for potential variation in therapist focus on specific components; thus it has been recommended that measures of *extensiveness*—frequency and thoroughness of coverage—may be a more sensitive alternative (Hogue, Dauber, et al., 2008). "Thoroughness" refers to the complexity, depth, and persistence of therapist coverage. Of course, when more than frequency or duration is considered, judgments of extensiveness may become less reliable. A good example of this approach is the Therapeutic Behavior Rating Scale–3 (Diamond, Hogue, Diamond, & Siqueland, 1998) which has been used to evaluate adherence to multidimensional family therapy for adolescent substance abuse. Despite the complexity of assessing the extensiveness of discrete interventions over the course of a session, good interrater reliability was attained for most items.

One promising observational system for assessing treatment adherence (and differentiation) across multiple types of therapy is the Therapy Process Observation Coding System—Strategies Scale (TPOCS-S; McLeod & Weisz, 2010). Originally developed to evaluate therapy process in usual clinical care, the TPOCS-S includes five subscales—Cognitive, Behavioral, Psychodynamic, Client-Centered, and Family—each with a specific set of relevant procedures. Initial results from a study of usual-care treatment of anxious or depressed youth showed good interrater reliability and internal consistency across subscales (McLeod & Weisz, 2010). Interrater reliability at the level of specific procedures was also quite sound. In regard to validity, the internal consistency of each subscale exceeded its correlation with other subscales, thus supporting construct validity. In a study of CBT versus usual care for child and adolescent anxiety (Southam-Gerow et al., 2010) and a study of CBT versus usual care for child and adolescent depression (Weisz et al., 2009), the TPOCS-S discriminated usual-care from CBT cases across multiple subscales. Again, high levels of interrater reliability were attained. Thus the TPOCS-S shows considerable psychometric strength and represents a promising method for characterizing and differentiating treatment procedures in clinical practice.

Participant Report of Principle-Consistent Strategies

The evaluation of therapist adherence in MST has been based on participant (parent, adolescent, and therapist) reports of therapist behavior that are consistent with MST principles (Henggeler & Borduin, 1992). Thus both the source and content of assessment differ from those of the traditional observational approach. Given that MST involves the integration of numerous strategies that can be delivered in a highly flexible manner based on an individual and family case formulation, a non-script-based approach to assessing adherence is indicated. The MST adherence measure (Henggeler & Borduin, 1992) contains 26 items that reflect therapist behaviors and strategies based on nine MST principles. Factor analyses have yielded somewhat different solutions for caregiver, youth, and therapist. For example, the youth scale includes four factors (Adherence, Family–Therapist Conflict, Therapist Attempts to Change Interactions, and Lack of Direction), whereas the caregiver report contains six factors (Adherence, Nonproductive Sessions, Therapist–Family Problem-Solving, Family–Therapist Conflict, Therapist Attempts to Change Interactions, and Lack of Direction). Overall, correlations across reporters have yielded small and mostly nonsignificant correlations for similar factors. Although relatively low consensus is often found across participant raters of process, the lack of shared variance raises questions about the convergent validity of these scales. Similarly, there is some question about the degree to which these ratings are distinct from ratings of other process constructs, such as the therapeutic alliance. The absence of research demonstrating relationships with observed therapist behavior leaves these issues unresolved.

Nevertheless, adherence ratings from caregivers, youth, and therapists have been shown to predict MST outcomes, and in fact provide some of the best evidence for predictive links between adherence and outcome in the youth literature (Henggeler, Schoenwald, Borduin, Rowland, & Cunningham, 2009; Schoenwald, Chapman, Sheidow, & Carter, 2009). For example, in one study, caregiver ratings of therapist adherence predicted reductions in delinquent behavior both directly and indirectly through changes in parental monitoring, family cohesion, and peer affiliation (Huey et al., 2000). Associations between youth- and therapist-rated adherence and other measures of change were also obtained. Such results might suggest that therapists can be used as valid reporters of treatment adherence; however, other research has found considerable divergence between therapists' reports of their own interventions and independent observers' ratings (Hurlburt et al., 2010).

Overall, then, the use of participant ratings of treatment adherence appears promising. Given the lack of convergence among participants' perspectives, however, it is not clear which source should be considered the "gold standard" for assessing adherence. Therapists appear to have the greatest stake in reporting high adherence, and the use of therapist ratings, especially alone, should be considered with great caution. Clinical supervision often relies exclusively on trainees' reports of therapy process. Interestingly, trainees may not have adequate therapy experience to evaluate delivery of interventions. Trainee or supervisor reviews of recorded sessions could be aided by the use of observation systems that target specific procedures or broad classes of intervention. Clearly, more work needs to be done in this area. Associations between participant ratings and observational ratings are sorely needed, and research on the convergence or divergence of participant ratings with ratings of other process variables (e.g., the alliance) is nonexistent.

Finally, we should note that the assessment of therapist competence has received scant attention in the child and adolescent literature. A noteworthy exception is the evaluation of therapist competence in the treatment of adolescent substance abuse (Hogue, Henderson, et al., 2008). Therapist competence with molar treatment tasks in CBT or family therapy was evaluated in different phases of treatment. Interrater reliability varied widely across items, with only a minority reaching an adequate level. Ratings of competence did not predict outcomes in either treatment condition. Thus the assessment of competence is, at best, at a very early stage of development for youth treatments.

APPLICATION TO THE CLINICAL CASES

Assessment of therapy processes and psychological predictors of process provides an empirical method for personalizing and adapting evidence-based treatments. The first task of all therapies is treatment engagement. All other therapeutic processes, as well as treatment outcomes, are contingent on treatment attendance and continuation. Attrition brings therapy to a halt; sporadic attendance limits treatment cohesion; and low levels of participation undermine therapeutic dose. In fact, early attrition and sporadic attendance may be among the most significant challenges to successful implementation of evidence-based treatments in community mental health clinics. The problem is serious, given early attrition estimates of 40–70% in community clinics (Armbruster & Kazdin, 1994). Thus, for both clinical cases, Sofia and Billy, our primary focus is on treatment engagement and alliance formation.

For both cases, we assume that therapists would collect and monitor treatment progress through the use of symptom checklists, targeted behavior charts, or idiographic ratings of problem severity (Weisz et al., 2011). As noted, ongoing assessment of progress is fundamental to evidence-based practice and is critical for determining whether an empirically supported treatment is having its intended effect. In addition, we assume that therapy for Sofia and Billy would be delivered by therapists who were under supervision. This assumption seems reasonable, insofar as estimates suggest that 40% of all child therapy is delivered by trainees or clinicians under supervision.

Complementing measures of progress, indicators of in-session process and pretreatment predictors of process can guide treatment adaptation. Because critical thresholds have been established for very few (if any) process indicators, we recommend a relatively conservative approach to interpreting pretreatment predictors and process scores. Although scores for alliance, involvement, and expectancies tend to be positively skewed (with means above the midpoint of most scales), in the absence of cutoff scores based on optimal sensitivity and specificity, we do not recommend significant modification of an existing protocol unless scores are two standard deviations below the scale mean *and* below the midpoint of the scale. Under such circumstances, significant adaptation—for example, through the addition of motivational interviewing at the start of treatment—seems justified. However, we recognize that such modifications have not been evaluated empirically and should be used only with those cases whose scores suggest serious risk for engagement failure. Of course, ratings of expectancies, barriers, and stages of change can be used qualitatively by alerting therapists to specific issues that could interfere with treatment delivery and require targeted problem solving. For example, parents who report the lack of reliable child care as a treatment barrier will be at risk for canceling sessions; consequently, a plan that addresses this issue will be essential for therapy continuity. Similarly, an adolescent who reports low expectancies should be given time to explore her or his personal motivation for treatment. Flexible adaptation of an evidence-based CBT protocol—for example, by providing depressed adolescents with additional time in the first session to relate their personal narratives or explore motives for treatment—has been shown to facilitate treatment involvement (Jungbluth & Shirk, 2009).

For measures of in-session process, alliance, involvement, and resistance, we recommend the use of *process trajectories*. Again, because critical thresholds have not been established, using a client as his or her own control by tracking *shifts* in alliance, involvement, or resistance represents an alternative method for gauging whether important dimensions of process are waxing or waning. Emerging research suggests that patterns or shifts in process, such as negative shifts in involvement (Chu & Kendall, 2004), are predictive of treatment outcome (Shirk, Karver, & Brown, 2011). For example, a specific pattern of resistance in parent training—an inverted-U shape—has been shown to be a better predictor of outcome than average resistance scores (Patterson & Chamberlain, 1994). The use of trajectories, then, can alert therapists to treatment deterioration that could signal risk for treatment failure.

Application to the Case of Sofia

Sofia was a 15-year-old Hispanic girl who had been previously treated for anxiety and school avoidance with CBT. Although treatment improved Sofia's school attendance and reduced her anxiety attacks, her chronic school absences had resulted in her falling significantly behind in her schoolwork. Retention in 10th grade had been recommended. Following this recommendation, Sofia again stopped attending school. The prospect of repeating 10th grade reignited her concerns about negative social evaluations. Of equal importance, Sofia now presented as highly demoralized and self-critical. A number of depressive symptoms had emerged, including social withdrawal, a marked increase in sleeping, and self-blame. Her view of the future seemed rather bleak. Sofia's mother appeared to be demoralized as well and had been accommodating Sofia's avoidance and withdrawal.

It should be noted that Sofia's initial "panic" attack had occurred shortly after a breakup with her boyfriend. Sofia noted that she was not comfortable with how "pushy" he was about sex, and she added that "guys don't always know when to stop." Although Sofia did not elaborate on events, it was possible that she had been a victim of sexual assault or date rape. Interpersonal trauma has been shown to diminish the effects of CBT for adolescent depression (Lewis et al., 2009; Shirk, Kaplinski, & Gudmundsen, 2009) and to interfere with adolescent alliance formation (Eltz, Shirk, & Sarlin, 1995). Therefore, an assessment of trauma history would be important for treatment planning.

Although specific diagnosis would require additional assessment, the intake pointed to residual symptoms of social anxiety and school avoidance, now complicated by significant symptoms of depression. Sofia's withdrawal, low energy, and pessimism were likely to interfere with her ability to engage actively in exposure-based CBT for anxiety. It was also possible that sexual trauma would undercut the effectiveness of CBT for adolescent depression. At present, there is no empirically supported treatment for depressed adolescents with a trauma history, though trauma-focused CBT has been shown to reduce depressive symptoms among victimized children (Cohen, Mannarino, & Deblinger, 2010). Treatment planning, then, would hinge on the results of the trauma assessment. If Sofia continued to avoid talking about the events that had precipitated the breakup with her boyfriend, symptoms of depression could be targeted with either CBT or interpersonal therapy. Given Sofia's social concerns, interpersonal therapy might be indicated. However, given her withdrawal and low energy, behavioral activation strategies might be particularly useful. As this example highlights, assessment involves more than reaching a diagnosis; it also involves an evaluation of the pathogenic processes that contribute to the disorder(s) (Shirk & Russell, 1996).

Given Sofia's (and her mother's) demoralization, a number of pretreatment process predictors seemed relevant. For Sofia, the Stages of Concern Questionnaire (SOCQ) was administered to determine her readiness to reengage in psychotherapy. Results of this assessment indicated that Sofia was primarily in the precontemplation stage, indicating less than optimal motivation to engage in therapy. Studies have shown that treatment specifically targeting the increase of client motivation leads to increased treatment participation and improved outcomes (see Miller & Rollnick, 2013; Prochaska & Norcross, 2002). Therefore, in order to facilitate engagement, treatment adaptation in the form of adding a motivational interviewing component (Miller & Rollnick, 2013) before the start of CBT was recommended. The primary aims of these initial sessions were to establish rapport with Sofia (particularly through the expression of empathy), to elicit talk of change from Sofia (particularly through developing discrepancies between her current state and how she would like things to be), and promote her confidence and commitment to change while acknowledging and accepting her reluctance to change.

Sofia's mother was administered the brief CEQ-P to evaluate her expectations about a second round of treatment for Sofia. Although her expectations were not extremely low, it was evident from the intake that she was stressed by Sofia's difficulties and in need of support. Given the language barrier, referral to a collateral support group for parents was not possible. However, the therapist planned to refer the mother to a Spanish-speaking school advocate to facilitate communication with the school. In addition, the mother's proficiency in English was adequate for the intake, and as a means of providing support, the therapist planned to meet with Sofia's mother for the last 10 minutes of each session.

Following two sessions focused on motivational interviewing, treatment shifted to target Sofia's depressive symptoms. Because of Sofia's low activity level and social withdrawal, the therapist introduced behavioral activation first, before cognitive restructuring. To assess the ongoing therapy process, Sofia was administered the TASC at the end of each session while the therapist met with her mother. Adolescent-reported alliance has been shown to predict treatment outcome with depressed adolescents (Shirk et al., 2008), and alliance trajectory could be used to index changes in Sofia's perceptions of therapy. For example, a deteriorating pattern could suggest a need for reevaluating goals or motivations.

Supervision of Sofia's case was aided by the use of an adherence checklist. Because the typical CBT sequence of components had been altered in order to personalize treatment to Sofia's primary symptoms, component adherence was emphasized. In addition, because the therapist also allocated time in each session to meeting with Sofia's mother, an important focus of supervision was on ensuring an adequate dose of specific interventions. A liability of simple adherence checklists is that they do not account for the extensiveness of interventions; consequently, the supervisor and therapist attempted to evaluate this parameter by consensus.

Application to the Case of Billy

Billy was a ten-year-old European American boy who presented with a mixed symptom picture. On the one hand, Billy's mother reported significant concerns about oppositional, negative, and defiant behavior, as well as peer relational problems at school. There was also some indication that Billy might have attention and behavior regulation problems that dated back to kindergarten. On the other hand, his mother also reported significant anxiety symptoms, including problems sleeping in his own bed, fear of the dark, and difficulties with being alone in the house or at play. Although the mother noted that Billy had been difficult to manage from an early age, his problems had escalated since the adjudication of his older brother. Although specific diagnosis would require additional assessment, the intake pointed to externalizing problems compounded by significant anxiety symptoms.

Most evidence-based treatments have been developed for specific disorders, and limited evidence is available for treatment sequencing in cases of comorbidity. (See Chorpita, Bernstein, & Daleiden, 2011, for additional discussion.) How, then, should Billy's therapist proceed, and how might measures of process inform this decision? In clinical trials, this decision is made by determining the primary disorder on the basis of severity, impact on functioning, or developmental ordering, and such considerations are certainly relevant. Alternatively, evidence on comorbidity and treatment response could be informative. In Billy's case, the therapist could consult the literature to determine whether collateral externalizing problems might complicate (predict poorer response to) the treatment of anxiety, or whether collateral anxiety symptoms might complicate or facilitate the treatment of externalizing problems. To the degree that disruptive problems were found to represent a "therapy-interfering" factor, then externalizing problems should be given treatment priority. Furthermore, because the treatment of child anxiety involves parent management of exposure trials, initially targeting parent management skills would be relevant to both sets of Billy's presenting problems.

From a process perspective, other issues would be worth considering. Evidence indicates that treatments often begin without a clear consensus on problem focus; in fact, Hawley and Weisz (2003) found that approximately 75% of therapist–caregiver–youth triads actually started therapy without consensus on a single problem, and nearly 50% did not agree on broad problem type (aggression vs. depression). Lack of consensus on targeted problems could compromise perceptions of treatment relevance (a dimension of treatment barriers), and result in early attrition. Billy's mother would be likely to view a treatment that failed to focus on the most pressing problem(s) as "off target" and an obstacle to engagement. Similarly, Billy's engagement would be likely to depend on identifying a problem whose change might bring personal benefits. Billy minimized his anxiety problems, externalized his peer difficulties, and blamed his mother for their conflicts, but hinted that he was troubled by lack of maternal availability. One might infer that Billy could be engaged by focusing on increasing his mother's availability through improving their relationship. The main point here is that client priorities should be considered in the process of treatment planning.

One useful way to assess client priorities is to systematically evaluate presenting problems from both the caregiver's and the youth's perspectives. Weisz et al. (2011) have developed and evaluated the Top Problems measure as a method for specifying presenting problems and evaluating their relative severity and importance. Following diagnostic assessment, youth and caregiver are asked to list the problems that concern them the most (e.g., "We argue too much"), and then each person rates the severity and importance of the problems. In Billy's case, one might find a number of problems, including "My mom and I fight too much," "Billy is afraid of the dark," and "Billy argues with me every day." Treatment priority, then, could be determined by consensus on the items receiving high importance ratings. In Billy's case, one area of some agreement revolved around mother–son conflicts. Severity ratings on this target problem were selected as one indicator of treatment progress.

The initial treatment plan targeted parent management skills plus collateral individual work with Billy on anger management and social problem-solving skills. Given that Billy's mother was a single parent, the BTPS was administered at the treatment-planning session in order to evaluate possible obstacles to engagement. The mother noted concerns about scheduling, especially if therapy required separate sessions for her and Billy each week. Given the availability of only one therapist, and the burden of attending two sessions, treatment sequencing was necessary. The therapist proposed that therapy begin with parent consultation and then shift to individual CBT for Billy.

Because parent alliance has been shown to be a significant predictor of treatment outcome in parent management training (Kazdin et al., 2005), the parent version of the TASC was selected for administration at the end of each session. Although alliance is not equivalent to resistance—another construct that is highly relevant to predicting outcomes in parent management training (Patterson & Chamberlain, 1994)—the low demand (and cost) of parent-reported alliance measurement made it more feasible than observational ratings.

As treatment shifted to focus on Billy in individual CBT, a new set of process measures became relevant. Child involvement, especially shifts in involvement, has been shown to be predictive of change in CBT for anxiety. In the absence of sound participant measures of involvement, and given the cost of coding involvement in clinical settings, few options are available. Youth ratings of treatment collaboration are not correlated with therapist ratings (Shirk & Saiz, 1992) or with observational ratings of collaboration (Shirk & Karver, 2003). Therapist ratings of collaboration are moderately associated with observational ratings; therefore, Billy's therapist was asked to rate the alliance on the TASC with particular attention to the Work scale items. By no means was such assessment ideal, but it was recommended to track potential shifts in Billy's in-session behavior, especially as more demanding exposure tasks were incorporated into treatment. Although exposure has not been shown to undermine alliance (Kendall et al., 2009), downward shifts at this stage could signal the need to improve involvement by modifying contingencies or breaking exposure trials into more manageable tasks. In Billy's case, initial alliance scores were relatively low, as Billy expressed reluctance to participate in sessions. In response, Billy's therapist elected to reinforce in-session involvement with a point system. After accumulation of sufficient points, Billy and his therapist could spend a portion of a session playing one-on-one basketball in a neighboring school yard. Billy's participation improved until the exposure phase of treatment was initiated. Therapist ratings of collaboration showed a sharp decline. At this point, the therapist coordinated more substantial reinforcement for exposure trials with Billy's mother.

Therapy supervision was aided in this case by review of audio recordings of treatment sessions. As part of supervision, Billy's therapist reviewed each session and assessed one component of integrity with the relevant checklist. Gaps in adherence were discussed in supervision, obstacles to implementation considered, and plans for administration discussed. Although such an approach is substantially different from methods used in clinical trials, therapist review of sessions guided with a checklist provides substantially more structure than simple narrative presentation. Supervisors can use the same method for reviewing sessions and can evaluate gaps in implementation as well as quality of therapist interventions. However, in the absence of sound measures of therapist competence, supervision will continue to rely on the individual expertise of supervisors.

As both of the foregoing cases illustrate, process assessment, either prior to the start of treatment or during its course, can provide therapists with feedback for treatment adaptation. Some preferred assessment methods (e.g., observation of treatment involvement and alliance) may not be feasible in community clinics where time and funds are scarce, and proxy measures may have to suffice. Similar constraints may limit the use of observation in supervision, but direct feedback on observed sessions should be part of therapist training, and this process would be enhanced by the development of user-friendly adherence and competence measures.

SUMMARY AND RECOMMENDATIONS

It has been our proposal that assessment of therapy process and predictors of process provide a method for *personalizing* evidence-based treatments for children and adolescents. Pretreatment assessment of expectancies, barriers, and readiness for change carry important implications for tailoring treatments in ways that optimize continuation and involvement. Ongoing assessment of alliance, involvement, and resistance can signal the need for therapeutic flexibility and the reevaluation of strategies. Therapy is far more than simply communicating the content of a manual to a client. Instead, therapy is predicated on mutual engagement of client and therapist; consequently, attending to unfolding processes is essential for treatment uptake. Of equal importance is the skillful delivery of core treatment components. Ongoing assessment of adherence and competence is critical for implementation of evidence-based treatments in service clinics.

A number of issues have emerged in our review of the literature. First, most measures of treatment process lack clinically meaningful thresholds for predicting process difficulties. Similarly, we simply do not know what level of adherence or competence is needed in order for evidence-based treatments to be effective. In fact, at this point, there is limited consensus about the nature of therapist competence. Thus considerable work remains to improve the clinical utility of process assessment.

At this point, the incremental validity of process assessment as a whole enterprise is not clear. Although research has demonstrated the usefulness of progress feedback for improving clinical outcomes (Shimokawa et al., 2010), comparable research on process feedback has not been conducted. It is possible that regular assessment and systematic feedback about client progress will be sufficient for optimizing outcomes, and that further information about ongoing process will add relatively little. However, process assessment could provide therapists with important information about *why* treatment is not progressing through monitoring specific (adherence) and nonspecific (alliance) factors. A randomized comparison of progress and process feedback, and their combination, relative to no feedback would begin to address this issue.

Our focus in this chapter has been on the assessment of therapeutic processes and not pathogenic processes—that is, those treatment targets that are typically viewed as change mechanisms (Kazdin & Nock, 2003).

Most therapeutic models are inherently mediational; the relation between specific therapeutic processes and treatment outcomes is conceptualized as running through modification of theory-specific treatment targets. For example, in the case of CBT for adolescent depression, cognitive restructuring is implemented to modify cognitive distortions. In turn, change in cognitions is presumed to account for symptom reduction. Clearly, the assessment of theory-specific change mechanisms and not just overt symptoms is critical for treatment process. For example, in order for therapists to gauge whether they have delivered interventions at a sufficient dose, change in the treatment target needs to be assessed. The absence of change in a specific target may signal the need for continued focus or a change in strategy. Typically, treatment manuals allocate fixed amounts of time to particular targets, and treatment moves forward regardless of change in specific mechanisms. A personalized treatment approach would involve both prioritization of treatment targets and customization of treatment dose.

In conclusion, the assessment of therapy process and predictors of process has the potential to improve outcomes of evidence-based treatments in clinical practice. Much work needs to be done to make process assessment "clinic-ready," however. Insofar as process research *and* assessment serve clinical outcomes, an important first step will be to demonstrate the clinical utility of process assessment.

REFERENCES

Armbruster, P., & Kazdin, A. E. (1994). Attrition in child psychotherapy. *Advances in Clinical Child Psychology, 16*, 81–108.
Auerbach, S. M., May, J. C., Stevens, M., & Kiesler, D. J. (2008). The interactive role of working alliance and counselor–client interpersonal behaviors in adolescent substance abuse treatment. *International Journal of Clinical and Health Psychology, 8*, 617–629.
Barber, J. P., Gallop, R., Crits-Christoph, P., Frank, A., Thase, M. E., Weiss, R. D., & Gibbons, M. (2006). The role of therapist adherence, therapist competence, and alliance in predicting outcome of individual drug counseling: Results from the National Institute Drug Abuse Collaborative Cocaine Treatment Study. *Psychotherapy Research, 16*, 229–240.
Bellis, J. (1994). The transtheoretical model of change applied to psychotherapy: A psychometric assessment of related instruments. *Dissertation Abstracts International, 54*, 3845B.
Bordin, E. S. (1979). The generalizability of the psychoanalytic concept of the working alliance. *Psychotherapy: Theory, Research and Practice, 16*, 252–260.
Borkovec, T. D., & Nau, S. D. (1972). Credibility of analogue therapy rationales. *Journal of Behavior Therapy and Experimental Psychiatry, 3*, 257–260.
Braswell, L., Kendall, P. C., Braith, J., Carey, M. P., & Vye, C. S. (1985). "Involvement" in cognitive-behavioral therapy with children: Process and its relationship to outcome. *Cognitive Therapy and Research, 9*, 611–630.
Chamberlain, P., Patterson, G., Reid, J., Kavanagh, K., & Forgatch, M. (1984). Observation of client resistance. *Behavior Therapy, 15*, 144–155.

Chiu, A. W., McLeod, B. D., Har, K., & Wood, J. J. (2009). Child–therapist alliance and clinical outcomes in cognitive behavioral therapy for child anxiety disorders. *Journal of Child Psychology and Psychiatry, 50,* 751–758.

Chorpita, B. F., Bernstein, A., & Daleiden, E. L. (2011). Empirically guided coordination of multiple evidence-based treatments: An illustration of relevance mapping in children's mental health services. *Journal of Consulting and Clinical Psychology, 74,* 470–480.

Chu, B. C., & Kendall, P. C. (2004). Positive association of child involvement and treatment outcome within a manual-based cognitive-behavioral treatment for children with anxiety. *Journal of Consulting and Clinical Psychology, 72,* 821–829.

Chu, B. C., & Kendall, P. C. (2009). Therapist responsiveness to child engagement: Flexibility within manual-based CBT for anxious youth. *Journal of Clinical Psychology, 65,* 736–754.

Cohen, J. A., Mannarino, A. P., & Deblinger, E. (2010). Trauma-focused cognitive-behavioral therapy for traumatized children. In J. R. Weisz & A. E. Kazdin (Eds.), *Evidence-based psychotherapies for children and adolescents* (2nd ed., pp. 295–311). New York: Guilford Press.

Cohen, P. J., Glaser, B. A., Calhoun, G. B., Bradshaw, C. P., & Petrocelli, J. V. (2005). Examining readiness for change: A preliminary evaluation of the University of Rhode Island change assessment with incarcerated adolescents. *Measurement and Evaluation in Counseling and Development, 38,* 45–62.

Colson, D. B., Murphy, T., O'Malley, F., Hyland, P. S., Cornsweet, C., McParland, M., & Coyne, L. (1990). Assessing difficulties in the hospital treatment of children and adolescents. *Bulletin of the Menninger Clinic, 54,* 78–89.

Constantino, M. J., Arnow, B. A., Blasey, C., & Agras, W. (2005). The association between patient characteristics and the therapeutic alliance in cognitive-behavioral and interpersonal therapy for bulimia nervosa. *Journal of Consulting and Clinical Psychology, 73,* 203–211.

Creed, T., & Kendall, P. C. (2005). Empirically supported therapist relationship building behavior within a cognitive-behavioral treatment of anxiety in youth. *Journal of Consulting and Clinical Psychology, 73,* 498–505.

Curry, J., Rohde, P., Simons, A., Silva, S., Vitiello, B., Kratochvil, C., & March, J. (2006). Predictors and moderators of acute outcome in the Treatment for Adolescents with Depression Study (TADS). *Journal of the American Academy of Child and Adolescent Psychiatry, 45,* 1427–1439.

Dennis, M. L., Ives, M. L., White, M. K., & Muck, R. D. (2008). The Strengthening Communities for Youth (SCY) initiative: A cluster analysis of the services received, their correlates and how they are associated with outcomes. *Journal of Psychoactive Drugs, 40,* 3–16.

Devilly, G. J., & Borkovec, T. D. (2000). Psychometric properties of the Credibility/Expectancy Questionnaire. *Journal of Behavior Therapy and Experimental Psychiatry, 31,* 73–86.

DeVet, K. A., Kim, Y. J., Charlot-Swilley, D., & Ireys, H. T. (2003). The therapeutic relationship in child therapy: Perspectives of children and mothers. *Journal of Clinical Child and Adolescent Psychology, 32,* 277–283.

Dew, S. E., & Bickman, L. (2005). Client expectancies about therapy. *Mental Health Services Research, 7,* 21–33.

Diamond, G. M., Hogue, A. T., Diamond, G. S., & Siqueland, L. (1998). *Scoring manual for the Therapist Behavior Rating Scale—3rd version* Unpublished manual.

Diamond, G. S., Liddle, H. A., Wintersteen, M. B., Dennis, M. L., Godley, S. H., & Tims, F. (2006). Early therapeutic alliance as a predictor of treatment outcome for adolescent cannabis users in outpatient treatment. *American Journal on Addictions, 15,* 26–33.

DiGiuseppe, R., Linscott, J., & Jilton, R. (1996). Developing the therapeutic alliance in child–adolescent psychotherapy. *Applied and Preventive Psychology, 5,* 85–100.

Ellis, M. L., Weiss, B., Han, S., & Gallop, R. (2010). The influence of parental factors on therapist adherence in multi-systemic therapy. *Journal of Abnormal Child Psychology, 38,* 857–868.

Eltz, M., Shirk, S., & Sarlin, N. (1995). Alliance formation and treatment outcome among maltreated adolescents. *Child Abuse and Neglect, 19,* 419–431.

Estrada, A. U., & Russell, R. L. (1999). The development of the Child Psychotherapy Process Scales (CPPS). *Psychotherapy Research, 9,* 154–166.

Faw, L., Hogue, A., Johnson, S., Diamond, G. M., & Liddle, H. A. (2005). The Adolescent Therapeutic Alliance Scale (ATAS): Initial psychometrics and prediction of outcome in family-based substance abuse prevention counseling. *Psychotherapy Research, 15,* 141–154.

Fjermestad, K., McLeod, B. D., Heiervang, E. R., Havik, O. E., Ost, L. G., & Haugland, B. S. M. (2012). Factor structure and psychometric properties of the Therapy Process Observational Coding System for Child Psychotherapy Alliance scale. *Journal of Clinical Child and Adolescent Psychology, 41*(2), 246–254.

Fitzpatrick, M. R., & Irannejad, S. (2008). Adolescent readiness for change and the working alliance in counseling. *Journal of Counseling and Development, 86,* 438–445.

Florsheim, P., Shotorbani, S., Guest-Warnick, G., Barratt, T., & Hwang, W. (2000). Role of the working alliance in the treatment of delinquent boys in community-based programs. *Journal of Clinical Child Psychology, 29,* 94–107.

Garcia, J. A., & Weisz, J. R. (2002). When youth mental health care stops: Therapeutic relationship problems and other reasons for ending youth outpatient treatment. *Journal of Consulting and Clinical Psychology, 70,* 439–443.

Garland, A. F., Hurlburt, M. S., & Hawley, K. M. (2006). Examining psychotherapy processes in a services research context. *Clinical Psychology: Science and Practice, 13,* 30–46.

Glueckauf, R. L., Liss, H. J., McQuillen, D. E., Webb, P. M., Dairaghi, J., & Carter, C. B. (2002). Therapeutic alliance in family therapy for adolescents with epilepsy: An exploratory study. *American Journal of Family Therapy, 30,* 125–139.

Gould, M. S., Shaffer, D., & Kaplan, D. (1985). The characteristics of dropouts from a child psychiatry clinic. *Journal of the American Academy of Child Psychiatry, 24,* 316–328.

Greenstein, D. K., Franklin, M. E., & McGuffin, P. (1999). Measuring motivation to change: An examination of the University of Rhode Island Change Assessment questionnaire (URICA) in an adolescent sample. *Psychotherapy: Theory, Research, Practice, Training, 36,* 47–55.

Guadiano, B. A., & Miller, I. W. (2006). Patients' expectancies, the alliance in pharmacotherapy, and treatment outcomes in bipolar disorder. *Journal of Consulting and Clinical Psychology, 74,* 671–676.

Gusella, J., Butler, G., Nichols, L., & Bird, D. (2003). A brief questionnaire to assess readiness to change in adolescents with eating disorders: Its application to group therapy. *European Eating Disorders Review, 11,* 58–71.

Hawley, K. M., & Garland, A. F. (2008). Working alliance in adolescent outpatient therapy: Youth, parent and therapist reports and associations with therapy outcomes. *Child and Youth Care Forum, 37,* 59–74.

Hawley, K. M., & Weisz, J. R. (2003). Child, parent, and therapist (dis)agreement on target problems in outpatient therapy: The therapist's dilemma and its implications. *Journal of Consulting and Clinical Psychology, 71,* 62–70.

Hawley, K. M., & Weisz, J. R. (2005). Youth versus parent working alliance in usual clinical care: Distinctive associations with retention, satisfaction, and treatment outcome. *Journal of Clinical Child and Adolescent Psychology, 34,* 117–128.

Hemphill, J. F., & Howell, A. J. (2000). Adolescent offenders and stages of change. *Psychological Assessment, 12,* 371–381.

Henggeler, S. W., & Borduin, C. M. (1992). *Multisystemic therapy adherence scales.* Unpublished instrument, Department of Psychiatry and Behavioral Sciences, Medical University of South Carolina.

Henggeler, S. W., Schoenwald, S. K., Borduin, C. M., Rowland, M. D., & Cunningham, P. B. (2009). *Multisystemic therapy for antisocial behavior in children and adolescents* (2nd ed.). New York: Guilford Press.

Hoberman, H. M. (1992). Ethnic minority status and adolescent mental health services utilization. *Journal of Behavioral Health Services and Research, 19,* 246–267.

Hogue, A., Dauber, S., Chinchilla, P., Fried, A., Henderson, C., Inclan, J., Liddle, H. A. (2008). Assessing fidelity in individual and family therapy for adolescent substance abuse. *Journal of Substance Abuse Treatment, 35,* 137–147.

Hogue, A., Henderson, C. E., Dauber, S., Barajas, P. C., Fried, A., & Liddle, H. A. (2008). Treatment adherence, competence, and outcome in individual and family therapy for adolescent behavior problems. *Journal of Consulting and Clinical Psychology, 76,* 544–555.

Horvath, A. O., & Greenberg, L. S. (1989). Development and validation of the Working Alliance Inventory. *Journal of Counseling Psychology, 36,* 223–233.

Huey, S. J., Jr., Henggeler, S. W., Brondino, M. J., & Pickrel, S. G. (2000). Mechanisms of change in multisystemic therapy: Reducing delinquent behavior through therapist adherence and improved family and peer functioning. *Journal of Consulting and Clinical Psychology, 68,* 451–468.

Hurlburt, M. S., Garland, A. F., Nguyen, K., & Brookman-Frazee, L. (2010). Child and family therapy process: Concordance of therapist and observational perspectives. *Administration and Policy in Mental Health and Mental Health Services Research, 37,* 230–244.

Jungbluth, N. J., & Shirk, S. R. (2009). Therapist strategies for building involvement in cognitive-behavioral therapy for adolescent depression. *Journal of Consulting and Clinical Psychology, 77,* 1179–1184.

Karver, M. S., Handelsman, J. B., Fields, S., & Bickman, L. (2006). Meta-analysis of therapeutic relationship variables in youth and family therapy: The evidence for different relationship variables in the child and adolescent treatment outcome literature. *Clinical Psychology Review, 26,* 50–65.

Karver, M. S., Shirk, S. R., Handelsman, J. B., Fields, S., Crisp, H., Gudmundsen, G., & McMakin, D. (2008). Relationship processes in youth psychotherapy: Measuring alliance, alliance-building behaviors, and client-involvement. *Journal of Emotional and Behavioral Disorders, 16*, 15–28.

Kavanagh, K., Gabrielson, P., & Chamberlain, P. (1982). *Manual for coding client resistance* (Technical Report No. a.2). Eugene: Oregon Social Learning Center.

Kazdin, A. E. (1979). Therapy outcome questions requiring control of credibility and treatment-generated expectancies. *Behavior Therapy, 10*, 81–93.

Kazdin, A. E. (1996). Dropping out of child psychotherapy: Issues for research and implications for practice. *Clinical Child Psychology and Psychiatry, 1*, 133–156.

Kazdin, A. E. (2000). Perceived barriers to treatment participation and treatment acceptability among antisocial children and their families. *Journal of Child and Family Studies, 9*, 157–174.

Kazdin, A. E., & Holland, L. (1991). *Parent Expectancies for Therapy Scale.* Unpublished manuscript, Yale University, Child Conduct Clinic, New Haven, CT.

Kazdin, A. E., Holland, L., & Crowley, M. (1997). Family experience of barriers to treatment and premature termination from child therapy. *Journal of Consulting and Clinical Psychology, 65*, 453–463.

Kazdin, A. E., Holland, L., Crowley, M., & Breton, S. (1997). Barriers to Treatment Participation Scale: Evaluation and validation in the context of child outpatient treatment. *Journal of Child Psychology and Psychiatry, 38*, 1051–1062.

Kazdin, A. E., Marciano, P. L., & Whitley, M. K. (2005). The therapeutic alliance in cognitive-behavioral treatment of children referred for oppositional, aggressive, and antisocial behavior. *Journal of Consulting and Clinical Psychology, 73*, 726–730.

Kazdin, A. E., & Mazurick, J. L. (1994). Dropping out of child psychotherapy: Distinguishing early and late dropouts over the course of treatment. *Journal of Consulting and Clinical Psychology, 62*, 1069–1074.

Kazdin, A. E., Mazurick, J. L., & Bass, D. (1993). Risk for attrition in treatment of antisocial children and families. *Journal of Clinical Child Psychology, 22*, 2–16.

Kazdin, A. E., & Nock, M. K. (2003). Delineating mechanisms of change in child and adolescent therapy: Methodological issues and research recommendations. *Journal of Child Psychology and Psychiatry, 44*, 1116–1129.

Kazdin, A. E., & Wassell, G. (2000). Predictors of barriers to treatment and therapeutic change in outpatient therapy for antisocial children and their families. *Mental Health Services Research, 2*, 27–40.

Kazdin, A. E., & Whitley, M. K. (2006). Pretreatment social relations, therapeutic alliance, and improvements in parenting practices in parent management training. *Journal of Consulting and Clinical Psychology, 74*, 346–355.

Kendall, P. C., & Chu, B. C. (2000). Retrospective self-reports of therapist flexibility in a manual-based treatment for youths with anxiety disorders. *Journal of Clinical Child and Adolescent Psychology, 29*, 209–220.

Kendall, P. C., Chu, B., Gifford, A., Hayes, C., & Nauta, M. (1998). Breathing life into a manual. *Cognitive and Behavioral Practice, 5*, 177–198.

Kendall, P. C., Comer, J. S., Marker, C. D., Creed, T. A., Puliafico, A. C., Hughes, A. A., & Hudson, J. (2009). In-session exposure tasks and therapeutic alliance across the treatment of childhood anxiety disorders. *Journal of Consulting and Clinical Psychology, 77*, 517–525.

Kronmuller, K. T., Hartmann, M., Reck, C., Victor, D., Horn, H., & Winkelmann, K. (2003). Therapeutic alliance in child and adolescent psychotherapy: Evaluation of a German version of the Therapeutic Scales for Children. *Zeitschrift für Klinische Psychologie und Psychotherapie, 32*, 14–23.

Krupnick, J. L., Sotsky, S. M., Simmens, S., Moyer, J., Elkin, I., Watkins, J., & Pilkonis, P. A. (1996). The role of the therapeutic alliance in psychotherapy and pharmacotherapy outcome: Findings in the National Institute of Mental Health Treatment of Depression Collaborative Research Program. *Journal of Consulting and Clinical Psychology, 64*, 532–539.

Lambert, M. J., & Shimokawa, K. (2011). Collecting client feedback. *Psychotherapy, 48*, 72–79.

Lane, T. W., & Strupp, H. H. (1987). *In pursuit of the obvious: Investigating the effects of patient qualities on process and outcome relationships in psychotherapy—a preliminary report.* Paper presented at the meeting of the Society for Psychotherapy Research, Ulm, West Germany.

Lewis, C. C., Simons, A. D., Silva, S. G., Rohde, P., Small, D. M., Murakami, J. L., & March, J. S. (2009). The role of readiness to change in response to treatment of adolescent depression. *Journal of Consulting and Clinical Psychology, 77*, 422–428.

Linscott, J., DiGiuseppe, R., & Jilton, R. (1993, August). *A measure of TA in adolescent psychotherapy.* Poster presented at the 101st Annual Convention of the American Psychological Association, Toronto, Ontario, Canada.

Littell, J. H., & Girvin, H. (2005). Caregivers' readiness for change: Predictive validity in a child welfare sample. *Child Abuse and Neglect, 29*, 59–80.

Maisto, S. A., Chung, T. A., Cornelius, J. R., & Martin, C. S. (2003). Factor structure of the SOCRATES in a clinical sample of adolescents. *Psychology of Addictive Behaviors, 17*, 98–107.

McConnaughy, E. A., DiClemente, C. C., Prochaska, J. O., & Velicer, W. F. (1989). Stages of change in psychotherapy: A follow-up report. *Psychotherapy: Theory, Research, Practice, Training, 26*, 494–503.

McConnaughy, E. A., Prochaska, J. O., & Velicer, W. F. (1983). Stages of change in psychotherapy: Measurement and sample profiles. *Psychotherapy: Theory, Research and Practice, 20*, 368–375.

McHugh, R., Murray, H. W., & Barlow, D. H. (2009). Balancing fidelity and adaptation in the dissemination of empirically–supported treatments: The promise of transdiagnostic interventions. *Behaviour Research and Therapy, 47*, 946–953.

McLeod, B. D., Southam-Gerow, M. A., & Weisz, J. R. (2009). Conceptual and methodological issues in treatment integrity measurement. *School Psychology Review, 38*, 541–546.

McLeod, B. D., & Weisz, J. R. (2005). The Therapy Process Observational Coding System—Alliance Scale: Measure characteristics and prediction of outcome in usual clinical practice. *Journal of Consulting and Clinical Psychology, 73*, 323–333.

McLeod, B. D., & Weisz, J. R. (2010). The Therapy Process Observational Coding

System for Child Psychotherapy Strategies Scale. *Journal of Clinical Child and Adolescent Psychology, 39*, 436–443.

Miller, W. R., & Rollnick, S. (2013). *Motivational interviewing* (3rd ed.). New York: Guildford Press.

Miller, W. R., & Tonigan, J. (1996). Assessing drinkers' motivations for change: The Stages of Change Readiness and Treatment Eagerness Scale (SOCRATES). *Psychology of Addictive Behaviors, 10*, 81–89.

Nock, M. K., & Ferriter, C. (2005). Parent management of attendance and adherence in child and adolescent therapy: A conceptual and empirical review. *Clinical Child and Family Psychology Review, 8*, 149–166.

Nock, M. K., Ferriter, C., & Holmberg, E. (2007). Parent beliefs about treatment credibility and effectiveness: Assessment and relation to subsequent treatment participation. *Journal of Child and Family Studies, 1*, 27–38.

Nock, M. K., & Kazdin, A. E. (2001). Parent expectancies for child therapy: Assessment and relation to participation in treatment. *Journal of Child and Family Studies, 10*, 155–180.

Nock, M. K., & Kazdin, A. E. (2005). Randomized controlled trial of a brief intervention for increasing participation in parent management training. *Journal of Consulting and Clinical Psychology, 73*, 872–879.

Nock, M. K., & Photos, V. (2006). Parent motivation to participate in treatment: Assessment and prediction of subsequent participation. *Journal of Child and Family Studies, 15*, 345–358.

O'Malley, S., Suh, C., & Strupp, H. (1983). The Vanderbilt Psychotherapy Process Scales: A report on scale development and a process–outcomes study. *Journal of Consulting and Clinical Psychology, 44*, 189–208.

Patterson, G. R., & Chamberlain, P. (1994). A functional analysis of resistance during parent training therapy. *Clinical Psychology: Science and Practice, 1*, 53–70.

Perepletchikova, F., & Kazdin, A. E. (2005). Treatment integrity and therapeutic change: Issues and research recommendations. *Clinical Psychology: Science and Practice, 12*, 365–383.

Perepletchikova, F., Treat, T. A., & Kazdin, A. E. (2007). Treatment integrity in psychotherapy research: Analysis of the studies and examination of the associated factors. *Journal of Consulting and Clinical Psychology, 75*, 829–841.

Peterson, E. L., Jungbluth, N. J., Siler, T. J., & Shirk, S. R. (2010). *Early predictors of client engagement in CBT for adolescent depression.* Poster presented at the annual convention of the Association for Behavioral and Cognitive Therapies, San Francisco.

Prinz, R. J., & Miller, G. E. (1994). Family-based treatment for childhood antisocial behavior: Experimental influences on dropout and engagement. *Journal of Consulting and Clinical Psychology, 62*, 645–650.

Prochaska, J. O., & DiClemente, C. C. (1982). Transtheoretical therapy: Toward a more integrative model of change. *Psychotherapy: Theory, Research and Practice, 19*, 276–288.

Prochaska, J. O., & Norcross, J. C. (2001). Stages of change. *Psychotherapy: Theory, Research, Practice, Training, 38*, 443–448.

Robbins, M. S., Liddle, H. A., Turner, C. W., Dakof, G. A., Alexander, J. F., & Kogan, S. M. (2006). Adolescent and parent therapeutic alliances as predictors of dropout in multidimensional family therapy. *Journal of Family Psychology, 20*, 108–116.

Sapyta, J. J., Karver, M. S., & Bickman, L. (1999) Therapeutic alliance: Significance in non-psychotherapy settings. In C. L. Liberton, C. Newman, K. Kutash, & R. M. Friedman (Eds.), *12th Annual Research Conference Proceedings, a system of care for children's mental health: Expanding the research base* (pp. 183–186). Tampa: University of South Florida Press.

Schoenwald, S. K., Carter, R. E., Chapman, J. E., & Sheidow, A. J. (2008). Therapist adherence and organizational effects on change in youth behavior problems one year after multisystemic therapy. *Administration and Policy in Mental Health and Mental Health Services Research, 35*, 379–394.

Schoenwald, S. K., Chapman, J. E., Sheidow, A. J., & Carter, R. E. (2009). Long-term youth criminal outcomes in MST transport: The impact of therapist adherence and organizational climate and structure. *Journal of Clinical Child and Adolescent Psychology, 38*, 91–105.

Shimokawa, K., Lambert, M. J., & Smart, D. W. (2010). Enhancing treatment outcome of patients at risk of treatment failure: Meta-analytic and mega-analytic review of a psychotherapy quality assurance system. *Journal of Consulting and Clinical Psychology, 78*, 298–311.

Shirk, S. R., Gudmundsen, G. R., Kaplinski, H. C., & McMakin, D. L. (2008). Alliance and outcome in cognitive-behavioral therapy for adolescent depression. *Journal of Clinical Child and Adolescent Psychology, 37*, 631–639.

Shirk, S. R., Jungbluth, N. J., & Karver, M. S. (2011). Change processes and active components. In P. C. Kendall (Ed.), *Child and adolescent therapy: Cognitive behavioral procedures* (4th ed., pp. 471–498). New York: Guilford Press.

Shirk, S. R., Kaplinski, H., & Gudmundsen, G. (2009). School-based cognitive-behavioral therapy for adolescent depression: A benchmarking study. *Journal of Emotional and Behavioral Disorders, 17*, 106–117.

Shirk, S. R., & Karver, M. (2003). Prediction of treatment outcome from relationship variables in child and adolescent therapy: A meta-analytic review. *Journal of Consulting and Clinical Psychology, 71*, 452–464.

Shirk, S. R., & Karver, M. (2006). Process issues in cognitive-behavioral therapy for youth. In P. C. Kendall (Ed.), *Child and adolescent therapy: Cognitive-behavioral procedures* (3rd ed., pp. 465–491). New York: Guilford Press.

Shirk, S. R., Karver, M., & Brown, R. (2011). The alliance in child and adolescent psychotherapy. *Psychotherapy, 48*, 17–24.

Shirk, S., & McMakin, D. (2007). Client, therapist, and treatment characteristics in evidence-based treatments for children and adolescents. In M. Roberts & R. Steele (Eds.), *Handbook of evidence-based therapies for children and adolescents* (pp. 457–472). New York: Springer.

Shirk, S. R., & Russell, R. L. (1996). *Change processes in child psychotherapy: Revitalizing treatment and research.* New York: Guilford Press.

Shirk, S. R., & Russell, R. (1998). Process issues in child psychotherapy. In A. Bellack & M. Hersen (Series Eds.) & T. Ollendick (Vol. Ed.), *Comprehensive clinical psychology: Vol. 5. Children and adolescents: Clinical formulations and treatment* (pp. 57–82). Oxford: Pergamon Press.

Shirk, S. R., & Saiz, C. S. (1992). Clinical, empirical, and developmental perspectives on the therapeutic relationship in child psychotherapy. *Development and Psychopathology, 4*, 713–728.

Siler, T. J., Crisostomo, P. S., & Jungbluth, N. J. (2010). *Therapeutic strategies to enhance involvement in emotional processing in cognitive behavioral therapy*. Poster presented at the annual convention of the American Psychological Association, San Diego, CA.

Southam-Gerow, M. A., Weisz, J. R., Chu, B. C., McLeod, B. D., Gordis, E. B., & Connor-Smith, J. K. (2010). Does cognitive behavioral therapy for youth anxiety outperform usual care in community clinics?: An initial effectiveness test. *Journal of the American Academy of Child and Adolescent Psychiatry*, 49, 1043–1052.

Stewart-Williams, S. (2004). The placebo puzzle: Putting together the pieces. *Health Psychology*, 23, 198–206.

Suh, C., O'Malley, S., Strupp, H., & Johnson, M. (1989). The Vanderbilt Psychotherapy Process Scale (VPPS), *Journal of Cognitive Psychotherapy*, 3, 123–154.

Tetzlaff, B. T., Kahn, J. H., Godley, S. H., Godley, M. D., Diamond, G. S., & Funk, R. R. (2005). Working alliance, treatment satisfaction, and patterns of posttreatment use among adolescent substance users. *Psychology of Addictive Behaviors*, 19, 199–207.

Tobon, J. I., Eichstedt, J. A., Wolfe, V. V., Phoenix, E., Brisebois, S., Zayed, R. S., & Harris, K. E. (2011). Group cognitive-behavioral therapy for anxiety in a clinic setting: Does child involvement predict outcome? *Behavior Therapy*, 42, 306–322.

Tryon, G., & Kane, A. S. (1995). Client involvement, working alliance, and type of therapy termination. *Psychotherapy Research*, 5, 189–198.

Weersing, V., Weisz, J. R., & Donenberg, G. R. (2002). Development of the Therapy Procedures Checklist: A therapist-report measure of technique use in child and adolescent treatment. *Journal of Clinical Child and Adolescent Psychology*, 31, 168–180.

Weisz, J. R., Chorpita, B. F., Frye, A., Ng, M., Lau, N., Bearman, S., & Hoagwood, K. E. (2011). Youth top problems: Using idiographic, consumer-guided assessment to identify treatment needs and to track change during psychotherapy. *Journal of Consulting and Clinical Psychology*, 79, 369–380.

Weisz, J. R., Southam-Gerow, M. A., Gordis, E. B., Connor-Smith, J. K., Chu, B. C., Langer, D. A., & Weiss, B. (2009). Cognitive-behavioral therapy versus usual clinical care for youth depression: An initial test of transportability to community clinics and clinicians. *Journal of Consulting and Clinical Psychology*, 77, 383–396.

Wierzbicki, M., & Pekarik, G. (1993). A meta-analysis of psychotherapy dropout. *Professional Psychology: Research and Practice*, 24, 190–195.

Windholz, M. J., & Silberschatz, G. (1988). The Vanderbilt Psychotherapy Process Scale: A replication with adult outpatients. *Journal of Consulting and Clinical Psychology*, 56, 56–60.

Wright, L., Everett, F., & Roisman, L. (1986). *Experiential psychotherapy with children*. Baltimore, MD: Johns Hopkins University Press.

Yen, C., Huang, Y., Chang, Y., & Cheng, C. (2010). Factor structure of the Chinese version of the University of Rhode Island Change Assessment in Taiwanese adolescents who abuse MDMA or methamphetamine. *American Journal of Drug and Alcohol Abuse*, 36, 114–117.

15

Diagnostic and Behavioral Assessment in Action

Amanda Jensen-Doss, Thomas H. Ollendick, and Bryce D. McLeod

The assessment of children and adolescents has made great strides in the past three decades. Numerous assessment tools now exist, and knowledge of how to apply these tools is growing. One of the most important recent advances is the evidence-based assessment movement. This movement has brought attention to the key role assessment plays in psychology. Moreover, the evidence-based assessment movement has led to the development of assessment guidelines that emphasize relying upon scientific findings to guide the assessment process.

Despite these advances, gaps still exist in our knowledge of how and when to use specific assessment tools. The purpose of this volume is to communicate how diagnostic and behavioral assessment principles and methods can be used to inform the treatment process from intake to termination for children and adolescents. In Part I of this volume, we have covered the overarching principles that guide our approach to diagnostic and behavioral assessment, whereas Part II has covered in detail the major diagnostic and behavioral assessment methods.

The purpose of the current chapter is to illustrate how the principles and methods covered in this volume can be used to formulate a case conceptualization. To achieve this goal, we return to the two sample cases presented in Chapter 4. In the following sections, we use each case to illustrate how diagnostic and behavioral assessment can be utilized to inform the treatment process for each case.

INTERNALIZING DISORDERS CASE EXAMPLE: SOFIA

The chapters in Part II of this volume have laid out recommendations for a variety of assessment strategies that could be used with Sofia and her family. However, following all of these excellent recommendations would lead to an assessment battery that would be too cumbersome to be practical for any one case, and the clinician would have to decide which ones to use. In the following description, we have therefore drawn from these recommendations to illustrate a sample battery that would be complete, yet feasible.

Initial Assessment

Before beginning treatment, Sofia and her mother, Adriana, participated in an intake evaluation. In the first session, the background information described in Chapter 4 was primarily obtained through unstructured interviews with Sofia and Adriana (focused on Sofia's presenting problem, family history, psychosocial stressors, family relationships, etc.). At the end of that session, as recommended by Achenbach in Chapter 6, the Achenbach System of Empirically Based Assessment (ASEBA) Youth Self-Report (YSR) and Child Behavior Checklist for Ages 6–18 (CBCL/6–18) (Achenbach & Rescorla, 2001) were used to gather child- and parent-reported symptom information. Sofia also completed the Children's Depression Inventory (CDI; Kovacs, 1985) and the Revised Children's Manifest Anxiety Scale (RCMAS; Reynolds & Richmond, 1978) to provide baseline data on her depression and anxiety symptoms, as recommended by Pina, Gonzales, Holly, Zerr, and Wynne in Chapter 13. Sofia and her mother were asked to take these measures home with them and to complete them between the first and second sessions. According to Pina et al.'s recommendations (Chapter 13), open-ended questions were used during the second session to assess cultural factors that might be influencing Sofia's or Adriana's reports.

To gather more information about Sofia's symptoms in order to generate a diagnosis, the Anxiety Disorders Interview Schedule for DSM-IV: Child and Parent Versions (ADIS-IV: C/P; Silverman & Albano, 1996) were administered in the second session to Sofia and her mother, as described by Marin, Rey, and Silverman in Chapter 5. Given that few diagnostic interviews currently have good support for use with Hispanic families (see Pina et al., Chapter 13), the ADIS-IV: C/P was chosen due to its strong support for assessing anxiety disorders in youth (Silverman & Ollendick, 2008).

After completion of all these measures, Sofia and Adriana were asked to complete some additional questionnaires at home to further inform the case conceptualization. Given evidence suggesting genetic risk for anxiety disorders (e.g., Eley, 2001; Hudziak, Rudiger, Neale, Heath, & Todd, 2000), the potential impact of parental modeling of anxious behavior (McLeod, Wood, & Weisz, 2007; Wood, McLeod, Sigman, Hwang, & Chu, 2003), and evidence suggesting Adriana had difficulty tolerating

Sofia's anxious behaviors (Tiwari et al., 2009), parental psychopathology was assessed with the Latin American Spanish version of the ASEBA Adult Self-Report (ASR; Achenbach & Rescorla, 2003). In addition, as recommended by La Greca, Lai, Chan, and Herge in Chapter 11, Sofia's social acceptance and areas of competence were assessed with the Self-Perception Profile for Adolescents (SPPA; Harter, 1985); as recommended by Hawes and Dadds in Chapter 12, parenting behavior and family relationships were assessed with the Children's Report of Parent Behavior Inventory (CRPBI-30; Schludermann & Schludermann, 1988) and the Conflict Behavior Questionnaire (CBQ; Prinz, Foster, Kent, & O'Leary, 1979). The parenting and family relationship measures were chosen to target specific risk factors for anxiety, including parental control (McLeod et al., 2007; Wood et al., 2003). As described by Shirk, Reyes, and Crisostomo in Chapter 14, Sofia also completed the Stages of Change Questionnaire (SOCQ; Lewis et al., 2009) to determine her readiness to engage in psychotherapy, and her mother completed the Credibility/Expectancies Questionnaire—Parent Version (CEQ-P; Nock, Ferriter, & Holmberg, 2007).

Finally, during the third session, a functional assessment of Sofia's school refusal behavior was conducted (see Ollendick, McLeod, & Jensen-Doss, Chapter 3). In addition to the ADIS-IV: C/P, the School Refusal Assessment Scale—Revised (SRAS-R; Kearney, 2002, 2006) was used to assess the function of Sofia's school avoidance behavior. In addition, as recommended by Reitman, McGregor, and Resnick in Chapter 7, Adriana was tasked with observing and recording the antecedents and consequences of Sofia's school refusal. As detailed by Cole and Kunsch in Chapter 8, Sofia was also asked to keep a diary of her school refusal, including its triggers, her thoughts and feelings about attending school, and the consequences of her refusal.

Case Conceptualization

Information obtained in the initial assessment was used to complete the case conceptualization worksheet presented in Figure 15.1. This worksheet follows the format of the blank worksheet we have provided in Chapter 4 (Figure 4.1).

Step 1: Identify Target Behaviors and Causal/Maintaining Factors

From the interview and rating scale data obtained during the intake, four possible target behaviors were identified: school refusal, panic attacks, social anxiety, and depression. The table under Step 1 in Figure 15.1 was used to delineate the cognitive, behavioral, and affective components of each target behavior, and to provide intensity ratings and descriptions of the frequency and duration of each target behavior. Through this process, it became clear that Sofia's school refusal behavior was related to both her panic attacks and her social embarrassment over her academic retention.

FIGURE 15.1. Worksheet for generating a case conceptualization: Sofia.

Step 1: Identify target behaviors and causal/maintaining factors.

What are the target behaviors? What are the cognitive, behavioral, and affective components of each target behavior? What is the frequency, intensity, and duration of each target behavior?

Target behavior	Cognitive	Behavioral	Affective	Intensity (1–10)	Frequency and duration
School refusal	• Believes that she will panic • Believes that peers will negatively evaluate her	• Avoidance of school	Anxiety	9	Daily; lasts until Adriana (her mother) gives her permission to stay home
Panic attacks	• Believes that she will die • Believes that peers will negatively evaluate her	• Avoidance of school and other situations where she might panic	Anxiety	3	Concern about panic happens daily; actual panic attacks in remission
Social anxiety	• Believes that peers will judge her for being retained	• Avoidance of school and peers	Anxiety	9	Daily; lasts until Adriana gives her permission to stay home from school
Depression	• Low self-esteem about academics • Negative view of the future • Guilt over conflict with father	• Sleeping • Social withdrawal • Conflict with father	Sad mood	9	Daily; lasts all day

What historical factors may be linked to one or more target behaviors?

• Genetic risk for anxiety and depression: Maternal self-reported history of both.

• Temperament: Adriana reports that Sofia was a timid child with early separation anxiety.

- Parenting behaviors: Adriana reports having difficulty setting limits around Sofia's avoidance; the father is described as critical of Sofia's academic performance.
- Cultural/familial pressures to achieve: Parents are immigrants who are very invested in their children's attending college and excelling in life.
- Trauma?: Sofia's description of her relationship with her ex-boyfriend suggests the possibility of a rape history, although she is unwilling to discuss it. Additional assessment is needed.

What causal factors may be linked to one or more target behaviors?
- Anxiety sensitivity: Sofia's history of panic attacks suggests that she tends to interpret bodily sensations as indicative of danger.
- Emotion regulation difficulties: Sofia appears to have poor coping and problem-solving skills.
- Cognitive distortions: Sofia describes anxious cognitions related to peers' perceptions of her, and depressive cognitions about her future and her relationship with her father.
- Social anxiety: Sofia's social anxiety is causing her to refuse to go to school because she fears that her peers will reject her.

What antecedents appear to precede the occurrence of one or more target behaviors?
- Cues to go to school: Sofia's anxiety and school refusal behaviors are triggered by cues that it is time to go to school.
- Fights with her father: Sofia's depression is triggered by conflicts with her father over school.

What factors appear to be maintaining one or more target behaviors?
- Avoidance of school: Sofia's avoidance maintains her anxiety, because she never learns whether her peers actually reject her, and she never learns to tolerate her anxiety.
- Social withdrawal: The social withdrawal resulting from Sofia's anxiety and depression also maintains these symptoms, because she never learns whether her peers will reject her, she never learns to tolerate her social anxiety, and she is not engaged in any positive social activities.
- Reduction in anxiety: The reduction in anxiety that results from Sofia's avoidance and social withdrawal serves to reinforce these behaviors (negative reinforcement).
- Adriana's anxiety: When Sofia refuses to go to school, Adriana becomes anxious about upsetting her and allows her to stay home.

(continued)

421

FIGURE 15.1. (*continued*)

Step 2: Arrive at a diagnosis.
Does the child meet diagnostic criteria for a DSM disorder?

300.23	Social phobia
296.22	Major depressive disorder, single episode, moderate
300.22	Agoraphobia
300.01	Panic disorder
V62.3	Academic or educational problem
V61.20	Parent–child relational problem

Step 3: Form the initial case conceptualization.
What are the treatment targets?
What historical factors may be linked to the treatment targets?
What causal factors are contributing to the treatment targets?
What role do contextual factors (antecedents, maintaining variables) play in the treatment targets?

Treatment targets	Historical factors	Causal factors	Antecedents	Maintaining factors
Sofia's anxiety-related school refusal	• Genetic risk for anxiety • Temperament • Parenting behaviors • Trauma?	• Cognitive distortions • Emotion regulation difficulties • Anxiety sensitivity • Social anxiety	• Cues to go to school	• Adriana's anxiety • Avoidance of school • Reduction in anxiety
Sofia's depression	• Genetic risk for depression • Cultural/family pressure for high academic achievement	• Cognitive distortions • Emotion regulation difficulties	• Fights with father	• Social withdrawal

Step 4: Proceed with treatment planning and selection.

List the hypotheses to be addressed in treatment, in order of treatment priority.
Identify therapeutic interventions that target those hypotheses.

Hypothesis	Intervention
1. Sofia's school refusal is being reinforced by her Adriana's inability to get her to go to school.	• Psychoeducation for Adriana about the relation between anxiety and avoidance • Behavioral parent training for Adriana aimed at changing the contingencies related to school attendance
2. Adriana's inability to tolerate Sofia's anxiety allows Sofia to avoid school.	• Affect management for Adriana
3. Sofia's social anxiety is being maintained by her school refusal.	• Exposure therapy
4. Sofia's anxiety and depression are being maintained by her social withdrawal.	• Exposure therapy • Behavioral activation
5. Sofia's anxiety and depression are being maintained by cognitive distortions.	• Cognitive restructuring
6. Sofia's anxiety and depression are increased by conflicts with her father over academic achievement.	• Cognitive restructuring • Family communication training

List evidence-based treatments designed to address the treatment targets.

1. Individual cognitive-behavioral therapy (CBT) + behavioral parent training for school refusal (King et al., 1998; Heyne et al., 2002)
2. Interpersonal psychotherapy (Mufson et al., 2004)

(continued)

FIGURE 15.1. (*continued*)

Step 5: Develop outcome-monitoring and evaluation strategies.
What measures will be used for ongoing assessment to monitor the target behavior and intervening variables?

Measure	Domain	Reporter	Frequency
Revised Children's Manifest Anxiety Scale (RCMAS)	Anxiety	Youth	Monthly
Children's Depression Inventory (CDI)	Depression	Youth	Monthly
Frequency of school refusal—self-monitoring	School refusal	Youth and parent	Monitored daily and brought to every session
Therapeutic Alliance Scale for Adolescents	Alliance	Youth	Every session

What measures will be used for treatment evaluation?

Posttreatment assessment battery

Measure	Domain	Reporter
Anxiety Disorders Interview Schedule for DSM-IV: Child and Parent Versions (ADIS-IV: C/P)	Diagnosis	Youth and parent
ASEBA Youth Self-Report (YSR) and Child Behavior Checklist for Ages 6–18 (CBCL/6–18)	Symptoms	Youth & parent
Revised Children's Manifest Anxiety Scale (RCMAS)	Anxiety	Youth
Children's Depression Inventory (CDI)	Depression	Youth
ASEBA Adult Self-Report (ASR)	Parental psychopathology	Parents
Self-Perception Profile for Adolescents (SPPA)	Social and other competencies	Youth
Children's Report of Parent Behavior Inventory (CRPBI-30)	Parenting behavior	Youth
Conflict Behavior Questionnaire (CBQ)	Family communication and conflict	Youth and parent

It was also apparent that the panic attacks were not the family's central concern at this point, given that the attacks themselves had remitted after Sofia's previous round of treatment. Thus her problems with anxiety and depression were given high priority.

The rest of Step 1 involved identifying historical and causal factors that might be linked to the target behaviors, as well as the antecedents and maintaining factors contributing to these behaviors. For example, Adriana's scores on the ASR Anxious/Depressed, Depressive Problems, and Anxiety Problems scales were elevated and consistent with her own self-reported history of anxiety and depression. These data suggested that one historical factor possibly related to Sofia's anxiety and depression was genetic risk for anxiety and depression (e.g., Eley, 2001; Hudziak et al., 2000). As described in detail in Figure 15.1, other historical factors included temperament, parenting behaviors, and cultural/familial pressures to achieve. A fifth possible historical factor was a trauma history. Sofia's discussion of her relationship with her ex-boyfriend indicated that she might have experienced unwanted sexual contact; however, her unwillingness to discuss this relationship precluded drawing firm conclusions about whether this was the case. The ADIS-IV: C included questions about trauma symptoms, and Sofia denied experiencing them. Despite this denial, Sofia's unwillingness to go into details about this relationship raised questions about whether she was avoiding these memories. This was therefore identified as an area in need of further assessment once rapport was established with Sofia.

A review of the developmental psychopathology literature and Sofia's self-reports suggested four possible causal factors for Sofia's difficulties. First, her description of her panic attacks suggested that she was experiencing high anxiety sensitivity. Defined as the degree to which an individual finds the symptoms of anxiety to be aversive, "anxiety sensitivity" has been proposed as a risk factor for panic and other anxiety disorders (e.g., Reiss, Silverman, & Weems, 2001). Second, consistent with literature suggesting that emotion regulation difficulties may be a risk factor for the development of youth psychopathology (e.g., Hannesdottir & Ollendick, 2007; Southam-Gerow & Kendall, 2002), Sofia seemed to have difficulty interpreting and managing negative emotion. Third, consistent with theories suggesting that cognitive schemas and automatic thoughts contribute to the development and maintenance of anxiety (e.g., Sweeney & Pine, 2004) and depression (e.g., Ollendick & Sander, 2012), Sofia was experiencing cognitive distortions. For example, in the absence of clear evidence that this would be the case, she believed that her peers would reject her because of her academic retention and that she would never achieve anything in her future. Finally, Sofia's social anxiety was conceptualized as a causal factor for her school refusal, since social fears appeared to be driving this avoidance of school.

Antecedents identified for Sofia's anxiety and depression included proximal cues that it was time to go to school (which triggered her anxiety and school refusal) and distal cues related to conflicts with her father (which triggered her depression). Maintaining factors included Sofia's avoidance of school, her social withdrawal, the reduction in anxiety that resulted from both of these behaviors, and her mother's anxiety, which made it difficult for her to set limits with Sofia. Figure 15.1, Step 1, details the rationale for selecting these maintaining factors.

Step 2: Arrive at a Diagnosis

The assessment data were used to generate DSM-5 diagnoses for Sofia. On the ADIS-IV: C, Sofia met criteria for *Diagnostic and Statistical Manual of Mental Disorders, Fourth Edition, Text Revision* (DSM-IV-TR) diagnoses of social phobia, panic disorder with agoraphobia, and major depressive disorder. In order to determine whether Sofia met criteria for DSM-5 diagnoses, additional questions were used where there were differences between DSM-IV and DSM-5 criteria (e.g., DSM-5 classifies panic disorder and agoraphobia separately, American Psychiatric Association, 2013). Sofia's difficulties with anxiety and depression were also apparent on her rating scales, as she reported elevated symptoms on the RCMAS, the CDI, and the Internalizing broad-band scale on the YSR, along with its associated subscales. The results of the SRAS-R also indicated that her school refusal was related to social anxiety rather than to oppositionality. On the ADIS-IV: P, Sofia also met criteria for panic disorder with agoraphobia; however, Adriana did not describe her daughter as depressed in this interview. Nevertheless, as Sofia indicated in her interview that she was making efforts to shield her mother from seeing just how depressed she was feeling about her school situation, and as Sofia also reported significant impairment associated with her depression, panic, and social anxiety, the clinician decided to assign all four diagnoses endorsed by Sofia, in order from most to least impactful (i.e., social phobia, major depressive disorder, agoraphobia, and panic disorder). In order to capture psychosocial and environmental factors that were affecting Sofia's symptoms and might have an impact on treatment, the DSM-5 codes for "Other Conditions That May Be a Focus of Clinical Attention" were used to document Sofia's academic difficulties (V62.3 Academic or Educational Problem) and her conflicts with her father (V61.20 Parent–Child Relational Problem).

Step 3: Form the Initial Case Conceptualization

Next, the target behaviors and diagnoses were used to identify treatment targets. Given the relationship between Sofia's social anxiety and her school refusal, the first target was the school refusal, which was conceptualized as a symptom of the social anxiety. The second treatment target was Sofia's depression. Using the table provided to assist in Step 3 (see Figure 15.1), the clinician linked the historical factors, casual factors, antecedents, and maintaining factors identified in Step 1 to these treatment targets. Figure 15.2 presents an integrated version of Sofia's initial case

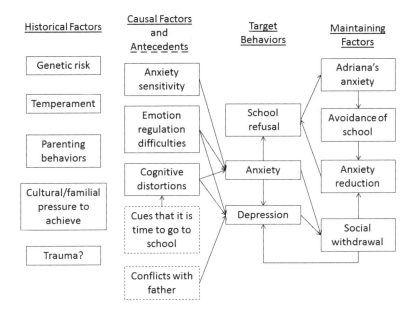

FIGURE 15.2. Case conceptualization for Sofia.

conceptualization. It should be noted that this was an initial case conceptualization that would be revised as new information became available throughout the course of treatment.

Step 4: Proceed with Treatment Planning and Selection

To facilitate treatment planning, the initial case conceptualization was used to form a list of hypotheses that could be examined during treatment (see Figure 15.1, Step 4). Because Sofia's school refusal was having a negative impact on her academic achievement, which in turn was contributing to her depression and her conflict with her father, the family agreed that addressing her school refusal was the most important treatment priority. Given that Adriana was having difficulty encouraging her daughter to attend school, it appeared that treatment would need to address Adriana's ability to manage her own anxiety (which was seemingly cued by Sofia's school refusal), as well as to provide her with parenting skills that would support her in setting limits with Sofia around her school attendance (see Wood & McLeod, 2008). Given the relationship between Sofia's school refusal and her social anxiety, it was determined that individual cognitive-behavioral therapy (CBT) to improve Sofia's coping skills and to address her negative cognitions would also be necessary. Because the CBT might also lead to improvements in Sofia's depression, the decision was made to treat Sofia's anxiety first, and then to consider other, depression-specific treatment strategies if her depression did not improve.

A review of the treatment literature suggested that for school-refusing, anxious adolescents like Sofia, the combination of individual CBT with behavioral parent training (Heyne et al., 2002; King et al., 1998) is a "possibly efficacious" treatment (Silverman, Pina, & Viswesvaran, 2008). No school refusal treatments were found that had greater research support. Some approaches were found that had more support for the treatment of social phobia (Silverman et al., 2008); however, these treatments either did not include a parent component, or were designed to be administered in a group format, so they were not a good fit to the case conceptualization and/or the treatment setting (which delivered individual therapy). The decision was therefore made to proceed with individual CBT plus parent training. However, interpersonal psychotherapy (Mufson, Dorta, Moreau, & Weissman, 2004) was selected as a second treatment option to be utilized if the CBT did not improve Sofia's depression. This treatment approach was deemed particularly relevant, given its focus on the role that social relationships play in depression, and its research support for use with adolescents in general and Hispanic adolescents in particular (e.g., Rosselló & Bernal, 1999).

Step 5: Develop Outcome Monitoring and Evaluation Strategies

Figure 15.1, Step 5, details the outcome-monitoring and treatment evaluation plans for Sofia. Frequent outcome monitoring focused on the behaviors being targeted in treatment: Sofia's anxiety, depression, and school refusal. Both Sofia and Adriana provided weekly ratings. In addition, as described by Shirk et al. in Chapter 14, Sofia provided weekly ratings of the alliance on the Therapeutic Alliance Scale for Adolescents (Shirk & Saiz, 1992). This outcome-monitoring strategy indicated that Sofia's school refusal decreased once her mother began to implement contingencies in the home to encourage her school attendance. In the fall, once Sofia began attending school more regularly and her ability to challenge her anxious cognitions improved, her social anxiety began to improve as well. Her improvements in school attendance also led to improvements in her relationship with her father. As Sofia began to notice these changes in her academic and family life, she reported feeling less depressed. Although the initial case conceptualization included a possibility that Sofia was experiencing symptoms of trauma, Sofia did not discuss her relationship with her boyfriend during treatment, and her symptoms improved without the incorporation of any trauma focus into the treatment plan. Once Sofia was attending school regularly, the family decided to terminate services.

At the end of treatment, the impact of treatment was evaluated by repeating most of the measures that were administered at intake. This assessment indicated that Sofia no longer met criteria for any DSM-5 diagnoses, and that her scores on the rating scales fell below the clinical cutoff in most domains. Sofia's ratings on the SPPA indicated that she was feeling much more competent in social and academic tasks, and she reported less family conflict on the CBQ. Given these assessment results, the therapist concurred with the family's decision to end services.

EXTERNALIZING DISORDERS CASE EXAMPLE: BILLY

As in the case of Sofia, the various chapters in this book provide rich commentary on many evidence-based assessment strategies that could have been used in the case of Billy; however, as noted, not all of them can be practically used with any one case. Still, the earlier chapters provide descriptions of these diverse strategies, as well as initial guidelines for when and with which clients they are appropriate. In the following description of Billy's case, we draw from these recommendations and illustrate a sample battery reflecting our approach to evidence-based case conceptualization, diagnosis, treatment planning, monitoring, and evaluation for a child with externalizing behavior.

Initial Assessment

Before treatment began, Billy's mother, Mary, was contacted by telephone to provide background information and to schedule their first appointment at the outpatient clinic. At this first appointment, Billy and Mary participated in an intake evaluation. This initial session is used to elaborate upon the presenting concerns and to determine suitability for treatment. Initially, a brief conjoint interview was conducted with Billy and Mary to have them elaborate on the "presenting complaints," followed by a brief developmental and social history obtained from Mary alone, and then a final interview with Billy alone. We follow this general procedure whenever possible—deliberately beginning with the parent and child together and ending with the child alone, so as to begin to form a good relationship and alliance with all parties (see Shirk et al., Chapter 14). This initial interview, as described in Chapter 4, resulted in concerns related to oppositionality, anxiety, attention, emotion regulation, and peer relationship difficulties for Billy, and concerns related to parenting practices and possible depression for Mary.

To gain more information about these various problems, the clinician requested permission from Mary (who was the custodial parent) to contact Billy's father (the parents had divorced about 6 years earlier, following their separation 8 years ago), his public school teacher, and his medical doctor. Along with a copy of this permission form and a brief cover letter, the CBCL/6–18 and Teacher's Report Form (TRF) from the ASEBA (Achenbach & Rescorla, 2001; see Achenbach, Chapter 6) were sent to Billy's father and teacher, respectively. A letter was also sent to his medical doctor requesting records related to Billy's history of earaches and enuresis, as well as any other medical problems that might be present. Mary was also given the CBCL/6–18 to complete. As was customary in the clinic, Mary was asked to complete the CBCL/6–18 during the week and to bring it to the next session, scheduled 1 week later. Were Billy 11 years of age or older, he would have also been asked to complete the YSR during the week; however, since he was only 10 years of age, this was not done in this instance.

As requested, Mary brought in her completed CBCL/6–18 for the second session. Mary also contacted the school and picked up the TRF from Billy's teacher on the way to the appointment. Unfortunately, Billy's father refused to complete the CBCL/6–18—stating to Mary on the telephone that "I really don't have any problems with Billy when he visits," and adding that he did not understand why Billy was being sent to see a "shrink." He attributed Billy's "problems" to Mary's inadequate and inconsistent parenting. On Mary's CBCL/6–18, Billy was reported to be in the clinical range for the Aggressive Behavior and Anxious/Depressed scales, and in the subclinical range for the Attention Problems and Social Problems scales. Billy's teacher did not endorse any TRF scales in the clinical range. However, she rated his Attention Problems, Aggressive Behavior, and Social Problem scales in the subclinical range. The Anxious/Depressed scale was in the average range on the TRF. His teacher also reported moderate difficulties in getting along with his peers, "not working up to his potential," and the need for a parent–teacher conference to discuss his problems at school. No additional medical problems were noted by his medical doctor.

In the second session, the ADIS-IV: C/P (Silverman & Albano, 1996; see Marin et al., Chapter 5) was administered separately to Billy and his mother. In addition to the strong support for use of the ADIS-IV: C/P in assessing anxiety disorders in youth (Silverman & Ollendick, 2008), Jarrett, Wolff, and Ollendick (2007) have shown that it provides reliable and valid diagnoses for youth with attention-deficit/hyperactivity disorder (ADHD), while Anderson and Ollendick (2012) have shown similarly strong psychometric properties for its use in diagnosing oppositional defiant disorder (ODD) in children and adolescents. Thus the ADIS-IV: C/P was determined to be an ideal diagnostic interview, since both internalizing and externalizing problems were hypothesized to be present in this case. On the basis of the ADIS-IV: P, Billy met diagnostic criteria for ODD and specific phobia of dark/being alone. He also showed subclinical but elevated symptoms of ADHD—combined type. On the basis of the ADIS-IV: C, Billy himself met diagnostic criteria for specific phobia of dark/being alone, and exhibited subclinical symptoms of ADHD-combined type and generalized anxiety disorder. When the composite scoring criteria for the ADIS-IV: C/P were employed (Silverman & Albano, 1996; see Marin et al., Chapter 5), Billy appeared to meet criteria for diagnoses of ODD and specific phobia of dark/being alone, as well as subclinical symptoms of ADHD—combined type. These "working" diagnoses paralleled the problems identified on the CBCL/6–18 and TRF.

After the second session, based on the information obtained in the first two sessions, Billy and his mother were asked to complete some additional questionnaires at home and to bring them to the third session. The available evidence suggests the role of both parental psychopathology and ineffective parenting practices in the onset and maintenance of both ODD (Kimonis & Frick, 2010; Murrihy, Kidman, & Ollendick, 2010) and anxious behaviors (McLeod et al., 2007; Ollendick & Benoit, 2012). In this case, parental psychopathology was assessed with the ASR (Achenbach & Rescorla, 2003; see Achenbach, Chapter 6), and parenting behaviors were assessed with the Alabama Parenting Questionnaire (APQ; Shelton, Frick, & Wootten, 1996; see Hawes & Dadds, Chapter 12). In addition, given Billy's problems with peer interactions and peer victimization, along with his seemingly ineffective behaviors in establishing social relationships and friendships, his social acceptance and areas of social competence were assessed with the Self-Perception Profile for Children (SPPC; Harter, 1985; see La Greca et al., Chapter 11). The SPPC Social Acceptance subscale, of particular interest for Billy, assesses children's perceptions of their peer acceptance. In addition, Billy was asked to complete two very brief questionnaires (10 items each) reporting on his perceived self-efficacy in making friends and the outcome expectancies associated with these actions (Ollendick & Schmidt, 1987). Finally, Billy was asked to complete the Fear Survey Schedule for Children—Revised (Ollendick, 1983). This 80-item measure taps the common fears of childhood: Danger and Death, The Unknown, Social Fears, Animal Fears, and Medical Fears. Collectively, these questionnaires took about 45 minutes for Mary and Billy to complete.

The questionnaires, returned at the beginning of the third session, revealed that Mary was experiencing moderate levels of depression on the ASR. She also reported that she engaged in very little positive parenting with Billy, and that her parenting was characterized by lax and inconsistent practices, together with insufficient monitoring of his activities. However, she also reported that she rarely if ever used corporal punishment. Billy indicated low levels of social acceptance, low levels of self-efficacy, and low levels of outcome expectancies in social situations. He also reported high levels of fear associated with danger and death and fear of the unknown. These types of fears characterize children with fear of the dark and being alone.

As recommended by Shirk et al. in Chapter 14, Billy completed the SCQ (Lewis et al., 2009) at the beginning of the third session to determine his readiness to engage in therapy, and his mother completed the CEQ-P (Nock et al., 2007), and the Barriers to Treatment Participation Scale (BTP; Kazdin, Holland, Crowley, & Breton, 1997; Kazdin, Holland, & Crowley, 1997). In addition, Billy completed a go/no-go task to tap his inhibitory processes and completed an interpretation bias task (see Lester & Field, Chapter 10). Finally, in Session 3, a functional analysis of Mary's parenting behavior was undertaken (see Ollendick, McLeod, & Jensen-Doss, Chapter 3), and Billy's compliance was assessed with a behavioral observation task (see Reitman et al., Chapter 7). Billy's fear of the dark/being alone was also assessed with a behavioral approach test (Ollendick, Allen, Benoit,

& Cowart, 2011). Although physiological assessment was not undertaken in this session because of practical constraints (see Patriguin, Scarpa, & Friedman, Chapter 9), it might have been desirable to do so—especially given the likely comorbidity of anxiety and oppositionality in this case, and the potential of physiological assessment to help sort out the relative impact of comorbid externalizing versus internalizing disorders (Drabick, Ollendick, & Bubier, 2010).

At the end of this session, as recommended by Reitman et al. in Chapter 7, Billy's mother was tasked with observing and recording the antecedents and consequences of Billy's oppositional behavior at home and his nighttime behaviors. For the latter target, she was also asked to record the time it took Billy to go to bed each evening, whether he slept in his own bed, and the types of avoidance behaviors in which he engaged (e.g., asking to have a snack, having to go to the bathroom multiple times, etc.). Finally, Billy too was asked to keep a diary of his nighttime behaviors (see Cole & Kunsch, Chapter 8).

Case Conceptualization

Information obtained in the initial assessment was used to complete the case conceptualization worksheet presented in Figure 15.3. Again, this worksheet follows the format of the blank worksheet in Chapter 4 (Figure 4.1).

Step 1: Identify the Target Behaviors and Causal/Maintaining Factors

From the assessment information obtained during the intake and assessment sessions, four possible target behaviors were identified for Billy: oppositionality, emotion regulation difficulties, peer relationship problems, and a phobia of the dark/being alone. The table under Step 1 was used to describe the cognitive, behavioral, and affective components of each target behavior, and to arrive at intensity ratings and descriptions of the frequency and duration of the target behaviors. Through this process, it became clear that Billy's oppositionality was the primary concern of the family and that it was closely intertwined with his poor emotion regulation skills and peer relationship problems, as well as his mother's inconsistent and lax parenting style. It also became clear that his phobia of the dark and of being alone was not the family's central concern at this time; as a result, the phobia was monitored but not specifically targeted for treatment, at least not initially.

The rest of Step 1 involved identifying historical and causal factors that might be linked to the target behaviors, as well as the antecedent and maintaining factors contributing to these behaviors. For example, Billy's father's family history of alcoholism and drug abuse, and his brother's incarceration for breaking and entering and for assaulting a police officer, suggested

FIGURE 15.3. Worksheet for generating a case conceptualization: Billy

Step 1: Identify target behaviors and causal/maintaining factors.

What are the target behaviors? What are the cognitive, behavioral, and affective components of each target behavior? What are the frequency, intensity, and duration of each target behavior?

Target behavior	Cognitive	Behavioral	Affective	Intensity (1–10)	Frequency and duration
Oppositional behavior	• Believes that he cannot manage his own behavior • Believes that Mary (his mother) is just out to get him because he is not the "good" child in the family • Believes that his father does not like him	• Oppositional, noncompliant, and negativistic	Anger, jealousy	9	Daily; more days than not in a typical week; lasts until Mary gives in and removes demands placed on him
Emotion regulation difficulties	• Believes that he cannot control his anger and jealousy • Believes that he is just like his father, who has impulse control problems	• Acts impulsively and sometimes violently around others	Anger, jealousy	9	Frequently reacts impulsively (this is his first reaction), but it usually lasts only a brief period of time, and then he is remorseful
Peer relationship problems	• Believes that other students do not like him • Possesses low self-efficacy and outcome expectancies for effective peer interactions	• Social interaction problems	Anger, jealousy, and some anxiety	7	Daily; results in strained peer interactions, sociometric rejection at some times, and sociometric neglect at other times

(continued)

433

FIGURE 15.3. (*continued*)

Phobia of dark/being alone	• "Someone will hurt me in the dark or when I am alone" • "A burglar will break into the house at nighttime and I will not see him" • "The sound outside is someone trying to break into the house"	• Unable to sleep alone in his own room • Unable to go to sleepovers because of fear of dark • Tired at school	Fear, anxiety, and some panic	8	Nightly; persists until either Mary comes into his room or he is able to sleep with her in her bedroom

What historical factors may be linked to one or more target behaviors?

• Genetic risk for conduct-related problems: Paternal family history of alcoholism and drug abuse; older brother incarcerated for assault.
• Temperament: Mary reports that Billy was a difficult child to soothe and comfort (including an insistence on co-sleeping); some early signs of overly active behavior, behavioral disinhibition.
• Parenting behaviors: Mary reports inconsistent/lax parenting and poor monitoring; she reports being overprotective and allowing Billy to co-sleep; father not involved in parenting; older brother is incarcerated, partially due to maternal overcontrolling behavior.
• Family stress: Mary is single parent, is mildly depressed, and has limited social support and income; brother is incarcerated.

What causal factors may be linked to one or more target behaviors?

• Social skills deficits: Mary reports that Billy has long-standing poor peer relationships; Billy reports few friends and rejection by classmates.
• Emotion regulation difficulties: Billy possesses poor emotion regulation skills, along with poor impulse control.
• Cognitive distortions: Billy reports threat cognitions related to peers' perceptions of him, and threat/anxious cognitions about his nighttime fear problems.

What antecedents appear to precede the occurrence of one or more target behaviors?

• Requests to comply at home or school, or even just to do ordinary chores around the home: Such requests trigger angry responses ("Why are you asking me? Why not Meredith [sister]?", "Why me and why not someone else in the classroom?", "Why are you always picking on me?").

- Arguments with students, sister, or father: Billy's poor emotion regulation skills are triggered by such events.
- Nighttime and turning out the lights to go to bed: Fears of the dark and being alone in his own room are triggered.

What factors appear to be maintaining one or more target behaviors?

- Inconsistent/lax parenting: Mary's problematic parenting maintains oppositional behavior, because Billy is negatively reinforced by her failure to follow through on requests; her parenting difficulties also maintain his anxiety, because she has difficulty setting limits for him about sleeping in his own bed.
- Mild maternal depression: Mary has difficulty with consistent parenting, due to low energy and poor self-efficacy related to her depression.
- Avoidance of peer interactions: Billy's social skills deficits and his threat-related cognitions about his peers are maintained by his avoidance of peer interactions; this avoidance serves to maintain poor interactions, because he never learns whether his peers really like him or not.
- Avoidance of sleeping alone: Billy's avoidance of sleeping alone maintains his anxiety, because he never learns that he is not in danger in the dark, and he never learns to tolerate his anxiety.
- Reduction in anxiety: The reduction in fear/anxiety that results from Billy's avoidance of sleeping in his own bed negatively reinforces his co-sleeping.

Step 2: Arrive at a diagnosis.
Does the child meet diagnostic criteria for a DSM disorder?

313.81	Oppositional defiant disorder
300.29	Specific phobia (dark/being alone)
V61.20	Parent–child relationship problem
V62.4	Social exclusion or rejection
V61.03	Disruption of family by separation or divorce

(continued)

FIGURE 15.3. (*continued*)

Step 3: Form the initial case conceptualization.

What are the treatment targets?

What historical factors may be linked to the treatment targets?

What causal factors are contributing to the treatment targets?

What role do contextual factors (antecedents, maintaining variables) play in the treatment targets?

Treatment targets	Historical factors	Causal factors	Antecedents	Maintaining factors
Billy's oppositionality (tied in with emotion regulation difficulties and poor peer relations)	• Genetic risk for conduct problems • Temperament • Parenting behaviors • Family stress	• Cognitive distortions • Emotion regulation difficulties • Social skills deficits	• Requests/commands • Arguments with sister, father, or classmates	• Inconsistent/lax parenting • Mild maternal depression • Avoidance of peer interactions
Billy's nighttime fears—phobia of the dark/being alone	• Temperament • Parenting behaviors • Family stress	• Cognitive distortions • Emotion regulation difficulties	• Nighttime • Turning lights out to go to bed	• Inconsistent/lax parenting • Avoidance of sleeping alone • Reduction in anxiety

Step 4: Proceed with treatment planning and selection.

List the hypotheses to be addressed in treatment, in order of treatment priority.

Identify therapeutic interventions that target those hypotheses.

Hypothesis	Intervention
1. Billy's oppositional behavior is being reinforced by Mary's inability/reluctance to get him to complete assigned tasks.	• Psychoeducation for Mary about the relations between oppositional behavioral and parenting • Behavioral parent training for Mary, designed to help her recognize antecedent events and provide consistent consequences for behavior

2. Billy's oppositional behavior is resulting partially from his poor emotion regulation skills and poor impulse control.	• Emotion regulation training
3. Billy's oppositional behavior is also resulting partially from poor social skills.	• Social skills training
4. Billy's oppositional behavior is also being maintained by cognitive distortions and social-cognitive deficits.	• Cognitive restructuring; social problem-solving training
5. Billy's specific phobia is resulting from lack of education about the dark and avoidance of dark cues.	• Psychoeducation about origins of fears/phobias; prolonged exposure; modeling and reinforcement
6. Billy's specific phobia is being maintained by Mary's attempts to protect Billy and to be a good parent.	• Psychoeducation for Mary about origins of fears/phobias, and work with her on her role in maintaining them

List evidence-based treatments designed to address the treatment targets.

1. Individual cognitive-behavioral therapy (CBT) + behavioral parent training for children with oppositional defiant disorder (Barkley, 1997; Kazdin, 2008; McMahon, Long, & Forehand, 2010; Ollendick & Greene, 2007)
2. Individual CBT for specific phobias (Davis et al., 2009; Ollendick et al., 2009, 2010; see also Silverman et al., 2008)

Step 5: Develop outcome-monitoring and evaluation strategies.

What measures will be used for ongoing assessment to monitor the target behavior and intervening variables?

Measure	Domain	Reporter	Frequency
Frequency of oppositional behaviors in the home/sleeping in own bed each night	Oppositional behavior	Parent	Daily; brought into each session weekly
Frequency of consistent parenting in response to requests/commands	Parenting behavior	Parent	Daily; brought into each session weekly

(continued)

FIGURE 15.3. (*continued*)

	Emotion regulation	Child and parent	Monitored weekly and brought into each session weekly
Frequency of emotion regulation difficulties			
Therapeutic Alliance Scale for Children	Alliance	Therapist	Every session

What measures will be used for treatment evaluation?

Posttreatment assessment battery

Measure	Domain	Reporter
Anxiety Disorders Interview Schedule for DSM-IV: Child and Parent Versions (ADIS-IV: C/P)	Diagnosis	Child and parent
ASEBA Child Behavior Checklist for Ages 6–18 (CBCL/6–18) and Teacher's Report Form (TRF)	Symptoms	Parent and teacher
ASEBA Adult Self-Report (ASR)	Parental psychopathology	Parent
Alabama Parenting Questionnaire (APQ)	Parenting practices	Parent
Self-efficacy and outcome expectancy scales	Social behavior	Child
Self-Perception Profile for Children (SPPC)	Social and other competencies	Child
Fear Survey Schedule for Children—Revised	Fear level	Child
Behavioral approach test	Phobic avoidance	Child

that one possible historical risk factor for Billy's behavior was a genetic risk for conduct-related problems. Billy's mother's description of his early behavior also suggested that temperament might be involved. Similarly, his mother's single-parent status and her overprotective, inconsistent, and lax parenting suggested that parenting behaviors were also likely to play a role. Finally, a host of family stressors was probably contributing to his problems, including his mother's level of depression, the demands of her job as an executive secretary, her low levels of social support, the family's financial stresses, and the brother's incarceration. A dynamic interplay among these various forces was obviously present. In other words, diverse historical factors were converging to cause and maintain the current problems in this family, including genetic risk factors, family system variables, parental psychopathology/poor parenting practices, and child characteristics. All of this is consistent with the developmental psychopathology literature (e.g., Hudziak et al., 2000; Kimonis & Frick, 2010; McLeod et al., 2007; Murrihy et al., 2010; Wolff & Ollendick, 2010).

A review of the developmental psychopathology literature and Billy's self-reports indicated three possible causal factors for his oppositionality and anxiety. First, Billy's description of his social problems at school, including his low peer acceptance and reported bullying, suggested that he lacked appropriate social skills and possessed low self-efficacy and outcome expectancies for appropriate social behavior. He was obviously experiencing peer rejection. Second, consistent with literature suggesting that emotion regulation difficulties may be a risk factor for the development of both conduct problems and anxiety in youth (e.g., Drabick et al., 2010; Greene, 2010), Billy seemed to have difficulty interpreting and managing negative emotion, and reported some difficulty experiencing positive emotions. Finally, consistent with theories suggesting that cognitive schemas and automatic thoughts contribute to the development and maintenance of both internalizing and externalizing problems (e.g., Lochman, Boxmeyer, Powell, & Wells, 2010; Ollendick & Schmidt, 1987; Rhodes & Dadds, 2010), Billy was experiencing cognitive distortions. Examples included his belief that nobody liked him; the belief that he, like his older brother, would never amount to anything in the future; and concerns about his safety at night.

Antecedents identified for Billy's oppositionality included proximal cues that his mother, teacher, or someone in authority expected him to do something (which triggered negative emotionality and subsequent behavioral refusal and noncompliance), and distal cues related to conflicts with his sister (whom he perceived as the "good" child in the family; moreover, his mother rarely asked her to do something, by his report), his peers, and his father (who would call or visit only occasionally, which triggered resentment and anger). Proximal cues for his anxiety included nighttime and turning out the lights for bed. Maintaining factors included his mother's inconsistent and lax discipline, his mother's depression, his avoidance of peer interactions, his avoidance of sleeping alone, and the reduction in anxiety that resulted from this avoidance. Figure 15.3, Step 1, describes the rationale for selecting these maintaining factors.

Step 2: Arrive at a Diagnosis

Assessment data were used to generate DSM-5 diagnoses for Billy. On the ADIS-IV: C/P, when composite criteria were used, Billy met DSM-IV-TR criteria for ODD and specific phobia of dark/being alone, and showed subclinical symptoms of ADHD—combined type. Follow-up questions suggested that these diagnostic impressions held when DSM-5 criteria were applied. Billy's difficulties with oppositionality were also apparent on the maternal CBCL/6–18 and subclinically on the TRF, as well as in reports from his teacher. They were also evident in the many examples provided by his mother and in his behavior during the assessment sessions. Although generally cooperative, he was noncompliant with some requests and actively refused others. As noted, these behaviors were hypothesized to be closely related to his victimization status at school, to Mary's inconsistent and lax parenting, and to his poor social skills and emotion regulation difficulties.

Although Billy was found to have subclinical symptoms of ADHD—combined type on the ADIS-IV: C/P, little support was obtained for this finding in the other assessment measures administered to Billy or his mother or teacher. Rather, it appeared that his occasional inattention and overactivity could be attributed to the lack of sleep associated with his specific phobia of the dark/being alone; to his vigilance to threat from other students at school; and to his general noncompliance with authority figures. Thus only the diagnoses of ODD and specific phobia were reported. Billy's conflicts with his mother (V61.20 Parent–Child Relational Problem), his social rejection (V62.4 Social Exclusion or Rejection), and his single parent family status (V61.03 Disruption of Family by Separation or Divorce) were also noted as psychosocial stressors that were affecting Billy's symptoms and might have an impact on treatment. This case nicely illustrates that even though a diagnostic interview is indispensable and the current "gold standard" for establishing diagnoses, it alone is insufficient for establishing final clinical diagnoses. Frequently, clinical experience and expert opinion must also be called upon.

Step 3: Form the Initial Case Conceptualization

Next, the target behaviors and diagnoses were used to identify treatment targets. Given the relationship among Billy's oppositionality, social skill deficits, and emotion regulation difficulties, the primary target was Billy's oppositional and noncompliant behaviors. The secondary treatment target was Billy's specific phobia of the dark/being alone. Using the table provided to assist in Step 3 (see Figure 15.3), the clinician linked the historical factors, casual factors, antecedents, and maintaining factors identified in Step 1 to each of these treatment targets. Figure 15.4 presents an integrated depiction of this initial case conceptualization. As in Sofia's case, it should be noted that this was an initial case conceptualization that could be revised as new information became available throughout the course of treatment.

Step 4: Proceed with Treatment Planning and Selection

To facilitate treatment planning, the initial case conceptualization was used to form a list of hypotheses that could be examined during treatment (see Figure 15.3, Step 4). Given that Billy's negativistic, oppositional behaviors were causing considerable conflict in the home and school, Billy (reluctantly) and his mother (wholeheartedly) agreed that these problems were the most important ones to address first in treatment. At the time of assessment, Mary was struggling with how to "parent" her son; she vacillated between being overly controlling (as she was with her older son, Mike) and being too lenient and permissive with Billy. As such, it was determined that treatment would need to include elements of parent management training that would help her identify and use the best parenting practices with Billy. It was also determined that treatment would need to address Mary's ability to manage her depression and to help her establish a social support network within her community. Given the literature on evidence-based interventions for children and families with these kinds of problems, it was determined that parent management training based on the work of Barkley (1997)

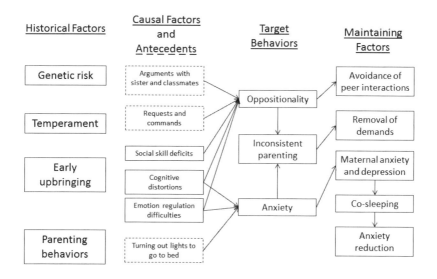

FIGURE 15.4. Case conceptualization for Billy.

and modified by several other authors (see Figure 15.3) would be implemented. This program also included a social skills training component and
addressed Billy's emotion regulation and cognitive processing difficulties.
In addition, the school was contacted to address problems with bullying in
that setting. Thus a comprehensive intervention was designed that involved
not only Billy, but also his family and his school. Initially, the clinician
elected not to address Billy's nighttime fears, so that treatment could concentrate on the primary presenting problems. Given the extant research on
treatment of specific phobias in children and adolescents, the clinician was
prepared to offer Billy and his family an intensive, exposure-based CBT
program developed by Ost, Ollendick, and colleagues (Davis, Ollendick, &
Ost, 2009; Ollendick et al., 2009; Ollendick, Ost, Reuterskiold, & Costa,
2010).

Step 5: Develop Outcome-Monitoring and Evaluation Strategies

Figure 15.3, Step 5, details the outcome-monitoring and treatment evaluation plans for Billy. Frequent outcome monitoring focused on the behaviors
being targeted in treatment: Billy's noncompliance, his mother's parenting skills, his peer relationships, and his cognitive distortions. In addition, as recommended by Shirk et al. in Chapter 14, Billy's therapist provided weekly ratings of the therapeutic alliance. Results from this weekly
monitoring revealed that Billy's noncompliance and oppositional behavior
diminished over the 12 weeks of intervention. These decreases appeared
to be related to his mother's learning to manage his negativistic behaviors
more effectively and to his own acquisition of emotion regulation strategies and cognitive strategies to help him manage his negative cognitions
surrounding threat. Although not directly monitored in the school, incidents of bullying also reportedly decreased over time. After 12 sessions of
treatment, both Billy and Mary were reporting a more harmonious relationship and working together on solving problems in the home and school
as they emerged. The problems with fear of the dark/being alone, however,
remained. Because the summer months were approaching and the family
was departing on an extended vacation, Mary and Billy elected not to
pursue these problems at that time. (However, it should be noted that they
did recontact the clinic at the end of the summer months and received the
intensive exposure-based CBT program for phobias. The treatment was
highly effective, at least partially because Billy was more compliant at this
time and his mother was able to assist him with the necessary exposure
exercises.)

   At the end of treatment, the impact of treatment was evaluated by
repeating the measures that were administered at the initial assessment.
This assessment indicated that Billy no longer met diagnostic criteria for
ODD; however, as just noted, the diagnosis of specific phobia was still
present (though it was subsequently treated successfully). Mary's ratings on
the CBCL/6–18 for aggressive behaviors were now in the subclinical range,

and the TRF ratings were now in the normal range. Billy's ratings on the SPPC indicated that he was feeling much more competent in social and academic tasks and feeling better about himself, and that other children were now more accepting of him. He also reported higher levels of self-efficacy and outcome expectancy regarding his ability to enact competent social behaviors with his peers. For herself, Mary reported less depression and enhanced parenting skills. Given these outcomes, the therapist concurred with the family's decision to end services for Billy's oppositional behaviors at that time, but, as noted above, also invited the family back to work on Billy's specific phobia after the summer months.

USING DIAGNOSTIC AND BEHAVIORAL ASSESSMENT TOOLS TO INFORM CLINICAL PRACTICE

As evidenced in our discussion of the two sample cases, numerous diagnostic and behavioral assessment methods are available for application to childhood disorders. Indeed, there is no shortage of assessment tools and methods for clinicians to choose from. Given the number of assessment methods available, determining when to use different methods to inform clinical practice can be a daunting task. In the absence of empirical guidelines to inform this process, we have presented a series of principles to guide child assessment. We have then used the sample cases to illustrate how these principles can be applied in clinical practice.

As repeated throughout this volume, it is important that child and adolescent assessment be guided by scientific findings. Unfortunately, little research currently exists to steer the assessment process. Many factors need to be carefully weighed and considered in conducting assessments with children and their families. Assessors need to consider developmental, cultural, and psychometric factors as they select and interpret tools. It is our hope that our assessment principles will help highlight those factors that need to be considered in child assessment and will provide clinicians with a framework to help them approach the assessment and treatment process.

FUTURE CONSIDERATIONS

Despite the many advances made in the assessment field over the past decade, much work remains to be done. Previous chapters have discussed directions for future research, so we will not go into depth here about possible next steps for the field. However, we do believe it is important to highlight one area that requires more attention: the judgmental heuristics that guide the selection and interpretation of assessment instruments. We hope that research will start to address this critical gap in our field. Establishing the psychometric properties of individual methods is important; however, we also need new research and conceptual models regarding the judgmental heuristics.

Several assumptions pervade child assessment. One such assumption is the need for a multimethod, multi-informant approach to assessment. Although this approach makes logical sense, we have very few empirical data to support this approach. What is the value of adding more assessment methods, or adding another informant? Does it benefit the client to gather more assessment data throughout treatment? The evidence-based assessment movement has focused increased attention upon the psychometric properties of individual assessment methods, which is very important. However, we believe that it is also vitally important to focus upon investigating how clinicians should consider assessment data and arrive at valid treatment decisions.

FINAL COMMENTS

In closing, our goal in producing this book has been to provide readers with the knowledge and skills needed to guide the assessment process for children and adolescents. We have covered critical areas of knowledge (e.g., psychometric theory), key skill areas (e.g., case conceptualization), and a host of assessment tools. We hope that this content, along with the assessment principles, will help prepare clinicians to critically apply, use, and interpret a variety of assessment methods throughout treatment.

REFERENCES

Achenbach, T. M., & Rescorla, L. A. (2001). *Manual for the ASEBA School-Age Forms & Profiles.* Burlington: University of Vermont, Research Center for Children, Youth, and Families.

Achenbach, T. M., & Rescorla, L. A. (2003). *Manual for the ASEBA Adult Forms & Profiles.* Burlington: University of Vermont, Research Center for Children, Youth, and Families.

Anderson, S. R., & Ollendick, T. H. (2012). The reliability and validity of the Anxiety Disorders Interview Schedule for the diagnosis of oppositional defiant disorder. *Journal of Psychopathology and Behavioral Assessment, 34,* 467–475.

Barkley, R. A. (1997). *Defiant children: A clinician's manual for parent training* (2nd ed.). New York: Guilford Press.

Davis, T. E., III, Ollendick, T. H., & Ost, L.-G. (2009). Intensive treatment of specific phobias in children and adolescents. *Cognitive and Behavioral Practice, 16,* 294–303.

Drabick, D. A. G., Ollendick, T. H., & Bubier, J. L. (2010). Co-occurrence of ODD and anxiety: Shared risk processes and evidence for a dual-pathway model. *Clinical Psychology: Science and Practice, 17,* 307–318.

Eley, T. C. (2001). Contributions of behavioral genetics research: Quantifying genetic, shared environmental and nonshared environmental influences. In M. W. Vasey & M. R. Dadds (Eds.), *The developmental psychopathology of anxiety* (pp. 45–59). New York: Oxford University Press.

Greene, R. W. (2010). Collaborative problem solving. In R. C. Murrihy, A. D. Kidman, & T. H. Ollendick (Eds.), *Clinical handbook of assessing and treating conduct problems in youth* (pp. 193–220). New York: Springer.

Hannesdottir, D., & Ollendick, T. H. (2007). The role of emotion regulation in the treatment of child anxiety disorders. *Clinical Child and Family Psychology Review, 10*(3), 275–293.

Harter, S. (1985). *Manual for the Self-Perception Profile for Children.* Denver, CO: University of Denver.

Heyne, D., King, N. J., Tonge, B. J., Rollings, S., Young, D., Pritchard, M., & Ollendick, T. H. (2002). Evaluation of child therapy and caregiver training in the treatment of school refusal. *Journal of the American Academy of Child and Adolescent Psychiatry, 41*(6), 687–695.

Hudziak, J. J., Rudiger, L. P., Neale, M. C., Heath, A. C., & Todd, R. D. (2000). A twin study of inattentive, aggressive, and anxious/depressed behaviors. *Journal of the American Academy of Child and Adolescent Psychiatry, 39,* 469–476.

Jarrett, M. A., Wolff, J. C., & Ollendick, T. H. (2007). Concurrent validity and informant agreement of the ADHD module of the Anxiety Disorders Interview Schedule for DSM IV. *Journal of Psychopathology and Behavioral Assessment, 29,* 159–168.

Kazdin, A. E. (2008). *The Kazdin method for parenting the defiant child.* Boston: Houghton Mifflin.

Kazdin, A. E., Holland, L., & Crowley, M. (1997). Family experience of barriers to treatment and premature termination from child therapy. *Journal of Consulting and Clinical Psychology, 65,* 453–463.

Kazdin, A. E., Holland, L., Crowley, M., & Breton, S. (1997). Barriers to Treatment Participation Scale: Evaluation and validation in the context of child outpatient treatment. *Journal of Child Psychology and Psychiatry, 38,* 1051–1062.

Kearney, C. A. (2002). Identifying the function of school refusal behavior: A revision of the School Refusal Assessment Scale. *Journal of Psychopathology and Behavioral Assessment, 28,* 235–245.

Kearney, C. A. (2006). Confirmatory factor analysis of the School Refusal Assessment Scale—Revised: Child and Parent Versions. *Journal of Psychopathology and Behavioral Assessment, 28*(3), 139–144.

Kimonis, E. R., & Frick, P. J. (2010). Etiology of oppositional defiant disorder and conduct disorder: Biological, familial and environmental factors identified in the development of disruptive behavior disorders. In R. C. Murrihy, A. D. Kidman, & T. H. Ollendick (Eds.), *Clinical handbook of assessing and treating conduct problems in youth* (pp. 49–76). New York: Springer.

King, N. J., Tonge, B. J., Heyne, D., Pritchard, M., Rollings, S., Young, D., Ollendick, T. H. (1998). Cognitive-behavioral treatment of school-refusing children: A controlled evaluation. *Journal of the American Academy of Child and Adolescent Psychiatry, 37*(4), 395–403.

Kovacs, M. (1985). The Children's Depression Inventory (CDI). *Psychopharmacology Bulletin, 21,* 995–999.

Lewis, C. C., Simons, A. D., Silva, S. G., Rohde, P., Small, D. M., Murakami, J. L., March, J. S. (2009). The role of readiness to change in response to treatment of adolescent depression. *Journal of Consulting and Clinical Psychology, 77,* 422–428.

Lochman, J. E., Boxmeyer, C., Powell, N. P., & Wells, K. C. (2010). Cognitive behavior therapy for the group-based treatment of oppositional youth. In R. C. Murrihy, A. D. Kidman, & T. H. Ollendick (Eds.), *Clinical handbook of assessing and treating conduct problems in youth* (pp. 221–244). New York: Springer.

McMahon, R., Long, N., & Forehand, R. L. (2010). Parent training for the treatment of oppositional behavior in young children: Helping the noncompliant child. In R. C. Murrihy, A. D. Kidman, & T. H. Ollendick (Eds.), *Clinical handbook of assessing and treating conduct problems in youth* (pp. 163–191). New York: Springer.

McLeod, B. D., Wood, J. J., & Weisz, J. R. (2007). Examining the association between parenting and childhood anxiety: A meta-analysis. *Clinical Psychology Review, 27,* 155–172.

Mufson, L., Dorta, K., Moreau, D., & Weissman, M. M. (2004). *Interpersonal psychotherapy for depressed adolescents* (2nd ed.). New York: Guilford Press.

Murrihy, R. C., Kidman, A. D., & Ollendick, T. H. (Eds.). (2010). *Clinical handbook of assessing and treating conduct problems in youth.* New York: Springer.

Nock, M. K., Ferriter, C., & Holmberg, E. (2007). Parent beliefs about treatment credibility and effectiveness: Assessment and relation to subsequent treatment participation. *Journal of Child and Family Studies, 16*(1), 27–38.

Ollendick, T. H. (1983). Reliability and validity of the Revised Fear Survey Schedule for Children (FSSC-R). *Behaviour Research and Therapy, 21,* 685–692.

Ollendick, T. H., Allen, B., Benoit, K., & Cowart, M. J. (2011). The tripartite model of fear in children with specific phobia: Assessing concordance and discordance using the Behavioral Approach Test. *Behaviour Research and Therapy, 49,* 459–465.

Ollendick, T. H., & Benoit, K. (2012). A parent–child interactional model of social anxiety disorder in youth. *Clinical Child and Family Psychology Review, 15,* 81–91.

Ollendick, T. H., & Greene, R. W. (2007). *Mediators and moderators of treatment outcomes for oppositional defiant youth.* Unpublished National Institute of Mental Health grant manuscript. (Available from T. H. Ollendick upon request)

Ollendick, T. H., Ost, L.-G., Reuterskiold, L., & Costa, N. (2010). Comorbidity in youth with specific phobias: Impact of comorbidity on treatment outcome and the impact of treatment on comorbid disorders. *Behaviour Research and Therapy, 48,* 827–831.

Ollendick, T. H., Ost, L.-G., Reuterskiold, L., Costa, N., Cederlund, R., Sirbu, C., & Jarrett, M. A. (2009). One-session treatment of specific phobias in youth: A randomized clinical trial in the United States and Sweden. *Journal of Consulting and Clinical Psychology, 77,* 504–516.

Ollendick, T. H., & Sander, J. B. (2012). Internalizing disorders in children and adolescents. In J. E. Maddux & B. A. Winstead (Eds.), *Psychopathology:*

Foundations for a contemporary understanding (3rd ed., pp. 473–498). New York: Routledge.

Ollendick, T. H., & Schmidt, C. R. (1987). Social learning constructs in the prediction of peer interaction. *Journal of Clinical Child Psychology, 16,* 80–87.

Prinz, R. J., Foster, S. L., Kent, R. N., & O'Leary, K. D. (1979). Multivariate assessment of conflict in distressed and nondistressed mother–adolescent dyads. *Journal of Applied Behavior Analysis, 12,* 691–700.

Reiss, S., Silverman, W. K., & Weems, C. F. (2001). Anxiety sensitivity. In M. W. Vasey & M. R. Dadds (Eds.), *The developmental psychopathology of anxiety* (pp. 92–111). New York: Oxford University Press.

Reynolds, C., & Richmond, B. (1978). "What I think and feel": A Revised Measure of Children's Manifest Anxiety. *Journal of Abnormal Child Psychology, 6,* 271–280.

Rhodes, T. E., & Dadds, M. R. (2010). Assessment of conduct problems using an integrated, process-oriented approach. In R. C. Murrihy, A. D. Kidman, & T. H. Ollendick (Eds.), *Clinical handbook of assessing and treating conduct problems in youth* (pp. 77–116). New York: Springer.

Rosselló, J., & Bernal, G. (1999). The efficacy of cognitive-behavioral and interpersonal treatments for depression in Puerto Rican adolescents. *Journal of Consulting and Clinical Psychology, 67*(5), 734–745.

Schludermann, E. H., & Schludermann, S. M. (1988). *Children's Report on Parent Behavior (CRPBI-108, CRPBI-30) for older children and adolescents (Technical Report).* Winnipeg, Manitoba, Canada: University of Manitoba, Department of Psychology.

Shelton, K. K., Frick, P. J., & Wootton, J. (1996). Assessment of parenting practices in families of elementary school-age children. *Journal of Clinical Child Psychology, 25,* 317–329.

Shirk, S. R., & Saiz, C. S. (1992). Clinical, empirical, and developmental perspectives on the therapeutic relationship in child psychotherapy. *Development and Psychopathology, 4,* 713–728.

Silverman, W. K., & Albano, A. M. (1996). *Anxiety Disorders Interview Schedule for DSM-IV: Child Version.* San Antonio, TX: Psychological Corporation.

Silverman, W. K., & Ollendick, T. H. (2008). Child and adolescent anxiety disorders. In J. Hunsley & E. J. Mash (Eds.), *A guide to assessments that work* (pp. 181–206). New York: Oxford University Press.

Silverman, W. K., Pina, A. A., & Viswesvaran, C. (2008). Evidence-based psychosocial treatments for phobic and anxiety disorders in children and adolescents. *Journal of Clinical Child and Adolescent Psychology, 37*(1), 105–130.

Southam-Gerow, M. A., & Kendall, P. C. (2002). Emotion regulation and understanding: Implications for child psychopathology and therapy. *Clinical Psychology Review, 22*(2), 189–222.

Sweeney, M. & Pine, D. (2004). Etiology of fear and anxiety. In. T. H. Ollendick (Ed.), *Phobic and anxiety disorders in children and adolescents: A clinician's guide to effective psychosocial and pharmacological interventions* (pp. 34–60). New York: Oxford University Press.

Tiwari, S., Podell, J. C., Martin, E. D., Mychailyszyn, M. P., Furr, J. M., & Kendall, P. K. (2009). Experiential avoidance in the parenting of anxious youth: Theory, research, and future directions. *Cognition and Emotion, 22,* 480–496.

Wolff, J. C., & Ollendick, T. H. (2010). Conduct problems in youth: Phenomenology, classification and epidemiology. In R. C. Murrihy, A. D. Kidman, & T. H. Ollendick (Eds.), *Clinical handbook of assessing and treating conduct problems in youth* (pp. 3–20). New York: Springer.

Wood, J. J., & McLeod, B. D. (2008). *Child anxiety disorders: A family-based treatment manual for practitioners.* New York: Norton.

Wood, J. J., McLeod, B. D., Sigman, M., Hwang, W. C., & Chu, B. C. (2003). Parenting and childhood anxiety: Theory, empirical findings, and future directions. *Journal of Child Psychology and Psychiatry, 44,* 134–151.

Author Index

The letter *f* following a page number indicates figure; the letter *t* indicates table.

Abbott, J., 118
Abbott, M., 118
Abela, J. R. Z., 226
Abidin, R. R., 328*t*, 331
Abikoff, H., 170
Aboud, F. E., 282
Abwender, D. A., 278, 285
Achenbach, T. M., 38, 41, 45, 118, 134, 135, 136, 137*f*, 138, 139*f*, 140, 141*t*, 142, 144*f*, 145*f*, 147, 149, 151*f*, 152, 153*f*, 154, 158, 171, 188, 288*t*, 291, 292, 418, 419, 429, 431
Acker, M. M., 189, 330
Adalio, C., 242
Adams, R. E., 278, 279, 281, 297
Adesso, V. J., 357*t*
Agran, M., 199
Agras, W., 379
Aikins, D. E., 228
Aikins, J. W., 287, 288*t*
Akers, R., 184
Albano, A. M., 22, 64, 68, 70, 107, 108*t*, 110, 111, 179, 355, 418, 430
Alberto, P., 166, 167, 168, 186
Alfano, C. A., 106, 258, 365
Algina, J., 358*t*
Allen, A., 10, 61
Allen, B., 70, 220, 431
Allen, J. L., 205, 206
Allen, J. P., 251
Almas, A. N., 319
Almquist, J., 41
Almqvist, F., 138, 147
Alper, S., 199
Altman, D. G., 59
Ambrosini, P. J., 108*t*, 109, 112, 115*t*, 116*t*

Amenta, S., 232
Amir, N., 264, 265
Amso, D., 258
Anastasi, A., 21
Anastopoulos, A. D., 133, 356, 358*t*, 364*t*
Anderson, D. A., 43
Anderson, S. R., 111, 430
Andreassi, J. L., 224, 225, 226
Andrews, R. K., 292
Angold, A., 21, 37, 39, 40, 44, 108*t*, 111, 112, 115*t*, 116*t*, 118, 127, 355
Angstadt, M., 222
Anthonysamy, A., 289*t*, 291
Apter, A., 207, 208
Archer, J., 284
Argulewicz, E. N., 358*t*
Armbruster, P., 389, 401
Armelius, K., 304
Armendariz, G. M., 177
Armstrong, I. T., 247
Armstrong, S. W., 202
Arnold, D. S., 189, 328*t*, 330
Arnow, B. A., 379
Arvanitis, P., 19
Ary, D., 23, 173, 174
Ascher, B. H., 355
Asendorpf, J. B., 253
Asher, S. R., 280, 281, 282, 288*t*, 289, 293, 294, 300, 303
Askew, C., 250, 259
Atkins, M. S., 19, 190
Atkinson, E., 325
Aucoin, K., 242
Auerbach, S. M., 394
Ayllon, T., 68, 69
Azenstzen, M., 242

B

Badanes, L. S., 226
Baer, D. M., 166, 168, 172, 175, 176, 181, 191
Baer, R. D., 350
Bagner, D., 298
Bagwell, C. L., 286, 292
Bailey, L., 285
Baker-Ericzén, M. J., 78
Bakermans-Kranenburg, M. J., 224, 242
Bakker, M. P., 323
Bal, E., 223, 230, 232, 233
Balconi, M., 232
Ballard, D., 210
Bambara, L. M., 198, 210
Bandura, A., 59
Banerjee, R., 250, 251, 264
Banks, W., 164
Bar-Haim, Y., 242, 248
Barajas, P. C., 385
Baranek, G. T., 228
Barber, B. K., 319
Barber, J. P., 385
Barkley, R. A., 12, 103, 104, 442
Barlow, D. H., 128, 305, 384
Barnes, V. A., 225
Barratt, T., 382
Barrett, P. M., 4, 18, 253, 254
Barrios, B., 10, 11, 20
Barrios, V., 118
Barry, C. T., 15, 16, 17, 165
Barry, L. M., 198
Basco, M. R., 41
Bass, D., 380
Bastain, T. M., 247
Basurto, F. Z., 110
Bathiche, M., 138, 147
Battaglia, M., 249, 255
Bauer, S., 205, 209
Baumeister, R. F., 165
Beals, J., 365
Beard, C., 264
Beauchaine, T. P., 224, 228, 231, 233
Becerra, I. G., 110
Bechtold, D. W., 365
Beck, A. T., 118, 342
Beck, J., 320
Becker, E. M., 7, 80
Beery, S. H., 278, 285
Beidel, D. C., 14, 204, 205, 206, 258, 302
Beiser, M., 356, 363t
Bell, M. A., 222
Bellis, J., 390
Bem, D. I., 10, 61
Benoit, K. E., 70, 220, 319, 431
Benoit, M. Z., 365
Bergeron, L., 355
Bergman, R. L., 118, 254
Berk, L., 258

Bernal, G., 367, 428
Bernhout, E., 208
Bernstein, A., 404
Bernstein, G. A., 35
Berntson, G. G., 220
Bérubé, R. L., 138, 140, 147
Best, M., 332
Beutler, L. E., 126
Bickman, L., 378, 379, 394
Bidaut-Russell, M., 355
Bierman, D., 258
Bigbee, M. A., 283, 284, 289t, 297, 299
Biggs, B. K., 356, 357t, 363t
Bilenberg, N., 138, 149
Bird, D., 381
Bird, H., 350n1
Birmaher, B., 35, 118
Black, J. L., 203
Blair, J., 242
Blanchette, I., 244
Blasey, C., 379
Blatter-Meunier, J., 205
Bluemke, M., 253
Boergers, J., 277
Bögels, S. M., 248, 253, 254, 264
Boggs, S., 334
Bohnert, A. M., 357t
Boivin, M., 277, 288t, 294
Bomyea, J., 264
Bongers, I. L., 104
Bonnet, M., 283
Bor, W., 335
Bordin, E. S., 382
Borduin, C. M., 399, 400
Borkovec, T. D., 378, 387
Boschen, M. J., 213
Boulton, M. J., 284
Bouwmeester, S., 255
Bowker, J. C., 279, 296, 297
Boxmeyer, C., 439
Boyajian, A. E., 199
Boyd, K., 200
Boykin, R. A., 203
Bradley, B. P., 242, 245
Bradshaw, C. P., 390
Brady, E. U., 125
Brady, M. P., 203
Braith, J., 383
Brambilla, F., 249
Brassard, M. R., 284
Braswell, L., 13, 383
Braver, S. L., 278
Bravo, M., 109, 352, 353t, 355, 366
Brendgen, M., 281, 282, 294, 296
Brennan, J., 319
Brennan, R. L., 22, 191
Brenner, S. L., 231
Brent, D., 118
Breton, S., 380, 388, 431
Briesch, A. M., 174, 176, 189, 197, 198

Brimacombe, M., 233
Broden, M., 196
Broeren, S., 255
Broks, P., 244
Broman-Fulks, J. J., 37
Brondino, M. J., 384
Brookman-Frazee, L., 78, 386
Brooks-Gunn, J., 16
Brosch, T., 244
Brosschot, J. F., 248, 249, 258
Brown Wright, L., 225
Brown, B. B., 280
Brown, J. S., 357t
Brown, L. M., 241
Brown, R., 36, 402
Brown, T. A., 128
Brown, T. J., 165
Bruchmüller, K., 45
Bruck, M., 197
Brukhardt, U., 259
Bubier, J. L., 432
Buckhalt, J. A., 223
Buhrmester, D., 277, 295
Bukowski, A. L., 280
Bukowski, W. M., 277, 278, 279, 280, 281, 282, 288t, 294, 297
Burns, B. J., 37, 41, 50, 127
Buskirk, A., 277
Bussing, R., 358t
Butler, G., 381
Byrne, B. M., 351

C

Cacioppo, J. T., 220, 222, 226, 227, 232
Calhoun, G. B., 390
Calhoun, K. S., 14
Cali, P. W., 360t
Calvo, M. G., 248
Calvocoressi, L., 331
Campbell, K. D. M., 365
Campbell, L., 266
Campbell, W., 112
Canino, G. J., 350n1, 352, 355, 365, 366
Carama, W. J., 5
Carapetian, S., 226
Cardoos, S. L., 292, 298
Carey, M. P., 383
Carr, S. C., 202
Carter, M. M., 359
Carter, R. E., 384, 400
Carthy, T., 207
Cartwright-Hatton, S., 263
Casas, J., 283
Casat, C. D., 354t, 355, 356, 358t, 364t
Caseras, X., 245
Cashel, M. L., 42, 105
Castellanos, F. X., 247
Cataldi, E. F., 284
Ceci, S. J., 197

Cerny, J. A., 56, 59, 63, 235
Chaffin, M., 332
Chafouleas, S. M., 166, 168, 169, 171, 172, 174, 189, 197, 198
Chaiyasit, W., 19
Chamberlain, P., 377, 383, 397, 402, 406
Chambers, W. J., 355
Chan, S., 285, 419
Chanese, J. A., 189
Chang, L. Y., 352
Chang, Y., 390
Chapman, J. E., 384, 400
Charlot-Swilley, D., 392
Chen, Y., 354t, 355
Cheng, C., 390
Chi, T. C., 16
Childs, K. E., 200
Childs, R. A., 5
Chiu, A. W., 395, 396
Chorpita, B. F., 41, 90, 91, 358t, 404
Christie, I. C., 232
Chu, B. C., 377, 383, 385, 396, 397, 402, 418
Chung, T. A., 381
Cicchetti, D., 13, 14, 226
Clark, L. A., 37, 127
Clarke, G. N., 208
Clarke, S., 200
Clerkin, S. M., 330
Cohen, D. J., 13, 14
Cohen, J. A., 35, 113
Cohen, P. J., 390, 403
Cohn, J. F., 232
Coie, J. D., 279, 280, 281, 286, 288t, 289
Cole, C. L., 196, 197, 210, 419, 432
Cole, D. A., 357t
Coleman, M., 198
Colson, D. B., 384
Cone, J. D., 10, 20, 22, 57, 59, 62, 63, 166, 167, 168, 169, 170, 172, 173, 174, 175, 176, 177, 178, 186, 190
Conger, R. D., 188
Conners, C. K., 133, 152
Connolly, J., 306
Connolly, S. D., 35
Connor, S., 233
Connor-Smith, J. K., 242
Conover, N. C., 17
Conroy, M. A., 185
Constantino, M. J., 379
Cook, C. R., 283, 285, 304
Cook, E., 264
Cooley, M. R., 365
Cooper, J. O., 172, 174, 190
Coric, V., 228
Cornelius, J. R., 381
Corwin, D., 112
Costa, N. M., 319, 442
Costello, A. J., 17, 352
Costello, E. J., 37, 108t, 111, 112, 115t, 116t, 118, 127

Cottler, L., 112
Cowan, P. A., 322
Cowart, M. J. W., 70, 220, 264, 265, 431
Coyne, S. M., 284
Craig, W., 306
Craske, M. G., 254, 264
Creed, T., 383, 392, 393
Creswell, C., 253, 255
Crick, N. R., 283, 284, 288t, 289t, 296, 297, 298, 299
Crisostomo, P. S., 7, 124, 383, 419
Crisp, H., 285, 298
Criss, M., 320
Crockett, L. J., 356, 360t, 362t
Cronbach, L. J., 11, 140, 173
Cronin, M. E., 198, 202
Croskerry, P., 39, 40
Cross, D. G., 332
Crowley, M., 380, 382, 388, 431
Cullerton-Sen, C., 299
Cunningham, P. B., 400
Curry, J., 379, 383, 386

D

D'Amato, R. C., 357t
Dadds, M. R., 16, 18, 70, 82, 178, 246, 247, 253, 318, 319, 320, 321, 325, 329t, 330, 333, 334, 335, 337, 419, 431, 439
Dagnone, M., 117
Dahlquist, L. M., 231
Daleiden, E. L., 90, 241, 255, 404
Dalgleish, T., 241, 248, 254, 259
Dalton, K. M., 222
Damsma, E., 255
Daniels, M., 233
Danner, G., 297
Dauber, S., 385, 398
Davanzo, P., 357t
David, C. F., 262t
David, F. J., 228
David-Ferdon, C., 357t
Davies, W. H., 357t
Davila, J., 277, 278, 285, 306
Davis, B., 208, 357t
Davis, T. E., III, 442
De Bruycker, E., 253
De Haas-Warner, S., 203
De Houwer, J., 242, 250, 252, 253
De Los Reyes, A., 16, 17, 25, 26, 142, 283, 284, 288t, 298
de Niet, J., 205
De Ruiter, K., 242
Dearing, E., 357t
Dearing, K., 254, 255
Deater-Deckard, K., 282
Deblinger, E., 403
Degnan, K. A., 319
Delfino, R. J., 200

DeLoache, J. S., 244
Demaray, M. K., 288t, 296
Demeersman, R., 224
Denckla, M. B., 247
Dennis, M. L., 393
Dennis, T. A., 232
Denys, D. A. J. P., 41
Derakshan, N., 248
Devany, J., 203
DeVet, K. A., 392
Devilly, G. J., 378
Dew, S. E., 378, 379
Deyhle, D., 357t
Diaferia, G., 249
Diamond, G. M., 382, 394
Diamond, G. S., 398
Diaz-Perez, M. J., 351
DiClemente, C. C., 381, 390
Dietz, L. J., 319
DiGiuseppe, R., 382
Dimoska, A., 259
Dinkes, R., 284
Dion, R., 356, 363t
Dionne, R., 357t, 358t
DiPerna, J. C., 170
Dishion, T. J., 171, 282, 283, 318, 320, 333, 335
Dobrean, A., 138, 149
Dodge, K. A., 279, 282
Donenberg, G. R., 385
Donkervoet, C., 41
Donnelly, N., 244, 248
Donohue, B. C., 204
Dorta, K. P., 302, 428
Dougherty, L. R., 44, 45
Dove, S., 297
Doxie, J., 222
Doyle, A. E., 124
Dozois, D. J. A., 264
Drabick, D. A. G., 432, 439
Drabman, R. S., 185
Driscoll, A. K., 356, 360t
Duax, J., 44
Dubois, D. L., 304
Dubow, E. F., 289t, 296
Duhig, A. M., 142
Duke, M., 334
Dulcan, M. D., 352
Dulcan, M. K., 17, 107, 355
Dumenci, L., 41, 138, 147, 149
Duncan, S., 258
Dunkel, S. B., 357t
Dunlap, G., 200, 202
Dunlap, L. K., 202
DuPaul, G. J., 133, 168

E

Eddy, J. M., 339
Eddy, M., 230

Edelbrock, C. S., 17, 71, 118, 138, 147, 152, 352
Edwards, A. W., 19
Edwards, B., 332
Edwards, P., 325
Edwards, S. L., 319
Eells, T. D., 7, 78, 79, 80, 84, 85
Egger, H. L., 353t, 355
Ehrenreich, J. T., 305
Eichstaedt, J., 253
Eisen, A. R., 89, 127
El Masry, Y., 246
El-Sheikh, M., 223
Eldar, S., 264
Elder, G. H., 357t
Eley, T. C., 138, 319, 418, 425
Elgar, F. J., 330
Elliot, A. J., 105
Elliot, C. M., 199
Elliot, S. N., 286, 288t, 289t, 300
Ellis, A. W., 244
Ellis, B. B., 149
Ellis, M. L., 379
Eltz, M., 402
Endicott, J., 113
Epstein, M. H., 197
Epstein, M. K., 142
Erath, S., 277
Erbaugh, J., 118
Erdley, C., 278
Erkanli, A., 37, 112, 127
Ernst, M., 246
Ervin, R. A., 168
Eschenbeck, H., 248, 259
Eslea, M., 284
Estell, D. B., 280
Esteves, F., 244
Estrada, A. U., 397
Evans, J. S. B. T., 39, 40
Everaerd, W., 249
Everett, F., 383
Ewell, K. K., 278, 285
Eyberg, S. M., 334, 337, 338, 358t
Eyde, L. D., 5
Eysenck, M. W., 248

F

Fabiano, G. A., 44, 120, 126, 166, 184
Farmer, E. M. Z., 37, 127
Faw, L., 382
Fazekas, H., 242
Fazio, R. H., 249
Fehm, L., 352
Ferdinand, R. F., 140
Ferrari, C., 232
Ferriter, C., 379, 386, 419
Ferro, J. B., 70
Festa, C., 293
Fetter, M. D., 280

Field, A. P., 242, 244, 248, 249, 250, 251, 255, 258, 259, 263, 431
Findling, R. L., 35
Fingerle, M., 251
First, M. B., 48, 49
Fischer, B., 259
Fisher, P. H., 107, 306, 352
Fisher, P. W., 21, 39, 40, 44
Fitch, D., 357t, 360t
Fitzgerald, D. A., 222
Fitzpatrick, M. R., 381, 393
Fjermestad, K., 382, 395, 396
Flessner, C. A., 331
Florin, I., 256
Florsheim, P., 382, 393, 394
Floyd, E. M., 358t
Flykt, A., 244
Follette, V. M., 11
Follette, W. C., 36
Forbes, C., 334, 338, 339
Forgatch, M., 166, 187, 397
Forman, L., 36
Foster, S. I., 166, 167, 168, 169, 170
Foster, S. L., 20, 22, 173, 174, 175, 176, 177, 178, 186, 188, 189, 190, 328t, 330, 419
Fox, E., 244
Fox, J. J., 185
Fox, N. A., 14, 319
Fradenburg, L., 166
Fraley, R. C., 37
Frances, A. F., 36, 48
Francis, S. E., 358t
Franco, F., 366
Franklin, M. E., 390
Freeman, C. M., 285
Freeman, K. A., 82
Freher, N. K., 256
Freitag, C. M., 226
French, C. C., 241, 248, 254
Freud, S., 164
Frick, P. J., 15, 16, 44, 45, 46, 104, 124, 125, 165, 167, 179, 242, 319, 329, 431, 439
Fried, A., 385
Friedberg, R., 19
Friedman, B. H., 220, 232, 432
Friese, M., 253
Friman, P. C., 168
Frisby, C. L., 19
Fristad, M. A., 44, 110, 118
Frith, G. H., 202
Frost, A. D. J., 319
Frost, S., 254
Fulcher, E. P., 246
Funder, D. C., 165
Furman, W., 277, 279, 280, 288t, 295, 306

G

Gabrielson, P., 397
Gadow, K. D., 133

Gallop, R., 379
Gamble, A. L., 246
Garb, H. N., 21, 39, 40
Garcia, J. A., 382
Gardner, F., 334
Gardner, K., 335
Garland, A. F., 385, 386, 394
Garner, M., 245
Garrido-Castillo, P., 366
Gatzke-Kopp, L., 233
Gaudet, N., 355
Geers, M., 256
Geffken, G. R., 317
Geldof, T., 253
Ghera, M. M., 14
Ghorpade, J., 350
Gifford, A., 377
Gifford, E. V., 11
Gifford-Smith, M., 282
Gilissen, R., 224, 225
Ginsburg, G. S., 293, 365
Girdwood, C. P., 7, 78
Girvin, H., 381
Gittelman, R., 170
Giuseppe, R., 393
Glaser, B. A., 390
Glasziou, P., 41, 47
Glazer, A. D., 189
Gleser, G. C., 11, 173
Glueckauf, R. L., 393
Goldner, E. M., 352
Goldstein, C. R., 305
Gonzales, N. A., 19, 60, 349, 367, 418
Gonzalez, A., 361t
Goodkind, J. R., 357t
Goodlin-Jones, B. L., 46
Goodman, R., 134, 140
Goodyer, I. M., 245
Goossens, F., 283
Gordon, B. N., 16
Gotlib, I., 254, 255
Gotowiec, A., 356, 363t
Gottman, J. M., 333
Gould, M. S., 389
Gould, T. D., 247
Gove, P., 138
Graham, S., 200
Granger, D. A., 226, 230
Gray, J. A., 227, 233
Green, S. M., 17, 320
Greenberg, L. S., 393
Greene, R. W., 124, 439
Greenstein, D. K., 390
Greenwald, A. G., 250
Gregory, A. M., 319
Gregoski, M. J., 225
Gresham, F. M., 166, 168, 172, 174, 185,
    186, 191, 286, 289t, 300
Griggs, L., 244
Grills, A. E., 104, 197

Grogan-Kaylor, A., 357t, 360t
Gross, A. M., 165
Gross, D., 356, 358t, 364t
Gross, J. J., 207, 232
Grotpeter, J. K., 288t, 289t, 296, 297
Grove, W. M., 40
Grumm, M., 251, 257, 258
Guadiano, B. A., 379
Guarnaccia, P. J., 350, 350n1, 365, 366
Guastella, A. J., 246
Gudmundsen, G., 402
Guerra, N. G., 283
Guest-Warnick, G., 382
Gullone, E., 18, 64
Gunnar, M. R., 226
Gusella, J., 381, 389
Guttmannova, K., 360t

H

Hadwin, J. A., 242, 244, 248, 254
Hagopian, L. P., 89
Hajcak, G., 232
Hall, R. V., 196
Halperin, J. M., 330
Hamby, R. S., 200
Hamby, S. L., 332
Hamill, S. K., 357t
Hamilton, J., 44
Hammerl, M., 246
Hammond, G., 254
Hampton, K. A., 247
Han, S., 379
Handwerk, M. L., 41, 124
Haney, C., 164
Hanf, C., 183
Hankin, B. L., 37, 226
Hannesdóttir, D. K., 222, 230, 231, 425
Har, K., 395
Harbin, H. T., 208
Hardin, M., 246
Harris, A., 358t
Harris, K. R., 200
Harrison, H. M., 277, 280, 282, 284, 285,
    290, 295
Harrison, R., 166
Hart, B., 178
Hart, E. L., 45
Harter, S., 289t, 290, 295, 296, 419, 431
Hartmann, D. P., 10, 11, 20
Hartup, W. W., 277, 280, 282
Harvey, A. G., 263
Harwell, J., 357t
Hasking, P. A., 319
Haslam, N., 37
Hastings, P. D., 230
Hattrup, K., 350
Hawes, D. J., 16, 82, 178, 318, 319, 320,
    321, 337, 419, 431
Hawker, D. S. J., 284

Hawkins, E. J., 186, 190
Hawkins, R. P., 70, 171, 179, 185, 187
Hawley, K. M., 4, 41, 45, 382, 385, 392, 393, 394, 405
Hawthorn, M. L., 210
Hay, L. R., 172, 203
Hay, W. M., 172
Hayes, C., 377
Hayes, S. C., 11, 71, 72, 190
Haynes, B., 41
Haynes, R. B., 47
Haynes, S. N., 57, 63, 64, 72, 78, 79, 85, 105, 167, 173, 177
Heath, A. C., 418
Hecht, D. B., 280
Heim-Dreger, U., 248, 259
Hein, S., 251
Heinrich, C. C., 278
Helzer, E. G., 242, 263
Helzer, J. E., 38, 39
Hembree-Kigin, T. L., 338
Hembrooke, H., 197
Hemphill, J. F., 390
Henderson, A., 357t
Henderson, C. E., 385, 400
Henderson, H. A., 14
Henggeler, S. W., 384, 399, 400
Henker, B., 200, 206, 210, 211, 212
Henry, D. B., 26
Henry, J., 242
Herald-Brown, S. L., 292
Herge, W., 285, 419
Herjanic, B., 112
Heron, T. E., 172
Hersen, M., 10, 15, 17, 20, 56, 57, 62, 71, 72, 79, 104, 125, 204
Hess, R. S., 357t
Hessel, E., 284
Hetherington, E. M., 322
Heward, W. L., 172
Heyman, R. E., 334, 339, 340
Heyne, D., 64, 428
Hiemstra, H., 256
Hietanen, J. K., 246
Hill, C. E., 23
Hill, N. E., 349, 351
Hilliard, A. M., 203
Hilt, L. M., 357t
Hinshaw, S. P., 16, 35, 126, 177, 277, 292, 298
Hintze, J. M., 170, 171, 173, 174, 175, 184
Hoagwood, K., 50
Hodges, E., 277
Hofstra, M. B., 138, 140
Hogan, S., 200
Hogue, A. T., 382, 385, 398, 400
Holland, L., 380, 382, 386, 388, 431
Holland, S., 242
Hollin, I., 213
Holly, L. E., 19, 60, 418

Holmbeck, G. N., 17
Holmberg, E., 379, 386, 419
Holton, A., 325
Hommer, D. W., 247
Hong, J., 224
Hooe, E. S., 262t
Hops, H., 208
Horder, P., 248
Horesh, N., 207
Horner, R. H., 185, 211
Hororitz, M., 80
Horselenberg, R., 256
Horsley, T. A., 247
Horvath, A. O., 393
Horvath, P. J., 230
Hough, R. L., 78
House, A. E., 59
Houts, A. C., 36
Howell, A. J., 390
Howell, C. T., 142, 152, 188
Hoyt, D. R., 357t
Hoza, B., 282, 286, 288t, 289, 294
Hsu, L., 352
Huang, Y., 390
Hubble, E., 172
Hudson, J. L., 318
Hudziak, J. J., 248, 418, 425, 439
Huey, S. J., Jr., 384, 400
Hufford, M. R., 204
Hughes, C. H., 198
Hui, H. C., 349
Huijding, J., 249, 250, 251, 258
Hunsley, J., 3–4, 20, 21, 22, 24, 35, 41, 57, 79, 104, 166, 178, 184, 190, 318, 332
Hunt, C., 241
Huntzinger, R. M., 89
Hupp, S. D. A., 168, 180, 186
Hurlburt, M. S., 78, 385, 386, 400
Hutchison, S. L., 8
Hwang, W. C., 382, 418
Hwu, H. G., 352
Hymel, S., 300

I

Iannotti, R. J., 277, 285
In-Albon, T., 245
Inderbitzen, H. M., 280
Ingersoll, R. G., 164
Ino, S., 352
Irannejad, S., 381, 393
Ireys, H. T., 392
Ishikawa, S. S., 211
Israel, M. E., 247
Ivanova, M. Y., 41, 135, 138, 147, 149
Ives, M. L., 393

J

Jaccard, J., 278, 358t
Jackson, A. P., 357t

Jackson, J. L., 11, 20, 21, 22, 23
Jackson, S., 226
Jacobs, J. R., 170, 171
Jacobson, N. S., 35
James, R. C., 18
James, W., 219
Jamner, L. D., 200, 210, 212
Jarrett, M. A., 111, 430
Jarrett, R. B., 71, 190
Jarzynka, J., 200
Jatrowski Mano, K. E., 357t
Jazbec, S., 246
Jelsone, L. M., 222
Jenkins, M. M., 41, 48, 78
Jennings, Y. R., 230
Jensen, A. L., 41
Jensen, P. S., 50, 117
Jensen-Doss, A., 4, 7, 25, 41, 45, 80, 85, 121,
    125, 128, 140, 178, 182f, 233, 240,
    279, 340, 366, 419, 431
Jewell, J., 41
Jilton, R., 382, 393
Johnson, P., 230
Johnson, S. B., 358t, 382
Johnston, C., 44, 45
Johnston, J. M., 11, 23, 173, 176
Johnstone, S. J., 259
Jones, G. V., 248
Julu, P., 233
Jungbluth, N. J., 377, 382, 383, 384, 397,
    401
Juvonen, J., 365

K

Kachnowski, S., 213
Kaholokula, J. K., 63, 78
Kalas, R., 17, 352
Kamarck, T., 230
Kamphaus, R. W., 15, 16, 134, 140, 165, 171
Kamphuis, J. H., 283
Kandel, D. B., 282
Kane, A. S., 383
Kanfer, F. H., 59
Kaplan, D., 389
Kaplinski, H., 402
Karatekin, C., 259
Kardes, F. R., 249
Karpinski, A., 253
Karver, M. S., 377, 382, 383, 386, 394, 396,
    402, 406
Kaslow, N. J., 208
Kaster-Bundgaard, J., 105
Kaufman, J., 118
Kavanagh, K., 397
Kazdin, A. E., 16, 17, 24, 26, 77, 89, 125,
    142, 232, 261t, 378, 379, 380, 382,
    384, 386, 387, 388, 389, 401, 405, 407,
    431
Kearney, C. A., 64, 67, 68, 180, 185, 419

Keeler, G. P., 37
Keeley, M., 317
Kellison, I., 317
Kelly, S. M., 19
Kendall, P. C., 72, 89, 125, 261t, 377, 383,
    385, 392, 393, 396, 397, 402, 406, 425
Kendler, K. S., 37
Kennedy, S., 319
Kent, R. N., 330, 419
Keogh, E., 241
Kern, L., 168, 199, 200
Kidman, A. D., 125, 431
Kiesler, D. J., 394
Kiesner, J., 283
Kilgore, K., 325
Kim, T. E., 283
Kim, Y. J., 392
Kimmel, H. D., 149
Kimonis, E. R., 242, 431, 439
Kindt, M., 248, 249, 256, 258
King, N. J., 59, 64, 66, 104, 197, 204, 428
King, P. S., 200
Kingery, J. N., 278, 279, 365
Kirkham, N., 258
Kistner, J. A., 262t, 357t
Klaric, S. H., 352
Klauer, K. C., 253
Klein, C., 259
Klein, D. N., 44, 228
Klein, R. G., 285, 306
Klein, R. M., 245
Klein-Tasman, B. P., 357t
Kleinhans, N. M., 222, 223
Klimes-Dougan, B., 230
Klumpp, H., 264, 265
Kneedler, B., 334
Knight, G. P., 349, 350, 351, 356, 359, 361t,
    362t, 367
Koch, G. G., 41, 113, 354t
Kogan, J. N., 8
Kohlmann, C. W., 248, 259
Koller, D., 248
Koot, H. M., 104, 140
Kordy, H., 205
Koslow-Green, L., 203
Kossowsky, J., 246
Kovacs, M., 118, 288t, 300, 418
Koverola, C., 332
Kowatch, R., 35
Kraemer, H. C., 38
Kramer, T. L., 41
Krasner, L., 58
Krishnamurthy, R., 4
Kronmuller, K. T., 392
Krueger, R. F., 38, 152
Krupnick, J. L., 379
Ku, H., 283
Kubany, E. S., 173
Kunsch, C., 419, 432
Kuntsi, J., 243

Kupersmidt, J. B., 279, 280, 281
Kupperbusch, C., 352
Kurth, S., 222
Kurtz, S. M., 186, 191
Kuttler, A. F., 277, 281, 282, 295
Kwok, O. M., 350

L

La Greca, A. M., 197, 277, 278, 279, 280,
    281, 282, 283, 284, 285, 286, 288*t*,
    289, 289*t*, 290, 291, 292, 295, 298,
    300, 306, 358*t*, 419, 431
Labouvie, E., 350
Lackritz, J. R., 350
Ladd, G. W., 277, 279, 280, 292
LaFromboise, T. D., 358*t*
Lahey, B. B., 37, 45, 320
Lai, B. S., 278, 284, 419
Laird, B., 226
Lamarche, V., 281
Lamb, D., 232
Lambert, M. J., 8, 23, 186, 190, 378
Lambert, S. F., 365
Lambiase, M., 230
Lamy, D., 242
Lance, C. E., 350
Landau, S., 278
Landis, J. R., 41, 113, 354*t*
Landoll, R. R., 277, 278, 279, 284, 285,
    288*t*, 298, 306
Lane, K. L., 70
Lane, T. W., 397
Lang, P. J., 179, 259
LaNoue, M. D., 357*t*
Lantz, J. F., 198
Laptook, R. S., 44
Lasker, A. G., 247
Last, C. G., 125
Lau, A. S., 357*t*
Lau, J. Y. F., 255, 319
Lawson, C., 254
Lawson, J., 250, 251
Lazovik, A. D., 179
Lebow, B. S., 40
LeBreton, J. M., 332
Lederer, A. S., 204
Lee, C. C., 358*t*
Lee, C. K., 352
Lee, S., 362*t*
Lefebvre, M., 332
Legerstee, J. S., 264
Lehey, B. B., 17
Lemanek, K. L., 197, 278, 286
Lenhart, A., 284, 306, 307
Leonard, I. J., 199
Leppanen, J. M., 246
Leser, M., 248
Lester, K. J., 242, 244, 258, 431
Leung, K., 352

Levenson, R. W., 232
Levine, L., 200
Lewin, A. B., 208
Lewinsohn, P. M., 208
Lewis, C. C., 381, 390, 402, 419, 431
Lewis, E. L., 359
Lewis, G. F., 232
Lewis-Fernández, R., 351, 366
Lewis-Palmer, T., 211
Li-Kelly, W., 284
Liaupsin, C. J., 70
Liberman, L., 250
Licht, M., 190
Lichtenstein, P., 138
Liddle, H. A., 382, 385
Liebert, D. E., 292
Linscott, J., 382, 393, 394
Linting, M., 224
Lipinski, D. P., 203
Lipp, O. V., 242, 244, 250
Littell, J. H., 381
Little, M., 351, 356, 359, 362*t*
Liu, J. F., 352
Lloyd, M. E., 203
LoBue, V., 244
Lochman, J. E., 439
Loeber, R., 17, 320
Loftin, R. L., 198
Lohre, A., 299
Lombart, K. G., 78, 79, 80, 84
Loney, B. R., 242
Longworth, S. L., 352
Lonigan, C. J., 24, 259, 262, 262*t*, 263
Lopez, C. M., 304, 357*t*
López, I., 350*n*1, 366
Lopez, M., 41
Lopez, N., 280, 282, 289*t*, 290, 300
Lorenz, F. O., 188, 189
Losoya, S., 351
Lucas, C. P., 41, 105, 107, 352
Luermans, J., 256
Luis, T. M., 357*t*, 363*t*
Luk, J. W., 277
Lumley, V., 105
Lunkenheimer, E. S., 188
Lustig, J. L., 278
Lydersen, S., 299
Lynch, A. D., 41
Lyneham, H. J., 114*t*, 118

M

MacDonald, V. M., 138
Mack, A. H., 36
Mackey, E. R., 280, 281, 290, 295
MacLeod, C., 266
Madrigal, L., 357*t*
Maehle, M., 299
Magee, E. A., 8
Mah, J. W. T., 44, 45

Mahon, N., 289t, 300
Maisto, S. A., 381, 389
Malecki, C., 288t, 296
Malloy, C. A., 184
Manion, I., 332
Mannarino, A. P., 403
Manning-Courtney, P., 184
Mansell, W., 263
Manson, S. M., 365
Marano, M. R., 351
March, S., 250
Marchand-Martella, N. E., 199
Marciano, P. L., 388
Marcovitch, S., 231
Marder, T. J., 199
Margraf, J., 45, 256
Marin, C. E., 44, 111, 301, 418, 430
Marks, D. J., 330
Marsh, P., 224
Marshall, K., 278
Marshall, P. J., 14
Martella, R. C., 199
Martin, C. S., 381
Martin, J. M., 357t
Martin, M., 248
Martinez, I., 366
Mash, E. J., 3–4, 12, 20, 21, 22, 24, 35, 41,
    56, 57, 59, 79, 103, 104, 166, 167, 178,
    184, 186, 188, 189, 190, 318
Masia-Warner, C. L., 284, 285, 298, 306
Massetti, G. M., 44, 166
Masten, A. S., 13
Mathews, A., 246, 264, 265, 266
Mathews, J. R., 179, 185, 190
Matson, J. L., 69
Matsumoto, D., 352
Matthews, W. J., 173, 175, 184
May, J. C., 394
Mayer, B., 256
Mayer, J. A., 66
Mazurick, J. L., 380
McAllister, R. A., 325
McBeath, B., 357t, 360t
McCall, C., 198
McCallum, K., 112
McClellan, J. M., 35, 355
McCloskey, D. M., 357t
McClure, E., 246
McClure, J., 19
McConaughy, S. H., 135, 142, 154, 171, 188
McConnaughy, E. A., 389, 390
McCord, J., 282
McCracken, J., 118
McDougall, D., 203
McDunn, C., 279
McElhattan, D., 199
McElroy, K., 200
McFall, R. M., 79
McFetridge, M., 200
McGhee, D. E., 250

McGonigle, J. J., 203
McGrath, J. J., 105
McGraw, K., 325
McGregor, 46, 69, 419
McGuffin, P., 390
McHugh, R., 384, 385
McKay, M. M., 19
McLaughlin, K. A., 357t, 358t
McLeod, B. D., 4, 7, 13, 23, 45, 80, 85, 121,
    125, 128, 140, 178, 182f, 233, 240,
    279, 318, 319, 340, 366, 385, 393, 395,
    396, 398, 399, 418, 419, 427, 431, 439
McLeod, C., 254, 264
McMahon, R. C., 183, 185
McMahon, R. J., 44, 45, 46, 104, 124, 125
McMakin, D., 378
McNaughton, N., 233
McNeil, C. B., 338
Mead, H., 233
Meadows, S. O., 357t
Mednick, S. A., 220
Medoff, L., 358t
Meehl, P. E., 40
Meester, C., 256
Mehta, M. A., 245, 259
Meichenbaum, D. H., 59
Melby, J. N., 188
Melnick, S., 177
Mendelson, M. J., 118, 282
Menneer, T., 244
Merkelbach, H., 255
Messer, J. J., 198
Mierke, J., 253
Milford, J., 357t
Milgram, S., 164
Milla, S., 166
Miller, C. A., 82
Miller, D. C., 358t
Miller, G. E., 380
Miller, I. W., 379
Miller, L. J., 200
Miller, O., 359
Miller, S. R., 200
Miller, T. L., 41
Miller, W. R., 381, 389, 403
Millsap, R. E., 349, 350
Milner, J. S., 329t, 331, 332
Miltenberger, R. G., 105, 168, 176, 178
Ming, X., 233
Minn, J. Y., 352
Minuchin, S, 320
Mischel, W., 10, 173
Mitchell, T., 184
Mitts, B., 196
Mock, J., 118
Moffitt, C., 358t
Moffitt, T. E., 138
Mogg, K., 242, 245
Molina, B. S., 286
Momper, S. L., 357t

Mooney, P., 197, 198
Moore, K. D., 247
Moore, L. A., 278
Moradi, A. R., 241, 248, 254
Morawska, A., 333
Moreau, D., 302, 428
Moreno, A. M. M., 110
Morgan, C. A., 228
Mori, L. T., 177
Morren, M., 248, 249, 256
Morris, T. L., 206, 302
Morris, T. M., 70
Mosk, J., 19
Mostofsky, S. H., 247
Mouchlianitis, E., 244
Mrug, S., 282
Muck, R. D., 393
Mufson, L., 302, 428
Mullane, J. C., 244
Mullen, K. B., 70
Mullins, M., 325
Mullins, S. M., 332
Mulvey, E. P., 351
Munoz, D. P., 247
Munoz, L., 242
Murdock, J. Y., 198, 202
Muris, P., 253, 255, 256
Murphy, G. C., 204
Murray, D. S., 184
Murray, H. W., 384
Murrihy, R. C., 125, 431, 439
Muthén, B., 351
Myers, K., 45

N

Naglieri, J. A., 134
Nanda, H., 11, 173
Nansel, T. R., 277, 284, 285
Napolitano, M., 319
Nash, G., 248
Nathan, J. S., 5
Nathan, P. J., 222
Nau, S. D., 387
Nauta, M., 377
Neal, A. M., 204
Neale, J. M., 292
Neale, M. C., 418
Neighbors, C., 366
Nelles, W. B., 111, 293
Nelson, C. A., 40, 246
Nelson, D. A., 283, 284, 288t, 296, 297
Nelson, M., 334
Nelson, R. O., 71, 172, 190, 196, 203
Nelson-Gray, R. O., 24, 35, 63, 65, 80, 166, 168, 186, 188
Nesdale, D. D., 279, 280, 304
Neshat-Doost, H. T., 241, 248, 254
Newcomb, A. F., 280, 289
Newman, B., 201

Nezu, A. M., 7, 78, 80, 85, 88
Nezu, C. M., 7, 78
Nguyen, K., 386
Nichols, K. E., 14
Nichols, L., 381
Nigg, J. T., 177
Nightingale, Z. C., 248
Nippe, G. E., 211
Nishina, A., 365
Nock, M. K., 186, 191, 379, 380, 386, 387, 389, 391, 407, 419, 431
Nolen-Hoeksema, S., 357t
Norcross, J. C., 381, 403
Norman, G., 39
Norton, H. J., 356, 358t, 364t
Novins, D. K., 365

O

O'Brien, W. H., 63, 78, 105
O'Connor, T. G., 253
O'Driscoll, G. A., 259
O'Leary, K. D., 329t, 333, 419
O'Leary, S. G., 189, 330
O'Malley, S., 397
O'Neill, R. E., 168, 178
Ocampo, K. A., 356, 361t
Odom, S. L., 198
Öhman, A., 244
Ojeda, V. D., 351
Okazaki, S., 349, 352
Oldehinkel, A. J., 323
Olino, T. M., 44
Ollendick, T. H., 4, 10, 15, 18, 20, 44, 45, 56, 57, 59, 62, 63, 64, 66, 69, 70, 71, 72, 85, 89, 104, 111, 121, 125, 128, 140, 178, 182f, 197, 200, 203, 204, 207, 220, 222, 231, 233, 240, 264, 265, 279, 319, 334, 340, 366, 418, 419, 425, 430, 431, 432, 439, 442
Olweus, D., 11, 61, 283
Ondersma, S. J., 332
Oosterlaan, J., 243, 248
Ormel, J., 323
Orobio de Castro, B., 247
Ortiz, C. D., 358t
Ost, L.-G., 442
Osterberg, L. D., 41
Ostrov, J. M., 284
Ouimet, A. J., 264
Ownby, R. L., 208
Ozonoff, S., 46

P

Paikoff, R. L., 16
Paquette, J., 297
Parker, J., 277, 278, 280, 281, 282, 288t, 289, 293, 294, 303
Parker, K. C. H., 117
Pasalich, D. S., 319, 337

Patel, U., 248
Patriquin, M. A., 220, 223, 432
Pattee, L., 280
Patterson, G. R., 59, 166, 171, 172, 187, 189,
    318, 333, 335, 377, 383, 397, 402, 406
Paulosky, C. A., 43
Paulsen, B., 299
Paulson, J. F., 63, 65
Pavlov, I. P., 164
Peacock, M. A., 7, 78
Peck-Stichter, J., 185
Peeke, L., 357t
Pekarik, E. G., 292, 380
Pelham, W. E., 44, 120, 126, 166, 167, 184,
    186, 187, 190, 191, 286
Peltola, M. J., 246
Penke, L., 253
Pennypacker, H. S., 11, 23, 173, 176
Pepler, D., 306
Pepper, C. M., 357t
Perepletchikova, F., 384
Perez-Olivas, G., 244
Pergamin, L., 242
Peris, T. S., 328t, 331
Perlmuter, L. C., 226
Perna, G., 248
Perrin, S., 125
Perryman, T. Y., 228
Petersen, D., 166
Peterson, E. L., 384
Petrocelli, J. V., 390
Petti, T., 50
Pfeiffer, S. I., 134
Phan, K. L., 222
Phares, V., 142
Phillips, D., 208
Phillips, J. S., 59
Phillips, S. D., 41
Photos, V., 389, 391
Piacentini, J. C., 118, 208
Piasecki, T. M., 152
Piazza, C. C., 185
Picard, R., 225
Pickrel, S. G., 384
Piesecki, T. M., 204
Pina, A. A., 19, 60, 106, 107, 118, 120, 351,
    355, 356, 359, 362t, 367, 418, 428
Pincus, H. A., 48
Pine, D. S., 242, 246, 425
Plude, D. J., 223
Pogge, D. L., 41
Policaro, K. L., 330
Poortinga, Y. H., 352
Porges, S. W., 220, 223, 232, 233
Porter, B., 329t, 333
Porzelius, L. K., 79
Poulin, F., 282, 283
Powell, M. B., 329t, 333
Powell, M. C., 249
Powell, N. P., 439

Power, T. J., 133
Prantzalou, C., 264
Prater, M. A., 200
Prenoveau, J. M., 362t
Prins, P. M. J., 72
Prinstein, M. J., 277, 278, 279, 280, 281,
    282, 283, 284, 286, 287, 288t, 289, 298
Prinz, R. J., 59, 292, 328t, 330, 331, 380,
    419
Prochaska, J. O., 381, 389, 390, 403
Prost, J. H., 349
Puente, A. E., 5
Punzo, R. P., 202
Purkis, H. M., 244

Q

Quay, H. C., 152
Quigley, K. S., 220
Quillivan, C. C., 210
Quinlan, P., 244

R

Raine, A., 220
Rajaratnam, N., 11, 173
Ramirez, R., 366
Randall, B. A., 356, 360t
Randall, E. T., 357t
Rao, U., 118
Rapee, R. M., 118, 246, 253, 256, 318, 319
Rathor, S., 306
Ray, W. J., 220
Rayfield, A., 358t
Raykov, T., 350
Reed, H., 211
Reed, M. A., 242
Rehm, L. P., 208
Reich, W., 108t, 112, 115t, 116t, 118
Reid, J. B., 171, 335, 397
Reid, R., 133, 196, 197, 198, 200, 356, 358t,
    364t
Reijntjes, A., 283, 285
Reise, S. P., 350, 351
Reiss, S., 425
Reitman, D., 46, 69, 80, 105, 168, 180, 183,
    185, 186, 419, 432
Renk, K., 142
Renshaw, P. D., 300
Rescorla, L. A., 14t, 38, 135, 136, 138, 140,
    145f, 147, 149, 151f, 152, 158, 418,
    419, 429, 431
Resnick, A., 46, 69, 419
Rettew, D. C., 41
Reuter, T., 278
Reuterskiold, L., 442
Rey, Y., 111, 301, 418
Reyes, 7, 124, 419
Reynolds, C. R., 19, 134, 140, 171, 350, 418
Reynolds, S., 37
Reynolds, W. M., 208

Rhodes, T. E., 70, 439
Ribera, J. C., 355
Richard, D. C. S., 173
Richards, A., 248, 254
Richards, H., 244
Richardson, W. S., 47
Richmond, B., 350, 418
Richters, J. E., 16, 105
Ridgeway, V., 264
Ridley, C. R., 19
Rieckmann, T. R., 357t
Rigby, K., 306
Riley, A. W., 59
Riley, J. L., 358t
Riley-Tillman, T. C., 166, 174, 189
Risley, T. R., 178
Rivera, M., 366
Robbins, J. M., 41
Robbins, M. S., 382
Roberti, J., 298
Roberts, J. E., 228
Roberts, M. W., 177
Roberts, N., 117
Roberts, R. E., 354t, 355
Robin, A. L., 328t, 330
Robins, E., 113
Rodrique, J. R., 317
Roemmich, J. N., 230, 231
Rogers, M., 68
Rogosch, F. A., 226
Roisman, L., 383
Rollnick, S., 381, 403
Rommelse, N. N. J., 247
Rooney, M. T., 44, 110
Roosa, M. W., 349, 356, 359, 361t, 367
Rosselló, J., 367, 428
Rothenberger, A., 259
Rothermund, K., 253
Rowe, P., 199
Rowland, M. D., 400
Rowley, G. L., 173
Roy, A. K., 242
Rozenman, M., 264
Rubin, K., 277, 281
Rubinstein, E. A., 36
Rubio-Stipec, M., 352, 353t, 355, 366
Rudiger, L. P., 418
Rudolph, K., 284
Ruetsch, C., 350
Russell, R. L., 379, 383, 386, 397
Russell, S. T., 356, 360t, 362t
Rutherford, E., 266
Rutter, M., 112
Ryan, J. B., 197
Ryan, S. M., 253, 356, 360t

S

St. Georges, M., 355
Saavedra, L. M., 106, 118, 355

Sadek, S., 283
Sahakian, B. J., 245
Saiz, C. S., 382, 383, 392, 406, 428
Salgado de Snyder, V. N., 351
Salmon, P., 118
Salvy, S. J., 230
Sameroff, A. J., 323
Samuel, D. B., 38, 39
San Pedro, E. M., 110
Sanbonmatsu, D. M., 249
Sanchez-Sosa, J., 357t, 363t
Sander, J. B., 425
Sanders, M. R., 321, 330, 334, 335
Santo, J. B., 278
Santos, R., 248
Sapyta, J. J., 394
Sarlin, N., 402
Sasso, G. M., 185, 191
Sassu, K. A., 189
Sbrocco, T., 359
Scahill, L., 361t
Scarpa, A., 220, 226, 432
Schecter, J., 44, 110
Scheuermann, B., 198
Schloss, P. J., 199
Schludermann, E. H., 328t, 330, 419
Schludermann, S. M., 328t, 330, 419
Schmidt, C. R., 431, 439
Schmidt, J., 284
Schmukle, S. C., 258
Schneider, S., 45, 205, 220, 245, 246, 256
Schniering, C. A., 318
Schoenwald, S. K., 384, 400
Schonberg, M., 320
Schotte, C. K. W., 41
Schouten, E., 256
Schroeder, C. S., 16
Schuengel, C., 283
Schwab-Stone, M. E., 107, 117, 355
Schwartz, E. B., 226
Schwartz, J. L. K., 250
Scott, S., 320
Scott, W. D., 357t
Scotti, J. R., 70
Sembi, S., 243
Sergeant, J. A., 247, 248
Setzer, N. J., 179
Shaffer, D., 105, 107, 108t, 109, 114t, 116t, 117, 352, 389
Shafran, R., 263
Shahar, G., 278
Shapiro, E. S., 170, 203
Shapiro, J. R., 196, 197, 210, 213
Sharma, D., 244
Sharpley, C. F., 332
Shavelson, R. J., 173, 351
Shaw, D. S., 320
Sheeber, L., 208, 357t
Sheehan, D. V., 44, 108t, 109, 110, 114t, 116t, 117

Sheffield, J., 330
Sheidow, A. J., 384, 400
Shelley, M. C., 357t
Shelton, K. K., 328t, 329, 431
Shen, Y., 356, 360t, 362t
Sherif, M., 164
Sherwood, A., 224, 231
Shiffman, S., 204
Shimokawa, K., 378, 407
Shirk, S. R., 7, 57, 124, 377, 378, 379, 381,
        382, 383, 384, 386, 392, 397, 401, 402,
        406, 419, 428, 429, 431, 442
Shotorbani, S., 382
Shrout, P. E., 306, 354t
Sidman, M., 173
Siedlarz, M., 226
Siegel, A. W., 208
Siegel, R. S., 277, 278, 284, 285, 298, 305,
        306
Siegrist, M., 258
Sigman, M., 19, 418
Sigvaldason, N., 330
Silberschatz, G., 397
Siler, T. J., 383, 384
Silk, J. S., 208
Silmere, H., 357t
Silverman, W. K., 18, 19, 22, 35, 44, 45, 64,
        67, 89, 104, 106, 107, 108t, 110, 111,
        114t, 116t, 118, 120, 121, 126, 127,
        204, 278, 293, 301, 334, 351, 355,
        358t, 362t, 418, 425, 428, 430
Simmel, C., 177
Singer, H. S., 247
Siqueland, L., 264, 398
Skinner, B. F., 59, 172
Skinner, C. H., 210
Sloman, S. A., 39
Slonje, R., 284
Smart, D. W., 378
Smith, D., 68
Smith, G., 57
Smith, J., 243
Smith, P. K., 284
Snitz, B. E., 40
Snyder, J., 325
Snyder, M. C., 197, 198
Sofronoff, K., 330
Solhan, M., 204
Solomon, M., 46
Solovitz, B. L., 354t, 355
Somers, J. M., 352
Sonuga-Barke, E. J. S., 242, 243
Sorbero, M. J., 8
Southam-Gerow, M. A., 90, 91, 385, 399,
        425
Southwick, S., 228
Spanier, G. B., 329t, 332
Spence, S. H., 242, 244, 250
Spencer, M. S., 357t, 360t
Spencer, S. V., 279, 281, 296, 297

Spitzer, R. L., 46, 47, 113
Sprafkin, J., 133
Sprague, J., 211
Stambaugh, E. E., 59
Stansbury, R., 365
Stark, K. D., 208
Starr, L. R., 278, 306
Staton, L., 223, 228
Steer, R. A., 342
Steffian, G., 228
Stein, B. D., 8
Stein, P., 224
Steinman, R. B., 253
Stemberger, R. T., 14
Stephens, C. L., 232
Stern, R. M., 220, 223, 227
Stevens, M., 394
Stevenson, J., 243, 244
Steward, C., 230
Stiffman, A. R., 357t
Stone, A. A., 204
Stone, W. L., 197, 208, 280, 286, 300
Storch, E. A., 284, 285, 297, 298, 317
Stormshak, E., 320, 333
Stouthamer-Loeber, M., 17
Strain, P. S., 200
Straus, M. A., 329t, 332
Straus, S. E., 47
Strosahl, K., 11
Stroufe, L. A., 18
Strupp, H., 397
Suchday, S., 359
Sue, D. M., 352
Sue, S., 349
Suen, H. K., 23, 173, 174
Suess, P. E., 223
Sugai, G., 166, 199
Suh, C., 397
Sulik, M. J., 349
Suppiger, A., 45
Susman, E. J., 226
Suwanlert, S., 19
Sweeney, M., 297, 425
Szanyi, J. M., 360t

T

Taghavi, M. R., 241, 248, 254
Talbot, E., 19
Tan, P. Z., 200, 207
Tanzer, N. K., 352
Tassinary, L. G., 220
Taub, J., 25
Taylor, E., 243
Teachman, B. A., 251
Teare, M., 118
Teasley, M., 356, 360t
Tein, J., 349, 350
Temple, E. P., 356, 358t, 364t
Tenney, N. H., 41

Terdal, L. G., 56, 59
Tetzlaff, B. T., 393
Thibodeaux, S., 335
Thomas, E., 211
Thomas, R., 337
Thompson, E., 333
Thrane, L. E., 357*t*
Timman, R., 205
Tingen, M. S., 225
Tipples, J., 244
Tiwari, S., 418
Tobon, J. I., 264, 397
Todd, R. D., 418
Tolan, P. H., 26
Tonge, B. J., 64, 66
Tonigan, J., 389
Toth, S. L., 226
Trammel, D. L., 199
Treanor, M., 254
Treat, T. A., 384
Treiber, F. A., 225
Triandis, H. C., 349
Troop-Gordon, W., 277, 284
Troutman, A., 166, 167, 168, 186
Truax, P., 35
Trull, T. J., 204
Tryon, G., 383
Turgeon, L., 282
Turner, S. M., 14, 206, 258, 302
Tyano, S., 208
Tyson, E. H., 356, 359, 360*t*

U

Uhing, B. M., 197
Ullman, D. G., 289*t*, 296
Ullmann, L. P., 58
Ulloa, R. E., 113
Umaña-Taylor, A. J., 349, 357*t*
Umbreit, J., 70
Umemoto, L. A., 358*t*
Underwood, M., 297
Unnewehr, S., 256
Updegraff, K. A., 357*t*
Ursprung, A., 205
Usher, B. A., 230

V

Valla, J. P., 355
Valvoi, J. S., 249
Van de Vijver, F., 352
van den Hout, M., 249
van der Ende, J., 104, 138, 140
Van der Schoot, M., 247
Van Der Stigchel, S., 247
Van Hasselt, V. B., 204
Van Hecke, A. V., 223, 232, 233
van IJzendoorn, M. H., 224, 242
van Kasteren, H., 249
van Megen, H. J. G. M., 41

van Mourik, R., 248
van Spauwen, I., 256
Vandenberg, R. J., 350
VanEerdewegh, M., 112
Varela, R. E., 356, 357*t*, 363*t*
Vasey, M. W., 24, 241, 255, 259, 262, 263
Vassilopoulos, S. P., 264
Vatten, L., 299
Velicer, W. F., 389, 390
Velting, O. N., 179, 185, 188
Venables, P. H., 220
Verhulst, F. C., 18, 104, 138, 140, 152, 323
Vermeulen, L., 256
Vernberg, E. M., 277, 278, 282, 284, 285, 286
Vervoort, L., 252, 259
Vidair, H. B., 156
Viding, E., 319
Villa, M., 105
Villalta, I. K., 19, 367
Virdin, L. M., 356, 361*t*
Visconti, K. J., 277
Visser, J. H., 140
Viswesvaran, C., 120, 428
Vitaro, F., 277, 281, 282
Vito, D., 332
Voerman, J. S., 255
Vogel-Farley, V. K., 246
Vohs, K. D., 165
Volpe, R. J., 170, 171, 172, 176
Vuchinish, S., 334
Vye, C. S., 383

W

Wadsworth, M. E., 357*t*
Wahler, R. G., 59
Wakschlag, L. S., 26
Walczak, S., 256
Waldman, I. D., 37
Walkup, J. T., 111
Walter, B. R., 19
Walters, K. S., 280
Walton, J. W., 358*t*
Wang, J. J., 277, 284, 285, 303
Wanner, B., 281
Waraich, P., 352
Ward, C. H., 118
Warnick, E., 361*t*
Warren, S. L., 18
Warren, W. L., 332
Waschbusch, D. A., 330
Washburn, J. J., 41
Wassell, G., 380, 388
Watamura, S. E., 226
Waters, A. M., 242, 244, 249, 254, 264
Watkins, E., 263
Watson, D., 37
Watson, L. R., 228
Watt, A. J., 259

Watts, S. E., 259
Webb, N. M., 173
Webber, J., 198
Weems, C. F., 259, 425
Weersing, V. R., 264, 361t, 385
Wei, J., 213
Weintraub, S., 292
Weiss, B., 19, 379
Weiss, R. L., 339
Weissman, M. M., 302, 428
Weisz, J. R., 4, 19, 41, 89, 90, 318, 319, 382,
    385, 392, 393, 395, 396, 399, 401, 405,
    418
Weller, E. B., 44, 108t, 110, 118
Weller, R. A., 44, 110, 118
Wells, K. C., 439
Wentura, D., 253
Werner, N. E., 284
Werry, J. S., 355
West, S. G., 165
Westenberg, H. G. M., 41
Whalen, C. K., 200, 206, 210, 211, 212
Wharton, T. A., 254, 264
Wheat, E., 7, 80
Wheeler, V. A., 280, 288t, 300
Whitaker, K., 278
Whitbeck, L. B., 357t
White, D., 210
White, M. K., 393
White, S., 242
Whitley, M. K., 382, 388
Whittingham, K., 330
Widaman, K. F., 349, 351
Widiger, T. A., 38, 39, 127
Wiers, R. W., 249
Wierzbicki, M., 380
Wilhelm, F. H., 220
Williams, K. R., 283
Williams, L. L., 241
Williams, T., 306
Wilmuth, M., 208
Wilson, E., 266
Wilson, K. G., 11
Wimalaweera, S., 246
Wimberley, R. C., 332
Windholz, M. J., 397
Winett, R. A., 59
Winters, N. C., 45
Witkow, M. R., 365
Wittchen, H., 352
Wojslawowicz, J., 277

Wolchik, S. A., 278
Wolf, M. M., 171, 187
Wolf, S., 222
Wolfe, C. D., 222
Wolfe, D. A., 332
Wolff, J. C., 111, 430, 439
Wolff, L. S., 189, 207, 208, 330
Wolff, R. P., 207, 208
Wolpe, S., 208
Wood, J. J., 118, 318, 319, 395, 418, 419,
    427
Wood, S. J., 198, 202
Woodbury-Fariña, M., 352, 353t
Woolston, J., 361t
Wootton, J., 329, 431
Wright, L. R., 305, 383
Wynne, H., 19, 60, 418

X

Xu, X., 188

Y

Yarcheski, A., 289t, 300
Yarcheski, T., 289t, 300
Yates, B. T., 25
Ybrant, H., 304
Yeh, E. K., 352
Yen, C., 390
Yiend, J., 264
Yim, L., 358t
Yoman, J., 63
Young, A. W., 244
Young, B., 279
Youngstrom, E. A., 4, 7, 13, 30, 41, 44, 48
Youngstrom, J. K., 41, 48
Yule, W., 241, 248, 254

Z

Zahn-Waxler, C., 230
Zald, D. H., 40
Zee, D. S., 247
Zelman, E., 297
Zerr, A. A., 19, 60, 359, 367, 418
Zigterman, D., 253, 254
Zimbardo, P., 164
Zimmer-Gembeck, M. J., 254, 289t, 291,
    337
Zinbarg, R. E., 259, 265
Zoccolillo, M., 125
Zupan, B. A., 177

Subject Index

The letter *f* following a page number indicates figure; the letter *t* indicates table.

A–B–C analysis, 168–169, 180
ABC (attributions bias context) model, 25–27
Acceptance–rejection, measures for assessing, 287*t*
Accuracy
defined, 22
validity and, 23
Achenbach System of Empirically Based Assessment (ASEBA), 38; *see also* Child Behavior Checklist for Ages 6–18 (CBCL/6–18); Youth Self-Report (YSR) (ASEBA)
Adult Self-Report of, 161
in externalizing disorders case example, 158–160, 431, 438*f*
in internalizing disorders, 135*t*, 156–158, 419, 424*f*, 425
Spanish version of, 156
alphas and test–retest reliabilities for, 140, 141*t*
Brief Problem Monitor of, 135–136
construct validity of, 140
cross-informant comparisons for, 142–146
methods for using, 143, 144*f*, 145*f*, 146
Direct Observation Form of, 171
domain, age, informant, 288*t*
in externalizing disorders case example, 430
assessing outcomes in, 160
assessing responses to interventions with, 159–160
initial client assessment with, 158–159
initial parent assessment with, 159

hierarchical model of, 136, 137*f*, 138, 139*f*, 140
instruments included in, 134, 135*t*
in internalizing disorder case example
assessing outcomes in, 157–158
assessing responses to interventions with, 157
initial client assessment with, 154–155
initial parent assessment with, 155–157
lay informants and, 134–136, 135*t*
method of, 134–136, 135*t*
minority youth and, 357*t*
multicultural norms for, 146–152, 161
constructing, 147, 148*t*–149*t*, 149–150
using, 150, 151*f*, 152
psychometric properties of, 140–152, 141*t*, 144*f*, 145*f*, 148*t*–149*t*, 151*f*
underlying theory of, 136, 137*f*, 138, 139*f*, 140
Youth Self-Report of, 135*t*, 136, 171, 187*t*, 188*t*, 291, 367*t*, 418, 424
ADHD Rating Scale–IV, 133, 160
Adolescent Symptom Inventory–4, 133
Adolescents, self-monitoring by, 198–199
Adult Behavior Checklist, 135*t*
Spanish version of, 156
Adult Self-Report (ASR) (ASEBA), 161
in externalizing disorders case example, 159–160, 431, 438*f*
in internalizing disorders case example, 135*t*, 156–158, 419, 424*f*, 425
Spanish version of, 156
Affectiva Q Sensor, 225, 235

Affective priming paradigm (APP), 249–250, 253, 258–259, 296
African American youth, population statistics for, 348
Aggression, measures for assessing, 287t
Agreement index, choosing, 174
Alabama Parenting Questionnaire (APQ), 329–330, 342
  description and reliability, 328t
  in externalizing disorders case example, 431
Ambiguous-vignettes paradigms, 253–256
American Psychiatric Association, diagnostic system of, 34–35
American Psychological Association Presidential Task Force on Evidence-Based Practice, 80, 126
American Psychological Association, ethics code of, 27–28
Analytic decision making, 40
Anecdotal observation, 168
Anxiety disorders; see also Internalizing disorders case example; School refusal
  behavioral/electronic diaries for monitoring, 204–207
  CBT for, 89
  dot-probe task for assessing, 241–242
  EAST and, 252–253
  go/no go task for assessing, 249
  interpretation bias and, 254
  peer assessment in, 304–306
  RED bias and, 255–256
  self-monitoring of, 205–207
  Stroop task and, 249
Anxiety Disorders Interview Schedule (ADIS) for DSM-IV, 67, 107, 110–111, 120, 301
  case examples using, 121–125
  characteristics of, 108t
  in externalizing diagnoses, 116t, 124–125, 430
  in externalizing disorders case example, 440
  in internalizing diagnoses, 114t, 121–123, 418
  in internalizing disorders case example, 425–426
  minority youth and, 355
  reliability and validity of, 118
  review of, 110–111
  Spanish version of, 108t, 111, 121, 123, 355
  treatment outcome and, 126
Asian American youth, population statistics for, 348

Assessment; see also Diagnostic and behavioral assessment; Evidence-based assessment
  disconnection from treatments, 4–5
  role in treatment, 3, 5–8, 6t
Assessment tools, 56; see also specific tools
  adult versus child/adolescent, 57–58
  for case conceptualization, 84
  choice of, 20–25, 87f
  for combining data, 46–47
  DSM differential diagnosis, 48–49
  evidence-based medicine approach, 47–48
  idiographic, 5, 10
  for informing clinical practice, 443
  LEAD standard, 47
  matching with client, 78
  nomothetic, 5, 10
  observational methods, 45–46
  practicality and cost of, 24–25
  psychometric criteria for, 4
  rating scales, 45
  standardized interviews, 43–45
  unstructured interviews, 42–43
Assessment training and practice, trends in, 4–5
Ataques de nervios, 350–351, 350n1
Attention-deficit/hyperactivity disorder (ADHD)
  direct observation in diagnosis of, 184
  dot-probe-type tasks for assessing, 243
  EEG assessment of, 222
  go/no go task for assessing, 249
  response inhibition in, 247
  self-monitoring and, 210–211
  visual-search tasks for assessing, 244–245
Attentional bias, 264–265
Attentional bias tasks, test–retest reliability of, 258
Attentional Network Task, 266
Attentional processes, measuring, 241–247
  with dot-probe task, 241–243
Attributions bias context (ABC) model, 25–27
Autism Diagnostic Observational Schedule (ADOS), 46
Autism-spectrum disorders (ASD)
  assessment of, 222, 223
  direct observation in diagnosis of, 184
Automatic associations, measuring, 249–253
Autonomic nervous system, assessment of, 227
Avoidance, experiential, 11

B

Barriers to Treatment Participation Scale (BTPS), 388–389, 405, 431
Bayesian method, 48
Behavior
in lab *versus* with parents, 26
operant model of, 58–59
Behavior Assessment System for Children (BASC), 134, 160, 171
minority youth and, 357*t*
Behavior Problem Index (BPI)
cross-ethnic measurement equivalence studies of, 360*t*
minority youth and, 357*t*
Behavioral approach system, 233
Behavioral approach test (BAT), 231
Behavioral assessment, 10–11, 56–76;
see also Diagnostic and behavioral assessment
developmental factors in, 56–57
diagnostic assessment *versus,* 12
direct observation in, 63
empirical validation of, 57
functional analysis in, 63–70
future directions for, 70–73
history of, 58–59
indirect methods in, 63
nomothetic *versus* idiographic distinction and, 62
principles of, 57–58
procedures in, 63
theoretical underpinnings of, 60–63
traditional approaches *versus,* 60–63
Behavioral avoidance test (BAT), 179, 186, 188
Behavioral challenge stressors, 231
Behavioral diaries, 204–207
Behavioral inhibition system, 233
Behavioral observation; *see* Direct observation
Behavioral skills, target behaviors and, 83*t*
Behaviors
descriptions of, 168
target (*see* Target behaviors)
Bias
attentional, 264–265
clinician, 39–40
interpretation, 254
method, ethnic minority youth and, 349–352
reasoning, 264
RED, 255–256
SDIs and, 43–44
Biofeedback, in school refusal treatment, 234–235

Biological factors, target behaviors and, 83*t*
Blended word paradigms, 254–255
Blood pressure
assessment of, 225–226
indices for, 221*t*
Blood-oxygen level-dependent (BOLD) method, 223
Brain, EEG assessment of, 221*t*, 222
Brief Problem Monitor, 135–136
Bullying, *versus* peer victimization, 283

C

Callous–unemotional (CU) traits, 319
Cardiography, impedance, functions of, 223–224
Case conceptualization, 77–100; *see also* Externalizing disorders case example, case conceptualization in; Internalizing disorders case example, case conceptualization in
clinical case examples of, 91–98
for externalizing disorders, 95–98
for internalizing disorders, 92–95
defined, 78
description of, 78–79
evidence-based approach to, 80
historical considerations in, 79–80
role in treatment, 6*t*, 7–8
steps in building, 81–91, 81*t*
1: identifying target behaviors contributing factors, 81–84, 81*t*, 83*t*, 86*f*
2: diagnosis, 81*t*, 84, 86*f*
3: initial conceptualization, 81*t*, 84–85, 86*f*–87*f*, 88
4: treatment planning and selection, 81*t*, 87*f*, 88–90
5: choosing assessment measures, 81*t*, 87*f*, 90–91
worksheet for generating, 86*f*–87*f*
CASSS; *see* Child and Adolescent Social Support Scale (CASSS)
Categorical model of classification, 36–39, 37–38
Center for Epidemiologic Studies Depression Scale (CES-D)
cross-ethnic measurement equivalence studies of, 360*t*–362*t*
minority youth and, 357*t*
Central nervous system, measures for assessing, 222–223
Checklists; *see* Rating scales
Child Abuse Potential Inventory (CAPI), 331–332, 342
description and reliability, 329*t*

Child and Adolescent Psychiatric Assessment
(CAPA)
   characteristics of, 108*t*
   reliability and validity of, 118
   reliability estimates for externalizing
      diagnoses, 116*t*
   reliability estimates for internalizing
      diagnoses, 115*t*
   review of, 111–112
   Spanish version of, 108*t*
Child and Adolescent Social Support Scale
   (CASSS), 296, 305
   domain, age, informant, 288*t*
Child Anxiety and Depression Scale–
   Revised; *see* Revised Child Anxiety and
   Depression Scale
Child Behavior Checklist for Ages 6–18
   (CBCL/6–18), 118–119, 135*t*, 136,
   137*t*, 138, 140, 171
   cross-ethnic measurement equivalence
      studies of, 360*t*
   cross-informant data and, 143
   in externalizing disorders case example,
      158–160, 302–303, 418, 429–430
   friendship assessment and, 292–293
   in internalizing disorders case example,
      154–158
   minority youth and, 356, 359
   multicultural norms for, 147, 148*t*–149*t*,
      149–150
   summary of, 287*t*, 288*t*
   test–retest reliabilities for, 141*t*
Child Involvement Rating Scale (CIRS),
   396–398
Child Psychotherapy Process Scales, 397
Child's Assessment by a Parent–ADHD
   (CAP–ADHD), cross-ethnic
   measurement equivalence studies of,
   363*t*
Child(ren)
   considerations for psychophysiological
      measurement, 227–228
   perspective of, on target behaviors, 16
   role of, 72
   self-monitoring by, 198–199
Childhood disorders, *DSM* and, 36
Children Sustained Attention Task, 266
Children's Depression Inventory (CDI),
   300
   cross-ethnic measurement equivalence
      studies of, 361*t*
   domain, age, informant, 288*t*
   in internalizing disorders case example,
      418
   minority youth and, 356, 357*t*

Children's Interview for Psychiatric
   Syndromes (ChIPS), 44
   characteristics of, 108t
   reliability and validity of, 117–118
   reliability estimates for internalizing
      diagnoses, 114*t*
   review of, 110
Children's Manifest Anxiety Scale–Revised
   (RCMAS); *see* Revised Children's
   Manifest Anxiety Scale (RCMAS)
Children's Report of Parent Behavior
   Inventory (CRPBI-30), 330–331, 341
   description and reliability, 328*t*
   in internalizing disorders case example,
      419
Children's Social Support, 296
Children's Stroop Test, 231
ChIPS; *see* Children's Interview for
   Psychiatric Syndromes (ChIPS)
Classical test theory, 172–173
Classroom Observation Code, 170–171
Classroom, direct observation in, 186
Client involvement/resistance, 383–384,
   396–398
Client Resistance Code (CRC), 397
Clinical judgment, in diagnosis, 39–41
Clinical utility, 24–25
Clinician, biases of, 39–40
Cognitive bias modification (CBM), 264
Cognitive deficits, role of, 240–241
Cognitive methodologies, 240–276
   advantages of, 257
   assessment method in, 240–256
      for measuring attentional processes,
         241–247
      for measuring automatic associations,
         249–253
      for measuring inhibitory processes,
         247–249
      for measuring reasoning processes,
         253–256
   child adaptations of, 257–258
   conceptual utility of, 260, 261*t*–262*t*
   conceptual validity of, 265
   diagnostic utility of, 260, 261*t*, 262–264
   in externalizing disorders case example,
      263, 264–265
   indirect utility of, 265–266
      versus direct utility, 260, 261*t*–262*t*,
         262
   in internalizing disorders case example,
      263–265
   laboratory-based (*see* Laboratory-based
      cognitive methodologies)
   miscellaneous, 266

monitoring utility of, 260, 261*t*
portable technologies for, 257
prevention utility of, 260, 261*t*, 265
psychometric properties of, 257–260
purpose-designed software and, 257
test–retest reliability of, 258
treatment planning and, 260–264,
    261*t*–262*t*
treatment utility of, 260, 261*t*
treatment/treatment-monitoring utility of,
    264–265
validational utility of, 261, 262*t*
Cognitive processes, target behaviors and,
    83*t*
Cognitive-behavioral therapy (CBT), 264
for anxiety and school refusal, 402–403
for child anxiety, 89
for depression, 408
in externalizing disorders case example,
    405–406
in internalizing disorders case example,
    427–428
Cognitively limited youth, 306
Cold-pressor paradigm, 231
Comorbidity
case conceptualization and, 89–90
interviewing and, 125–126
Conceptual utility, 260, 261*t*–262*t*
Conduct problems, dot-probe-type tasks for
    assessing, 242–243
Configural invariance, 350
Conflict Behavior Questionnaire, 330–331
description and reliability, 328*t*
in internalizing disorders case example,
    419
Conflict Tactics Scales (CTS), 332
description and reliability, 329*t*
Conners Continuous Performance Test–II,
    266
Conners Rating Scale, 133, 160
minority youth and, 358*t*
Conners Teacher Rating Scale, 171
cross-ethnic measurement equivalence
    studies of, 364*t*
Consequences
punishing, 66
reinforcing, 66
Consequent stimuli, 66
Construct validity, 23–24
Construct validity equivalence, 351
Content validity, 22–23
Contextual factors, 4, 10–11, 14–15, 24–27,
    59, 61, 64, 66, 104
in case conceptualization, 82–83, 85–86
in interviewing, 104

in school refusal, 67
unstructured interviews and, 43, 105
Controlled Oral Word Association Test, 266
Cortisol, salivary, assessment of, 226–227
Cost–benefit analysis, treatment planning
    and, 88
Credibility/Expectancies Questionnaire–
    Parent Version (CEQ-P), 419
Cultural factors, 18–19
ASEBA norms and, 147–152, 148*t*–149*t*,
    151*f*
Cultural norms, in ethnic minority youth
    assessment, 365
Culture, defined, 19
Cyber Victimization Scale for Adolescents,
    298
domain, age, informant, 288*t*
Cyber-victimization, 284

D

Data collection
for case conceptualization, 84
for direct observation, 167–168
Decade of Behavior campaign, 164
Decision making
dual-processing, 39–40
heuristic (System 1) *versus* analytic
    (System 2), 40
Depression, self-monitoring of, 208
Developmental factors, 18, 56–58
future focus on, 70–71
in target behaviors, 83*t*
Developmental issues, normative–
    developmental perspective and, 104
Developmental psychopathology, 13–14
Devereux Scales of Mental Disorders, 134,
    160
Diagnosis
in case conceptualization, 84
clinical judgment in, 39–41
clinician *versus* algorithmic standardized
    interviews, 40–41
direct observation and, 184
in externalizing disorders case example,
    435*f*, 440
in internalizing disorders case example,
    422*f*, 426
interview schedules and, 107
OED definition of, 34
role in treatment, 6*t*, 7
Diagnostic and behavioral assessment
in action, 417–448 (*see also* Externalizing
    disorders case example; Internalizing
    disorders case example)
behavioral component of, 10–11

Diagnostic and behavioral assessment
  (*continued*)
  child's perspective in, 16
  choosing methods and interpretation
    processes, 17–18
  combining, 12
  combining data from, 25–27
  diagnostic component of, 9–10
  ethics and standards of, 27–28
  future considerations for, 443–
    444
  goals of, 9*t*
  methods of, 9*t*
  parents' perspective in, 16–17
  peers' perspective in, 17–18
  principles of, 12–25, 13*t*
  psychometric principles in, 9*t*
  rationale for focus on, 9–12
  teachers' perspective in, 17
  treatment phases and, 9*t*
  uses of, 9*t*
*Diagnostic and Statistical Manual of Mental
    Disorders*
  childhood disorders and, 36
  medical model of, 50, 119
  reliability and validity of, for ethnic
    minority youth, 352, 355
*Diagnostic and Statistical Manual of Mental
    Disorders* (DSM-I), 36
*Diagnostic and Statistical Manual of Mental
    Disorders* (DSM-II), 36
*Diagnostic and Statistical Manual of Mental
    Disorders* (DSM-III), 37
*Diagnostic and Statistical Manual of Mental
    Disorders* (DSM-IV)
  differential diagnosis and, 48–49
  structured and semistructured interviews
    and, 106
*Diagnostic and Statistical Manual of Mental
    Disorders* (DSM-IV-TR)
  differential diagnosis approach of, 48–
    49
  structured and semistructured interviews
    and, 106
*Diagnostic and Statistical Manual of Mental
    Disorders* (DSM-V)
  changes in, 119–120
  classification models of, 36–37, 38–
    39
Diagnostic assessment, 34–55; see also
    Diagnostic and behavioral assessment
  behavioral assessment *versus,* 12
  categorical *versus* dimensional
    classification in, 36–39, 50
  clinical judgment in, 39–40
  evidence-based, 40–42 (*see also* Evidence-
    based diagnosis)
  future directions for, 49–50
  historical roots of, 36–42
  process of, 42–49
  purposes of, 34–35
  tools for, 42–49 (*see also* Assessment
    tools)
Diagnostic Interview for Children and
    Adolescents (DICA)
  characteristics of, 108*t*
  reliability and validity of, 118–119
  reliability estimates for externalizing
    diagnoses, 116*t*
  reliability estimates for internalizing
    diagnoses, 115*t*
  review of, 112
Diagnostic Interview Schedule for Children
    (DISC)
  ethnic minority youth and, 352, 355
  reliability and validity for ethnic
    minorities, 353*t*–354*t*
  Spanish version of, 108*t*, 109, 353*t*, 355
Diagnostic process, 42–49
Diagnostic systems, 34–35
Diagnostic tools, uses of, 10
Diagnostic utility, 260, 261*t*, 262–264
Diaries, behavioral/electronic, 204
Differential diagnosis, *DSM,* 48–49
Dimensional model of classification, 36–39,
    50
Direct behavior ratings (DBRs), 189
Direct observation, 164–195
  accuracy of, 176
  alternatives to, 189
  assessment method for, 166–172
    event-based recording, 169
    formal systems in, 170–171
    limitations of, 171–172
    narrative recording, 168–169
    steps in, 167–168
    time-based recording, 169–170
  classical test theory and, 172–173
  decline in use of, 164–165
  diagnostic use of, 184
  of discrete procedures, 398–399
  in externalizing disorders case example,
    180–183
  factors in choosing, 166–167
  in family/parent assessment, 333–340
    coding systems for, 337–340
    planning for, 334–335, 337
    procedures for, 336*t*
  generalizability of, 175–176, 177–178
  IDEA and, 191

in internalizing disorders case example, 178–180
psychometric properties of, 174–178
recommendations for, 190–191
reliability of, 174–175
self-reports/rating scales and, 188–190
summary of, 187–190
treatment outcomes and, 190
treatment planning and, 187–188
treatment planning/outcomes evaluation and, 183–187
underlying theory of, 172–173
validity of, 177–178
Direct Observation Form, 171
DISC; see Diagnostic Interview Schedule for Children (DISC)
DISC-IV; see National Institute of Mental Health Diagnostic Interview Schedule for Children, Version IV
Discriminative stimuli, 66
Dominic-R: A Pictorial Interview, 355
Dot-probe task, 241–243, 257
Dyadic Adjustment Scale (DAS), 332
description and reliability, 329t
Dyadic Parent–Child Interaction Coding System (DPICS), 334, 335, 337–338
Dynamic Affect Recognition Evaluation, 232
Dysfunctional Attitude Scale, cross-ethnic measurement equivalence studies of, 362t

E

Ecological momentary assessment (EMA), 204, 207–209
Elaborative validity, 22
Electrocardiography (ECG)
functions of, 223–224
indices for, 221t
Electrodermal activity (EDA)
assessment of, 224–225
considerations in children, 228
indices for, 221t
Electroencephalography (EEG)
functions of, 222
indices for, 221t
Electromyography, index for, 221t
Electronic diaries, 204–209
ADHD and, 210–211
Electrooculography (EOG), indices for, 221t
Emotional expression tasks, 255
Emotional reasoning, 256
Emotional responses, measuring, 251
Emotional stimuli, 232
Emotionally valenced stimuli, responses to, 242, 246

Emotions, self-monitoring of, 208
Environmental factors, in behavioral approach, 60–61
Epidemiologic Studies Depression Scale (CES-D), minority youth and, 356
Equifinality principle, 14
Ethical issues, 27–28
future focus on, 72–73
Ethnic minority youth, 348–376
assessment issues for, 359, 365–366
assessment tools for, 352, 353t–354t, 355–356, 357t–358t, 359, 360t–364t
additional needs for, 366
cross-ethnic measurement equivalence studies of, 360t–364t
cultural norms and, 365
in internalizing disorder case example, 366–367
theoretical context of, 359, 365
Census Bureau statistics on, 348
DSM diagnoses and, 352, 355
measurement equivalence and, 349–352
method bias and, 349–352
nonequivalent cross-ethnic information and, 349
variations among, 349
Evaluation strategies, 90–91
Event-based recording, 169
Evidence-based assessment, 3, 57, 165
call for, 41–42
influence of, 28–29
of parenting and family, 317–319
Evidence-based medicine, in assessment, 47–48
Evidence-based treatments, 89–90
matching with client, 78
therapy process assessment and, 377–378
Exogenous Cueing Task, 266
Experience sampling, 204
Experiential avoidance, 11
Explicit effective Simon task (EAST), 250, 252–253
Externalizing disorders case example, 95–98, 429–443
assessment of therapy processes in, 402–404
case conceptualization in, 432–443, 441f
step 1, 432–435, 439–440
step 2, 435f, 440
step 3, 436f, 441
step 4, 436f–437f, 441–442
step 5, 437–438f, 442–443
cognitive methodologies and, 264–265
direct observation in, 180–183
eye-tracking methodologies and, 246–247

Externalizing disorders case example
    (*continued*)
  family/parent assessment in, 341–342
  go/no go task and, 249, 259–260
  IAT and, 251–252
  initial assessment in, 429–432
  interview schedules for, reliability
    estimates of, 116t
  interviewing strategies in, 123–125
  parenting issues in, 318–319
  parenting self-reports and, 329–330
  peer victimization and, 284–285
  physiological assessment in, 235
  self-monitoring of, 210–212
  target behaviors in, 432, 433f–435f
  treatment outcome monitoring in,
    437f–438f, 442–443
  treatment planning in, 441–442
Eyberg Child Behavior Inventory
  cross-ethnic measurement equivalence
    studies of, 364t
  minority youth and, 358t
Eye-tracking tasks, 245–247
  internal consistency of, 259

F

Family Accommodation Scale–Parent Report
  (FAS-PR), 328t, 331
Family Observation Schedule, 335
Family Problem Solving Code (FAMPROS),
    334, 335, 338–339, 341, 342
Family Process Code, 335
Family system, structural model of, 320–321
Family violence, screening for, 326
Family, defined, 316–317
Family/parent assessment, 316–347
  child focus in, 323–324
  definitions for, 316–317
  evidence-based, 317–319
  in externalizing disorder case example,
    341–342
  facilitating discussion in, 324–325
  family/parent issues in, 323–325
  functions of, 317
  historical aspects in, 322–323
  initial interview in, 321–326
  in internalizing disorder case example,
    340–341
  marital relationship in, 326
  observational procedures in, 333–335,
    336t, 337–340
  parent focus in, 324
  preliminary process issues in, 319–321
  presenting problem in, 321–322
  recommendations for, 325–326, 342–343

self-report inventories in, 327, 328t–329t,
    329–333
Fear Survey Schedule for Children–Revised
  in externalizing disorders case example,
    431
  minority youth and, 357t
Feelings, as target behaviors, 64–65
FQM; *see* Friendship Qualities Measure
    (FQM)
FQQ; *see* Friendship Quality Questionnaire
    (FQQ)
Friendship Qualities Measure (FQM), 294,
    297, 303
  domain, age, informant, 288t
Friendship Qualities Scale, 294
  domain, age, informant, 288t
Friendship qualities, self-reports of, 293–295
Friendship Quality Questionnaire (FQQ),
    293–294, 302, 303
  domain, age, informant, 288t
Friendships
  aspects of, 281–283
  close, measures of, 287t, 293
Functional analysis, 63–70, 186
  appropriate use of, 188
  assessment of behavior functions in,
    66–68
  behavioral consequences and, 66
  in naturalistic and simulated settings,
    68–70
  operant and respondent conditioning and,
    66
  target behavior description and, 64–66
Functional assessment, 168–169, 180, 183
Functional Assessment Interview, 178
Functional equivalence, 351
Functional magnetic resonance imaging
    (fMRI)
  functions of, 222–223
  index for, 221t

G

G theory; *see* Generalizability theory
Galen, 79
Generalizability theory, 11, 172–173
  method and, 177–178
  observers and, 175
  reliability and, 22
  settings and, 177
  time and, 175–176
Generalized anxiety disorder (GAD), 107
Genetic factors, target behaviors and, 83t
Go/no go task, for measuring inhibitory
    processes, 249
Goals, diagnostic/behavioral, 9t

H

Health risk behaviors, peer crowds and, 280–281
Heart rate variability, assessment of, 223–224
Heuristic decision making, 40
Hippocrates, 79
  dimensional model of, 36
Hispanic/Latino youth; *see also* Spanish versions of assessment tools
  population of, 348
Homophily, 282
Homophone/homograph tasks, 254, 257–258
Hypothesis testing, 14–15

I

Idiographic approach, in traditional *versus* behavioral assessment, 62
Idiographic assessment tools, 5, 10
  in case conceptualization, 84
  outcome-monitoring/evaluation strategies and, 90–91
  psychometric concepts and, 20
  reliability of, 22
  response class and, 10–11
  target behaviors and, 10–11
  validity of, 23
Impedance cardiography, functions of, 223–224
Implicit association test (IAT), 249–253
  advantages of, 257
  convergent validity of, 259
  internal consistency of, 259
In-session constructs, 381–386
  measurement of, 392–400
    client involvement and resistance, 396–398
    therapeutic alliance, 392–396
    treatment integrity, 398–400
Individualized target behavior evaluation (ITBE), 189–190
Individuals with Disabilities Education Act (IDEA), 167, 191
Informant discrepancies
  ASEBA assessment of, 160
  ASEBA documentation and comparison of, 142–146, 144f, 145f
Informants
  combined data on, 25–27
  inter- and intraobserver reliability and, 174–175
  nonprofessional, 185–186
  norm validity and, 147

perspectives of, 16–18
Inhibitory processes, measuring, 247–249
Insurance providers, diagnosis and, 35
Internal consistency, 21
Internalizing disorders case example, 92–95
  ambiguous-vignettes paradigm and, 256
  ASEBA and, 152–158, 153f
  assessment of therapy processes in, 402–404
  case conceptualization in, 419–429, 427f
    step 1, 419–421, 425–426
    step 2, 422, 426
    step 3, 422, 426–427
    step 4, 423, 427–428
    step 5, 424, 428–429
  cognitive methodologies and, 264–265
  diagnosis in, 422, 426
  direct observation in, 178–180
  emotional Stroop task and, 248
  ethnic minority youth considerations in, 366–367
  eye-tracking methodologies and, 246
  family/parent assessment in, 340–341
  initial assessment in, 418–419
  interview schedules for, reliability estimates of, 114t–115t
  interviewing strategies in, 121–123
  parenting issues in, 318–319
  parenting self-reports and, 330–331
  peer assessment in, 302–306
  peer victimization and, 284–285
  physiological assessment in, 233–235
  self-monitoring in, 204–209
    case example of, 210–211
  target behaviors in, 419–421, 425–426
  treatment monitoring in, 424f, 428–429
  treatment planning in, 423f, 427–428
International Affective Picture System, 232
International Statistical Classification of Diseases and Related Health Problems, 10th revision
  classification system of, 36
  structured and semistructured interviews and, 106
Interobserver reliability, 174–175
Interpersonal Psychotherapy for Adolescents, 302
Interpretation bias, 253–256
Interrater reliability, 22
Interview-based interviews (IBIs), 44
Interviewing
  age-related concerns in, 104
  clinical expertise and, 120
  DSM-5 changes and, 127–128

Interviewing (*continued*)
  in externalizing disorder case example,
    124–125
  in family/parent assessment, 321–326
  future research on, 127–128
  in internalizing disorder case example,
    121–123
  limitations of, 126–127
  medical model and, 119
  purpose of, 120
  reliability of, 127
  role of, 103
  selection factors in, 120–121
  theory underlying, 119–120
  time factors in, 120
  treatment outcome and, 126
  treatment planning and, 125–126
Interviews, 103–132
  appropriate use of, 57
  contextual considerations in, 104
  developmental considerations in, 103–104
  interviewer-based, 44
  respondent-based, 44
  standardized, 43–45, 84
  structured and semistructured, 105–119
    (*see also* Semistructured interview
      schedules; Semistructured interviews;
      Structured interview schedules;
      Structured interviews)
  unstructured, 42–43, 105
Intraobserver reliability, 174–175
Issues Checklist (IC), 330
  description and reliability, 328*t*

L

Laboratory-based cognitive methodologies;
  see Cognitive methodologies
LEAD standard, 46–47
Learning processes, target behaviors and, 83*t*
Loneliness Scale, 288*t*, 300

M

Magnetic resonance imaging, functional,
  221*t*, 222–223
Marital relationship
  assessment of, 326
  self-report assessment of, 329*t*, 332–333
Measurement equivalence, 349–352
Measurement equivalence studies,
  limitations of, 365
Mediators, 7
Medical history, target behaviors and, 83*t*
Mental disorders, historical documentation
  of, 36

Method bias, 349–352
Metric invariance, 350–351
Mini International Neuropsychiatric
  Interview for Children and Adolescents
  (MINI-KID), 44
  characteristics of, 108*t*
  reliability and validity of, 117
  reliability estimates for externalizing
    diagnoses, 116*t*
  reliability estimates for internalizing
    diagnoses, 114*t*
  review of, 109–110
Momentary time sampling, 200
Motivation
  Gray's theory of, 233
  low, 381
Multicultural norms
  constructing, 147, 148*t*–149*t*, 149–150
  using, 150, 151*f*, 152
Multidimensional Anxiety Scale for
  Children, minority youth and, 357*t*
Multifinality principle, 14
Multimethod approach, 15–16, 57–58, 63,
  71–72
Multisystemic therapy (MST), 379, 384,
  399–400

N

Narrative recording, 168–169
National Institute of Mental Health
  Diagnostic Interview Schedule for
  Children, Version IV
  characteristics of, 108*t*
  reliability and validity of, 117
  reliability estimates for externalizing
    diagnoses, 116*t*
  reliability estimates for internalizing
    diagnoses, 114*t*
  review of, 107, 109
  treatment outcome and, 126
Naturalistic settings; *see also* Contextual
  factors
  behavioral assessment in, 68–70
Nervous system, components and functions
  of, 220–222
Networks of Relationships Inventory–
  Revised (NRI), 294–295, 302, 305
  domain, age, informant, 288*t*
Nomothetic assessment tools, 5, 10–11
  in case conceptualization, 84
  psychometric concepts and, 20
  reliability of, 21–22
  in traditional *versus* behavioral
    assessment, 62
  validity of, 22–23

Normative–developmental perspective, 104
Norms
    ASEBA, 146–152, 161
        constructing, 147, 148t–149t,
            149–150
        multicultural, 150, 151f, 152
    quality of, 21
    validity of, 146–147
NRI; see Networks of Relationships
    Inventory–Revised (NRI)

O

O'Leary–Porter Scale, 333
    description and reliability, 329t
Observation; see also Direct observation
    anecdotal, 168
Observation of Discrete Procedures,
    398–399
Observational methods, 45–46
Obsessive–compulsive disorder (OCD)
    Family Accommodation Scale and, 331
    self-monitoring of, 207–208
Open-ended inquiries, 325–326
Operant conditioning, functional analysis
    and, 66
Operant model of behavior, 58–59
Oppositional defiant disorder (ODD)
    direct observation in diagnosis of, 184
    interpretation bias and, 254
    Stroop task and, 248
Outcome-monitoring strategies, 90–91

P

Panic disorder, self-monitoring of, 207
PAPA; see Preschool Age Psychiatric
    Assessment (PAPA)
Paraprofessionals, in direct observation,
    185–186
Parent Expectancies for Therapy Scale–
    Parent Version (PETS-P), 386–388,
    403, 419, 431
Parent Problems Checklist (PPC), 329t, 333
Parent reports
    for assessing peer victimization, 299
    in peer relationship assessment, 292–293
Parent–child relationship, self-report
    assessment of, 328t
Parent(s); see also Family/parent assessment
    defined, 316–317
    influences of, 83t
    perspective of, 16–17
    physiological assessments and, 229
Parental stress, self-report assessment of,
    328t–329t, 331–332

Parenting practices, self-report assessment
    of, 328t
Parenting Scale (PS), 330
    description and reliability, 328t
Parenting Stress Index (PSI), 328t, 331
Parenting, role of, 318–319
Partial-interval recording form, 181, 182f
PCQ; see Peer Crowd Questionnaire (PCQ)
Peer acceptance, 279–281
Peer assessment, 277–315, 285–300
    with acceptance–rejection measures,
        286–289
        peer reports, 286–287, 289
    developing strategy for, 286
    in externalizing disorder case example,
        302–304
    in internalizing disorder case example,
        304–306
    measures for, 287t, 288t–289t
    with measures of close friendships,
        293–297
    with measures of peer victimization,
        297–299
    of miscellaneous areas, 299–300
    treatment planning/outcome evaluation
        and, 300–302
    underlying theory and research on,
        279–285
Peer crowd affiliation, 280–281
Peer Crowd Questionnaire (PEQ), 288t,
    290–291, 293, 305
Peer Experiences Questionnaire (PEQ), 288t,
    298, 301, 305
Peer nominations, 286–287, 288t, 289,
    296–297
Peer relationships
    key aspects of, 279–285
        acceptance/social status, 279–281
        friendships, 281–283
        victimization, 283–285
    role of, 278–279
    technological impacts on, 306–307
Peer reports
    for assessing peer relationships, 286–287,
        289
    for assessing peer victimization, 298–300
Peer victimization, 283–285
    assessment measures for, 297–299
    versus bullying, 283
    impacts of, 277–278
    measures for assessing, 287t
Peers, perspective of, on target behaviors,
    17–18
PEQ; see Peer Experiences Questionnaire
    (PEQ)

Peripheral nervous system, assessment measures for, 223–227
Personality
traditional views of, 60–61
traits *versus* situational factors in, 61
Physiological assessment, 219–239
adaptations for children, 227–230
for CNS, 222–223
eliciting physiological reactivity and, 230–232
in externalizing disorders, 235
fun adaptations of, 228–229
in internalizing disorders, 233–235
method of, 220–232
multimodal measures in, 227
parents in, 229
for PNS, 223–227
recommendations for, 235
resources on, 220
underlying theory of, 232–233
Physiological measures, properties of, 220–222, 221t
Physiological reactivity
baseline, 230–231
paradigms for eliciting, 230–232
Plato, categorical model of, 36
Polar Heart Rate Monitor, 224, 234
Polyvagal theory, 232–233
Popularity, 279–281
Pre-ejection period (PEP), 224, 231
Preschool Age Psychiatric Assessment (PAPA)
minority youth and, 355
reliability and validity for ethnic minorities, 353t
Pretreatment constructs, 378–381
measurement of, 386–392
readiness for change, 389–392
treatment barriers, 388–389
treatment expectancies, 386–388
readiness for change, 381
treatment barriers, 379–381
treatment expectancies, 378–379
Prevention utility, 260, 261t, 265
Prognosis, role in treatment, 6t, 7
Protective factors, 14
Psychometric properties
of ASEBA, 140–152
clinical utility, 24–25
diagnostic/behavioral, 9t
of direct observation, 174–178
of laboratory-based cognitive methodologies, 257–260
for nomothetic *versus* idiographic instruments, 20
norms, 21

reliability, 21–22
standardization, 20–21
of structured and semistructured interview schedules, 113, 114t–116t
validity, 22–24
Psychometric support, 20
Psychopathology
categorical classification of, 127–128
categorical *versus* dimensional models of, 37–38, 50
developmental principles of, 13–14
parenting factors in, 319
Psychotherapy, case conceptualization and, 79–80

R

Rapid Marital Interaction Coding System (RMICS), 334, 335, 339–340, 341
Rating scales, 45, 133–163
broad-band, 133–134
direct observation correspondence with, 188–190
narrow-band, 133
Reaction times, age and, 258
Readiness for change, 381, 389–392
Reasoning biases, CBT and, 264
Reasoning processes, measuring, 253–256
Reasoning, emotional, 256
Recording devices, for self-monitoring, 200–201
Reduced evidence for danger (RED) bias, 255–256
Referral complaints, avoiding dependence on, 154
Reliability
for idiographic instruments, 22
intraobserver/interobserver, 174–175
for nomothetic instruments, 21–22
Reporting practices, cultural factors in, 19
Representative validity, 22
Resistance, client, 383–384, 392–396
Respiration, index for, 221t
Respondent conditioning, functional analysis and, 66
Respondent-based interviews (RBIs), 44
Response class, defined, 10–11
Response inhibition, in ADHD, 247
Response modes, 82
Responses to interventions (RTIs), ASEBA assessment of
in externalizing disorder example, 159–160
in internalizing disorder example, 157
Revised Child Anxiety and Depression Scale, minority youth and, 358t

Revised Children's Manifest Anxiety Scale (RCMAS), 350–351
  cross-ethnic measurement equivalence studies of, 362t, 363t
  ethnic minority youth and, 366–367
  in internalizing disorders case example, 418, 426
  minority youth and, 358t
Revised UCLA Loneliness Scale, 300
Reynolds Adolescent Depression Scale, minority youth and, 358t

S

Salivary cortisol, assessment of, 226–227
Scalar equivalence, 351
Schedule for Affective Disorders and Schizophrenia for School-Age Children (K-SADS), 108t, 109–110, 112–113, 117, 120
  minority youth and, 355
  reliability and validity of, 119
  reliability estimates for externalizing diagnoses, 116t
  reliability estimates for internalizing diagnoses, 115t
  review of, 112–113
  treatment outcome and, 126
School Observation Coding System–Revised Edition (REDSOCS), 170–171
School refusal; see also Internalizing disorders case example
  case example of, 92–95, 121–123
    direct observation in, 178–180
    self-monitoring in, 209–210
  family/parent assessment in, 340–341
  functional analysis of, 66–67
  peer assessment in, 304–306
  physiological assessment in, 233–235
School Refusal Assessment Scale–Revised (SRAS-R), 68, 419, 426
School settings, direct observation in, 186
Scorer generalizability, 175
Screen for Child Anxiety Related Emotional Disorders, Parent and Child Report (SCARED), cross-ethnic measurement equivalence studies of, 361t
Screening
  peer assessment and, 301
  role in treatment, 6, 6t
Self-monitoring, 196–218
  accuracy of, 202–203
  assessment with, 196–198
  by children and adolescents, 198–199
  defined, 196
  description of, 198–202

of externalizing behaviors, 210–211
  case example of, 210–211
future directions for, 212–213
information collected by, 199–200
of internalizing behaviors, 204–209
  case example of, 209–210
for interventions, 196–198
procedures for, 199
prompts for, 201
reactivity of, 203
recording devices for, 200–201
technological enhancements of, 212–213
  (see also Electronic diaries)
training for, 201–202
Self-Perception Profile for Adolescents (SPPA), 290, 305
  domain, age, informant, 289t
  in externalizing disorders case example, 431, 438
  in internalizing disorders case example, 419, 428
Self-Perception Profile for Children (SPPC), 290, 301, 303
  domain, age, informant, 289t
Self-report inventories, in family/parent assessment, 327–333, 328t–329t
Self-reports
  for assessing peer relationships, 286
  for assessing peer victimization, 297–298
  for case conceptualization, 84
  direct observation correspondence with, 188–190
  for friendship qualities, 293–295
  in peer assessment, 290–291
  of social support, 295–296
Semistructured interview schedules
  psychometric properties of, 113, 114t–116t, 117–119
  reliability estimates for externalizing diagnoses, 116t
  reliability estimates for internalizing diagnoses, 114t–115t
  for resistant youth, 124
  review of, 110–113
    Anxiety Disorders Interview Schedule for DSM-IV: Child and Parent Versions, 110–111
    Child and Adolescent Psychiatric Assessment, 111–112
    Diagnostic Interview for Children and Adolescents, 112
    Schedule for Affective Disorders and Schizophrenia for School-Age Children, 112–113

Semistructured interviews
  description of, 106–107
  DSM-IV and DSM-IV-TR and, 106
  interviewer-based nature of, 105–106
Separation Anxiety Daily Diary, Child
    Version (SADD-C), 205–206
Separation anxiety disorder (SAD), 107
  DSM-IV-TR criteria for, 65
Sexual minority youth, 306
Simulated settings, behavioral assessment in,
    69–70
Situational specificity, 11
Skin conductance level, 224
Skin potential level, 224
Smart phones, self-monitoring and, 204–205
Social Anxiety Scale for Adolescents, 300
  domain, age, informant, 289t
Social Anxiety Scale for Children, 300
  domain, age, informant, 289t
Social Effectiveness Therapy for Children,
    302
Social Experiences Questionnaire, 289t, 301
Social Experiences Questionnaire–
    Peer Report, 298–299
Social Experiences Questionnaire–
    Self-Report, 297–298
Social Experiences Questionnaire–
    Teacher Report, 299
Social networking sites, cyber-victimization
    and, 284
Social Phobia and Anxiety Inventory for
    Children, minority youth and, 358t
Social Skills Rating System, 300, 304
  domain, age, informant, 289t
Social status, 279–281
Social support
  measures for assessing, 287t
  self-reports of, 295–296
Social Support Scale for Children and
    Adolescents, 295
  domain, age, informant, 289t
Society for Psychophysiological Research
    (SPR), website of, 231, 235
Spanish versions of assessment tools
  ADIS-IV, 108t, 111, 121, 123, 355
  Adult Behavior Checklist, 156
  ASEBA Adult Self-Report, 156, 419
  CAPA, 108t
  CB/CL 6–18, 154
  ChIPS, 108t, 110
  interview schedules, 120
  NIMH DISC-IV, 108t, 109, 353t, 355
  YSR, 154
Special education services, diagnosis and, 35
Spot-checking, 200

SPPA; see Self-Perception Profile for
    Adolescents (SPPA)
SPPC; see Self-Perception Profile for Children
    (SPPC)
Stages of Change Questionnaire (SOCQ), in
    internalizing disorders case example,
    419
Standardized diagnostic interviews (SDIs)
  categories and uses of, 43–45
  versus clinician diagnoses, 40–41
  LEAD standard and, 47
State–Trait Anxiety Inventory for Children,
    minority youth and, 358t
Strengths and Difficulties Questionnaire
    (SDQ), 134, 160
Stroop task, 247–249, 260
Structured interview schedules
  reliability estimates for externalizing
    diagnoses, 116t
  reliability estimates for internalizing
    diagnoses, 114t
  review of, 107–110
    Children's Interview for Psychiatric
      Syndromes, 108t, 110
    Mini International Neuropsychiatric
      Interview for Children and
      Adolescents, 108t, 109–110
    National Institute of Mental Health
      Diagnostic Interview Schedule for
      Children, Version IV, 107, 108t, 109
Structured interviews, 105–110
  description of, 106–107
  DSM-IV and DSM-IV-TR and, 106
  respondent-based nature of, 105
Survey of Children's Social Support, domain,
    age, informant, 289t
Sutter–Eyberg Student Behavior Inventory,
    171
  minority youth and, 358t
Symptom expression, cultural factors in, 19

T

Target behaviors, 4, 56
  antecedent and consequent events and,
    65–66
  in case conceptualization, 81–83, 81t
  child's perspective on, 16
  consequences of, 66
  context of, 58
  defining, response modes in, 82
  description of, 58
  for direct observation, 167
  expanded concept of, 63
  in externalizing disorders case example,
    181, 432, 433f–435f, 439–440

in family direct observation, 334
family-based, 320
functional analysis and, 64–70
historical events and causal factors in, 82, 83*t*
in internalizing disorders case example, 419, 420*f*–421*f*, 425–426
maintaining factors in, 84
multiple, 15–16
operationalizing, 86*f*
parents' perspective on, 16–17
peers' perspective on, 17–18
self-monitoring of, 199–200, 202–203
teachers' perspective on, 17
thoughts and feelings as, 64–65
topography of, 64
treatment priority for, 82
Teacher nominations, 291–292
domain, age, informant, 289*t*
Teacher Report Form, 135*t*, 171, 287*t*, 288*t*, 292
Teacher reports
for assessing peer victimization, 299
in peer assessment, 291–292
Teachers, perspective of, on target behaviors, 17
Telephone checklist, 189
Temporal instability, 11
Test battery approach, 57
Test-criterion relationships, 23–24
Test–retest reliability, 21–22, 258
Texting
peer relationships and, 306–307
peer victimization and, 284
self-monitoring and, 205, 213
Therapeutic alliance, 382–383, 392–396
Therapeutic Alliance Scale for Children (TASC), 392–393, 403, 406, 428
Therapist, competence of, 385
Therapy Process Observation Coding System–Strategies Scale (TPOCS-S), 399
Therapy Process Observational Coding System–Alliance Scale (TPOCS-A), 395–396
Therapy processes, 7
assessment constructs and, 378–386
in-session, 381–382
involvement and resistance, 383–384
readiness for change, 381
therapeutic alliance, 382–383
treatment barriers, 379–381
treatment expectancies, 378–379
treatment integrity, 384–386
assessment instruments and, 386–400

for measuring in-session constructs, 392–400
for measuring pretreatment constructs, 386–392
assessment of, 377–413
in clinical cases, 400–407
in externalizing cases, 404–407
in internalizing cases, 402–404
recommendations for, 407–408
Thoughts, as target behaviors, 64–65
Threat stimuli, 222, 234, 241–242, 244, 246, 248–251, 254–256, 263–265
Threshold invariance, 351
Time-based recording, 169–170
Trail Making Test, 266
Trauma, target behaviors and, 83*t*
Treatment
assessment's role in, 5–8, 6*t*
disconnection from assessment, 4–5
families' perceptions of, 380–381
family issues in, 317 (*see also* Family/parent assessment)
history of, 59
personalized, 377–378, 407
premature termination of, 379–380
prescriptive approach to, 89–90
Treatment barriers, measurement of, 379–381, 388–389
Treatment evaluation, role in treatment, 6*t*, 8
Treatment expectancies, 378–381
measurement of, 386–388
Treatment integrity, 384–386
discrete procedures and, 398–399
measurement of, 398–400
and participant report of principle-consistent strategies, 399–400
Treatment monitoring
role of, 6*t*, 8
utility of, 260, 261*t*
Treatment outcomes
ASEBA assessment of
in externalizing disorder example, 160
in internalizing disorder example, 157–158
assessment and, 4
diagnosis and, 35
direct observation and, 186–187, 190
interviews and, 126
monitoring
in externalizing disorders case example, 437*f*–438*f*, 442–443
in internalizing disorders case example, 424*f*, 428–429
peer relationships and, 302

Treatment outcomes (*continued*)
  therapeutic alliance and, 382–383
  treatment integrity and, 384–386
Treatment phases, diagnostic/behavioral, 9*t*
Treatment planning/selection, 87*f*
  in case conceptualization, 88–90
  cognitive measures and, 260–266
  diagnosis and, 35
  direct observation and, 183–186,
    187–188
  in externalizing disorders case example,
    441–442
  in internalizing disorders case example,
    423*f*, 427–428
  interviews and, 125–126
  peer assessment and, 300–302
  role in treatment, 6*t*, 8
  for school refusal, 180
Treatment priorities, setting, 82
Treatment sensitivity, 24
Treatment utility, 260, 261*t*, 264–
  265
Treatment-monitoring utility, 264–
  265
Trier Social Stress Test for Children,
  225

U

UCLA Loneliness Scale–Revised, 300
  domain, age, informant, 289*t*

V

Validational utility, 260, 262*t*
Validity, 22–24, 72
Validity generalization, 24
Vanderbilt Psychotherapy Process Scales,
  Patient Participation subscale of, 397
Victimization; *see* Peer victimization
Violence, family, screening for, 326
Visual-search tasks, 243–245

W

Working Alliance Inventory (WAI), 393–394
World Health Organization (WHO),
  diagnostic system of, 34–35

Y

Youth Self-Report (YSR) (ASEBA), 135*t*,
  136, 171, 187*t*, 188*t*, 291, 367*t*, 418,
  424, 426